DISEASES OF EAR, NOSE AND THROAT

Dr. Kashieca Yap

ALLIED HEALTH PRESS

Diseases of Ear, Nose and Throat

Author: **Dr. Kashieca Yap**

Allied Health Press
4164 Lakeshore Road
Burlington ON L7L 1A4
Canada
www.alliedhealthpress.com
Email: orders@arclereducation.com

ISBN: 978-1-77956-226-5

General Disclaimer:

This book is a summation of information from different sources and encompasses a wide range of medical conditions, the latest therapy methods, principals and techniques that are used in current practice, at the time of publication. This book offers general information with educational purposes, it is not to be applied or relied on for any diagnostic or treatment purposes. Please do not use the data/matter as a substitute for professional diagnosis and treatment. Please consult your healthcare provider or a licensed physician before making any healthcare queries or treatment choices. The medical information and research findings presented in this book are for educational purposes only and should not be used for the treatment of specific individual patients, as individual cases may vary. The author(s), editors(s) and publisher cannot be held accountable and make no guarantees that the information provided in this book will apply to each and individual patient. This book is meant to serve as a basic guideline and other relevant literature sources should be used for more specific information. This text can be a vital resource for students, trainees, and practitioners, covering essential topics. This book encompasses a wide range of medical conditions and the latest therapy options used in current practice. Through the utilization of many different medical studies this book provides the basics of different medical conditions, which can be used as a basic guide from where medical students, trainees and practitioners can extract necessary information. Further, some of the books have graphic images to explain anatomy for medical/educational purposes only. Hence, the book is intended for students or teachers/staff or individuals with a mature outlook looking to learn or enhance their knowledge.

Allied Health Press publishes wide variety of books and eBooks. For more information about Allied Health Press and its products, visit our website at www.alliedhealthpress.com

ABOUT THE AUTHOR

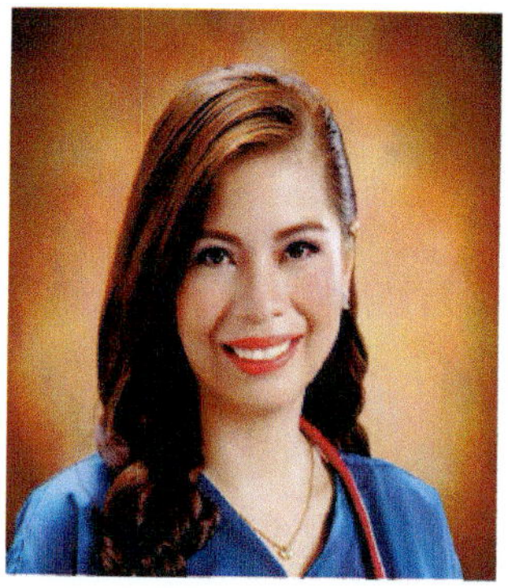

Kashieca Yap, M.D., is a devoted medical doctor and medical writer. She currently works as a general practice physician in a rural town, where she handles adult and pediatric cases, infectious diseases, and chronic medical conditions. Kashieca also lectures on mental health, clinical pharmacology, physiology, and psychiatry and is an enthusiastic researcher and medical writer. She obtained her medical degree from Cebu Doctor's University College of Medicine and further developed her clinical skills at a large public hospital. Alongside her professional endeavors, Kashieca dedicates her time to volunteering at NGOs and medical missions, reaching out to people in geographically isolated areas. Her unwavering passion for medicine and her strong desire to serve people is a testament to her compassion and skill as a healthcare professional.

Word Roots, Prefixes, and Suffixes by Chapter

Chapter 1 Diseases of the Ear

Ab- away from
Ante- before
Anti- opposite, against
Bi- two
Calc- relating to calcium

Chapter 2 Diseases of Nose and Paranasal Sinuses

anti- against
ante- before
bi- two, both
dys- painful, difficult
dors- back
endo- inside

Chapter 3 Diseases of the Oral Cavity and Salivary Glands

-algia pain
arth- joint
dent- tooth or teeth
-ectomy excision
-emia blood
endo-within

Chapter 4 Diseases of the Pharynx

aden- glands
adren- the adrenal glands
angi- blood vessels
arteri- arteries
arthr-, articul- joints
bronch(i)- the lungs

Chapter 5 Diseases of the Larynx and Trachea

bio- life
chem- chemistry
cyt- cell
-blast bud, germ
fibr-, fibro- fiber
gluco- glucose, sugar
hydr-, hydro- water

Chapter 6 Thyroid Gland and Its Disorders

Angi- Blood vessel
Brachi- Arm
Bronch- Airways or windpipe
Carcin/o- Cancer
Cardi/o- Heart
Carp- Wrist

Chapter 7 Diseases of the Esophagus

Ectomy to cut out or remove
gram the image (X-ray)
tachy- fast
trans- across or through
Vaso- blood vessel

Chapter 8 Recent Advances

Anti- Against
Auto- Self
Bio- Life
Chem/o- Chemistry
Contra- Against
Necr/o- Death
Neo- New

Chapter 9 Clinical Methods in ENT and Neck Masses

-ectomy to cut out or remove
-gram the image (X-ray)
-scopy/-scopic to look, observe
Melan/o- Black

Chapter 10 Operative Surgery

-ectomy Removal (excision)
-ostomy A new opening
-otomy Cutting into (incision)
-oplasty Surgical repair

Table of Contents

7 Diseases of the Esophagus 279

8 Recent Advances 325

LIST OF FIGURES

LIST OF TABLES

PREFACE

According to the World Health Organization, over 5% of the world's population (approximately 430 million people) require rehabilitation services for disabling hearing loss, indicative of the prevalence and impact of ear diseases alone.

Ear diseases are diverse, including conditions like otitis media (middle ear infection), which is particularly prevalent among children. The Centers for Disease Control and Prevention (CDC) estimates that by the age of three, over 80% of children will have experienced at least one episode of otitis media, highlighting its significance as a public health concern. Another common condition, tinnitus, characterized by a ringing or buzzing in the ears, affects about 15% of people, according to the American Tinnitus Association.

Nose-related conditions also significantly impact health and quality of life. Rhinitis, an inflammation of the nasal mucous membrane, affects a large portion of the population, with allergic rhinitis alone affecting approximately 20% of Americans, as reported by the American College of Allergy, Asthma, & Immunology. Sinusitis, another widespread condition, afflicts about 31 million Americans every year, leading to a substantial economic burden due to healthcare costs and lost productivity.

Throat disorders encompass a variety of diseases such as pharyngitis (throat infection), tonsillitis, and laryngitis. Pharyngitis, commonly caused by viral infections, is a leading cause of doctor visits, with millions of cases reported annually in the United States. Tonsillitis and laryngitis also contribute significantly to morbidity, with their viral and bacterial causes necessitating careful diagnosis and treatment.

ENT diseases are not only prevalent but also carry substantial economic, health, and social implications. Advances in medical science have led to better diagnostic and treatment options, improving outcomes and quality of life for many affected individuals. However, prevention, timely diagnosis, and access to effective treatments remain crucial in managing the global burden of these conditions. Public health initiatives aimed at reducing exposure to risk factors, such as smoking cessation and vaccination programs, play a key role in preventing and controlling ENT diseases.

This book "Diseases of Ear, Nose, and Throat" serves as a comprehensive and authoritative guide to the diagnosis, treatment, and management of ENT disorders. It will equip medical students, ENT specialists, general practitioners, and healthcare professionals with in-depth knowledge and practical insights into the wide range of conditions affecting the ear, nose, and throat. The book is written to bridge the gap between theory and clinical practice, offering detailed explanations of disease mechanisms, symptomatology, diagnostic procedures, and contemporary treatment options, including both surgical and non-surgical approaches. Presenting up-to-date research, case studies, and evidence-based practices, the book aims to enhance the reader's understanding of ENT diseases, improve patient care outcomes, and encourage the development of skills necessary for effectively addressing the challenges encountered in otolaryngology. Furthermore, it attempts to raise a multidisciplinary approach to patient care, recognizing the importance of collaboration among various healthcare disciplines in the treatment of complex ENT conditions.

Chapter 1

DISEASES OF THE EAR

Contents

Introduction

The ear is a sophisticated and sensitive sensory organ. It is linked to the organ of balance and gives people the ability to hear. Therefore, ear diseases can have far-reaching consequences. In particular, painful chronic ear conditions are frequently the root cause of hearing loss. Hearing and balance disorders are frequently symptoms of other illnesses rather than being their own distinct diseases. Widespread tinnitus, for instance, is a symptom rather than an illness. Signs of what are thought to be ear diseases can also be brought on by injuries and stress. A doctor must provide clarification on each patient's specific health issues and problems when it comes to diseases of the ears.

Orientation and Directional Terms

Term	Definition	Illustration
Otitis media	An inflammation of the inner ear caused by a bacteria or virus that causes fluid to accumulate behind the eardrum. When treated correctly, there is less recurrence and complications.	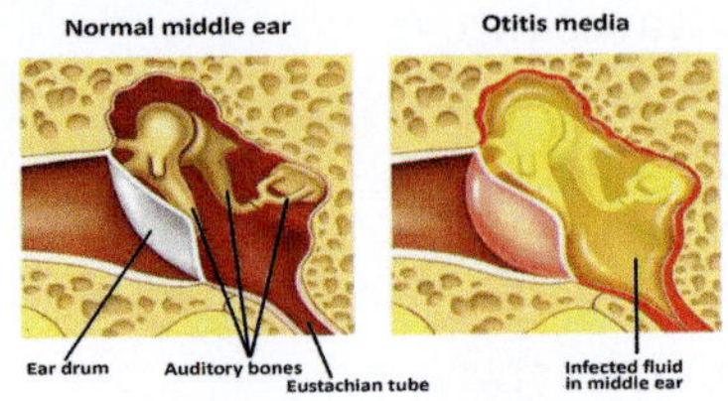
Otosclerosis	Abnormal growth of the small bones in the middle ear. It is one of the most common causes of gradual hearing loss, but hearing can be recovered with surgery.	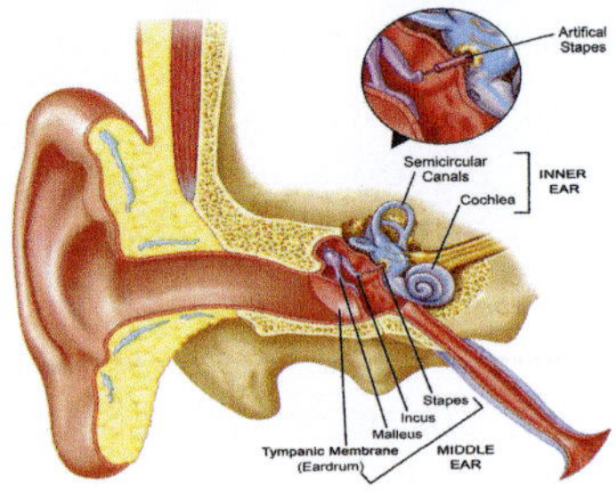
Tinnitus	A sensation of constant ringing or buzzing without an actual source of the noise. There is currently no specific cure for this condition.	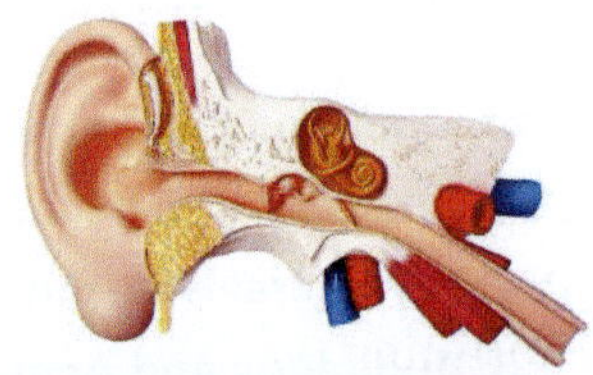
Presbycusis	This is the gradual loss of hearing in adults as they grow older. It is usually bilateral and symmetrical.	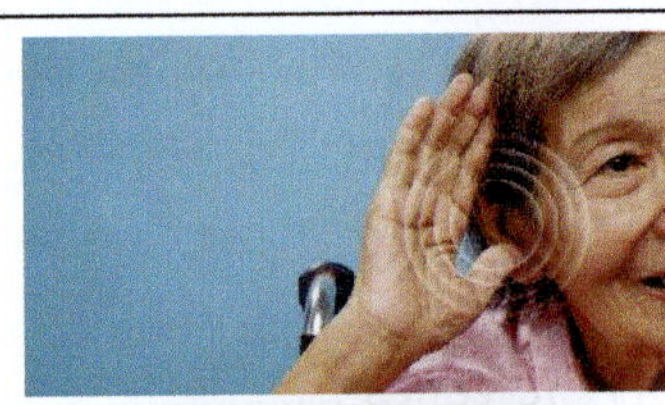
Perichondritis	An infection of the skin and tissue covering the cartilage of the external part of the ear. It results in redness, pain and fever.	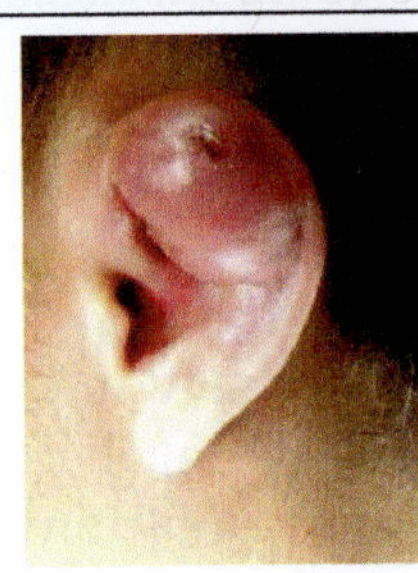

1.1. Anatomy of Ear

The human ear is an organ of balance and hearing that uses transduction—the conversion of sound waves into electrochemical impulses—to detect and analyze sound and preserve equilibrium. Similar to other mammal ears, the human ear is composed of sense organs that have two distinct purposes: hearing and maintaining postural balance and head and eye coordination. The outer, middle, and inner ear are the three distinct anatomical sections of the ear. The external auditory canal, whose inner end is sealed off by the tympanic membrane, also known as the eardrum, and the visible part of the ear known as the auricle, or pinna, which protrudes from the side of the head, make up the outer ear. Sound waves are collected and directed toward the tympanic membrane by the outer ear. Within the temporal bone is a small, air-filled cavity that houses the middle ear. It is supported by a chain made up of three small bones known as the auditory ossicles: the malleus (hammer), incus (anvil), and stapes (stirrup). The inner ear also referred to as the labyrinth since Galen's time from around 2nd century CE. It receives sound waves from the tympanic membrane through this ossicular chain. It is a complex network of cavities and passageways filled with fluid that is situated deep within the temporal bone's petrous layer. The vestibular apparatus, which includes the vestibule and semicircular canals and houses the sensory organs of postural equilibrium, and the cochlea, which resembles a snail shell and houses the sensory organ of hearing, make up the two functional units of the inner ear. The vestibulocochlear nerve, also known as the eighth cranial nerve, is the highly specialized end of the sensory organs. Knowing the components of the auditory system is necessary before we can comprehend how the ear functions. The middle ear, inner ear, eardrum, and outer ear are the four main components of the ear. Let's take a closer look at each of these.

1.1.1. Outer Ear

The structure of the outermost part of the ear, the auricle, is where the human ear differs most dramatically from the ears of other mammals. Located near the side of the head, the auricle in humans is a nearly primitive, immobile shell. The thin yellow elastic cartilage plate that makes up its surface is covered in tightly fitting skin. An irregular shallow funnel is formed by the cartilage being molded into distinct hollows, ridges, and furrows. The term concha refers to the lowest depression that goes straight to the acoustic meatus, also known as the external auditory canal. The tragus, which resembles a tongue, and the antitragus, which is located behind, partially uncover it. The helix, a noticeable ridge that starts from the concha's floor and continues as the upper portion of the auricle's incurved rim, is located above the tragus.

A groove known as the scapha, or the fossa of the helix, divides the helix from the antihelix, an inner, concentric ridge that encircles the concha. Darwin's tubercle, a small protrusion identified as the remnant of a distant human ancestor's folded-over ear point, can be seen in some ears along the upper, posterior section of the helix.

The only portion of the outer ear devoid of cartilage is the lobule, the fleshy base of the auricle. Several tiny, primitive muscles on the auricle also serve to secure it to the scalp and skull. While some people can deliberately activate these muscles to produce limited movements, most people cannot use them. The external auditory canal is a blind tube that begins at the tympanic membrane and curves slightly inward from the floor of the concha. The outer third of the canal wall is made of cartilage, while the inner two-thirds are made of bone. Skin covers the outside surface of the tympanic membrane and lines the passage for its whole length of 24 mm, or nearly 1 inch.

Insects are kept out of the canal by fine hairs pointing outward and modified sweat glands that create cerumen, or earwax.

1.1.2. Tympanic Membrane and Middle Ear

1.1.2.1. Tympanic Membrane

Stretched obliquely across the end of the external canal is the thin, semitransparent tympanic membrane, also known as the eardrum, which serves as the divide between the middle and outer ears. Its diameter ranges from 8 to 10 mm, or 0.3 to 0.4 inches, and its shape is a flattened cone with an inward-pointing apex. Its exterior is therefore somewhat concave. The membrane's edge thickens and is connected to a groove in the tympanic annulus, an incomplete ring of bone that nearly encircles and stabilizes the membrane. The pars flaccida, or uppermost small area where the ring is open, is slack, but the pars Tensa, or much larger portion, is tightly stretched. The appearance and mobility of the tympanic membrane are critical in the diagnosis of middle ear disease, which is particularly prevalent in young children. The healthy membrane appears translucent and pearl-gray under the otoscope, occasionally exhibiting a hint of pink or yellow.

Three layers are making up the entire tympanic membrane. The skin's ouster layer and the external canal are one and the same. The tympanic cavity of the middle ear lining and the inner layer of mucous membrane are continuous. The layer of fibrous tissue that lies between these layers gives the membrane its tension and stiffness. It is composed of radial and circular fibers. Due to the membrane's abundant blood vessels and sensory nerve fibers, it has a high pain threshold (Figure 1.1).

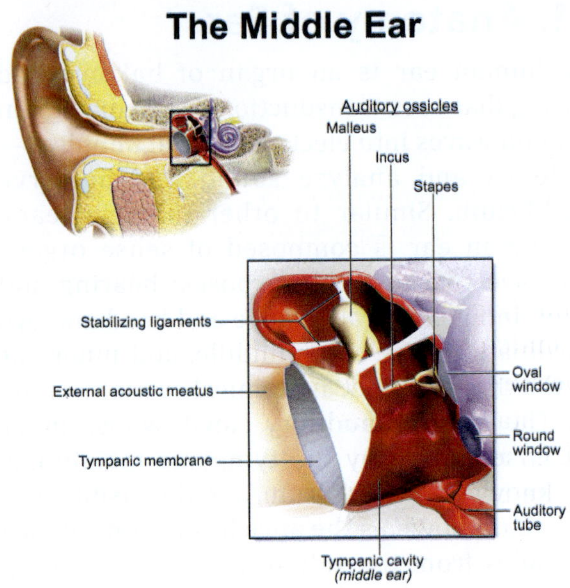

Figure 1.1. *The middle ear.*

Source: By Bruce Blaus, Own work, CC BY 3.0, https://commons.wikimedia.org/w/index.php?curid=29025010.

1.1.2.2. Middle-Ear Cavity

The middle ear cavity is a small, air-filled space. It is separated into an upper and a lower chamber, the epitympanum above and the tympanum (tympanic cavity) proper below, by a slight constriction. These rooms are also known as the attic and the atrium, in that order. An approximately rectangular room with four walls, a floor, and a ceiling is what the middle-ear space looks like. The tympanic membrane forms the outer (lateral) wall of the middle-ear space. The middle ear cavity is isolated from the cranial cavity and brain above by the ceiling, also known as the superior wall. It is a thin plate of bone. Similar to the inferior wall, the floor is a thin bony plate that divides the middle ear cavity from the carotid artery and jugular vein below.

Part of the back wall (posterior wall) divides the middle ear cavity from the mastoid antrum, but this wall has an opening that leads to both the antrum and the small air cells of the mastoid process, the slightly protruding, roughened part of the temporal bone located directly behind the auricle and the external auditory canal. The eustachian tube, also known as the auditory tube, opens in the front (anterior) wall and joins the middle ear to the nasopharynx. A component of the bony otic capsule of the inner ear is the inner (medial) wall, which divides the labyrinth, or middle ear, from the inner ear. It has two tiny apertures, one above the other, called fenestrae. The stapes footplate closes the oval window, which is located on top. The circular window at the bottom is shielded by a thin membrane.

1.1.2.3. Auditory Ossicles

The middle ear has auditory ossicles and the supporting structures. The short ossicular chain, made up of three small bones, connects the tympanic membrane to the oval window and inner ear by crossing the middle ear cavity. They are the malleus (hammer), incus (anvil), and stapes (stirrup) from the outside in. The incus resembles an unevenly rooted premolar tooth more than an anvil, while the malleus more closely resembles a club than a hammer. Ligaments hold these bones in place, allowing the chain to freely vibrate and transfer sound from the tympanic membrane to the inner ear.

The handle and head make up the malleus. From the center (umbo) to the upper border, the handle is securely fastened to the tympanic membrane. Three tiny ligaments attach the head of the malleus to the walls and roof of the epitympanum, where it is suspended slightly above the upper rim of the tympanic annulus. The head of the malleus and the body of the incus are firmly joined. The short process (crus) of the incus is fixed in a shallow depression in the cavity's back wall known as the fossa incudis by another minute ligament. The head of the stapes and the long process of the incus form a loosely ligament-enclosed joint where the incus is bent near its end and bears a small bony knob. The smallest bone in the body is the stapes. Its length is approximately 3 mm (0.01 inch), and its weight is hardly 3 mg (0.0001 ounces). It is positioned at an almost horizontal angle, perpendicular to the incus process. Its base, or footplate, is free to vibrate in order to transmit sound to the labyrinth, but it fits neatly in the oval window and is encircled by the elastic annular ligament.

1.1.2.4. Muscles

The middle ear is made up of two tiny muscles. The eustachian tube opening is where the longer muscle, known as the tensor tympani, emerges from a bony canal. It changes direction, running backward and then outward while crossing a bone projection that resembles a pulley. This muscle's tendon is joined to the upper portion of the malleus handle. The tensor tympani pulls the malleus inward when it contracts and keeps the tympanic membrane taut or makes it more so. The stapedius, a shorter and stouter muscle, originates from the middle ear cavity's back wall, extends forward, and joins the stapes head's neck. As if to yank it out of the oval window, the stapes tends to tip backward due to its reflex contractions. As a result, it selectively attenuates sounds that enter the inner ear, particularly those with lower frequencies.

1.1.2.5. Nerves

The facial nerve, the seventh cranial nerve, travels through the facial canal in the petrous portion of the temporal bone in a somewhat roundabout manner en route from the brainstem to the facial muscles responsible for expression. Emerging from the canal into the middle ear cavity, the chorda tympani nerve is a small but significant branch that runs forward along the inner surface of the pars tensa of the membrane, between the malleus handle and the long process of the incus. Currently, the tympanic mucous membrane is the only covering, giving the impression that it is completely exposed. The sensory fibers for taste are brought to the anterior two-thirds of the tongue, and parasympathetic secretory fibers are brought to the salivary glands as it continues along the anterior bone wall.

1.1.2.6. Eustachian Tube

The nasopharynx, which is located above the soft palate and behind the nasal passages, is reached by the eustachian tube, which is approximately 31–38 mm (1.2–1.5 inches) long. It descends and inwards from the tympanum. The tube is narrow and has bone all around it at the top. It widens and turns cartilaginous as it approaches the pharynx. The cilia, which resemble tiny hairlike projections and cover the mucous lining of the tympanum and middle ear, are responsible for the rapid drainage of mucous secretions from the tympanum into the pharynx through rhythmic sweeping motions.

Maintaining equal air pressure on both sides of the tympanic membrane and aiding in middle ear ventilation are the functions of the eustachian tube. To enable minor pressure changes to be adjusted without conscious effort, the tube is closed when at rest and opens during swallowing. The tube may stay securely closed during an airplane's fast descent or underwater dive. A forced expiration with the mouth and nostrils tightly closed can usually be used to relieve the discomfort that arises with an increase in external pressure. The Valsalva maneuver is named for the Italian physician-anatomist Antonio Maria Valsalva (1666–1723), who advocated it for removing pus from an infected middle ear. This maneuver increases the air pressure in the pharynx and causes the tube to open.

1.1.3. Inner Ear

The membranous labyrinth inside the bony labyrinth is one of the two inner ear labyrinths, which exist in reality. The vestibule, a central chamber, the three semicircular canals, and the spirally coiled cochlea make up the bony labyrinth. A matching segment of the membranous labyrinth is contained within each structure, taking up only a small percentage of the available space: the vestibule houses the utricle and saccule, each semicircular canal its semicircular duct, and the cochlea its cochlear duct. The watery substance known as perilymph fills the empty space around the membranous labyrinth. It is made from blood plasma and is similar to, but distinct from, the aqueous humor of the eye and the brain's cerebrospinal fluid. The membranous labyrinth, like the majority of hollow organs, is lined with epithelium, a layer of specialized cells that covers both internal and external body surfaces.

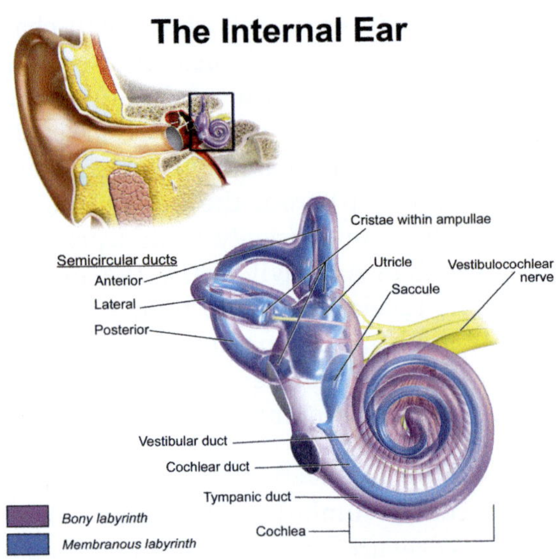

Figure 1.2. *The outer ear receives sound, transmitted through the ossicles of the middle ear to the inner ear, where it is converted to a nervous signal in the cochlear and transmitted along the vestibulocochlear nerve.*

Source: By BruceBlaus- Own work, CC BY 3.0, https://commons.wikimedia.org/w/index.php?curid=29025011.

It is filled with a fluid known as endolymph, which differs significantly from perilymph in terms of ionic composition. The endolymph and perilymph do not mix because the membranous labyrinth is a closed system (Figure 1.2).

1.1.4. Vestibular System

The inner ear system responsible for balance is called the vestibular system. It is made up of the vestibule and the semicircular canals, two bony labyrinth structures, as well as the membranous labyrinth structures that are housed within them.

1.1.4.1. Vestibule

The otolith organs are the two membranous sacs of the vestibule, the saccule and the utricle. They are also known as gravity receptors because of their ability to react to gravitational fields. A single, roughly 2 mm (0.08 inch)-diameter patch of sensory cells known as a macula is located on the inner surface of each sac. The macula tracks the head's orientation with respect to the vertical. The macula in the utricle extends from the tubular sac's anterior wall and is mostly located in the horizontal plane. The bone of the inner wall of the vestibule is directly overlaid by the macula, which is positioned in the vertical plane in the saccule. It has an elongated shape that is similar to the letter J. A basement membrane, nerve fibers and nerve endings, underlying connective tissue, and the neuroepithelium, a layer composed of supporting and sensory cells, make up each macula. The hair-like cilia that protrude from the apical ends of the sensory cells—both the flexible motile kinocilia and the stiff nonmotile stereocilia—are what give these cells their name, hair cells. The vestibulocochlear nerve's superior, or vestibular, division is where the nerve fibers originate. They puncture the basement membrane and, depending on the kind of hair cell, either terminate at the cell's basal end or create a calyx, or cup-shaped structure, around it.

A hair bundle, made up of one motile kinocilium and roughly 100 fine, nonmotile stereocilia of varying lengths, atop each hair cell of the vestibular organs. At the apex of the cell, the stereocilia are fixed in a dense cuticular plate. At one side of the cuticular plate, the single kinocilium—which is longer and larger than the stereocilia—emerges from a noncuticular region of the cell membrane. The stereocilia that are closest to the kinocilium are the longest; as they move farther away from the kinocilium, their lengths gradually decrease. Little filamentous threads connect the shafts and tips of nearby stereocilia. When the strands of hair are bent—e.g., due to a head tilt, the hair cells are stimulated to change the frequency of the nerve impulses they continuously send to the brainstem via the vestibular nerve fibers. The otolithic, also known as statolithic, membrane is a delicate acellular structure that covers the entire macula. This membrane has a fibrillar pattern, but it is sometimes described as gelatinous. Rhombohedral crystals, also known as statoconia or otoconia, which are composed of calcium carbonate in the form of calcite, cover the membrane's surface. With a specific gravity nearly three times that of the membrane and the endolymph, these crystalline particles, with lengths ranging from 1 to 20 μm (1 μm = 0.000039 inches), contribute a significant amount of mass to the membrane because they are denser than it.

There are two types of vestibular hair cells: type II cells have a cylindrical body with nerve endings at the base, and type I cells have a rounded body surrounded by a nerve calyx. On the maculae's surface, they resemble a mosaic, with the cylindrical cells encircling the periphery and the type I cells predominating in a curvilinear region (the striola) close to the macula's center. Although the significance of these patterns is unclear, they might make minor head tilts more sensitive.

1.1.4.2. Semicircular Canals

The superior, horizontal, and posterior semicircular canals make up the bony labyrinth, and their names correspond to their respective positions. The vertical diagonal planes in which the superior and posterior canals cross at right angles are home to them. The vestibule is accessible through the ampulla, the enlarged end of each canal. The ampullae of the posterior canal opens on the opposite side of the vestibule from the ampullae of the horizontal and superior canals, which are located slightly above the oval window. The superior and posterior canals come together to form a common stem known as the crus, which also opens into the vestibule. The vestibular aqueduct canal's mouth, which leads into the brain cavity, is located nearby. A separate entrance into the vestibule is located at the opposite end of the horizontal canal. The vestibule, then, completes the circle for every semicircular canal.

A membranous semicircular duct with a much smaller diameter and its own ampulla is enclosed by each of the three bony canals and their respective ampullas. With their entrances into the utricle and a common crus for the superior and posterior ducts, the membranous ducts and ampullae resemble the canals and ampullae of the bony labyrinth. Similar to the remaining sections of the membranous labyrinth, they are encircled by perilymph and contain endolymph. The vestibular aqueduct allows the narrow endolymphatic duct, which carries extra endolymph to be absorbed by the endolymphatic sac, to exit the utricle and enter the cranial cavity.

The sensory end organ known as the crista, which spans the side-to-side length of each membranous ampulla, is a saddle-shaped ridge of tissue. The neuroepithelium that surrounds the crista is made up of supporting and hair cells. A gelatinous structure called the cupula rises from this ridge and divides the interior of the ampulla into two roughly equal sections. It reaches the roof of the ampulla directly above it. Hair bundles extend from the apices of the cristae hair cells, just like those of the maculae hair cells. The kinocilium and longest stereocilia occupy fine parallel channels that extend far up into the cupula's substance. The cupula is thus free to incline toward or away from the utricle in response to even the smallest endolymph flow or change in pressure, even though it is attached at its base to the crista. The direction in which the tufts of cilia bend affects how quickly the vestibular nerve fibers carry nerve impulse discharges to the brainstem. These tufts of cilia move in tandem with the cupula.

1.1.5. Cochlea

1.1.5.1. Structure of the Cochlea

The sensory organ of hearing is found in the cochlea. It is remarkably similar to a snail's shell, so much so that the Greek word for it inspired the name. The modiolus, a hollow central pillar, is the center of a spiral tube that makes two and a half rotations around the cochlea. It is shaped into a cone that is 5 mm tall and 9 mm (0.35 inch) in diameter at the base. The spiral tube has a length of about 30 mm when it is extended. It tapers until it ends blindly at the apex, where it is the widest (2 mm) where the basal coil opens into the vestibule. The cochlear artery and vein, as well as the twisted trunk of cochlear nerve fibers, are located in the otherwise hollow center of the modiolus. The internal meatus, an opening in the petrous part of the temporal bone, is where this nerve, a division of the very short vestibulocochlear nerve, enters the base of the modiolus from the brainstem. The cochlear nerve's spiral ganglion cells are located in a bony spiral canal that encircles the core.

The modiolus is encircled by a thin bony shelf called the osseous spiral lamina, which resembles a screw thread. The structure protrudes approximately halfway through the cochlear canal, partially bifurcating it into two sections: the scala vestibuli, which is the upper chamber, and the scala tympani, which is the lower chamber (tympanic ramp). The helicotrema, or opening at the apex of the cochlea, is visible if the cochlea is cut longitudinally down the middle. It serves as a communication channel between the perilymph-filled scala vestibuli and scala tympani. The vestibule and the scala vestibuli open at the basal end, close to the middle ear. The scala tympani's basal end abruptly ends below the circular window. The perilymphatic duct passes through the nearby opening of the narrow cochlear aqueduct. This duct joins the subdural space in the posterior cranial fossa, or the back part of the cranial cavity floor, with the interior of the cochlea.

The cochlear part of the membranous labyrinth is a smaller scala known as the cochlear duct (scala media), which is located between the larger vestibular and tympanic scalae. Filled with endolymph, the cochlear duct ends blindly at both ends—i.e., below the round window and at the apex. This cross-section of the duct has a right triangle-like shape. The basilar membrane and the osseous spiral lamina, which divide the cochlear duct from the scala tympani, form its base. The organ of Corti, which is perched on the basilar membrane, is home to the hair cells that generate nerve signals in response to acoustic vibrations. Two tissues that border the cochlea's bony wall—the fibrous spiral ligament, which sits between the stria and the bony wall—are what make up the triangle's side. The stria vascularis lines the cochlear duct's outer wall. The stria is bounded by a layer of flat cells that keeps it apart from the spiral ligament. The transparent vestibular membrane, also known as the Reissner membrane, forms the hypotenuse and is made up of just two layers of flattened cells. On the edge of the osseous spiral lamina lies a low ridge known as the spiral limbus. The Reissner membrane extends from the inner edge of the limbus to the upper border of the stria.

In the scala vestibuli, the spiral ligament touches the perilymph and extends above the point where the Reissner membrane attaches. Reaching down below the basilar membrane's insertion, it makes contact with the scala tympani's perilymph. It has a large number of robust fibers that serve as anchors for the basilar membrane as well as connective tissue cells. The spiral ligament's structure is denser behind the stria than it is in the vicinity of the upper and lower margins. Similar to the nearby stria, the spiral ligament has an abundant supply of blood vessels. It is the recipient of the radiating arterioles that exit the modiolus through the bony channels of the scala vestibuli. Above the junction with the Reissner membrane, branches from these vessels form a network of capillaries that may play a major role in the formation of the perilymph from the blood plasma. A few more branches go through the stria, and yet more go past it and reach the spiral prominence. Little veins that descend beneath the basilar membrane's attachment gather blood from these disjointed capillary networks and transfer it to the spiral vein in the scala tympani's floor.

The spiral prominence, a low ridge running parallel to the basilar membrane and home to a unique collection of longitudinally directed capillary vessels, is located at the lower edge of the stria. It is the outer sulcus below the prominence. Cells of epithelial origin line the floor of the outer sulcus, and some of these cells project long projections into the spiral ligament's matrix. Capillary vessels emerge from the spiral ligament and descend between these so-called root cells. This region might be involved in clearing waste products from the endolymph because it seems to have an absorptive rather than a secretory function. The basilar membrane in humans has a length of roughly 30 to 35 mm. Its width increases toward the apex to 0.5 mm from less than 0.1 mm near its basal end. Stiff elastic fibers that are joined at their basal ends in the modiolus span the basilar membrane. They are able to vibrate because their distal ends are inserted into the membrane but are not genuinely attached. From the base of the cochlea, which is near the middle ear, to the apex, the fibers become longer and less caliber, resulting in a notable decrease in the overall stiffness of the basilar membrane. In addition, compared to the apex, the osseous spiral lamina, stria vascularis, and spiral ligament are all wider at the basal end. On the other hand, the mass of the Corti organ is highest at the apex and lowest at the base. As a result, the cochlear duct's structure and contents have some degree of tuning. The basal end has more stiffness and less mass, which makes it more sensitive to higher-frequency sounds. Lower frequencies are more responsive to the apical end due to its increased mass and decreased stiffness.

The acellular ground substance of the basilar membrane is located beneath its fibrillar layer. One layer of spindle-shaped mesothelial cells, with long processes arranged longitudinally and parallel, covers each layer in turn. These cells face the scala tympani and form the tympanic lamella, which is in contact with the perilymph. Capillary blood vessels are located beneath the limbus's tympanic lip and, in certain species, such as humans and guinea pigs, within the basilar membrane, below the tunnel. Although these spiral-shaped vessels do not enter the organ of Corti, it is believed that they provide the majority of the oxygen and other nutrients that the organ's cells require. The outer spiral vessel is present in the human fetus even though it is uncommon in adult members of some species, like the dog, cat, and rat, and it is not present in every adult human's basilar membrane. Its remarkable diameter in the developing fetus indicates that it serves as a vital blood supply channel to the organ of Corti.

1.1.5.2. Organ of Corti

Neatly arranged in rows on the surface of the basilar membrane are sensory hair cells that respond to sound vibrations by generating nerve impulses. These cells, along with their supporting cells, make up a complex neuroepithelium known as the basilar papilla or organ of Corti. The name of the organ of Corti comes from Italian anatomist Alfonso Corti, who first identified it in 1851. An important feature of the organ of Corti is the arch, or tunnel, formed by two rows of pillar cells. These cells provide crucial support for the structure and separate a single row of larger inner hair cells from several rows of smaller outer hair cells. The inner hair cells are surrounded by inner phalangeal cells, which rest on the tympanic lip of the spiral limbus. The inner hair cells and their supporting cells are bordered by a curved furrow called the inner sulcus, lined with cuboidal cells.

A phalangeal cell of Deiters, also known as a supporting cell, holds the base of each outer hair cell in a cup-shaped depression. A projection rises from each Deiters' cell to the reticular lamina, a stiff membrane covering the organ of Corti. The lamina firmly holds the top of the hair cell in place, but the body is suspended in a fluid that occupies the Corti tunnel and the Nuel space. Its composition is believed to be similar, if not identical, to that of the perilymph, despite the fact that it is occasionally referred to as cortilymph. Three additional types of epithelial cells lie beyond the hair cells and the Deiters' cells. These cells are commonly referred to as the Hensen, Claudius, and Boettcher cells after the 19th-century anatomists who first described them. Although their exact role is unknown, it is thought that through ion transport and absorptive activity, they contribute to the maintenance of the composition of the endolymph.

Actin filaments make up the cytoskeleton of each hair cell, giving the structures it resides in their characteristic stiffness. A dense cuticular plate made of actin filaments atop the hair cell supports a tuft of stiffly erect stereocilia that are also made of actin and are arranged in a staircase pattern with varying lengths. The cuticular plate is firmly anchoring the rootlets of this so-called hair bundle. 40 to 60 stereocilia are arranged in two or more asymmetrically parallel rows on the top of the inner hair cells. Approximately 100 stereocilia form a W pattern on the outer hair cells. The plate is incomplete at the W notch; only a thin cell membrane is present. The basal body of a kinocilium lies beneath the membrane, but unlike the hair cells of the vestibular system, there is no a motile ciliary (hairlike) portion there.

The stereocilia range in length from 3 to 5 µm. The longest come into contact with the tectorial membrane but do not pass through it. This membrane is a thin fibrillar layer covering the top of the spiral limbus. It is an acellular gelatinous structure that thickens as it extends outward over the reticular lamina and the inner sulcus. Radially and somewhat obliquely, its fibrils extend until they terminate at its lateral border, directly above the point where the Hensen cells and the reticular lamina converge. The membrane border in the upper turns of the cochlea terminates in finger-like projections that touch the stereocilia of the outermost hair cells. From the modiolus, the myelin-ensheathed vestibulocochlear nerve fibers fan out spirally to enter the canal of Rosenthal, which is located close to the root of the osseous spiral lamina. The spiral ganglion is made up of the bipolar cell bodies of these neurons. Their distal processes continue radially beyond the ganglion, through the habenula perforata, a collection of tiny pores directly beneath the inner hair cells in the bony lamina beneath the limbus. It is at this point that the fibers abruptly shed their multiple myelin coats and continue into the organ of Corti as slender, clear, and unmyelinated fibers. A longitudinally directed bundle of some fibers runs beneath the inner hair cells, and another bundle is formed just inside the tunnel, above the inner pillar cells. About 95% of the fibers in an adult human ear terminate on the inner hair cells. The rest emerge as longitudinal bundles beneath the rows of outer hair cells, where they eventually come to an end.

There are two different kinds of nerve fiber endings located beneath the hair cells. Many tiny vesicles, or liquid-filled sacs, containing neurotransmitters, which mediate impulse transmission at neural junctions, are found in the larger and more numerous endings. These ends are a part of a unique bundle of nerve fibers that originate in the brainstem and form the cochlea's efferent system, also known as the feedback loop. There are fewer vesicles and other cell structures in the smaller, less numerous endings. These are the ends of the cochlear nerve's afferent fibers, which send impulses from hair cells to the brainstem.

It has been estimated that the cochlea contains 12,000 outer hair cells overall and 3,500 inner hair cells. The cochlear nerve has roughly 30,000 fibers, but the innervation of the outer hair cells overlaps significantly. Numerous hair cells may receive their endings from a single fiber, sharing a "party line" in the process. Additionally, several fibers can send nerve endings to a single hair cell. Though the precise distribution of nerve fibers within the organ of Corti is unknown, it is known that the majority of afferent fiber endings reach the inner hair cells, which do not share or overlap fibers like the outer hair cells. When viewed from above, the reticular lamina, which covers the organ of Corti, creates a distinct mosaic design. In humans, the outer hair cells are arranged in three distinct and orderly rows in the basal turn of the cochlea. However, in the higher turns of the cochlea, the arrangement becomes slightly irregular as scattered cells form the fourth or fifth row. Phalangeal plates, which are irregularly shaped extensions of the supporting cells, occupy the spaces between the outer hair cells. The inner and outer pillar cells' double row of head plates divides the inner from the outer hair cells and covers the tunnel. Both of these cell groups are not included in the reticular lamina, which stretches from the inner border cells close to the inner sulcus to the Hensen cells. Aging, illness, or noise-induced injury can cause a hair cell to degenerate and eventually disappear. In this case, the adjacent phalangeal plates quickly cover the missing hair cell and enlarge to form a distinctive "scar."

1.1.5.3. Endolymph and Perilymph

The composition of the perilymph, which fills the area inside the bony labyrinth that encircles the membranous labyrinth, is similar to that of other extracellular bodily fluids, such as cerebrospinal fluid, but distinct. Like other extracellular fluids, the perilymph has a high concentration of sodium ions (roughly 150 milliequivalents per liter) and a low concentration of potassium ions (roughly 5 milliequivalents per liter). Similar to these fluids, it appears that transport mechanisms that permit certain substances to pass through capillary walls selectively form the perilymph locally from the blood plasma. Experimental research suggests that it is unlikely that the cerebrospinal fluid is involved in the normal production of perilymph, even though it is anatomically possible for it to enter the cochlea through the perilymphatic duct.

The endolymph that fills the membranous labyrinth is distinct from other extracellular bodily fluids, such as perilymph, in that it has a higher potassium ion concentration (approximately 140 milliequivalents per liter) than sodium ion concentration (about 15 milliequivalents per liter). Uncertainties still exist regarding the endolymph's formation and the maintenance of the ionic composition gap between it and the perilymph. Between the two fluids, the Reissner membrane creates a selective barrier. There also seem to be blood-endolymph and blood-perilymph barriers, which regulate the flow of chemicals, including medications, from the blood to the inner ear. There is evidence that the endolymph is not directly produced from the blood, but rather from the perilymph via selective ion transport via the Reissner membrane's epithelial cells. It is believed that the stria vascularis, a secretory tissue located in the cochlear duct's lateral wall, is crucial to preserving the endolymph's high potassium-to-sodium ion ratio. It is also believed that maintaining the ionic composition of the endolymph involves other cochlear tissues and the dark cells of the vestibular organs, which need to produce their own endolymph. Since the membranous labyrinth is a closed system, the endolymph's removal and flow are also significant issues. Even though this seems to be only part of the story, it is believed that the endolymph is reabsorbed from the endolymphatic sac. Additional cochlear and vestibular tissues may play significant roles in controlling the inner-ear fluids in terms of volume and composition.

1.2. Peripheral Receptors and Physiology of Auditory and Vestibular Systems

The pathway of hearing transmits auditory information from the receptors in the inner ear's organ of Corti (cochlear hair cells) to the central nervous system through the vestibulocochlear nerve (CN VIII). This pathway culminates in the primary auditory cortex for conscious perception, while also allowing for unconscious processing of auditory information to occur simultaneously.

1.2.1. Components of the Auditory Pathway

The auditory pathway is complicated because information diverges and converges at various points in time.

There are two main components of the auditory pathway:

i. The primary pathway: also known as the lemniscal pathway, is the primary means by which auditory information gets to the primary auditory cortex (A1).
ii. Non-lemniscal pathway: mediating auditory reflexes, emotional response, and attention, among other unconscious perceptions.

1.2.1.1. Primary Pathway

1.2.1.1.1. Spiral Ganglion

The first order neuronal cell bodies are located in the spiral ganglion (ganglion is a term used to describe a grouping of cell bodies that are not part of the central nervous system). These neurons move within the osseous spiral lamina and receive information from hair cells in the Organ of Corti. The primary structure of the cochlear nerve is made up of its central axons. When the vestibular and cochlear nerves converge at the internal acoustic meatus, they are referred to as the vestibulocochlear nerves. Because lesions to this nerve typically cause symptoms in both the vestibular and auditory domains, this closeness is clinically significant. The nerve passes through the internal acoustic meatus of the skull and then goes to the cerebellopontine angle, where it enters the brainstem after a brief (approximately 1 cm) journey. It is at the ipsilateral cochlear nuclei where the first order neurons synapses.

1.2.1.1.2. Cochlear Nuclei

Information is transmitted to the cochlear nuclei on either side of the brainstem by means of bifurcating cochlear nerve fibers. The region where the nerve enters the brainstem is home to the ventral (anterior) cochlear nucleus. The inferior cerebellar peduncle is situated in front of the dorsal (posterior) cochlear nucleus. The auditory tubercle, a tiny bulge on the brainstem's surface, is the result of it.

The majority of the fibers ascend in the contralateral lateral lemniscus after crossing the midline from the dorsal cochlear nucleus. In the ipsilateral lateral lemniscus, additional fibers ascend. Certain fibers also ascend bilaterally in the lateral lemniscus from the ventral cochlear nucleus. Nonetheless, in an area referred to as the trapezoid body, the majority of fibers from the ventral cochlear nucleus decussate to the contralateral superior olivary nuclei. Certain fibers synapse at the ipsilateral superior olivary nucleus, despite the ventral cochlear nuclei neurons decussating at the trapezoid body. The trapezoid body and the superior olivary nucleus are adjacent to each other. Additionally, it extends through the lateral lemniscus upward.

In conclusion, certain fibers in the ventral and dorsal nuclei decussate while others do not. As a result, each lateral lemniscus receives information bilaterally from both ears. The reason for this is that supranuclear lesions, or i.e., above the level of the cochlear nucleus) won't cause significant hearing loss. Thus, hearing issues are rarely central but can be conductive or sensorineural.

1.2.1.1.3. Inferior Colliculus and Medial Geniculate Body

The inferior colliculus is where all of the auditory information-carrying fibers that ascend from the superior olivary and cochlear nuclei congregate after passing through the lateral lemniscus. Remember that vision is relayed on the lateral geniculate body. These fibers project to the ipsilateral medial geniculate body (MGB) in the thalamus. The MGB mediates the refining of the incoming information and has reciprocal connections with the auditory cortex, so it functions as more than just a simple relay center. The primary auditory cortex is the next location for projections coming from the medial geniculate body.

1.2.1.1.4. Primary Auditory Cortex

Situated directly beneath the lateral fissure in the superior temporal gyrus is the primary auditory cortex (A1).

1.2.1.2. Non-Lemniscal Pathways

These are not the routes that lead to the primary auditory cortex. They include attention, reflexes, emotional reactions, and multisensory integration.

1.2.2. Physiology of Vestibular System

The vestibular system is an intricate network of neural pathways and structures that performs a multitude of tasks that support our sense of equilibrium and proprioception. Orientation and head acceleration in any direction, along with the corresponding adjustments to posture and eye movement, are among these functions. Vestibulo-ocular and vestibulospinal reflexes are the names given to these reflexes, respectively. The brain's neural pathways, which are part of the central vestibular system, react to afferent input from the peripheral vestibular system in the inner ear to produce efferent signals that enable these reflexes. According to available research, the vestibular system may also be involved in consciousness. Cognitive deficiencies pertaining to learning, navigation, and spatial memory can result from vestibular system dysfunction.

1.2.2.1. Cellular Level

The vestibular system is made up of a huge number of afferent and efferent cellular connections. The peripheral vestibular system, which is housed in the inner ear within the petrous temporal bone, is the primary source of afferent nerve signals. Both a membranous and a bony labyrinth are found in the inner ear. Perilymph, a fluid that drains into the subarachnoid space and is similar to cerebrospinal fluid, fills the bony labyrinth. The membranous labyrinth, which is suspended inside the bony labyrinth, is home to endolymph, a fluid with a distinct composition because of its high potassium ion concentration. Similar to the Stria vascularis of the cochlea, the Vestibular Dark Cells in the vestibular system produce endolymph. The sensory epithelium is surrounded by endolymph in the membranous labyrinth, which also interacts with hair cells in the vestibular apparatus to provide a high potassium gradient that aids in hair cell depolarization and afferent nerve transmission. The utricle, saccule, and superior, posterior, and lateral semicircular ducts make up the vestibular apparatus. The macula is the sensory neuroepithelium found in the utricle and saccule, and the crista ampullaris is the sensory neuroepithelium found in the semicircular ducts. Hair cells are specialized mechanoreceptor cells found in both neuroepithelial structures. Many stereocilia, or cross-linked actin filaments, are found inside hair cells and are joined at the tips by "tip links."

The stereocilia are arranged in rows according to length and have cation channels at their apex. The tallest stereocilium is connected to an immobile kinocilium. The unique 9 + 2 microtubule arrangement is found in the kinocilium, the only real cilium. Type 1 and Type 2 hair cells are the two subtypes of hair cells. Type 2 hair cells have a low resting discharge variability compared to Type 1 hair cells' high resting discharge variability. Depending on which way the inertial drag is moving, the movement of stereocilia due to endolymph acceleration causes either depolarization or hyperpolarization. As the tip links move in the direction of the kinocilium, they pull open the cation channels, causing depolarization and an influx of potassium ions. Neurotransmission to the vestibular ganglion and glutamate to afferent nerve receptors are released by the depolarized hair cell. Stereocilia converge when movement occurs in the opposite direction of the kinocilium, which closes the cation channels through tip links. The hair cell becomes hyperpolarized and the afferent nerve's ability to release glutamate is inhibited when there is insufficient potassium influx. Thousands of bipolar neurons found in the vestibular ganglion, also called the Scarpa ganglion, process sensory information from hair cells in the macula and crista ampullaris. The vestibular nerve is formed by the union of afferent axons from the vestibular ganglion. After that, the vestibular and cochlear nerves combine to form the vestibulocochlear nerve, also known as cranial nerve VIII. The central vestibular system of the brain then interprets the afferent nerve signals that the vestibulocochlear nerve carries. The peripheral signals from the two ascending pathways are combined by the central vestibular system to produce motor responses in the body, head, and eyes that regulate orientation and balance.

1.2.2.2. Development

The third week marks the start of the peripheral vestibular system's development when surface ectoderm forms the otic placodes. When they are encircled by embryonic mesoderm in the fourth week, the otic placodes transform into the otic pits. Subsequently, the otic pits grow into otic vesicles. As the vestibular apparatus, the upper part of the otic vesicle develops. A division takes place between the ventral saccular portion and the dorsal utricular portion of the otic vesicle as it lengthens. The dorsal utricular portion forms the utricle and semicircular canals, while the ventral saccular portion becomes the adult saccule and cochlear duct. With the exception of the vestibular aqueduct's internal aperture, which develops until birth, the system ossifies starting at 19 weeks of gestation and reaches adult size by 25 weeks. At seven weeks, otoconia and hair cells begin to develop. Between 11 and 13 weeks, Type 1 and Type 2 hair cells differentiate.

1.2.2.3. Function

The vestibular system plays a crucial role in detecting head position and movement in space, enabling coordination of eye movements, posture, and balance. It consists of the inner ear's vestibular apparatus, which sends nerve signals to the brain. The utricle and saccule within the vestibular apparatus detect linear acceleration, gravitational forces, and head tilting. The macula in these structures provides feedback on horizontal and vertical motion, aided by tiny calcium carbonate crystals called otoliths. Three semicircular ducts sense head rotation in different planes, with each containing an ampulla housing the crista ampullaris. The crista ampullaris, covered by a gelatinous substance called the cupula, aids in hair cell response. Unlike the macula, it does not contain otoliths. The central vestibular system processes and interprets signals, allowing for a coordinated response to head movements.

The vestibulo-ocular reflex is one example of an efferent signal that enables the eyes to stay fixed on an object while the head moves. This is achieved by synchronizing movement of the parapontine reticular formation in both eyes, which outputs to different extraocular eye muscles through the abducens and oculomotor nerves. By coordinating head movement and spinal musculature, the vestibulospinal reflex preserves posture and balance. Though many of these neural pathways remain unknown, established neural pathways underpin cognitive functions involving the central vestibular system. The vestibulo-thalamo-cortical tract, the nucleus reticularis pontis oralis to hippocampus tract, and the dorsal tegmental nucleus to entorhinal cortex tract are among the recognized central vestibular connections. These tracts connect in a complex way and are involved in self-motion perception, object recognition memory, spatial navigation, and spatial memory.

1.2.2.4. Mechanism

The acceleration of endolymph within the various vestibular apparatus structures is the mechanism underlying the peripheral vestibular system's function. This acceleration that causes the stereocilia of hair cells to be stimulated is caused by head movement in different directions. Hair cells return to their baseline position when the head stops accelerating, enabling them to react to additional variations in endolymph acceleration. The inertial drag of the endolymph pushes the stereocilia in the direction of acceleration or away from the fixed kinocilium. Tip links pull open cation channels when the hair cell moves in the direction of the kinocilium, which depolarizes the hair cell by bringing in potassium ions. Moving away from the kinocilium causes the afferent firing rates to decrease, hyperpolarization to occur, and the cation channels to close. The opening of calcium channels is the outcome of depolarization. Neurotransmitters are released across the synaptic cleft as a result of calcium channel opening, which causes nerve transmission to the vestibular ganglion. Nerve signals travel along the vestibular nerve after passing through the 20,000 bipolar neurons in the vestibular ganglion. At the pontomedullary junction, the vestibular nerve connects to the cochlear nerve and enters the brainstem. The vestibular nucleus complex, which stretches from the rostral medulla to the caudal pons, is the main processor of vestibular signals. In order to process and modify efferent signals to postural or ocular muscles, the vestibular nucleus sends a multitude of signals to the thalamus, cortex, or cerebellum. Notably, the hippocampal region is crucial for spatial memory, which includes orientation and navigational processes.

1.2.2.5. Related Testing

To ascertain whether the vestibular system is operating correctly, numerous tests are available. Using vestibular system reflexes, the oculocephalic reflex is a straightforward test that can be used to assess if a patient in a comatose state has an intact brainstem. The vestibular system on the ipsilateral side of rotation should be stimulated when a patient's head is rotated horizontally during the test. If the brainstem is still intact, this causes the patient's eyes to gradually veer to the side opposite to head movement. The eyes will follow the head's movement to the ipsilateral side if the brainstem is damaged. Caloric testing is a diagnostic procedure that uses temperature variations to identify acoustic nerve damage. One of your ears is softly administered a tiny bit of cold water or air. There should be an involuntary movement in your eyes known as nystagmus. After that, they ought to slowly turn away from that ear and return. In the event that water is used, the ear canal is allowed to empty. After that, the same ear is gently given a tiny amount of warm water or air. Again, nystagmus should be visible in your eyes. They should then slowly turn back toward that ear.

The most popular vestibular function test, videonystagometry, is one of the more specialized assessments for vestibular function components. The examination consists of three sections: positional testing, calorie testing, and ocular motor testing. Video head impulse testing (VHIT) and rotation tests are additional diagnostic modalities. These two tests assess the vestibulo-ocular reflex integrity by using devices to track eye movements when the head is rotated in different directions.

1.2.2.6. Clinical Significance

Vestibular dysfunction can cause vertigo, nausea, vomiting, visual disturbances, hearing abnormalities, and a range of cognitive deficits as symptoms. Although the vestibular system's relationship to cognition is poorly understood, many patients with vestibular dysfunction show impairments in their ability to learn, remember, navigate spatially, and recognize objects. Peripheral or central pathophysiology can be used to describe vertigo. Three of the most frequent causes of peripheral vertigo are viral labyrinthitis, Meniere's disease, and benign paroxysmal positional vertigo. Peripheral vertigo is more common than central vertigo.

Peripheral vertigo is most commonly attributed to benign paroxysmal positional vertigo (BPPV), which can last anywhere from a few seconds to several minutes. The pathophysiology of the majority of cases is thought to be caused by displaced otoconia in the posterior semicircular canal, which results in an inappropriate sensation of movement. Based on a detailed medical history and the results of the Dix-Hallpike test, BPPV is diagnosed along with associated nystagmus and vertigo symptoms. The Epley maneuver is frequently mentioned as one of the most useful movement techniques for treating brain pressure partial encephalopathy (BPPV). The method involves shifting displaced otoconia in the inner ear by tilting and rotating the head and body in different directions. Anti-vertigo drugs are recommended for acute, severe BPPV exacerbations in order to aid in symptom management. Meniere's disease is a peripheral vertigo condition that can cause episodes lasting for hours, along with symptoms like hearing loss and tinnitus. It is caused by an increase in the volume of endolymph fluid in the inner ear's membranous labyrinth, affecting both the vestibular apparatus and cochlea. This expansion of fluid in the cochlear duct can lead to hearing issues that set it apart from BPPV. Diagnosis is based on clinical criteria, and there are currently no known cures for Meniere's disease. However, symptoms can be managed with medications to reduce vertigo, following a low-salt diet, and in severe cases, surgical decompression of the endolymphatic sac may be considered.

Another condition that can cause peripheral vertigo is viral labyrinthitis, also referred to as vestibular neuritis. This condition is caused by inflammation of the vestibular nerve as a result of a viral infection. One of the symptoms, which can linger for days or weeks, is a simultaneous loss of hearing and balance in the afflicted ear. Antivertigo drugs are used as a form of treatment, and symptoms usually go away in one to three weeks. Apart from the disorders mentioned, vestibular function in the elderly has been thoroughly investigated as a potential contributor to lightheadedness and unsteadiness that result in falls. This is brought on by the substantial loss of Type 1 and Type 2 hair cells, which is most noticeable in the 65–70 age range. Salicylate, or aspirin, has the ability to cause hearing loss by reversibly removing the electromotility of outer hair cells. Salicylate reversibly inhibits electromotility by competitively binding to the motor protein. Aspirin toxicity can also cause vomiting, tinnitus, hyperpnea, nausea, and disorientation. Quinines, aminoglycosides, furosemide, and cisplatin are a few more common ototoxicants.

1.3. Audiology and Acoustic

One type of energy that can be moved from one location to another is sound. A pressure wave produced by objects vibrating is called sound. In our daily lives, sound is used extensively and carries energy. Audiology is the study, evaluation, treatment, and prevention of balance and hearing impairments. Assessing how the human ear functions, which influences hearing sensitivity and balance, is the main focus of clinical audiology. Characterizing particular hearing or balance losses helps with impairment diagnosis and allows for the creation of efficient treatment or management strategies.

1.3.1. Hearing Sensitivity

The human ear has a wide dynamic range, from the threshold of hearing (sound just detectable) to the threshold of discomfort (sound uncomfortably loud). The difference in level between these two extremes is over six orders of magnitude. The human ear can hear frequencies of vibration from 20 to 20,000 Hz, with some reduction in the upper limit as we age.

For a long time, it has been known that frequency and the dynamic range of hearing are generally correlated. Research on the lowest audible level of hearing has used stimuli that are either presented to both ears simultaneously or individually (usually through an earphone and loudspeaker, respectively). The two methods yielded similar, though not identical, results, indicating that human hearing is most sensitive in the 500–10,000 Hz range. As a baseline reference level, the typical values obtained at individual frequencies in a group of young, healthy individuals are used to compare listeners suspected of having a hearing impairment.

1.3.2. Pure-Tone Audiometry

Pure-tone audiometry is the most popular evaluation method in clinical audiology. On a graph known as a pure-tone audiogram, the listener's hearing threshold level, or hearing level, is plotted in decibels (dB). The hearing level is plotted on the ordinate (vertical axis) as a function of signal frequency on the abscissa (horizontal axis). In a traditional clinical audiogram, the abscissa is closer to the raised levels (reduced hearing) and the top of the chart is occupied by low dB values (normal hearing). As a result, on the pure-tone audiogram chart, higher hearing levels are plotted lower, signifying decreased hearing.

On the audiogram chart, the 0 dB hearing level line is represented by the reference baseline, also known as audiometric zero. For instance, if a listener's hearing threshold for a given signal is 60 dB, then the listener's hearing threshold is 60 dB higher than the median value found in a sample of young, healthy individuals who are normally distributed. It is generally accepted that the normal hearing range is within ±20 dB of the zero line; however, not every young adult in good health has a hearing threshold level that is on the 0 dB line. The hearing threshold is typically measured for discrete frequencies between 500 Hz and 8,000 Hz for clinical purposes. The measurement is reported in 5 dB step sizes and occurs at octave or half-octave intervals. A traditional measurement technique called the method of limits is used to choose which signals to show the listener. The listener's job is to react each time he or she detects a signal in a series of signals that are presented in an ascending or descending run (from loud to quiet, or vice versa). There is a level above which the pure tone is always heard and a level below which the tone is never heard, just like with any psychophysical measurement. When a signal is detected at least 50% of the time, it is said to be at the threshold of hearing. Because a host of extrinsic and intrinsic factors can influence the measurements (e.g., ambient noise level and duration of the test signal, respectively), clearly defined procedures have been developed for clinical testing.

While it might seem like a simple process to measure hearing thresholds from each ear independently, sound can travel from one side of the head to the other. For instance, if the listener's hearing is poor in the ear being tested, the signal might be strong enough to pass through the skull and be picked up by the better-hearing ear on the other side. To avoid the test signal being cross-heard in those situations, a masking noise is played for the nontest ear. The when and how of masking have been standardized through the development of procedures. Insufficient masking can allow the nontest ear to continue detecting the test signal; excessive masking can lead to cross-masking, which raises the test ear's hearing threshold unnaturally.

The severity of hearing loss can vary by frequency, but is typically categorized as mild, moderate, severe, or profound based on average hearing threshold levels. The ability to understand speech is impacted by the degree of hearing loss. Mild impairment (26–40 dB) can make it challenging to hear speech, especially in noisy environments. Moderate impairment (41–60 dB) can make speech difficult to hear without a hearing aid. Severe (61–80 dB) or profound (81 dB or greater) impairment may make conversational speech completely inaudible without assistance. Some individuals may require a cochlear implant to hear speech effectively. The Speech Intelligibility Index can be used to measure the proportion of speech that is audible and understandable for a listener with or without a hearing aid. At high volume levels, the test signal may be perceived as a vibration, especially for low-frequency sounds, which can make it difficult to distinguish between auditory and vibrotactile perception.

1.3.3. Air-Conduction and Bone-Conduction Testing

In general, there are two types of hearing loss: sensorineural and conductive. When something wrong with the middle or outer ear stops sound from getting to the inner ear's cochlea, it results in conductive hearing loss. A malfunction with the cochlea's sensory transducer cells or, less frequently, the brain's neural pathway can cause sensorineural hearing loss. The term "mixed hearing loss" refers to the situation where conductive and sensorineural hearing loss coexist. Sensorineural hearing loss is typically irreversible, but conductive hearing loss is frequently treatable with surgery and is more common in children. The audiologist must differentiate between the two conditions as a result.

Comparing the air-conduction and bone-conduction hearing threshold levels can help distinguish between conductive and sensorineural hearing loss. This entails using two distinct kinds of earphones to measure hearing sensitivity. An earphone or loudspeaker is used to present a pure tone during the air-conduction test. The signal passes from the middle ear to the cochlea in the inner ear via the air in the outer ear. In the bone-conduction test, the skull is implanted with an electromechanical earphone in place of an earphone. This makes it possible to mechanically vibrate the skull to stimulate the cochlea while barely stimulating the middle and outer ears. The hearing threshold for both air and bone conduction is usually near 0 dB in people with normal hearing. People with auditory pathway hearing disorders in general have low air-conduction thresholds. Since abnormalities of the conduction mechanism have relatively little effect on bone-conduction measurements, poor air-conduction threshold is the primary indicator of conductive hearing loss. The thresholds for both bone and air conduction are impacted in sensorineural hearing loss, resulting in an air-bone gap that is almost zero (bone conduction less air conduction). An air-bone gap indicates conductive hearing loss.

The difference in sound levels between the threshold of hearing and the level of discomfort is typically around 100 dB for people with normal hearing. Individuals with sensory hearing loss may have higher hearing thresholds, but their sensitivity to loud sounds is similar to that of individuals with normal hearing. Those with sensory hearing impairment often have a smaller dynamic range and may experience loudness recruitment, which is an abnormal increase in loudness for a small increase in sound intensity. This can impact the design of hearing aids, as nonlinear amplification – where soft sounds are amplified more than loud sounds – may be necessary. However, while this type of amplification can help with soft sounds, it cannot fully address issues such as difficulty in distinguishing frequencies, leading to continued challenges with background noise for many individuals.

1.3.4. Pediatric Assessment Procedures

The preferred measurement method between the ages of six months and two or three years is typically visual reinforcement audiometry. This is associating a head-turn in response to auditory stimuli with an engaging visual reward, like a flashing light or an animated plush animal. After this classical conditioning is established, operant conditioning occurs, where a correct sound triggers a head turn that results in a visual reward. Using this method, one can ascertain the lowest response level necessary to cause a head turn. While ear-specific measurements are typically attempted on children, there are situations when earphones are intolerable and the signal must be presented through a loudspeaker; this is referred to as sound field audiometry. In general, babies are more likely to be sensitive to high-frequency sounds than low-frequency sounds; it is unclear whether this is because of physiological development or other factors, like infant-directed speech, which is partly typified by high-frequency pitches.

Behavioral testing is not very helpful in determining hearing threshold levels before six months. Nonetheless, the healthy cochlea produces a tiny amount of sound, known as otoacoustic emission, which can be detected in the ear canal using a tiny, sensitive microphone. A clinical procedure that can be used to screen a newborn's hearing is based on the typical response from a healthy ear. Event-related potentials, or the brain activity resulting from a sensory or cognitive response to a stimulus, can be utilized to estimate hearing sensitivity in the absence of otoacoustic emission recordings. This entails using scalp-attached recording leads to measure electrical potentials. Since it can be obtained while the baby is sleeping, the auditory brainstem response is the preferred method. Starting at a high level and lowering it until the evoked response is no longer detectable is a common protocol. The tester's subjective analysis of the waveform determines whether a response is present. When adult participants in pure-tone audiometry are unable or unwilling to provide accurate information, event-related potentials can also be used to estimate hearing sensitivity. If a newborn's initial hearing test is unsuccessful, they may go through auditory steady state response testing, which measures the baby's brain activity while they sleep by exposing them to tones with varying frequency and intensity. Statistics are used to determine whether a steady state response is present.

Tympanometry is a widely used procedure that gives information about the health of the middle ear and the tympanic membrane (eardrum). When assessing the eardrum in kids who are susceptible to ear infections—a condition where fluid builds up in the middle ear space that is normally filled with air—tympanometry is often utilized. Using a handheld device, the air pressure inside the ear is altered while a pure tone is produced. Based on the idea that some sound enters the ear canal and is reflected back from the eardrum, the procedure measures the amount of reflected sound using a sensitive microphone. The air pressure in the ear canal rises when the eardrum is stiff, which causes the eardrum to reflect sound more often. Several middle ear disorders are linked to eardrum stiffening.

1.3.5. Vestibular Assessment

The vestibular system of the inner ear is responsible for the perception of motion and balance. Rotatory vertigo, the sensation that the surroundings are spinning, can be brought on by abrupt abnormalities in the vestibular organ's function. Observing eye movements during specific visual and vestibular stimulation can provide valuable insights into vestibular function. The audiologist is especially interested in the existence of nystagmus, a slow, rapid oscillation of the eyes. Following a shift in vestibular function, this eye movement will occur on its own and may last for several days or weeks until the brain has had time to adjust. Changes in body posture, such as getting out of bed in the morning, can also cause nystagmus. A caloric test can be used to compare the sensitivity of the left and right vestibular organs. In this test, hot or cold water is irrigated into the external ear canal to elicit a response. Body sway can be measured using a force platform in vestibular assessment, which can reveal details about how the visual, vestibular, and proprioceptive systems are used for postural control and balance function.

Exercises for the head and eyes are commonly used in rehabilitation procedures to support the central compensation mechanism. Surgery might be considered in extreme situations. In order to treat vestibular disorders, surgery is typically performed in two ways: either destructively, removing the portion of the inner ear structures that are causing the patient's condition, or correctively, trying to stabilize inner ear function. Endolymphatic sac decompression is one type of corrective procedure that relieves pressure on the vestibular system, especially in cases of Ménière disease. Labyrinthectomy, which involves removing the inner ear's balance and hearing organs, and vestibular nerve section, which involves chopping the vestibular nerve to stop the brain from receiving balance information, are two examples of harmful surgeries.

1.4. Assessment of Hearing

A hearing evaluation establishes an individual's threshold for various frequencies of sound. Pure tone audiometry, a piece of equipment known as an audiometer, is used to conduct the assessment. The patient is given a button to hold and has earphones put in their ears. Each time the sound is played, the patient is instructed to press the button. The patient will be required to sit in a soundproof booth for this evaluation. The test takes around depending on the degree of hearing loss. 15 or 20 minutes. A middle ear function test will be performed to evaluate middle ear function using a tympanometer to conclude the hearing evaluation. Any middle ear abnormalities the patient may have will be revealed by this test. A tiny probe is inserted into the ear for a brief period of time during this quick, easy test. We will be able to provide a clear picture of any hearing loss to help with the diagnosis of hearing/tinnitus and balance disorders, along with the hearing assessment and middle ear function test.

1.4.1. Ear Examination

The patient's ears are typically examined with an otoscope before the hearing test to ensure that there is no wax buildup, the eardrum is undamaged, the ears are not infected, and there is no fluid in the middle ear, which could indicate a middle ear infection.

1.4.2. Pure Tone Audiometry

Pure tone audiometry is the most common and standard type of hearing test. It measures the air and bone conduction thresholds in each ear at eight standard frequencies ranging from 250 Hz to 8000 Hz. Either supraural headphones or a pair of foam inserts connected to an external audiometer are used for the test, which is performed in a sound booth. An audiogram diagram that plots a person's hearing sensitivity at the tested frequencies is the test's result. The softest threshold heard in the left ear at each particular frequency is represented by an "x" plot on an audiogram, while the softest threshold heard in the right ear at each specific frequency is represented by an "o" plot. In certain situations, a high-frequency version of the test that measures frequencies above 8,000Hz to 16,000Hz may be used.

1.4.3. In-Situ Audiometry Using Mobile Applications

New audiologic diagnostic techniques that enable people to determine their level of hearing loss on their own have emerged as a result of the accessibility of stereo headphones and smartphones or tablets with sound reproduction systems. Audiometric hearing testing is made possible for users of these mobile devices through a variety of applications. Additionally, there are applications for hearing aids that include a built-in hearing test for adjusting the devices.

Initial hearing thresholds of tone signal perception on various frequencies (audiogram) are determined during a hearing test using specialized applications. Hearing thresholds are established on a standard range of frequencies from 125 Hz to 8 kHz, much like with traditional audiometry and with a specific application. Additionally, a feature for evaluating the applicability of perceiving distinct sounds and intelligibility figures under varied acoustic circumstances can be integrated into an application.

The following blocks make up the hearing test application technically:

- a program module that generates tone signals at the necessary frequency.
- graphic interface options (to adjust the user's response when the threshold for tone perception is exceeded);
- interpreter of both text and graphic test results;
- database containing hearing age norms parameters and past exam results.

For the following reasons, the results of a hearing test performed by an audiologist and those obtained through the application will differ:

- the application of specific, calibrated apparatus
- soundproofing the space used for the hearing test
- heterogeneity of sound-recording system parameters in tablets, smartphones, and headphones or headsets
- noise masking effect of tone signals

The ability to perform the audiometry test independently and the availability of a specialized application or hearing aid application are benefits of this type of testing. The ability to perform the hearing test independently and the accessibility of hearing testing are unquestionably beneficial features of hearing testing with a special application or hearing aid application, even in the event that diagnostic results contain errors. Researchers propose that mobile applications for hearing tests can be used for both screening and diagnosis of hearing disorders.

1.4.4. Weber and Rinne

A thorough assessment of hearing also includes several additional tests. A bone conduction hearing test is used to identify the type of hearing loss that is present. A vibrating tuning fork is positioned on the mastoid process, behind the ear, for this test. The tuning fork is held in front of the ear until the patient can no longer feel or hear the vibration; at that point, the patient should hear a ringing sound once more. In the event that they are unable to, that ear has conductive hearing loss. The tuning fork is also positioned on the forehead. The patient is then questioned about whether the sound is more intense in one ear or if it is concentrated in the middle of the head. The affected ear will probably be louder if conductive hearing loss is present, and quieter if sensorineural hearing loss is present. This test aids the audiologist in determining whether the hearing loss is neural—caused by an issue in the brain's auditory pathways or cortex—sensorineural—caused by issues in the cochlea, the sensory organ of hearing—or conductive—caused by issues in the outer or middle ear.

1.4.5. Hearing in Noise

The Hearing in Noise Test (HINT) assesses a person's capacity to understand speech both in noisy and quiet environments. During the test, the patient has to repeat sentences in a quiet setting as well as when there is competing noise coming from various directions. In more detail, the conditions are as follows: (1) no competing noise in the sentences; (2) competing noise in the sentences presented directly in front of the patient; (3) noise presented at a 90° angle to the patient's right; and (4) noise presented at a 90° angle to the patient's left. For the patient to repeat the sentences correctly 50% of the time, the test determines the signal-to-noise ratio for each condition, or how loud the sentences must be played above the background noise.

1.4.6. Words-in-Noise Test

Monosyllabic words are used in the Words-in-Noise Test (WIN) at seven different signal-to-noise ratios along with masking noise, which is usually speech spectrum noise. The WIN test will provide a score indicating an individual's capacity to comprehend speech in a noisy environment. The WIN test may offer a more practical assessment of a person's hearing in an environment that is likely to arise than a pure-tone audiogram.

1.4.7. Modified Rhyme Test

"Methods for Measuring the Intelligibility of Speech Over Communication Systems," an American National Standard (ANSI S3.2), defines the Modified Rhyme Test (MRT). 50 sets of six monosyllabic words with different initial or final consonants (e.g., not, rave, rake, race, raze, rate, got, pot, hot, lot, or ray. Usually, one of the couplet's words is presented to the listener first, followed by the sentence "You will mark the word ___." The listener chooses what they think is the right answer out of the six rhymes that are presented. The US Air Force uses the MRT extensively to evaluate various communication systems, many of which have a noise interference component. An acceptable performance level is typically reached if a condition receives 80% or more of the correct answers.

1.4.8. Other Tests

The patient repeats words that they hear during speech tests administered by the audiologist or hearing instrument specialist. Furthermore, a tympanogram test is typically performed.

This test involves inserting a tiny probe into the ear canal and adjusting the air pressure within. The results of this test indicate to the audiologist how well the middle ear's eardrum and other structures function. The volume of the ear canal suggests whether or not there may be a tympanic membrane (eardrum) perforation. If there is any fluid in the middle ear space, it can be determined by measuring the middle ear pressure (also called glue ear or otitis media with effusion). The ossicles, or three ear bones, and the eardrum movement are measured for compliance.

An acoustic reflex test is the last examination the audiologist could conduct. This test involves inserting a probe into the ear to produce a loud tone that is higher than 70 dBSPL. The test measures the stapedius muscle's reflexive contraction, which is crucial for shielding the ear from loud noises like speech, which can have a decibel level of 90 dBSPL at the eardrum. This test can be used to reveal details about the facial and vestibular nerves and show whether a lesion might be present.

1.5. Common Types of Ear Diseases

While most people are aware of hearing loss, the ears can also be affected by a wide range of other conditions. While some are just inconvenient, others may be painful. Additionally, the effects of these illnesses may cascade into your hearing, aggravating any pre-existing hearing loss you may have. It is critical to understand the disorders that may impact your ears. The most prevalent ear illnesses are listed below. This section addresses the more significant conditions affecting the middle, outer, and inner ears.

1.5.1. Outer Ear

Disorders affecting the skin, cartilage, glands, and hair follicles within the outer ear canal are referred to as diseases of the outer ear. When earwax (cerumen), tumors, or infectious materials fill the ear canal, sound cannot travel to the tympanic membrane or eardrum, impairing the outer ear's ability to transmit sound. These paragraphs provide a brief description of the most common outer ear diseases.

1.5.1.1. Infections and Injuries

- **Frostbite:** The outer ear is the body part most commonly affected by freezing, or frostbite, due to its exposed position. Frostbite is more likely to occur in situations where the temperature is below freezing, as well as in conditions involving humidity, exposure time, and—above all—wind. The upper and outer edges of the ear are where the frozen area starts. It appears yellow-white and waxy, feels cold and hard to the touch, and loses skin sensation as it becomes numb. In order to treat frostbite, the victim is placed in a warm room as soon as possible. However, until the frozen part of the ear gradually thaws from within, the frozen part is kept cool by applying ice that is wrapped in a towel. Avoid massaging the frozen ear as this could cause skin damage. Blood in the blood vessels may clot if heat is applied to the frozen area before circulation is established. This can then cause dry gangrene, which is the death of that portion of the ear that eventually turns black and falls off.
- **Hematoma:** An external ear injury may result in bleeding between the skin and cartilage, which can form hematomas, which are smooth, non-tender purple swellings. A

surgeon removes the clot of blood because, if left, it will turn into scar tissue and result in cauliflower ear, a permanent irregular thickening of the outer ear that is common in boxers and wrestlers whose ears are frequently injured.

- **Perichondritis:** Perichondritis, an uncommon infection of the outer ear cartilage, can result from an injury or swimming in contaminated water. Pseudomonas aeruginosa is the specific microorganism responsible for it. The outer ear affected becomes dusky red, tender, and two to three times thicker than usual. A musty or foul-smelling discharge comes from the outer ear canal. It is imperative to receive prompt antibiotic treatment in order to avoid permanent deformity of the outer ear.
- **External Otitis:** Molds and other microorganisms can infect the outer ear canal, particularly in warm, humid climates and in swimmers. The ear canal becomes tender and itchy, and a thin, frequently odorous substance appears to drain from it. Hearing loss may result from the swelling and drainage clogging the canal. To treat the infection, a doctor's careful and comprehensive cleaning of the outer ear canal, the use of antiseptic or antibiotic eardrops, and refraining from swimming are recommended.
- **Boil in the Ear (Furuncle):** A boil, sometimes known as a furuncle, is an infection of a hair follicle anywhere on the body. This can happen in an outer ear canal hair follicle, particularly if the skin surrounding the canal is infected. It is always caused by a specific kind of bacteria called Staphylococcus. A boil in the ear canal is particularly painful, accompanied by swelling, redness, and tenderness, but usually without fever because the skin of the ear canal is closely attached to the underlying cartilage. Applying heat to the outer ear with an electric pad or hot-water bottle encourages the infection to intensify and start to drain. To stop the infection from spreading to other hair follicles, treatment with a systemic and local antibiotic is needed.
- **Erysipelas of the Outer Ear:** A specific strain of streptococcus bacteria causes erysipelas, a skin infection that is characterized by a gradually developing red, slightly tender skin thickening. It might start at the ear and move to the neck and face. Erysipelas epidemics caused serious, frequently fatal infections centuries ago. One of the worst erysipelas epidemics ever happened in AD 1089. The illness was known as St. Anthony's fire as a result of people who prayed to Saint. Anthony is reported to have recovered, while others did not and died. Nowadays, erysipelas is typically a mild infection that is relatively uncommon and goes away quickly with antibiotic treatment.
- **Leprosy:** Leprosy was another ancient scourge that occasionally affected the outer ear but is now uncommon outside of the tropics. Mycobacterium leprae, the leprosy

bacillus, is the cause. It causes the affected tissues to thicken and distort painlessly over time. The leprosy bacilli, which resemble the bacilli that cause tuberculosis in appearance, are found by looking under a microscope at a small sample of the infected tissue. Thankfully, antibiotics that were once effective against tuberculosis are also effective today at halting the progression of leprosy.

- **Osteoma of the Bony Ear Canal:** A bony bump that develops near the tympanic membrane is called an osteoma of the bony ear canal, and it is more common in people who frequently swim in cold water. Unless the bony overgrowth grows to the point where it blocks the ear canal, it is not dangerous and does not need to be removed.
- **Cyst of the Ear:** A sac containing liquid or semisolid material is called a cyst. A gland that lubricates the skin behind the earlobe, and less frequently at the entrance of the ear canal, is the most common cause of an ear cyst. The lubricating fatty material builds up as a soft, rounded nodule in the skin if this gland's duct becomes blocked. When the cyst becomes infected, a tender abscess forms and begins to drain. If surgery is not performed to remove the cyst entirely, it will return. Another kind of cyst can develop in the space directly in front of the outer ear, above the ear canal, or, less frequently, in the neck behind and below the ear. This is a piece of the early embryo's primitive gill, a reminder of our distant fish ancestors. It could be as small as a pit that occasionally leaks a little bit of moisture, or it could become a cystic swelling that needs to be surgically removed if the pit's opening closes.
- **Keloid of the Ear:** A thicker raised area on a scar known as a keloid can result from excessive growth of scar tissue from any type of skin injury or incision in people with dark skin. When earlobes are pierced for earrings, it can occasionally cause a large, painless nodular keloid enlargement of the earlobe that is unsightly but harmless. Keloids are surgically removed.

1.5.1.2. Deformities

- **Absence of the Outer Ear:** The absence of the outer ear canal frequently coexists with a congenital deformity, which is the absence of the outer ear, typically on one side but occasionally on both. In rare cases, this failure of the primitive gill structures to properly develop into the normal outer and middle ear is hereditary. It is often due to unknown reasons. In certain instances, it can be linked to congenital rubella syndrome when a pregnant woman is exposed to rubella during the first trimester. In most cases, hearing is preserved because the inner ear, equilibrium, and hearing nerves originate from the otic vesicle, which is independent of the gill structure. When sound conduction fails to reach the inner ear's hearing nerve, hearing can often be restored through surgery that creates a new ear canal and tympanic membrane.

- **Lop Ear:** A more common but less severe deformity of the outer ear is called lop ear, which is an excessive protrusion of the ear from the side of the head. Repositioning the ears to a more natural and unobtrusive position may require surgery.

1.5.1.3. Other Ailments

- **Eczema:** Like eczema elsewhere, eczema of the outer ear causes itching, scaling redness, and occasionally even tears on the affected skin. It frequently results from an allergy to a food or chemical that comes into contact with the skin, like hairspray. The best course of action is to identify the allergen and stay away from it. Applying cortisone ointment topically may provide momentary symptom relief.
- **Impacted Earwax:** Normally, the waxy material secreted by the glands in the outer ear canal's skin migrates slowly to the skin's outer layers. Overproduction of wax can lead to accumulation, which fills the outer ear canal completely and prevents sound from reaching the tympanic membrane, impairing hearing painlessly. A doctor may suction or remove larger plugs of earwax. Smaller quantities may be diluted with a few drops of mineral oil, left overnight, and then syringed out with an infant ear syringe made of soft rubber.

1.5.1.4. Cancer of the Outer Ear

The most common cause of outer ear cancer is prolonged exposure to direct sunlight over a long period of time. A tiny, initially painless ulcer that has a dry scab covering it and gradually grows larger and deeper could be a skin cancer. A tiny sample of tissue is taken from the edge and examined under a microscope to make the diagnosis. To effect a cure, the cancerous tissue needs to be completely removed through radiation therapy or surgery. Ear canal cancer is more dangerous because it has the potential to spread to the bone before it is discovered. After that, removal therapy becomes more challenging. While cancers of the outer ear skin are more common and more easily treated with excision, cancers of the ear canal are relatively uncommon.

1.5.2. Middle Ear

The eustachian tube, which runs from the upper region of the pharynx to the middle-ear cavity, provides air to the air-filled cavity and the air cells in the mastoid bone that extend backward from it. The mastoid and middle ear air spaces are directly above and behind the brain cavity, which is only separated from them by very thin bone plates. The middle ear cavity and the mastoid bone are both traversed by the nerve that supplies the facial expression muscles; only a thin layer of bone separates them. The facial nerve may occasionally rest directly against the mucous membrane lining the middle ear and mastoid air cells due to an incomplete bony covering. This mucous membrane, which lines the upper part of the throat and nose, is an extension of a similar mucus-producing membrane. It passes through the eustachian tube and into the middle ear and mastoid. It is vulnerable to the same infections and allergic responses that affect the nasal passages. Thus, the middle ear and mastoid air cells may be affected by an acute head cold or another infection of the nose and throat, such as measles or scarlet fever, which can spread through the eustachian tube. Because of the close proximity of the brain cavity to the mastoid air cells, an infection has the potential to cause meningitis, or inflammation of the brain's covering, or a brain abscess if left untreated. The mastoid bone is crossed by the large vein that drains blood from the brain en route to the jugular vein in the neck. This vein may become infected if the middle ear infection spreads, leading to "blood poisoning" (also known as septicemia, or infection of the bloodstream). Other potential consequences of middle-ear infection include facial nerve paralysis and infection spreading from the middle ear into the inner ear labyrinth. The specific location of the middle ear cavity, which is small but crucial, gives rise to all these possibilities.

1.5.2.1. Acute Middle-Ear Infection

Fortunately, bacteria that are sensitive to antibiotics are almost always the cause of acute middle ear infections, also known as acute otitis media. Consequently, it is now uncommon for an acute infection of the mastoid air cells to exacerbate an acute infection of the middle ear cavity and lead to a dangerous mastoid abscess that may cause meningitis, a brain abscess, septicemia, an infection of the labyrinth, or facial nerve paralysis. Mastoid abscess and other acute middle ear infection complications are most common in isolated areas and nations where people lack access to adequate healthcare and nutrition. Although severe and potentially fatal acute infections of the mastoid air cells and middle ear have become uncommon, chronic infections—discussed below—and another form of middle ear disease, secretory otitis media, are still common.

1.5.2.1.1. Secretory Otitis Media

The middle ear cavity fills with a clear, pale yellowish fluid that is not infected when one has secretory otitis media. The condition arises from insufficient middle ear ventilation via the eustachian tube. When the middle ear's supply of air is no longer supplied by this tube, the mucous membrane gradually absorbs the air and replaces it with fluid. Eventually, fluid—rather than air—completely fills the middle ear cavity. The fluid impairs the tympanic membrane's and the ossicular chain's ability to vibrate, which results in a painless hearing loss (Figure 1.3).

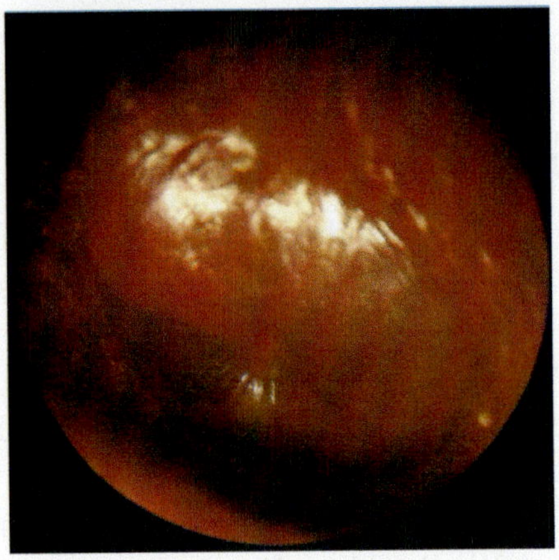

Figure 1.3. *Otitis media acuta.*

Source: By B. Welleschik – Own work, CC BY-SA 3.0, https://commons.wikimedia.org/w/index.php?curid=1514419.

The common causes of secretory otitis media include an allergic reaction to substances in the eustachian tube, an enlarged adenoid (a lymphoid tissue nodule) obstructing the eustachian tube's entrance, and an acute cold accompanied by swelling of the tube's membranes. If the middle ear fluid does not go away on its own in a week or two, the condition can be cured by identifying and eliminating the cause. The fluid must be expelled by forcing air through the eustachian tube after the tympanic membrane has been punctured. Antibiotics are not required if there is no fever or middle ear infection because they could compromise the middle ear's natural immune defenses. To help restore normal middle-ear ventilation in situations where an allergic reaction is not the underlying cause of the condition, a tiny plastic tube may need to be inserted through the membrane. This plastic tube is taken out after a while, once the middle ear and hearing have recovered. The tympanic membrane's tiny hole heals swiftly.

1.5.2.1.2. Aero-Otitis Media

An inability to stabilize the air pressure in the middle ear cavity during a sudden altitude change, such as during a fast descent in an inadequately pressurized aircraft, can cause aero-otitis media, a painful form of hearing loss. A person's ability to equalize—which is achieved by yawning or swallowing to open the eustachian tube—may be hampered by allergies or a cold that already exists. When the air pressure inside the throat increases relative to the outside, the tympanic membrane contracts sharply, and the air pressure in the throat presses the tube's opening firmly shut, making it impossible to open the tube by swallowing. Pain and a loss of hearing are associated with an intense feeling of pressure in the ear. The pressure differential between the tympanic membrane's two sides can occasionally cause it to burst. Usually, the discomfort doesn't go away until the middle ear fills with fluid or the membrane is surgically perforated. Aero-otitis media produced during flight is typically transient and goes away on its own.

1.5.2.2. Chronic Middle-Ear Infection

When the tympanic membrane is permanently perforated, dust, water, and bacteria from the outside world can enter the middle ear cavity and cause a chronic middle ear infection. As a result, there is persistent middle ear drainage via the outer ear canal. There are two different kinds of chronic middle ear infections: one is relatively benign, while the other is brought on by a risky bone-invading process that can cause major complications if left untreated. A stringy, odorless mucoid discharge that emerges from the surface of the mucous membrane lining the middle ear is indicative of the benign form of chronic middle-ear disease. Applications of powdered boric acid as part of medical treatment will stop the chronic drainage. After that, the membrane perforation may be sealed, returning the ear's normal structure and functionality along with hearing restoration.

A bone-invading process beneath the mucous membrane causes a foul-smelling discharge, which is often sparse and identifies the dangerous type of chronic middle-ear drainage. Cholesteatoma of the middle ear is the most common cause of these cases. This is a skin ingrowth from the outer ear canal that develops into a middle ear cyst. A cholesteatoma cyst infection grows slowly but steadily, progressively eroding bone until the cyst reaches the brain cavity, the nerve supplying the facial muscles, or an inner ear semicircular canal. A major consequence resulting from the infected material inside the cyst is either meningitis or brain abscess, facial nerve paralysis, or infection of the inner ear labyrinth with vertigo, all of which have the potential to cause complete deafness.

Thankfully, middle ear cholesteatomas are rarely ignored enough to allow a major complication to arise. The diagnosis of the bone-eroding cyst can be made by closely inspecting the tympanic membrane perforation and using X-ray studies. The cyst can then be surgically removed before it causes significant damage. This procedure is referred to as a modified radical mastoid or a radical mastoid. Tympanoplasty, or plastic reconstruction of the middle ear cavity, is the name given to the procedure if the ossicular chain is repaired and the tympanic membrane perforation is closed during the same procedure.

1.5.2.3. Ossicular Interruption

An infection or a forceful blow to the head can damage the ossicular chain, which is necessary to transfer sound waves from the tympanic membrane to the fluid that fills the inner ear. Where the incus joins the stapes is usually its weakest point. A partial separation results in a mild hearing impairment; a complete separation results in a severe hearing loss. A hearing test shows that while the inner ear's nerve of hearing is operating normally, sound is not being conducted from the tympanic membrane to the inner ear. Tympanoplasty corrects the malfunctioning ossicular chain ensuring that sound can once again be conducted to the inner ear.

1.5.2.4. Otosclerosis

The most common cause of progressive hearing loss in early and middle adulthood is "otosclerosis." This is affects the outer layer of bone that encircles the inner ear labyrinth. The name is misleading because the diseased nodule is softer than the ivory-hard bone it replaces when it is still in its early stages of expansion. "Otospongiosis" is a more appropriate term that is occasionally used, but tradition is so strong that the older name, applied before the process was fully understood, has stuck.

The softened otosclerotic bone nodule's underlying cause is unknown. Half of the cases occur in families where one or more relatives have the same condition, indicating a certain familial tendency. It affects black people 10 times more frequently than white people and twice as frequently in women as in men. During late childhood or early adulthood, the softened otosclerotic bone nodule initially manifests itself. Luckily, it stays small and benign most of the time, causing no symptoms, and only becoming apparent when the ear bones are extracted after death and examined under a microscope. Based on available data, it is estimated that by middle adulthood, 1 in 5 white adult women and 1 in 10 white adult men will have such an otosclerotic bone nodule (Figure 1.4).

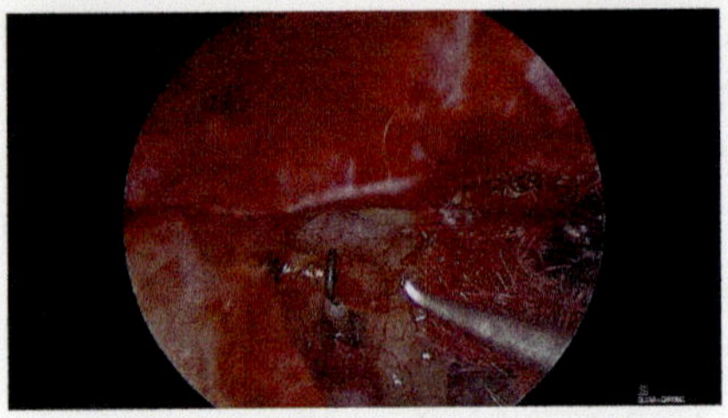

Figure 1.4. *Endoscopic view of the ear with the piston inserted into the stapedotomy.*

Source: By Mustafakapadiya – Own work, CC BY-SA 4.0, https://commons.wikimedia.org/w/index.php?curid=105133269.

A softened bone nodule that reaches the oval window containing the stapes footplate (stirrup) occurs in approximately 12% of cases of otosclerosis. The tympanic membrane's ability to vibrate in response to sound waves is hindered by the expanding nodule's increasing pressure. People who are affected gradually and covertly start to lose their hearing acuity. Initially, their capacity to perceive low-pitched sounds diminishes, followed by difficulty understanding whispered words, challenges in following conversations over a distance, and ultimately, their ability to hear and comprehend spoken words is limited to loud or near noises. One feature of hearing loss resulting from otosclerosis-induced stirrup fixation is the ability to hear a phone call by pressing the receiver against the head, which allows bone conduction to transmit sound waves to the inner ear. One more feature of this kind of hearing impairment is that it seems to get better when driving, traveling by plane, or taking a train. This is because people with normal hearing raise their voices involuntarily in response to the low-pitched roar of motors, but those with stirrup fixation are unable to detect this sound, so they hear better and take pleasure in the raised voices around them.

The diagnosis of stirrup fixation due to otosclerosis is based on a patient's history of gradual hearing loss, and the lack of a middle ear infection or tympanic membrane perforation. The results from hearing tests would indicate a functioning inner ear auditory nerve but sound is not reaching it properly. Audiometry or tuning fork tests would show that bone conduction is better than air conduction. Surgically exploration findings of an immobile stapes due to an osseous nodule is definitive for otosclerosis. To demonstrate that otosclerosis has spread to the stapes footplate, an ear X-ray using computed tomography may be taken.

Surgery can be used to correct stapes fixation. In 1956, it was discovered that in situations where the fixed stapes could not be mobilized, they could be removed and swapped out for a plastic or wire. Currently, the most common procedure for correcting stapes fixation due to otosclerosis is stapedectomy. The auditory nerve gradually deteriorates as a result of the osteosclerotic bone disease expanding in certain cases to the cochlea of the inner ear. This progressive deafness of the nerves can occur either before or after the stapes becomes fixed. It can sometimes happen without the stapes becoming fixed.

Although the exact causes of otosclerosis are unknown, the absence of fluoride in drinking water has been linked to the condition. There is evidence that augmenting the fluoride intake could encourage the softened nodule of the osteosclerotic bone to harden, thereby stopping or delaying its growth. This may help to postpone the progressive loss of auditory nerve function that frequently results from stapes fixation. Numerous nations have lowered the incidence of otosclerosis by fluoridating their water supplies.

1.5.3. Inner Ear

The vestibular nerve, also known as the nerve of equilibrium, and the auditory nerve, which are branches of the vestibulocochlear, or eighth cranial, nerve, are located in the labyrinth of the inner ear. The semicircular canals and otolithic membranes in the vestibule are supplied by the vestibular nerve ends. The cochlea is supplied by the auditory nerve. Disorders pertaining to the labyrinth of the inner ear can impact not only the vestibular nerve, which causes vertigo but also the auditory nerve, which results in hearing loss.

1.5.3.1. Nerve Deafness

1.5.3.1.1. Congenital Nerve Deafness

Congenital nerve deafness is a defect of the cochlea's auditory nerve that can develop during or shortly after birth, or it can be present from birth. When congenital nerve loss occurs, the inner ears are typically affected to a similar extent, and hearing is usually severely impaired, though it can occasionally be moderately impaired.

The rubella (German measles) virus, which infected the mother during the first three months of her pregnancy and stopped the development of the embryo's vesicle, has been linked to numerous cases of congenital nerve deafness. During a rubella epidemic, this can occur even in cases where the mother shows no signs of infection. Most of the time, the outer and middle ear structures are unaffected, and the vestibular nerve is either completely unaffected or only slightly affected. In developed nations, the incidence of congenital nerve deafness has decreased since the rubella virus vaccine became accessible in 1969.

Congenital nerve deafness that develops at birth or shortly after may be caused by anoxia, or inadequate oxygen, during a difficult and drawn-out delivery, or by kernicterus, a condition in which the baby becomes jaundiced due to an incompatibility between maternal and fetal blood groups. Congenital nerve deafness can occasionally be inherited as a result of improper cochlear development. Without specialized training, speech acquisition is impossible in cases of severe hearing loss. Children who are severely deaf are required to attend special classes or schools where they can learn sign language, lipreading, and speech. Utilizing the residual hearing that is typically present in such cases, electrical hearing aids can be useful, particularly in the classroom.

A cochlear implant is an additional option that is controversial among the deaf community but can be helpful in situations where there is significant hearing loss or complete deafness when the nerve responsible for hearing is present. An electrode is surgically inserted during this procedure to directly stimulate the auditory nerve, which connects the brain to the ear.

1.5.3.1.2. Viral Nerve Deafness

At any age, viral infections have the potential to cause severe sensorineural hearing loss in one or both ears. Severe sensorineural hearing loss in one ear is frequently caused by the mumps virus. The influenza and measles viruses are less frequent culprits. If a virus has damaged your hearing, there is no reliable medical or surgical cure.

1.5.3.2. Effects of Injury and Trauma

1.5.3.2.1. Ototoxic Drugs

Drugs classified as ototoxic (damaging to the ears) can impair auditory nerve function temporarily or occasionally permanently. When taken in sufficient quantities, salicylates like aspirin can cause ringing in the ears followed by a transient loss of hearing that goes away when the patient stops taking the medication. Quinine can have a similar effect, but in some cases, it can cause permanent impairment of the function of the auditory nerve. A number of antibiotics, including neomycin, kanamycin, dihydrostreptomycin, and streptomycin, have the potential to permanently harm auditory nerve function. Individual differences exist in the susceptibility to ototoxic drug-induced damage to the auditory nerve. Most of the time, the more resilient and less prone to damage vestibular nerve is unaffected, except for situations in which streptomycin is administered. More so than the auditory nerve, the vestibular nerve is impacted by streptomycin.

1.5.3.2.2. Skull Fracture and Concussion

The auditory and vestibular nerves can function less normally in cases of skull fracture and concussion from a severe blow to the head. The most severe hearing loss occurs when a skull fracture completely destroys the labyrinthine structure of the inner ear.

1.5.3.2.3. Exposure to Noise

The duration and intensity of the noise determine how it affects hearing. The results could last a short while or a lifetime. Hearing loss can be severe and irreversible after just one exposure to an extremely loud sound, like an explosion. Frequent exposure to noise levels above 80 to 90 dB may lead to a progressive loss of hearing by causing the inner ear's hair cells to die, potentially resulting in the degeneration of nerve fibers. Rock bands usually produce noise levels that are higher than 110 dB. Snowmobiles, power mowers, and farm tractors can produce noise levels of up to 100 dB. According to US law, employees who spend eight hours a day in environments where noise levels are higher than 90 decibels must be provided with a protective device, such as earmuffs or earplugs.

The likelihood that noise exposure will cause hearing loss varies from person to person. The effects of noise exposure may not be apparent until the hearing loss spreads to the lower frequencies of 1,000 to 2,000 hertz because hearing loss usually starts at the higher frequencies of 4,000 to 6,000 hertz. If given within a few hours of excessive noise exposure, 20 minutes of inhaling carbogen—a mixture of 5% carbon dioxide and 95% oxygen—will hasten hearing recovery.

1.5.3.3. Inflammation and Tumor

- **Labyrinthitis:** An infection resulting from meningitis, syphilis, acute otitis media and mastoiditis, or chronic otitis media and cholesteatoma can cause labyrinthitis, an inflammation of the inner ear labyrinth. In the afflicted ear, hearing and balance are both lost. Sometimes the damage is stopped by prompt antibiotic treatment, which makes partial inner ear function recovery possible.
- **Acoustic Neuroma:** An acoustic neuroma is a benign tumor on the auditory nerve that develops close to the point where it enters the inner ear labyrinth. One side experiences a progressive and gradual loss of vestibular and auditory nerve function due to the tumor. Ultimately, the tumor spreads into the brain, resulting in paralysis and headaches. Death and blindness could ensue if it is not removed. Thankfully, an acoustic neuroma can typically be detected early on with magnetic resonance imaging (MRI) and removed before it causes significant problems.

1.5.3.4. Ménière Disease

Ménière disease, also known as endolymphatic hydrops, is a fairly common disorder of the inner ear labyrinth that affects the auditory nerve, which results in hearing impairment, and the vestibular nerve, which causes vertigo attacks. It was initially reported by the French physician, Prosper Ménière, in 1861. It is now understood that the inner ear's excess endolymphatic fluid is the source of the symptoms. The endolymphatic duct and sac, which are responsible for resorbing endolymphatic fluid from the inner ear, frequently malfunction, though the exact cause of the excess endolymphatic fluid is not always known. A food allergy may also be the cause of the illness.

The symptoms include recurrent episodes of vertigo (often accompanied by nausea and vomiting), fluctuating degrees of hearing impairment with distorted sound in the affected ear, and a feeling of fullness or pressure in the ear. Confirmation of the diagnosis can be achieved by hearing tests, electrocochleography (to assess inner-ear pressure), and electronystagmography (to track eye movements indicative of nystagmus, an involuntary response to head positions that elicits symptoms and is caused by abnormal inner-ear function). The goal of treating Ménière disease is to identify the source of the excess endolymphatic fluid and bring it under control. Surgery might be required if non-medical therapy is unable to stop the vertigo episodes that keep happening. Some patients may experience a reduction in symptoms when pressure pulses are delivered to the ear canal via a minimally invasive Meniett device.

1.5.3.5. Presbycusis

Presbycusis is the age-related, progressive loss of hearing. Because it happens to different people at different ages and at different rates, it is comparable to other aging processes. Hearing is gradually diminished and eventually lost as a person ages due to a gradual loss of cochlear hair cells, which starts at the basal end of the organ of Corti. This loss occurs first for the highest audible frequencies (roughly 20,000 hertz) and then progressively for sounds of lower frequency. Typically, hearing loss does not start to gradually worsen until after the age of 60. The affected person experiences a growing inability to hear high-pitched sounds and comprehend spoken words. The progressive hearing loss may be stabilized by treating a zinc, coenzyme Q10, or possibly vitamin A nutritional deficiency. The doctor needs to confirm that the patient's condition cannot be fixed, such as buildup of earwax, secretory otitis media, or stirrup fixation due to otosclerosis. Some people find that an electrical hearing aid is very helpful, while others find that it only makes voices louder and less clear.

1.6. Rehabilitation

A deaf child or one with severe hearing loss cannot learn to speak through normal means; instead, they need to attend special classes or a school specifically designed for the deaf in order to learn lipreading and speech. The majority of these kids still possess some hearing, which they can use in their education by using devices that boost sound. A child with a moderate or mild hearing impairment can learn to speak on their own, although it will take them a little longer than a child with normal hearing. To improve diction, speech-correction instruction is typically necessary. For adults and children who are completely deaf or have hearing loss so severe that hearing aids are ineffective, cochlear implants may be a viable option. A deaf child can acquire speech with the help of implants, and a deaf adult can communicate more successfully.

Thanks to technological advancements in hearing aids, a greater number of people with hearing impairments can now reap significant benefits from amplification. For those with sensori-neural (or nerve-type) hearing loss, choosing the right hearing aid can be challenging and time-consuming. However, research has shown time and time again that wearing the right kind of hearing aid can greatly improve a listener with sensorineural hearing loss's ability to understand speech at conversational levels. When used in conjunction with lipreading, a hearing aid can help people with severe speech distortions comprehend more speech than they would be able to with lipreading alone. For those with conductive hearing loss, on the other hand, choosing a hearing aid is frequently a simpler process. To guarantee that the greatest amount of speech understanding is possible in noisy environments, careful selection is required. The person with hearing loss should speak with qualified specialists like audiologists, who are skilled in assessing the advantages of using a hearing aid.

Even those with normal hearing use lipreading, which really involves paying close attention to the entire facial expression rather than just the movements of the lips, as a means of supplementing their hearing in noisy environments with visual cues. Lipreading, or perhaps more accurately called speechreading, becomes more and more useful and significant as hearing starts to deteriorate. By closely observing a speaker of the language, a hearing-impaired person who is conversant in spoken language can learn lipreading. For individuals with hearing impairments who have not yet learned to speak a spoken language, formal lipreading instruction from a teacher either one-on-one or in a classroom setting is required. Lipreading becomes increasingly important as hearing loss increases, necessitating good lighting. As a communication tool, the hearing-impaired can also be taught a sign language like American Sign Language.

Speech-correction training becomes essential for an adult who unexpectedly loses all hearing in both ears, just as it does for children with significant hearing impairments. When one is profoundly deaf, their speech starts to sound flat and toneless, as they lose the monitoring effect of hearing their own voice.

A Closer Look

Tinnitus

Ear ringing or buzzing is known as tinnitus. About 10 to 15% of people suffer from chronic tinnitus, and one-third of adults are thought to have experienced tinnitus at some point in their lives. Tinnitus comes in two types: subjective, which is the most prevalent type, and objective, which is comparatively uncommon. Subjective tinnitus is a condition where noise perception is limited to the affected individual. A doctor can hear the ringing, buzzing, or clicking sound in objective tinnitus.

Tinnitus is characterized by a perceived ringing sound in the ears that can be caused by a variety of ear conditions, such as inflammation of the eardrum membrane, the middle ear, or the inner ear, or by earwax clogging the external auditory canal (cerumen). In addition, exposure to noise, high dosages of specific medications (like aspirin or the malaria medication chloroquine), and prolonged phone use can all cause tinnitus. It could be present in conjunction with hearing loss, especially high-frequency hearing. In addition, tumors pressing on blood vessels in the head or neck, such as cranial nerves (acoustic neuromas), atherosclerosis (the buildup of fat and cholesterol in the inner layer of arteries), and hypertension (unusually high blood pressure) can also result in tinnitus. Vertigo (dizziness) can occasionally be accompanied by ringing in the ears. For most people with tinnitus, there is no known cause despite these known factors. When someone is tired, tinnitus may become more severe, and it is frequently more noticeable at night than during the day.

Tinnitus can be treated with simple measures like getting rid of extra earwax or stopping drugs that can aggravate the condition. Tinnitus-causing vascular disorders may require surgery to treat. To reduce the noticeableness of the ringing or buzzing sound, one may utilize hearing aids, noise suppression equipment, and comparable techniques. It has been demonstrated that some people's perception of the loudness of chronic tinnitus can be lessened by music therapy, which involves the patient listening to music that does not contain notes that are equivalent in frequency to the ringing sound they experience. Drugs like amitriptyline and alprazolam may be prescribed in severe cases to lessen tinnitus symptoms.

Summary

- The human ear is an organ of balance and hearing that uses transduction—the conversion of sound waves into electrochemical impulses—to detect and analyze sound and preserve equilibrium.
- The structure of the outermost part of the ear, the auricle, is where the human ear differs most dramatically from the ears of other mammals.
- The membranous labyrinth inside the bony labyrinth is one of the two inner ear labyrinths, which exist in reality. The vestibule, a central chamber, the three semicircular canals, and the spirally coiled cochlea make up the bony labyrinth.
- The inner ear system responsible for balance is called the vestibular system. It is made up of the vestibule and the semicircular canals, two bony labyrinth structures, as well as the membranous labyrinth structures that are housed within them.
- The pathway of hearing transmits auditory information from the receptors in the inner ear's organ of Corti (cochlear hair cells) to the central nervous system through the vestibulocochlear nerve (CN VIII).
- One type of energy that can be moved from one location to another is sound. A pressure wave produced by objects vibrating is called sound.
- In general, there are two types of hearing loss: sensorineural and conductive. When something wrong with the middle or outer ear stops sound from getting to the inner ear's cochlea, it results in conductive hearing loss.
- A hearing evaluation establishes an individual's threshold for various frequencies of sound. Pure tone audiometry, a piece of equipment known as an audiometer, is used to conduct the assessment.
- New audiologic diagnostic techniques that enable people to determine their level of hearing loss on their own have emerged as a result of the accessibility of stereo headphones and smartphones or tablets with sound reproduction systems.
- Disorders affecting the skin, cartilage, glands, and hair follicles within the outer ear canal are referred to as diseases of the outer ear.
- The eustachian tube, which runs from the upper region of the pharynx to the middle-ear cavity, provides air to the air-filled cavity and the air cells in the mastoid bone that extend backward from it.
- The vestibular nerve, also known as the nerve of equilibrium, and the auditory nerve, which are branches of the vestibulocochlear, or eighth cranial, nerve, are located in the labyrinth of the inner ear.
- A deaf child or one with severe hearing loss cannot learn to speak through normal means; instead, they need to attend special classes or a school specifically designed for the deaf in order to learn lipreading and speech.

References

1. Fine, D. M., & Waheed, S. (2017). *Renal Complications*. Oxford University Press. http://dx.doi.org/10.1093/med/9780190493097.003.0042.
2. Lehnhardt, E. (2011). *Clinical Aspects of Inner Ear Deafness*. Springer.
3. Smouha, E. E. (2010). *Cholesteatoma*. Thieme.
4. Swanepoel, D., & Louw, B. (2009). *HIV/AIDS Related Communication, Hearing and Swallowing Disorders*. Plural Publishing.
5. Wiet, R. J. (2005). *Ear and Temporal Bone Surgery: Minimizing Risks and Complications*. Thieme.

Chapter 2

DISEASES OF NOSE AND PARANASAL SINUSES

Contents

Introduction

Over 20 million outpatient visits are made annually in the United States for nose and sinus issues. These visits are often related to nasal congestion, sinus problems such as infections and inflammation, as well as symptoms like pain and pressure. Other common complaints include allergic rhinitis, nasal sores, and nosebleeds. Healthcare providers can provide treatment for many nose and sinus problems, but the recommended care varies depending on the cause and severity. In some cases, specialty care from an ENT specialist, allergist, or pulmonologist may be necessary.

Orientation and Directional Terms

Term	Definition	Illustration
Congenital deformities	These include cleft palate, nasal mass or weakness in the structure of the nose that were present at birth.	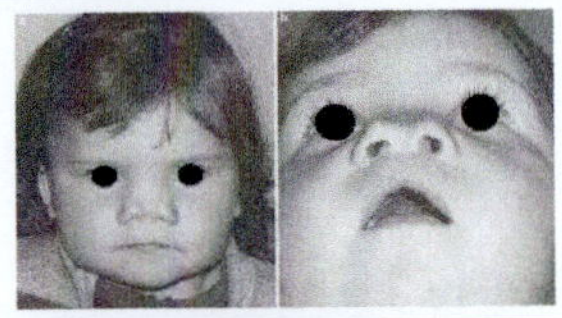
Enlarged adenoids	Adenoids are lymph glands found at the back of the nose. When they become enlarged, they can block the airway and cause sleep apnea.	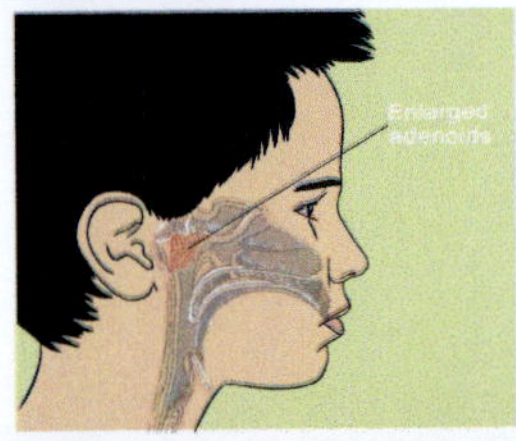
Enlarged turbinates	There are three turbinates, or baffles, on the side of each nostril that clean and humidify the air before it goes to your lungs. Swollen turbinates can interfere with breathing through the nose.	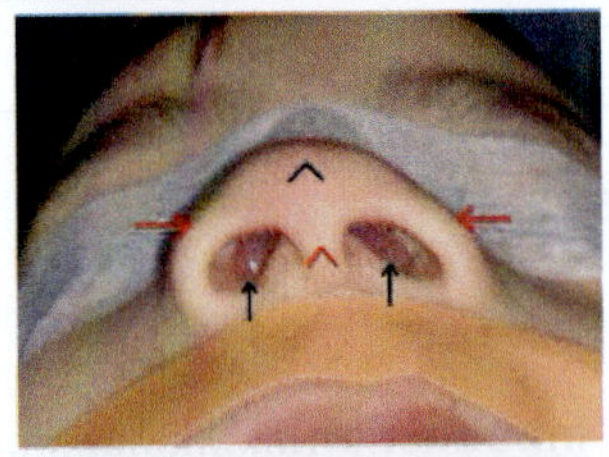
Deviated septum	This is when the wall of cartilage between your nasal passages is malformed or bent to one side. A deviated septum can be congenital or caused by trauma.	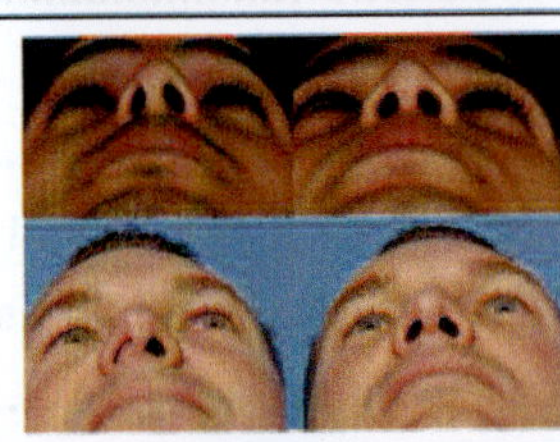
Saddle nose	Sometimes known as a boxer's nose, the saddle nose has an extremely flat or concave bridge. It is associated with trauma, cocaine abuse or certain diseases.	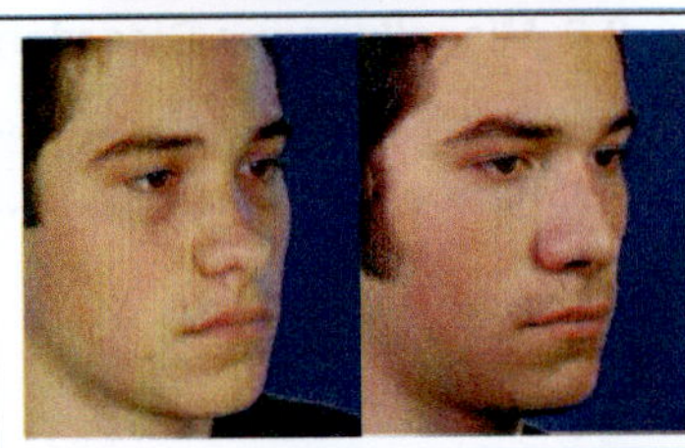

2.1. Anatomy of Nose

The nose, separated by the nasal septum, serves as the organ of smell and is divided into two parts. It filters out contaminants like pollen and dirt with tiny hairs in the nostrils, while also bringing humidified air to the lungs. Nerves in the upper nasal cavity play a role in influencing taste. Despite differences in shapes and sizes, the basic nasal anatomy remains consistent for all individuals (Figure 2.1).

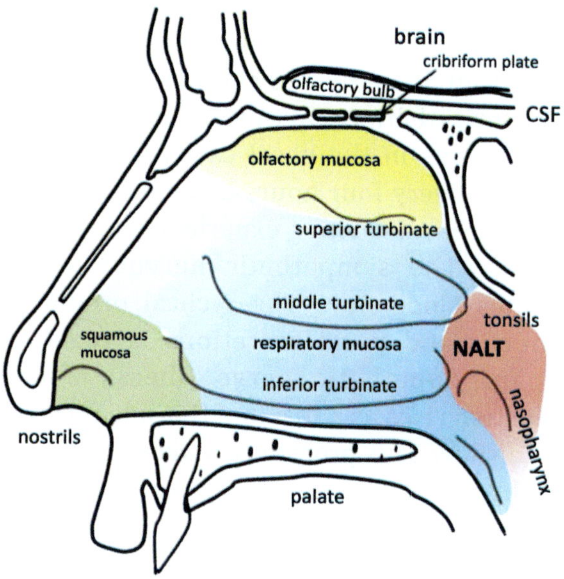

Figure 2.1. *Anatomy of the nasal cavity. Nasal-associated lymphoid tissue labeled NALT.*

Source: Gänger S, Schindowski K. (2018). Tailoring formulations for intranasal nose-to-brain delivery: A review on architecture, physico-chemical characteristics and mucociliary clearance of the nasal olfactory mucosa. Pharmaceutics,10(3), 116. https://doi.org/10.3390/pharmaceutics10030116.

2.1.1. External Nasal Structure

The nose appears pyramid-shaped from the outside, with the nasal root connecting to the forehead. The apex, located at the lower part of the nose, contains the openings of the nostrils (nares). The nose is composed of the nasal bone, flexible cartilage, and fatty tissue on the exterior. Some facial expressions are controlled by small muscles that connect to the external nose.

2.1.2. Nasal Cavity

The structure of the nose includes the nasal cavity, which is lined with respiratory cells. The vestibule, located just inside the nostrils, is lined with mucus-secreting cells in the respiratory region. The olfactory region is responsible for the sense of smell, with millions of receptors helping the brain interpret various scents. The nasopharynx, located above the soft palate at the back of the nose, connects the nose to the mouth and also connects to the middle ear through a tube.

2.1.3. Mucous Membrane

Air that has just been inhaled travels through the throat, nose, and lungs. This air is warmed, moistened, and filtered by a number of tiny structures in your nose before it enters your lungs. In particular, the mucous membrane—a thin, moist layer of tissue—is responsible for warming and moistening the air you breathe. This area of the nose produces snot, which is a sticky material that collects dust and other particles. Sneezing is an involuntary air expulsion that also clears the nose of unwanted particles.

2.1.4. Sinus Cavities

Sinus cavities are small tunnels or spaces located around or near the nose. The largest of these hollow cavities is approximately one inch in diameter.

- Your nose's sphenoid sinuses are situated behind it.
- Your eyes are separated by the ethmoid sinuses.

- Your forehead's center is home to the frontal sinuses.
- Your cheekbones contain the maxillary sinuses.

The middle meatus, a drainage pathway, allows the majority of these sinus cavities to empty into the nose. The nose is not a standalone organ. For example, a sore throat may occur if you have sinusitis, an infection of the sinuses. Eustachian tubes, which connect the back of the nose and throat to the middle ear, can be compressed by nasal allergies, which frequently cause discomfort in the throat. In the end, there are numerous vital tasks that the nose, ears, and throat are meant to collaborate on.

2.2. Physiology of Nose

The nose's typical duties include breathing, sinus drainage, conditioning inspired air, vocal resonance, smell, nasal resistance, and protection of the lower airway (Figure 2.2).

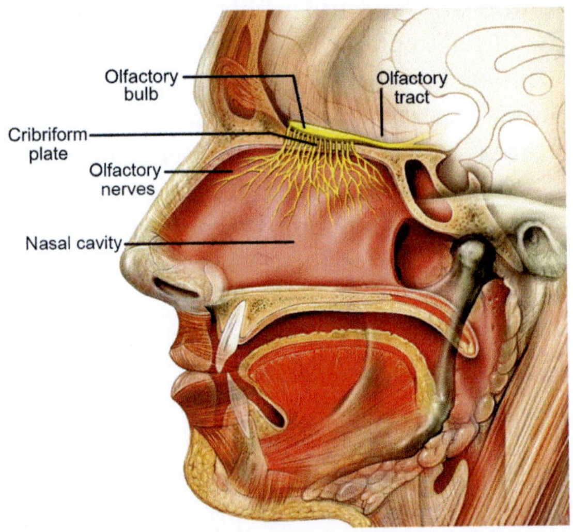

Figure 2.2. *Cross-section of the interior of a nose showing parts involved in smell (olfaction).*

Source: By Patrick J. Lynch, medical illustrator – Patrick J. Lynch, medical illustratorFile:Head_olfactory_nerve.jpg, CC BY 2.5, https://commons.wikimedia.org/w/index.php?curid=68370471.

2.2.1. Respiration

One of the body's natural channels for breathing (perspiration) is the nose. Humans breathe through their noses most of the time for basic respiration. Breathing in causes the nose to function as an air conditioner. To help with gas exchange in the lungs, it warms, humidifies, and filters the air. Humidity rises to 85% when water evaporation from the mucosa (the lining of the nose) occurs. The air is also brought to body temperature (37°C) by the mucosa.

The process of warming and humidifying inspired air is known as the nasal cycle. It is characterized by a rhythmic enlargement of blood vessels in the nasal cavity's turbinates, or ridges. Every four hours on average, the left and right nasal cavities experience alternating swelling. The sympathetic nervous system regulates blood flow. The cyclical production of mucus and nasal secretions is regulated by parasympathetic nerve fibers. Mucous production rises as a result of the side receiving more airflow. This procedure makes inspired air more humid. Patients typically are not aware of their nasal cycle, which is ordinary. If a patient does experience alternating nasal obstruction, further testing might be necessary.

2.2.2. Vocal Resonance

Speech is also influenced by the nose. The hollow, air-filled cavities known as the sinuses serve as resonance chambers. The palate stays open when phonating the letters M, N, and NG. This permits sound and air to travel up through the nose and nasopharynx. Speech quality can be affected by conditions that obstruct the sinuses or nose, leading to hyponasality.

2.2.3. Olfaction

The unique olfactory neuroepithelium is responsible for smell. These particular nerve cells are located in the olfactory cleft, which is high in the nasal cavity. The superior part of the nasal septum and turbinates is where the olfactory cleft is situated. A tiny amount of air enters the nasal cavity and makes its way to the olfactory cleft. Odorant molecules attach to the nerve receptors there. The brain receives signals from this process that give rise to the sense of smell. Our taste sense is also derived from smell. Complex flavors are produced when the five basic tastes—sweet, salty, bitter, sour, and umami—are combined with scent. Thus, a loss of taste can arise from an impairment of the sense of smell. The sense of smell can be diminished by conditions that impair or damage the olfactory nerve cells. As people age, olfactory dysfunction—a diminished sense of smell—becomes more prevalent. 50% of adults over 65 suffer from olfactory dysfunction. It is also commonly observed in patients with sinus and nasal diseases including chronic sinusitis. Olfactory dysfunction in sinusitis is probably caused by inflammation-induced olfactory nerve damage in addition to a physical obstruction of nasal airflow.

2.2.4. Filtration of the Airway

The nose is continually in contact with germs, viruses, and fungi that are inhaled. To fend off this attack, the respiratory system has evolved multiple defense mechanisms. The nasal vibrissae, or nose hairs, which are located at the nose's entrance (nostrils), capture large particles. One of the first barriers to the airway is the nasal mucus, which traps small particles. The purpose of mucus is to capture inhaled particles, including microorganisms. After being moved down the nose and into the throat, the mucus and trapped debris are swallowed. The stomach's acidic environment destroys microorganisms. Sneezing and coughing can also occasionally clear mucus. These shields aid in preventing particulates from entering the lungs.

2.2.5. Cilia

Mucus is transported to the throat by the cilia, which are minuscule hair-like structures that beat rhythmically. The airways are lined by cilia (Figure 2.3).

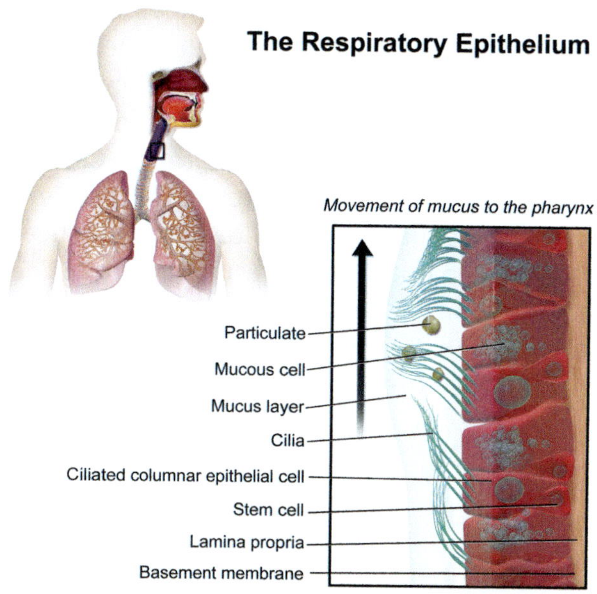

Figure 2.3. *Representation of cilia in the upper respiratory system.*

Source: https://en.wikipedia.org/wiki/File:Blausen_0766_RespiratoryEpithelium.png.

The sinuses and nose have cilia that are programmed to beat in unison in a particular direction. An ostium, or entryway from the sinus into the nasal cavity, is present in every sinus. The mucus produced by the sinuses is transported by the cilia into and through the ostium. The nasal cavity, which is the main hallway, is reached by this naturally occurring drainage channel. Here, mucus is forced toward the back of the nose by the beating of the cilia together. After passing through the nasopharynx, it enters the throat and is eventually swallowed. We refer to this procedure as mucociliary clearance. Because ciliated cells are equipped with sensors, they can react to environmental changes. An increase in mucous thickness, for instance, will cause the cilia to beat more quickly. The cilia can now continue to remove the thick mucus as a result. The mucous clears more quickly in response to an irritating stimulus. Mucociliary clearance does not happen normally when these cilia's beating is compromised. One known cause of sinus disease is impaired mucociliary clearance. Patients with cystic fibrosis experience this issue. Some microbiological infections also show impaired mucociliary clearance. Certain microorganisms can produce toxins that paralyze cilia. This reduces mucus flow and enhances the environment conducive to infection. The body's response to fighting the microbes is inflammation. Regrettably, cilia damage or loss may also result from this inflammation (Figure 2.4).

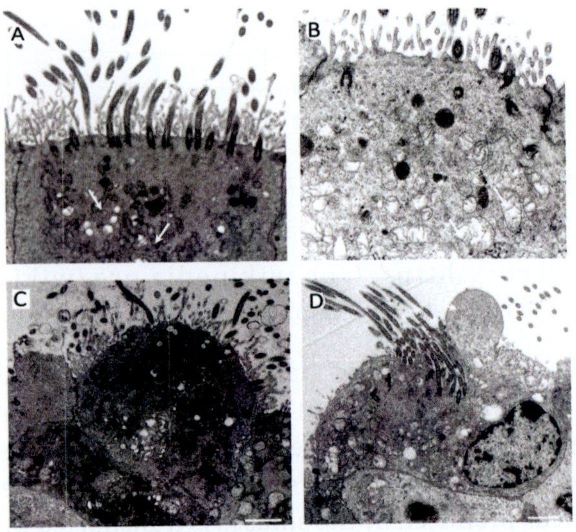

Figure 2.4. *Loss of cilia due to microbial toxins and the resulting inflammation.*

Source: Lee, SL., O'Callaghan, C., Lau, YL. et al. (2020). Functional analysis and evaluation of respiratory cilia in healthy Chinese children. Respir Res., 21, 259. https://doi.org/10.1186/s12931-020-01506-w.

These factors could potentially put a patient at risk for recurring infections and persistent rhinosinusitis. Fortunately, cilia can regenerate and resume normal mucus movement if the bacteria are eliminated and the inflammation is under control. Some patients develop chronic rhinosinusitis after recovering from an upper respiratory infection, although most patients recover. A number of factors are thought to be responsible for this. Inflammatory response, microbiological exposure, and the anatomy of the patient probably play a role. To comprehend the diseases that can arise in the nose and sinuses, it is essential to have an understanding of physiology.

2.3. Diseases of External Nose and Nasal Vestibule

As it protrudes over and provides entry into the nasal cavity, the external nose is a visible feature of the face. A sinus infection (nasal vestibule) is referred to as nasal vestibulitis. Excessive blowing or picking of the nose is usually to blame. The area around your nose's opening may scab and crust over time. Antibiotic creams, tablets, or oral medications are used as treatments.

2.3.1. Cellulitis

A red, swollen, and tender nose may result from a streptococcal or staphylococcal infection of the nasal skin. Occasionally, the infection extends from the nasal vestibule. Analgesics, hot fomentation, and systemic antibacterials are the methods of treatment.

2.3.2. Nasal Deformities

A nasal deformity is a deviation in the structure and look of the nose that can lead to problems with breathing, loss of smell, and other issues.

Individuals who have a nasal deformity may also be more susceptible to sinus infections, nosebleeds, dry mouth, chronic sinusitis, and snoring and noisy breathing. These problems are frequently accompanied by dissatisfaction with the nose's form and appearance.

2.3.2.1. Deviated Septum

A physical condition of the nose involving the displacement of the nasal septum is known as nasal septum deviation. 80% of people experience some degree of displacement, most of them without realizing it (Figure 2.5).

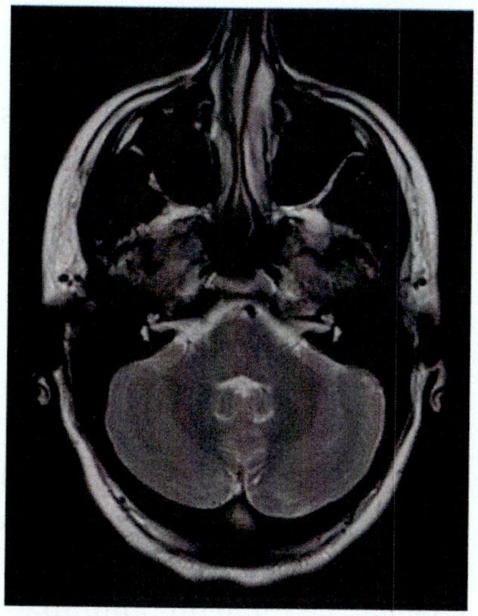

Figure 2.5. *An MRI image showing a congenitally deviated nasal septum, bowed to the left between the eye sockets.*

Source: By Ptrump16 – Own work, CC BY-SA 4.0, https://commons.wikimedia.org/w/index.php?curid=71206585.

2.3.2.1.1. Signs and Symptoms

The bone and cartilage in the nose that divides the nasal cavity into the two nostrils is called the nasal septum. The maxillary crest, vomer, and the perpendicular plate of the ethmoid are among the bones that make up the septum. The cartilage is referred to as the quadrangular cartilage. Since the septum usually lies in the middle, the nasal passages are symmetrical. The top of the cartilaginous ridge tilts to the left or right in a deviated septum, which is an abnormal condition that obstructs the nasal passage in question.

Nasal septa frequently stray from the precise centerline; a deviation from this line is only deemed to be significant or problematic. On its own, a deviated septum can remain undiagnosed for years without requiring correction. A deviated septum can cause sinus infections, sleep apnea, snoring, frequent sneezing, facial pain, nosebleeds, mouth breathing, breathing difficulties, and a mild to severe loss of smell. Breathing problems are the only signs of a deviated septum that need medical attention in more serious cases.

2.3.2.1.2. Causes

Impact trauma, such as a blow to the face, is the most common cause. It might also be a congenital condition brought on by the nose being compressed during childbirth. Genetic connective tissue diseases like Marfan syndrome, homocystinuria, and Ehlers-Danlos syndrome are linked to deviated septum.

2.3.2.1.3. Diagnosis

Nasal obstruction most commonly results from deviation of the nasal septum. There is frequently a history of trauma to the nose, including microfractures or trauma sustained during childbirth. An otorhinolaryngologist (a doctor of the ears, nose, and throat) or other medical professional usually makes the diagnosis after obtaining a complete medical history and doing a physical examination. The diagnosis can also occasionally be aided by imaging of the nose.

2.3.2.1.4. Treatment

Whenever possible, medical treatment using nasal sprays—such as decongestants, antihistamines, or nasal corticosteroid sprays—is attempted prior to exploring surgical options for nasal septum deviation. Medication treats the symptom but doesn't address the underlying cause. Nasal strips can also be used for non-medical relief.

Septoplasty, a minor surgical procedure, is a treatment option for symptoms associated with septal deviations. The procedure takes about an hour, and there are no visible scars or changes to appearance afterward. In the initial days following surgery, nasal congestion, pain, drainage, or swelling are possible side effects. It could take two days to four weeks for full recovery following the procedure. Septal bones do not grow back. Recurring symptoms are not connected to deviations. Mucosal metaplasia of the nose could be the cause of resurfacing symptoms. Sometimes, though, the surgery may not be successful and the symptoms may still persist.

2.3.2.2. Enlarged Adenoids

The pharyngeal tonsil, sometimes referred to as the nasopharyngeal tonsil or adenoid, is the tonsil on the superior aspect of the body. It is a mass of lymphatic tissue that is situated in the roof of the nasopharynx, which is the area where the throat and nose meet, behind the nasal cavity. It often takes the shape of a soft mound in children's nasopharynx, which is located directly above and behind the uvula on the back wall and roof. The abnormal growth of the pharyngeal tonsils, known as adenoid hypertrophy, is also referred to by the term "adenoid."

2.3.2.2.1. Structure

The adenoid is a lymphatic tissue mass situated in the roof of the nasopharynx, the area where the throat and nose meet, behind the nasal cavity. The adenoid has pseudostratified epithelium, in contrast to the palatine tonsils. The palatine, lingual, and tubal tonsils are also a part of the lymphoid tissue known as the Waldeyer ring, which also contains the adenoids.

- **Development:** Following the 16th week of embryonic life, lymphocytes infiltrate the epithelium to form adenoids. Enlargement starts at birth and lasts for five to seven years.
- The function of adenoids is to identify and trap pathogens, including bacteria and viruses, as a component of the immune system. Adenoid glands produce T and B cells in response, aiding in the body's immunologic memory by battling infection and assisting in the synthesis of IgA immunoglobulins.
- **Microbiome:** By the time a child is six months old, bacteria species like actinomycosis, Fusobacterium species, lactobacilli, and anaerobic Streptococci are typically present. Alpha-hemolytic Streptococci, Enterococci, Corynebacterium species, coagulase-negative Staphylococci, Neisseria species, Haemophilus species, Micrococcus species, and Stomatococcus species are among the normal flora found in the adenoid.

2.3.2.2.2. Clinical Significance

Enlargement: Adenoid hypertrophy, or enlarged adenoid, can grow to almost the size of a ping pong ball and obstruct airflow through the nasal passages. Even though the enlarged adenoid is not large enough to physically block the back of the nose, it can still impede airflow to the point where breathing through the nose is uncomfortable and inhaling through the open mouth instead. Additionally, the enlarged adenoid would impede nasal airflow to the extent that voice quality would be compromised without complete cessation (Figure 2.6).

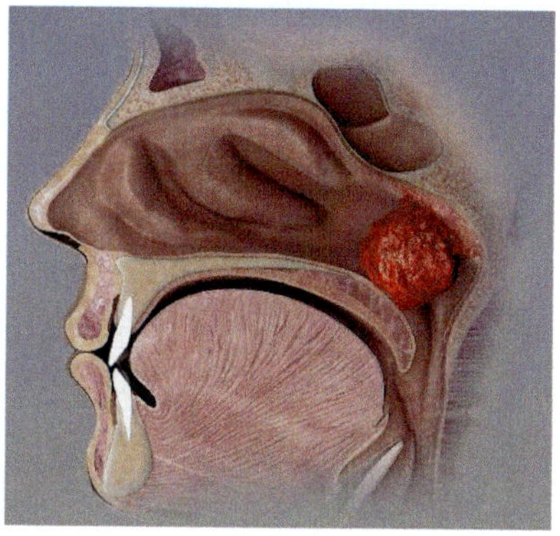

Figure 2.6. *3D still showing adenoid hypertrophy.*

Source: By www.scientificanimations.com – http://www.scientificanimations.com/wiki-images/, CC BY-SA 4.0, https://commons.wikimedia.org/w/index.php?curid=64473889.

Snoring, nasal airway obstruction, and breathing obstruction during sleep are all possible due to symptomatic enlargement, which is common between the ages of 18 and 24 months. When kids get older and start school, it is reasonable to assume that this will decrease and that it will gradually shrink from there.

- **Adenoid Facies:** Enlargement of the adenoid gland, particularly in children, results in an unusual facial appearance that is commonly known as adenoid facies. Mouth breathing, an extended face, prominent incisors, a hypoplastic maxilla, a short upper lip, elevated nostrils, and a high-arched palate are characteristics of adenoid facies.
- **Removal:** An adenoidectomy is the surgical removal of the adenoid. Excessive mucus production is one symptom of an adenoid infection that can be treated by clearing it out. Research has indicated that up to 19% of cases experience adenoid regrowth following removal. Adenoidectomy, which is performed through the mouth under a general anesthetic (or less frequently a topical), entails curetting, cauterizing, lasing, or otherwise ablating the adenoid. The palatine tonsils are frequently extracted along with the adenoid.

2.3.2.3. Swollen Turbinates

The nasal passageway's structures are called turbines. There are three turbinates in each nostril, and they are composed of both soft and hard tissue. The inferior, middle, and superior turbinates are these three types of turbinates. These structures are located close to the septum, the bone and cartilage partition that divides the nostrils. Along with the turbinates, the mucosal lining covering the septum contributes to the preservation of moisture and warmth in the air passing through the nose. As the turbinates are located right inside the nasal passages, enlargement may result in breathing obstructions. Inflammation can cause one or more of the three turbinates in the nostrils to enlarge. Seasonal allergens can cause the turbinates to enlarge in certain cases. Environmental irritants can occasionally lead to enlargement. The turbinates may become chronically swollen due to chronic sinusitis, which is characterized by ongoing inflammation in the nasal passages.

2.3.2.3.1. Symptoms of Enlarged Turbinates

The enlargement (hypertrophy) of the inferior turbinate is frequently the cause of persistent nasal obstruction or a stuffy nose. A clogged nasal blockage can make it difficult for a patient to breathe normally, which often interferes with daily activities. Since the nasal airway is the typical breathing pathway during sleep, enlarged turbinates and nasal obstruction can also aggravate headaches and sleep disorders like obstructive sleep apnea and snoring.

2.3.2.3.2. Causes of Enlarged Turbinates

Common causes may be:

- Allergies
- Sinusitis
- Irritants in the environment (like cigar or cigarette smoke).
- Pregnancy or other hormonal changes
- Aging process
- Congenital variations

2.3.2.3.3. How Are Enlarged Turbinates Treated?

Treatment plans are customized for each patient with persistently enlarged turbinates. Proper medication, such as nasal corticosteroid sprays or antihistamine sprays, may help some patients manage this issue. These drugs provide a transient reduction in swelling. In cases where nasal obstruction and trouble breathing through the nose are caused by enlarged turbinates, surgery might be a better course of action. A physician specializing in otology may take into account various methods to decrease the size of the turbinates. Submucosal reduction and radiofrequency ablation are two popular choices.

- **Radiofrequency Ablation (RFA):** This outpatient office procedure gently heats the submucosal lining between the turbinate and the septum, which causes the turbinate to shrink. This is accomplished by inserting a tiny probe through the nostril and using low-power radiofrequency energy to target the tissue. The actual RFA procedure takes no more than 10 minutes, although it may take a few minutes for the local anesthetic to completely numb the nasal passages.
- **Submucosal Reduction (SMR):** Under general anesthesia, Submucosal Reduction is an outpatient procedure carried out in a surgical center. It might take place in tandem with a surgical septoplasty to enhance breathing even more. A thin tube with a light at the end is called an endoscope, and it is used to perform the procedure. The surgeon created a tiny incision in the mucosal lining of the inferior turbinate by using the endoscope to view this structure. A tiny tool may be used to thin the tissue surrounding the turbinate after the underlying bone is removed. As an alternative, this tissue may be cauterized with radiofrequency or electrical current, which will cause shrinkage.

2.3.2.3.4. Special Considerations

- **Septal Deviations:** It is not unusual for patients to have blockages on both sides of the nose when they have a septal deviation. One side of the nose being blocked by inferior turbinate hypertrophy and the other by a deviated septum is a common occurrence.
- **Allergies:** Allergies can enlarge the body, which frequently results in turbinate hypertrophy.

- **Colds and Infections:** Enlarged turbinates caused by a cold or infection can lead to congestion. Typically, the turbinates will shrink back to their normal size once the illness has passed. However, in cases of chronic sinusitis, the enlargement may become permanent.

In certain instances, swollen turbinates may be treated without surgery. Among the suggested tactics are:

- **Avoid Smoking:** Smoking irritates the body as a whole, including the nasal passages. This habit can make breathing more difficult even though it might not cause the turbinates to enlarge.
- **Use saline Nasal Lavage:** Mucus and bacteria can build up in the nasal passages. Many rinse their nasal passages with saline nose drops to wash away substances. One teaspoon of baking soda, one teaspoon of salt, and two cups of distilled water can be combined to create a solution. The fluid can be sprayed into the nose using a bulb syringe or neti pot after this solution is added. To keep bacteria from growing inside the syringe or neti pot, excellent maintenance is required. Guidelines for cleaning and maintenance must be closely adhered to.
- Maintain proper nasal lubrication in rooms by using a vaporizer or humidifier.
- Use prescription drugs and over-the-counter nasal sprays as prescribed. Excessive use of some medications can exacerbate nasal blockage.

2.3.2.4. Saddle Nose

A collapsed nasal bridge or a loss of nasal height is referred to as a saddle nose deformity. The term "saddle" in the condition's name refers to the appearance of the nose's midsection, or "mid vault region," which is said to be sagging (Figure 2.7).

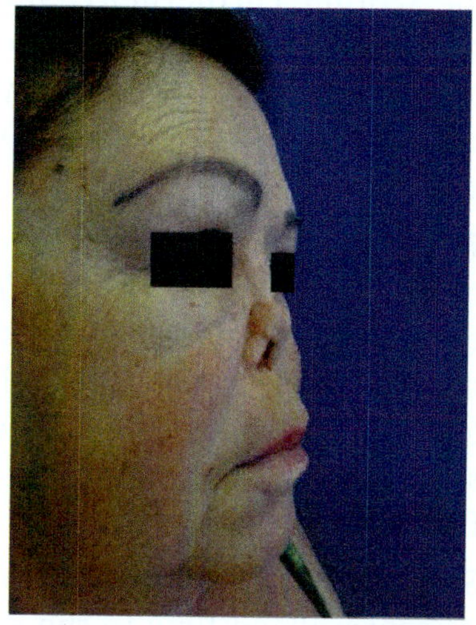

Figure 2.7. *Lateral view of the face with a saddle nose deformity far up on the bridge due to granulomatosis with polyangiitis from using a nasal prosthesis.*

Source: Kawabata, S., Hirono Hotta, P., E Dias, R., Camara Mattos, B. Wegener Granulomatosis: Case Report of Facial Prosthetic Rehabilitation. Journal of Medical Cases, North America, 5, nov. 2014. Available at: <https://www.journalmc.org/index.php/JMC/article/view/2036/1374>.

2.3.2.4.1. Causes a Saddle Nose Deformity

Loss of nasal height can be caused by a variety of factors. The nose's structural integrity is largely dependent on the nasal septum. It provides most of the structural stability of the nose, acting as its central pillar. A collapsed nose can result from any condition that affects the nasal septum. No matter what causes it, the nose will frequently appear sunken in the end.

- **Previous Surgery:** A saddling of the nose may result from a previous septoplasty or septorhinoplasty. Over time, the nose may weaken and possibly collapse if an aggressive septoplasty is carried out, removing the majority of the septum. Furthermore, any septoplasty operation done on a patient who is too young may cause the nose to saddle as the patient grows.
- **Trauma:** The most common cause of nasal saddling is trauma. Any type of nose trauma can cause the nose to sag or saddle. Nasal height loss can occur from weakened septum, which is caused by fractures.
- **Septal Hematoma and Septal Abscess:** Blood flow to the septum may be compromised, leading to nasal saddling, if there is a collection of blood or pus in the septum as a result of trauma, surgery, or septal manipulation.
- **Autoimmune and Vascular Disorder:** These conditions have the potential to cause vasculitis, or inflammation of the blood vessels, in the septum. Due to reduced blood flow to the septum caused by this inflammation, tissue necrosis and loss may occur. Declining nasal height and weakening of the septum are the results of disease progression. Wegener's Granulomatosis and Relapsing Polychondritis are two examples of disorders.
- **Cocaine Use:** Long-term or chronic cocaine use also reduces blood flow to the nasal septum, which leads to tissue loss and necrosis. In the end, this causes the nasal septum to shrink and the nasal height to decrease.
- **Infections:** Persistent infections like syphilis can also weaken blood circulation to the nose and septum, resulting in nasal deformities.

2.3.2.4.2. Symptoms of a Saddle Nose Deformity

The most common symptom is an external nose deformity that gives the appearance of being sunken. However, you might also have trouble breathing through one or both of your nostrils due to the location of the deformity and the possibility that inadequate healing played a role in its development. Nasal septal perforation, persistent crusting, nosebleeds, and nasal discomfort are possible additional symptoms.

2.3.2.4.3. Treatment

Generally speaking, surgery is the best option when using an open rhinoplasty technique to treat a saddle nose deformity. Secondary rhinoplasty surgery may be required if the problem stems from an excessively aggressive prior rhinoplasty or septoplasty. Correction of the deformity frequently requires the use of grafting material, such as rib grafts.

2.3.2.5. Nasal/Dorsal Hump

The dorsal hump is a natural irregularity of cartilage and bone on the nose, causing a bump or hump in its appearance instead of a straight slope from the bridge to the tip. While generally not harmful, some individuals may feel self-conscious about these humps and opt for dorsal hump removal through cosmetic rhinoplasty.

2.3.2.5.1. Symptoms of Dorsal Humps

Dorsal humps primarily manifest as bumps or pimples in or on the nose, but there are additional related symptoms as well, such as nasal swelling, pain in the nostrils, redness in or around the nose, tenderness in or around the nose, and a foreign body sensation.

An infection could develop if there is an irritation or obstruction of the hair that lines the inside of the nose. Additionally, an infection may cause your nose to swell, turn red, or feel sensitive to the touch. A lump called a dorsal hump may result from severe infections. A bump inside the nostril can also result from acne on the nose.

2.3.2.5.2. Causes Dorsal Humps

The bone and cartilage structure that joins your nose to your face is called the nasal "dorsum." The majority of us call it the nose's "bridge." There are various reasons why the dorsum can get humps.

- **Genetics:** Dorsal humps can be inherited by certain individuals. This indicates that due to the structure of the nose, they have a predisposition to have a bump on them from birth. Genetically caused dorsal humps don't always show up in childhood; they can also show up during puberty when the nose is still growing.

Various parts make up your nose, and any of the following areas could have bumps.

  - **Nostrils:** Smells are taken in through the entrance of the nasal cavity.
  - **Septum:** The septum, which divides the nostrils, is composed of cartilage toward the tip and bone at the top.
  - **Nasal Cavity:** The area behind your nose is this. It is attached to your throat, but your palate keeps it apart from your mouth.

- **Trauma or Injury:** A dorsal hump can also arise from trauma or injury to the nose. A dorsal hump may develop from a broken or bruised nose if the bone and cartilage heal unevenly. Dorsal humps caused by injuries are frequently self-inflicted. Irritation from things like picking your nose, pulling hair from the inside of your nostrils, or even getting a nose piercing can result in an infection from bacteria or fungus. There could be swelling and redness, and a dorsal bump could result from serious infections.
- **Medical Causes:** Dorsal humps can occasionally be caused by severe allergies. Furthermore, uncomfortable growths called polyps can encase the sinuses and cause pain. Boils are infections of the hair follicles brought on by a particular kind of bacteria known as *Staphylococcus aureus*, or "staph."
- **Infectious Causes:** An infection may arise from an obstruction in the follicles or from bacteria or fungi getting past the hair follicles lining the nostrils. Certain infections worsen to the point where a dorsal bump develops.

2.3.2.5.3. Dorsal Hump Removal Options

The surgical procedure known as rhinoplasty and the nonsurgical procedure known as nonsurgical rhinoplasty are the options for removing a dorsal hump (Figure 2.8).

- **Open Rhinoplasty:** The most popular technique for permanently eliminating a dorsal hump is an open rhinoplasty, also known as a traditional rhinoplasty. During this procedure, which calls for general anesthesia, a plastic surgeon makes a tiny incision through which they can see all of the bone and cartilage beneath your skin. After that, your surgeon reshapes and sands down the nose's contour, which might entail breaking and realigning the nasal bones for a better fit. You may have a cast or splint on your nose for up to a week following an open rhinoplasty. An average recovery can take up to three weeks.
- **Closed Rhinoplasty:** During a closed rhinoplasty, your plastic surgeon makes no visible incisions on the nose bridge; instead, they operate through your nostrils. Also necessary for this procedure is general anesthesia. The bone and cartilage above your nasal passages are altered by your surgeon as they operate beneath your nostrils. With a closed rhinoplasty, recovery is typically quicker, taking one to two weeks to complete.
- To improve the shape of the dorsal hump, the surgeon may break and realign the nasal bones in both open and closed rhinoplasty procedures. The majority of the bruising and swelling following rhinoplasty is caused by these fractures. If this is done, you will probably have a plaster or metal splint on the outside of your nose for a week or more in order to help the bones heal properly.
- **Nonsurgical Rhinoplasty:** Also referred to as a liquid rhinoplasty, nonsurgical rhinoplasty yields results that typically endure for two years to six months. This takes approximately 30 minutes to complete and calls for topical anesthesia. Your plastic surgeon will use dermal fillers to smooth out the areas of your nose around the start of the dorsal hump. Your nose's bridge may appear smoother as a result of this. Compared to a rhinoplasty, this procedure is much less expensive, has fewer potential complications, and requires little to no recovery time before returning to your normal activities.

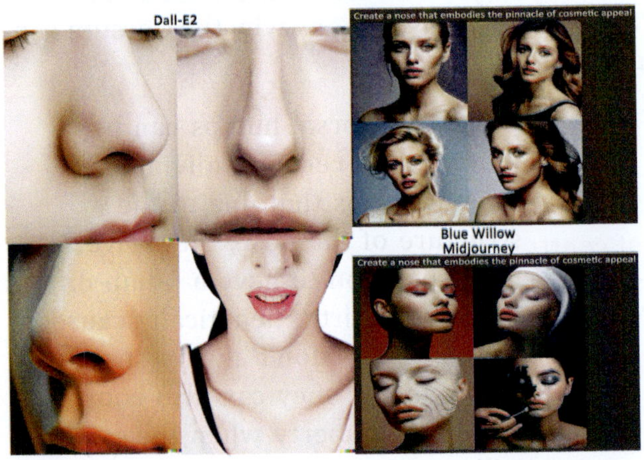

Figure 2.8. *Dorsal hump reduction before and after.*

Source: Lim B, Seth I, Kah S, Sofiadellis F, Ross RJ, Rozen WM, Cuomo R, (2023). Using generative artificial intelligence tools in cosmetic surgery: a study on rhinoplasty, facelifts, and blepharoplasty procedures. Journal of Clinical Medicine, 12(20), 6524. https://doi.org/10.3390/jcm12206524.

2.3.3. Tumors

An abnormal growth of tissue in the nose is called a nasal tumor. The majority of nasal tumors are benign. Nasal tumors are uncommon and usually affect adults over the age of 40.

2.3.3.1. Types of Nasal Tumors

Most tumors in the nose are not malignant. Nasal tumors that are not cancerous are among the more prevalent types, such as inverted papilloma and juvenile nasopharyngeal angiofibroma.

These are a few of the more typical malignant nasal tumors:

- neuroblastoma esthesionique (also known as olfactory neuroblastoma);
- squamous cell carcinoma; and
- adenocarcinoma.

These tumors can develop in the sinuses, which are hollow spaces in the skull that link to the nasal passages, or in the nose. Anasal tumors are tumors that arise in the sinuses surrounding the nose.

2.3.3.2. Nasal Tumor Causes

When aberrant cells proliferate and grow out of control, tumors are created. The reason why some people get nasal tumors and others don't is unknown to experts. Among the risk factors are:

- smoking and being in the company of smokers.
- extended exposure to allergens and chemicals at work, including formaldehyde, glue fumes, and wood dust; and.
- Human papillomavirus (HPV) infection is a common sexually transmitted illness.

2.3.3.3. Nasal Tumor Symptoms

Common symptoms for people with a nasal tumor include:

- trouble breathing through your nose, particularly if it is unilateral;
- double vision;
- pressure, edema, or pain in the face (especially if one-sided);
- frequent nosebleeds;
- loss of sense of smell; and
- a runny nose.

2.3.3.4. Treatment Plans for Nasal Tumors

When appropriate, the rhinologist will discuss your care with colleagues in radiation oncology, pathology, medical oncology, or radiology. By doing so, an ideal treatment plan can be created for you.

Before completing your treatment plan, the rhinologist might discuss the need for:

- Obtaining a biopsy of the growth to enable laboratory testing (the biopsy may be performed in an operating room or clinic, depending on the tumor's location);
- Imaging tests, like magnetic resonance imaging (MRI) and computed tomography (CT); and
- appointments with radiation oncologists, neurosurgeons, and other tumor specialists who may be involved in your care.

Your rhinologist will discuss with you the results of your biopsy, imaging studies, and recommended course of treatment for your particular tumor. This conversation can take place over the phone or in a follow-up meeting.

2.3.3.5. Nasal Tumor Surgery

Most patients who have a nasal tumor require surgery to remove it. If the tumor is malignant, you might also receive treatment from radiation or oncologists, among other cancer specialists. Your treatment plan may include radiation therapy and/or surgery, either on their own or in conjunction with chemotherapy. The rhinologist will collaborate with other cancer specialists to determine the most appropriate course of treatment based on the type, location, and growth stage of your tumor.

- **Endoscopic Surgery to Remove Nasal Tumors:** Most surgeries to remove a tumor in the nose can be performed using a minimally invasive technique. Using endoscopes that are inserted into your nose, the surgeon will access your nasal passages during this procedure. No skull bones need to be removed or external incisions made to perform endoscopic surgery. Compared to patients who have open surgery, patients typically recover more quickly, feel less pain, and leave the hospital sooner.
- **Open Surgery to Remove Nasal Tumors:** The rhinologist may choose to perform an open procedure if the tumor is very big or has spread into the tissues of your brain or eyes. This may entail creating incisions next to the eye, beneath the lip, or beside the nose in order to reach the tumor and extract as much of it as feasible. A craniotomy, or temporary removal of a portion of the skull to allow the surgeon to access the tumor, may be necessary in certain cases for the open surgery.

2.3.3.6. Follow-Up Treatment for People with Cancer

You will see the rhinologist and other members of the cancer team for follow-up if your nasal tumor is cancerous. To guarantee that you receive care that is well-coordinated, these specialists will collaborate. Further testing will be performed to determine the success of your treatment after you finish your initial course of treatment, which may include radiation therapy, chemotherapy, and/or surgery. To make sure the tumor hasn't returned; you will have follow-up appointments for the next five years or so. Nasal tumors that are not cancerous can regrow as well. Your rhinologist will discuss with you the need for imaging tests and follow-up visits over the next few years, just to be sure.

2.3.4. Furuncle or Boil

A boil in the nasal vestibule caused by a hair follicle infection is known as nasal furunculosis.

- marked by a sudden, localized infection of the hair follicle in the nasal vestibule's lining skin.
- lesion/lesions are usually small and tender, commonly infected with *Staphylococcus aureusylococcus aureus*
- occurs as painful, swollen, red nodules over the tip of the nose, frequently accompanied by pustules.
- It can be a primary infection or develop as a secondary condition due to chronic rhinorrhea, upper respiratory infections, and nose picking.

Treatment is typically conservative and consists of applying warm compresses to the affected area or intranasal topical mupirocin. In certain cases, topical or systemic antibiotics are used in addition to over-the-counter pain relievers. Abscess formation, ophthalmic vein thrombosis, cavernous sinus thrombosis, orbital abscess, and progression to septal hematomas (due to abscess development) are uncommon but serious complications.

Patients should be aware that nasal vestibulular involvement may develop or present.

- usually present with painful swelling in the vestibule
  - There may be a visible boil in the nostril and tense, red skin surrounding the nose.
  - If the condition is not adequately managed, the patient may experience sequelae such as facial cellulitis and cavernous sinus thrombosis, which manifests as fever, headache, chemosis, proptosis, and palsies of the cranial nerves III, IV, V, and VI.
  - Patients who have problems frequently need to be admitted to the hospital, have their boils drained, and receive intravenous antibiotics.

2.3.5. Vestibulitis

The diffuse dermatitis of the nasal vestibule is known as nasal vestibulitis. *Staphylococcus aureus*, persistent rhinorrhea, nose picking, and viral infections are the common causes.

- **Causes:** Constant blowing of the nose, picking at the nose, pulling out nasal hairs, getting nose piercings, and getting objects stuck in the nose are among the causes. It can also result from the common cold, herpes simplex, shingles, or persistent runny nose.
- **Symptoms:** Skin that has acute vestibulitis is tender, swollen, and red. Crusting and induration of the vestibular skin are observed in chronic vestibulitis. Additional symptoms include nose pain, swelling, discoloration, itching, bleeding, scabbing, and crusting around the nose opening.
- **Complications:** In severe cases, boils may form inside the nostrils, leading to cellulitis at the tip of the nose, even though the disease is easily treatable. The reason the condition gets serious is that there are veins leading to the brain in that area of the face. If bacteria enter the brain through these veins, it can cause a potentially fatal brain infection called cavernous sinus thrombosis. Encephalitis and nasal septal abscess are further complications.
- **Treatment:** In addition to oral antibiotics, antibiotic steroid ointment can be beneficial at times. Silver nitrate can be used to cauterize persistent fissures. The nasal boils may need to be surgically drained if antibiotics are not effective. The illness lasts for three to four days after treatment.
- **Prevention:** Hand washing, refraining from blowing one's nose too much, picking at nasal hairs, popping pimples close to the nose, and nose picking are some preventative measures.

2.3.6. Stenosis and Atresia of the Nares

A congenital condition known as choanal atresia causes the formation of nasal choanae (i.e., paired openings that connect the nasal cavity with the nasopharynx), soft tissue or a mix of both. This occurs as a result of the nasal fossae's failure to recanalize during fetal development. When unilateral, it manifests as mucopurulent discharge. However, it is a critical condition when it is bilateral. Without nasal openings, the neonate cannot breathe. Since newborns only breathe through their noses, opening their airway is an otolaryngologic emergency.

2.3.6.1. Etiology

The development of nasal choanae occurs during the third and seventh weeks of embryonic life, after the disruption of the vertical epithelial fold that separates the olfactory groove from the primary oral cavity's roof (stomodeum). The persistence of the buccopharyngeal membrane and nasobuccal membrane of Hochstetter, the incomplete resorption of the nasopharyngeal mesoderm, and the local misdirection of neural crest cell migration are some theories that have been put forth.

2.3.6.2. Epidemiology

This deformity affects between 1:5,000 and 1:8,000 live births. More often than not, it is unilateral (60% vs. 40%) and happens more often in females than in males (ratio 2:1).

2.3.6.3. Pathophysiology

The infant is an obligatory nasal breather, except when crying. This results from the newborn's higher laryngeal position relative to the adult. The larynx locks between the side of the nasopharynx and the soft palate during a newborn's swallowing motion. The newborn sucks their tongue during inspiration, creating a vacuum in the oropharynx that aids in pushing the soft palate's floor of the mouth upward and backward. The oral airway becomes obstructed during expiration due to the soft palate pushing forward against the tongue and soft tissue in the mouth due to the pressure in the airway. Consequently, when the mouth is closed, particularly during sleep or feeding, the baby with bilateral choanal atresia suffers from episodes of asphyxia and extreme distress in quiet respiration. When the child opens their mouth wide, releasing the air blockage, the infant will no longer be cyanotic and will cry or gasp in relief.

2.3.6.4. Histopathology

According to earlier reports, the deformity consisted of 10% membranous tissue and 90% bony tissue. About 30% of cases of pure bone atresia and 70% of cases of mixed membranous and bone atresia—that is, no purely membranous anomalies—are seen in the CT workup and histologic specimens.

2.3.6.5. History and Physical

Choanal atresia can present clinically as either a unilateral or bilateral abnormality, ranging from acute life-threatening airway obstruction to chronic recurrent nasal discharge on the affected side. Affected infants with bilateral choanal atresia experience episodes of acute respiratory distress with cyanosis that are relieved by crying and return to cyanosis with rest (a condition known as paradoxical cyanosis). Due to their inability to breathe and feed at the same time, infants who have difficulty feeding may present with progressive airway obstruction and choke episodes during feeding. This can be the first warning sign of a feeding difficulty. Rarely does a newborn experiencing respiratory distress exhibit unilateral choanal atresia. A history of chronic sinusitis and/or purulent nasal discharge and obstruction on the affected side are the most typical presentations. Because unilateral nasal obstruction symptoms are nonspecific, in certain cases the correct diagnosis is not made until adulthood. CHARGE syndrome, which includes coloboma, heart disease, atresia choanae, growth and mental retardation, genital hypoplasia, and ear abnormalities, is the most common combination of anomalies that can be linked to choanal atresia (Figure 2.9).

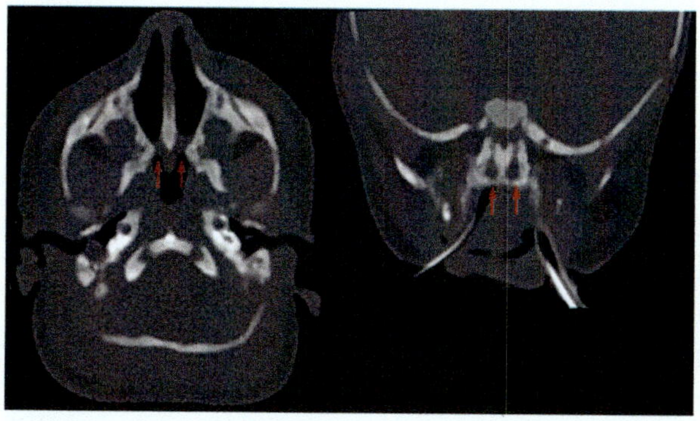

Figure 2.9. *Bilateral membranous choanal atresia in CT scan.*

Source: By Hellerhoff – Own work, CC BY-SA 3.0, https://commons.wikimedia.org/w/index.php?curid=61572218.

2.3.6.6. Evaluation

This condition needs to be diagnosed as soon as the baby is born. To check for fogging, a laryngeal mirror is placed under each nostril during the initial clinical evaluation. A suction catheter is then inserted through each nostril and into the child's oral cavity. When a newborn has undergone the appropriate preparations, such as nasal decongestion and mucous suctioning, the clinical suspicion of choanal atresia can be verified through examination with a flexible nasal endoscope, which enables direct visualization of the potential obstruction in the nasal passage. A CT scan should be performed to further define the features of the malformation, such as the anatomy of the atretic area, including the thickness of the atretic plate and the presence and thickness of a bony plate, to confirm the diagnosis of choanal atresia. CT helps distinguish choanal atresia from other causes of nasal obstruction in addition to defining the type and severity of the condition. Pyriform aperture stenosis, nasolacrimal duct cysts, turbinate hypertrophy, septal dislocation and deviation, antrochoanal polyp, or nasal neoplasm are examples of differential diagnoses.

2.3.6.7. Treatment / Management

Choanal atresia is primarily treated surgically. Restoring choanal patency, minimizing invasiveness, preventing recurrences, and not interfering with the patient's normal craniofacial development are the goals. When a child reaches school age and the anatomy of the affected area more closely resembles that of an adult, surgical treatment for unilateral choanal atresia can wait. It must, nevertheless, be continuously observed for any indications of a breathing issue. Maintaining the nasal passage clear can also be aided by using a nasal saline spray. When there is no other option, a McGovern nipple—an intraoral nipple with a large opening made by cutting off the end and securing it in the mouth with ties around the infant's occiput—may be used to maintain an adequate oral airway for the acute care of infants with bilateral choanal atresia in asphyxia. This is followed by perforation of the atresia plate. There have been five distinct surgical approaches suggested: transpalatal, transeptal, transantral, and transnasal. Up until the endoscopic endonasal approach became popular in recent decades, the transpalatal approach was the most widely used method. Many surgeons are using the endoscopic endonasal technique more frequently for the repair of choanal atresia due to the growing experience with both instrumentation and technique in endoscopic sinus surgery. This approach has produced better results and fewer surgical complications than traditional procedures. In the management of choanal atresia, the use of choanal stenting and mitomycin C as adjunct therapy to prevent restenosis is a contentious issue because the efficacy of stents or mitomycin after choanal atresia repair is not well established.

2.4. Nasal Septum and Its Diseases

The nasal septum divides the two nostrils and keeps the left and right airways of the nasal cavity apart. The depressor septi nasi muscle depresses it.

2.4.1. Structure

The columella, also known as the columella nasi, is the fleshy external end of the nasal septum. It is composed of soft tissue and cartilage. Hyaline cartilage and bone can be found in the nasal septum. It typically has a thickness of 2 mm.

Four structures make up the nasal septum:

- Maxillary bone (the crest)
- Perpendicular plate of ethmoid bone
- Septal nasal cartilage (i.e., quadrangular cartilage)
- Vomer bone

The length of the septum is represented by the narrow strip of bone at its lowest point, which protrudes from the maxilla and palatine bones. The maxillary crest is the name given to this bone segment, which articulates with the vomer at the back and the septal nasal cartilage at the front. The anatomy of the nasal septum describes the maxillary crest as having both a maxillary and a palatine component.

2.4.1.1. Development

The *ethmovomerine cartilage*, a plate of cartilage, makes up the early portion of the septum of the nose. The vomer is ossified in the membrane covering its posteroinferior part, while the posterosuperior part of this cartilage is ossified to form the perpendicular plate of the ethmoid. Its anteroinferior portion remains as the septal cartilage. The vomer is mainly made up of two lamellae because two ossification centers, one on each side of the middle line, form in this area of the membrane around the eighth week of fetal development.

These come together below around the third month, creating a deep groove where the cartilage is deposited.

The lamellae's union grows forward and upward as growth continues, and the cartilage plate that lies between them absorbs cartilage at the same time.

The lamellae nearly unite to form a median plate by puberty, but the groove on the anterior margin and the everted alae of the upper border of the bone show signs of the bone's bilaminar origin.

2.4.2. Clinical Significance

Trauma-induced deviation of the nasal septum from the nose's center line is referred to as this condition. It is typical to have a small skew to one side, though. Up until roughly the age of seven, the septum usually remains in the midline; after that, it frequently deviates to the right. A septoplasty is a procedure to realign the nasal septum. An ulcer, trauma from an inserted object, prolonged exposure to welding fumes, and cocaine use can all result in a perforated nasal septum. For people with a perforated septum, there is a procedure that may be helpful. To seal the open sore, place a silicone button inside the opening. Both benign tumors like fibromas and hemangiomas as well as malignant tumors like squamous cell carcinoma can affect the nasal septum.

2.4.3. Fractures of Nasal Septum

Because of their outward projection on the face and relative weakness, the nasal bones are the most commonly fractured bones in the maxillofacial area. From 42% to 96% of cases have nasal septal fractures that are connected to nasal bone fractures. Nasal airway function is affected by nasal bone and septal fractures in addition to looking bad. Cartilage, bone, and skin make up the majority of the nose's structural support. The frontal bone superiorly and the frontal processes of the maxillae laterally, at the nasofrontal and nasomaxillary suture lines, respectively, are where the paired nasal bones are associated. Above the level of the medial canthus, the nasal bones are typically denser. The nasal septum is made up of cartilage in the front and bone in the back. The bony septum is composed of the vomer inferiorly and the perpendicular plate of the ethmoid bone superiorly. These unite with the quadrangular cartilage, constituting the nasal septum's anterior segment. From the keystone region to the supratip of the nose, the nasal dorsum is supported by the quadrangular cartilage. This keystone region, which makes up the 10–15 mm bony-cartilaginous septal junction directly inferior to the rhinion, is a major structural support of the middle third of the nose. The dorsal margin of the cartilaginous septum, which is firmly adherent to the perpendicular plate of the ethmoid bone, is attached to the upper lateral cartilages, which articulate with the caudal edges of the nasal bones at the keystone level. The nasal spine on the anterior side and the nasal crest of the maxilla and palatine bones on the posterior side of the septum connect to the nasal floor, respectively.

2.4.3.1. Etiology

Numerous injuries to the maxillofacial skeleton can result in fractures of the nasal bones. Worldwide, motor vehicle accidents, sporting accidents, falls, and acts of interpersonal violence are the leading causes of nasal bone fractures. More nasal bone fractures occur in traffic accidents in North America than in acts of interpersonal violence. Depending on the source, athletic or auto accidents are typically the most frequent cause of injuries in children. Fascinatingly, compared to fighting-related sports, ball-related sports like rugby, basketball, baseball, and soccer have a higher rate of nasal bone fractures.

2.4.3.2. Epidemiology

Compared to women and girls, men and boys experience nasal bone and septal fractures far more frequently. This has been linked to the greater frequency of male-to-male interpersonal violence. Nostril fractures are most common in the second and third decades of life. Rates of nasal bone and other facial fractures have been rising in the US since 2000, but rates of repair have stayed the same. This could indicate a rise in the frequency of nonoperative fracture patterns, a move toward more conservative care, and a rise in the use of computed tomography (CT) imaging to help guide treatment.

2.4.3.3. Pathophysiology

A fracture of the nasal bones and/or nasal septum is generally more likely to result from a frontal or lateral blow to the nose. Greenstick, comminuted, unilateral, bilateral, nondisplaced, and severely depressed fractures are all possible. In more severe injuries with higher energy impacts, fractures can involve the nasal bones, nasal cartilage, septal cartilage, and even the surrounding facial skeleton.

2.4.3.4. History and Physical

Prior to treating patients with trauma to the maxillofacial region, a primary trauma survey that addresses breathing, circulation, airway, and disability should be completed. A comprehensive history and subsequent physical examination might be carried out once life-threatening conditions have been resolved. Determining the mechanism causing the trauma to the maxillofacial region is crucial first. Higher energy impact traumas, such as those that occur in car crashes, have the potential to cause more serious injuries and even several facial fractures. In order to gain a better understanding of the underlying fracture pattern, the direction of impact might be crucial. Impacts directed straight onto the nasal dorsum typically result in splaying outfractures of the bilateral nasal bones, whereas lateral blows typically cause an infracture on the impacted side and an outfracture on the opposite side. Gaining an understanding of premorbid appearance is also crucial. Patients ought to be questioned about any glaring differences or deformities from their pre-injury state. Breathing difficulties through either side of the nose should be evaluated because they may indicate intranasal edema or damage to the nasal septum. It is important to inquire about any previous nasal trauma or surgeries the patient may have had. Telecanthus, diplopia, vision loss, clear rhinorrhea, malocclusion, facial weakness, and facial numbness are symptoms that could point to more serious injuries. An extensive evaluation of the head and neck should be part of the physical examination, including intraoral, intranasal, skin, eye, and ear exams. A rigid endoscope or nasal speculum, in addition to a headlamp, should be used to perform a thorough examination of the nasal dorsum and nasal cavity. It is important to examine the outside of the nose carefully to check for cuts and exposed bone or cartilage. Documentation is necessary for any deviations from the bony nasal pyramid. An increased intercanthal distance following trauma indicates the possibility of a nasoorbitoethmoid fracture. In order to determine whether the nasal dorsum is properly supported, the nasal tip should be palpated. If there is a saddle nose deformity, this could mean a significant fracture or dislocation of the septum. A septal hematoma, which manifests as a fluctuant red or blue discoloration along the nasal septum, should be ruled out first with an intranasal examination. Incision and drainage of this submucoperichondrial blood collection must be done quickly to avoid abscess formation and/or septal cartilage necrosis, which can happen in as little as 24 hours. The consequent cartilage necrosis may eventually result in saddle nose deformity and/or septal perforation. Not only should significant septal dislocations be recorded, but also any intranasal cuts or disruptions of the mucosa. It is important to look for signs of clear rhinorrhea, which could indicate a CSF leak.

2.4.3.5. Evaluation

Simple fractures of the nasal bones usually do not require imaging. Usually not very helpful are plain film X-rays. The best method for assessing bony trauma in the maxillofacial region, should more extensive facial injuries be suspected, is a CT scan performed without intravenous contrast of the facial bones. Imaging studies should be prompted by concerning symptoms, as previously mentioned. While ultrasonography has been studied more recently, it has not yet shown to be as effective as CT scanning in helping to diagnose nasal bone fractures. If the patient has a simple nasal bone fracture or septal hematoma, laboratory testing is usually not necessary. For patients with epistaxis who have lost a significant amount of blood or who take anticoagulant medication, coagulation studies and complete blood counts may be necessary. To help determine whether or not a CSF leak is present, patients with persistent clear rhinorrhea may choose to have fluid collected and sent for beta-2-transferrin testing.

2.4.3.6. Treatment / Management

Controlling epistaxis and, if feasible, suturing any cuts on the external skin or inside the nose lining should be the first steps in treatment. By applying conservative pressure to the nasal alae and pressing them against the septum, epistaxis can be managed. Neural packing or cauterization may be necessary for more severe epistaxis. For patients without a noticeable cosmetic deformity or nasal obstruction, observation without surgical intervention is advised. Until local edema goes down, conservative measures like icing the area and elevating the head are advised. Patients should be closely monitored for a follow-up examination in three to five days, as the resolution of edema may reveal nasal deviation.

For fractures that result in nasal deviation or obstruction of the airway, closed reduction of the nasal bone and septal fractures is usually advised. Although general anesthesia is frequently preferred due to improved airway protection and overall patient comfort, the procedure can be carried out under local anesthesia or with minimal sedation. The literature differs in its reporting of when closed reduction should be carried out; some sources recommend early intervention within five to seven days, while others say that edema should fully resolve and closed reduction should be carried out one to two weeks after injury. Two weeks in, there is a significant decline in patient satisfaction with the cosmetic results. Because the fractured segments will have started to heal in place, later intervention runs the risk of callus formation and difficulty reducing nasal bones to their premorbid location. Osteotomies can be used to accomplish an endonasal or percutaneous reduction in these situations. Typically, a postoperative splint is placed on the nasal dorsum after a flat, broad instrument, like a Boies or Sayre elevator, is introduced endonasally to reduce the fractured bony segments. With an Asch forceps or Boies elevator, closed reduction on the nasal septum can also be carried out. Some authors support open septoplasty in the acute setting if adequate reduction of the nasal septum cannot be achieved in a closed manner, noting that patients experience a notable improvement in nasal obstruction after surgery. After reduction, intranasal splints or packing may also be used to maintain the alignment of the septum, but these are usually not inserted until after a septoplasty. A significant disruption of the mucosa along the septum precludes the use of septoplasty due to the possibility of postoperative septal perforation.

Since nasal trauma frequently coexists with lacerations on the nose or disruptions of the cartilage, open septorhinoplasty is generally avoided in the acute setting. In the acute situation, further dissecting these cartilages could devascularize them, and cartilage grafts used in rhinoplasty might be more prone to infection, extrusion, or absorption. Therefore, it is frequently advised to postpone septorhinoplasty for three to six months following an injury. Another helpful adjunct that has been mentioned is the placement of osteotomies using CT guidance in the healed fracture lines to aid in reduction months or years after the injury.

2.4.3.7. Differential Diagnosis

Injuries to the surrounding skeletal structure of the face should be considered as a differential diagnosis for nasal bone fractures. They consist of the following:

- **Nasoorbitoethmoid (NOE) Complex Fracture:** These are fractures of the nasal bones that affect the medial canthus of one or both eyes and extend posteriorly into the ethmoid air cells. Traumatic telecanthus is the defining feature of this illness. All LeFort type III midface fractures also involve nasoorbitoethmoid fractures.
- **Orbital Fracture***:* Ecchymosis or periorbital edema may indicate an orbital fracture. Patients may experience hypoesthesia in the cheek or restricted eye movements in the event of an orbital floor fracture.
- **Skull Base Fracture:** The base of the skull fractures can be caused by high-speed collisions. In addition to postauricular ecchymosis, also referred to as "Battle's sign," patients may exhibit the distinctive bilateral periorbital ecchymosis, also known as "raccoon eyes." CSF leaks and spinal fractures are more

common in patients with fractures to the base of the skull.

2.4.3.8. Prognosis

After reducing nasal bone fractures, patients usually recover well, but surgical interventions vary significantly in their effectiveness. Nasal deformity remains present in 9% to 50% of patients after closed reduction. Treating nasal septal fractures or deviations as soon as possible after injury can improve the results. With septorhinoplasty, residual deformity or nasal obstruction can be treated gradually. If a nasal deformity or obstruction existed before the nasal bone or septal fracture, patients would be more likely to require revision surgery.

2.4.3.9. Complications

After nasal bone reduction and septal fractures, residual nasal deformity is often present in varying degrees. Septal perforations and saddle nose deformity can develop following severe septal injury, septoplasty, or septal hematoma formation. Disturbances in smell are comparatively frequent, impacting as many as one-third of individuals suffering from nasal bone fractures. The olfactory neuroepithelium, which is situated on the superior and/or supreme turbinate, may have been altered during closed reduction, which could account for this.

2.4.3.10. Postoperative and Rehabilitation Care

Within a week, both the internal and external nasal splints should be taken out. To prevent toxic shock syndrome, patients are frequently given oral antibiotics if true nasal packing is inserted. In the acute context, physical activity that could cause additional trauma to the nose should be avoided, and strenuous activity is discouraged. Saline spray nasal hygiene is recommended to stop recurrent epistaxis. It is crucial to closely monitor any nasal deformity or obstruction that may persist and require revision surgery.

2.4.3.11. Consultations

In patients with nasal bone and septal fractures, early involvement by a surgeon skilled in managing a wide range of facial trauma is recommended. Usually, a plastic surgeon, oral surgeon, or otolaryngologist will handle this.

2.4.3.12. Deterrence and Patient Education

Ahead of reducing nasal bone fractures, it is imperative to establish realistic expectations with patients due to the possibility of residual deformity or nasal obstruction. Teaching patients that close monitoring is required and that the first surgery should ideally be done shortly after the injury is also crucial. In order to stop more nasal trauma, there should be more instruction on how to use seatbelts and protective gear during sporting events.

2.4.3.13. Pearls and Other Issues

- The maxillofacial region's most commonly fractured bones are the nasal bones.
- Injuries to the nasal septum are common in patients with nasal bone fractures, though they may go unnoticed.
- Imaging studies should be avoided in cases of isolated nasal bone fractures unless there is evidence of more extensive injuries from the physical examination or the history.
- For better cosmetic results, closed reduction of the nasal bones should be done before two weeks.
- When there is only a small amount of mucosal damage and a severely

deviated or fractured septum, septoplasty should be taken into consideration.

- In order to give lacerations and cartilaginous injuries time to heal, septorhinoplasty for nasal obstruction or residual deformity should be postponed for three to six months.

2.4.3.14. Enhancing Healthcare Team Outcomes

Common injuries that can have a long-term impact on a patient's nose's appearance and functionality are nasal bone fractures. These patients need to be referred to facial trauma surgeons right away. Early closed reduction therapy may prevent the need for later, more involved surgery. These patients usually see emergency room doctors or primary care physicians as their first clinicians; identifying concerning symptoms and getting in touch with facial trauma specialists early on may help these patients receive better care.

2.4.4. Septal Abscess

A condition affecting the nasal septum where pus accumulates between the mucoperichondrium and septal cartilage is known as a nasal septal abscess.

- **Signs and Symptoms:** Fever, a general malaise, and nasal pain, including soreness over the nose's dorsum, are other possible symptoms of this illness. There might also be a persistent nasal obstruction on one side.
- **Complications:** A nasal septal abscess may result in saddle deformity from cartilage necrosis, septal perforation, or cavernous sinus thrombophlebitis.
- **Cause:** A secondary bacterial infection of a nasal septal hematoma often results in a nasal septal abscess.
- **Treatment:** Treatment for other bacterial infections is comparable to that for a nasal septal abscess. Once the affected area has been cleared of fluid, aggressive broad-spectrum antibiotics may be administered.

2.4.5. Perforation of Nasal Septum

A nasal septum full-thickness defect is known as a nasal septal perforation. The three-layer divider between the right and left nasal cavities is made up of bilateral mucoperichondrial leaflets and a structural middle layer (quadrangular cartilage, perpendicular plate of ethmoid, or vomer). Most frequently, septal perforation happens along the anterior cartilaginous septum. Nasal blockage, whistling, epistaxis, crusting, pain, rhinorrhea, chronic rhinosinusitis, and bad odor are some of the symptoms.

2.4.5.1. Etiology

The causes of nasal septal perforations include neoplastic, infectious, autoimmune, and fungal diseases (such as syphilis, tuberculosis, and Granulomatosis with polyangiitis, or GPA). People with weakened immune systems may be more vulnerable to opportunistic infections like fungal infections. Iatrogenic septal perforation may happen following elective septoplasty, cautery for epistaxis, or patient self-manipulation. After septoplasty, the incidence of reported cases of septal perforation varies from 0.5 to 3.1%. Steroid nasal spray, vasoconstrictor nasal spray, and intranasal drug abuse are some additional causes.

2.4.5.2. Epidemiology

There is an increased risk in some professions. In the past, exposure to the offending chromic mist caused inflammation, erosion, and perforation in chrome platers. Nowadays, the risk of intranasal carcinoma is increased for metalworkers and woodworkers who are exposed to nickel dust.

2.4.5.3. Pathophysiology

The maxillary artery (sphenopalatine artery and greater palatine artery), the ophthalmic artery (anterior and posterior ethmoid arteries), and the superior labial artery (a branch of the facial artery) provide the nasal septum's blood supply. The mucoperichondrial leaflets that cover each side of the septal cartilage receive the majority of their blood supply from branches of the maxillary artery. Any danger to these leaflets' vascularity puts the underlying cartilage's viability in danger and increases the risk of septal perforation. Septal perforations change the direction of airflow in the nose, causing turbulence that dries out the mucosa and increases the risk of crusting and epistaxis. Subjective nasal obstruction or audible whistling that is audible during rest, sleep, or exercise can also result from disturbances in laminar airflow.

2.4.5.4. Histopathology

Analysis of a nasal septal biopsy may reveal vasculitis symptoms, infectious organisms, or tumors, all of which may help determine the etiology and facilitate treatment.

2.4.5.5. History and Physical

Thoroughly assessing a patient's medical history can reveal the underlying causes of a septal perforation. This should include information about past nasal injuries, use of nasal drugs (prescription, over-the-counter, and illicit), nasal hygiene practices, respiratory and kidney symptoms, as well as autoimmune diseases. Collecting data should involve understanding when symptoms started, how long they have been present, how severe they are, and previous treatments. During a physical examination, the size of the septal perforation should be measured both horizontally and vertically using a headlight, nasal speculum, and cotton-tipped applicator. The height of the septum is important for determining the amount of tissue available for repair. The presence of a saddle deformity should be noted, as it can affect nasal structure. Inflammation can cause tissue growth or excessive crusting, and signs of foreign substances may suggest substance abuse. An intraoral exam can confirm if the palate is involved, and examining the ear or temporal region can help identify potential donor sites for repair if needed.

2.4.5.6. Evaluation

The clinical scenario dictates the workup for a septal perforation. For instance, a biopsy and laboratory workup are typically not recommended in patients who have had a prior history of septoplasty, following which a perforation was discovered.

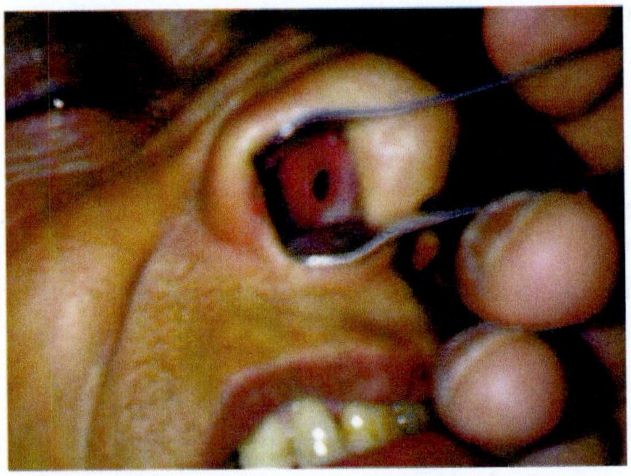

Figure 2.10. *Nasal septum perforation.*

Source: By Dr. J. S. Bhandari, India – Own work, CC BY-SA 3.0, https://commons.wikimedia.org/w/index.php?curid=6736314.

On the other hand, a biopsy of the perforation is done and sent to pathology for permanent sectioning when the cause is less obvious. It is important to advise the patient that the biopsy will inevitably result in an expansion of the perforation. The posterior edge is the region that is typically biopsied since repair options are typically unaffected by horizontal enlargement. This blood analysis includes FTA-ABS, ACE, RF, ANCA, ANA, ESR, and CRP. Imaging, such as a sinus CT scan or CXR, may be necessary. PPD testing or other tuberculosis testing may be necessary if tuberculosis is suspected (Figure 2.10).

2.4.5.7. Treatment / Management

Medical and surgical management are two possible treatments for nasal septal perforation. To reduce discomfort, crusting, and epistaxis, medical management involves applying emollients and humidification to the inside of the nose. To reduce aspiration and the risk of lipoid pneumonia, care should be taken when using petroleum-containing products inside the nose. Water- and saline-based gels are generally less dangerous. Nasal septal prostheses are options for patients who might not be good candidates for formal repair or general anesthesia. These are typically made of medical-grade synthetic material and mechanically cover the perforation. It is beneficial to continuously humidify the prosthesis because tolerance to it varies. Overall, the rate of infection with prostheses is low.

Numerous surgical repair methods have been reported for nasal septal perforations. Acellular dermis graft, staged inferior turbinate flap, auricular cartilage interposition, bilateral mucoperichondrial flap repair with an interpositional graft, and facial artery musculomucosal (FAMM) flap are a few of these. It should come as no surprise that larger than 20 mm septal perforations have a higher failure rate following repair than smaller ones. Resection of the posterior wall of the perforation, or posterior septal resection, may be beneficial for patients who are not good candidates for repair or who have large perforations in an effort to lessen symptoms. There is a need for caution if there is an autoimmune disease.

2.4.5.8. Differential Diagnosis

The three most important primary causes to rule out following a diagnosis of septal perforation are neoplasm, infectious disease, and autoimmune disease. All of these are examples of curable systemic diseases that call for more thorough evaluation and care than just symptomatic relief or repairs.

2.4.5.9. Surgical Oncology

Referrals are essential if a biopsy reveals a neoplasm in the nasal septum, with squamous cell carcinoma being the most common type. Other types of neoplasms in this area include adenocarcinoma and malignant melanoma. The primary treatment is surgical removal with wide margins, and radiation therapy may be considered if necessary. Any reconstructive surgery following the removal of nasal septal carcinoma should be carefully discussed with a head and neck oncologist or oncologic surgeon.

2.4.5.10. Radiation Oncology

If the biopsy reveals a neoplasm and the conditions call for adjuvant treatment, appropriate referrals may be made.

2.4.5.11. Pertinent Studies and Ongoing Trials

One clinical trial for nasal septal perforation repair is currently recruiting participants worldwide. The trial, which is based in China, evaluates the safety and effectiveness of a collagen membrane combined with clinical-grade human umbilical cord mesenchymal stem cells that are transplanted between the leaflets of the septum mucosa.

2.4.5.12. Medical Oncology

Similar to radiation oncology, if the biopsy reveals a neoplasm and the circumstances call for adjuvant treatment, the right referrals must be made.

2.4.5.13. Staging

A "graduated approach" to repair has garnered support for small (less than 0.5 cm), medium (0.5 – 2 cm), and large (greater than 2 cm) perforations, with the goal of systematically classifying this heterogeneous entity, despite the lack of a formal or widely-accepted staging system for septal perforations.

2.4.5.14. Prognosis

Perforation enlargement, epistaxis, nasal pain, bad odor, and loss of dorsal nasal support (saddle nose deformity) are all possible consequences of persistent crusting caused by septal perforation. The quality of life of the patient may suffer as a result of these symptoms. Perforations can be treated medically and kept stable for years with consistent humidification procedures.

2.4.5.15. Complications

Care would be delayed if a neoplasm or systemic illness were not diagnosed. Constant perforation, donor site scar, epistaxis, wound breakdown, nasal obstruction, need for revision, ozena, worsening symptoms, crusting, or whistling are among the complications from septal perforation repair.

2.5. Rhinitis

A reaction that results in runny nose, itchy, and congested nasal passages is called rhinitis. The majority of rhinitis types are brought on by inflammation and manifest as symptoms in the throat, ears, or eyes. Rhinitis occurs in various forms. Typically brought on by a viral infection, allergic or seasonal rhinitis, and nonallergic or year-round rhinitis are the most prevalent types. When allergens in the air cause the body to release histamine, allergic rhinitis results. Itching, swelling, and fluid accumulation in the delicate linings of the sinuses, eyelids, and nasal passages are all brought on by histamine.

2.5.1. Allergic Rhinitis

According to ARIA, allergic rhinitis is a well-defined endotype. It is described as a type 1 hypersensitivity reaction mediated by IgE to a variety of inhaled environmental allergens. The symptoms of allergic rhinitis include anterior or posterior rhinorrhea, nasal congestion or blockage, nose itching, and sneezing that lasts for more than an hour on two or more days in a row. Based on the length of symptoms (intermittent and persistent) and severity (mild–moderate and severe), ARIA classifies allergic rhinitis. Proteins from airborne particles such as pollens, dust mites, insect feces, animal dander, and molds are known allergens linked to allergic rhinitis. Asthma and conjunctivitis are frequent comorbidities linked to allergic rhinitis. The theory of the unified airway, which maintains that upper and lower airway inflammation share common pathophysiologic mechanisms and coexist and communicate via the systemic circulation, may help to explain its strong correlation with asthma. A series of immunological and biochemical processes culminate in the disease's clinical manifestation. After being inhaled, allergens adhere to nasal mucus and permeate into the nasal tissues. After breaking down antigens into antigenic peptides, antigen-presenting cells (APCs) move to lymph nodes and present the peptides to $CD4^+$ T lymphocytes (T cells) that are still naïve.

Certain surface T-cell receptors interact with allergen MHC class II complexes on APCs to initiate the activation of $CD4^+$ T cells. DCs and antigen-presenting signals aid in the differentiation of naïve T helper cells into Th1 or Th2 cells. B-cells produce IgE antibodies as a result of Th2 lymphocytes stimulating the production of particular cytokines. The surface of dendritic cells has high-affinity receptors that IgE antibodies can bind to; monocytes, macrophages, and B lymphocytes have low-affinity receptors; mast cells and basophils have high-affinity tetrameric receptors called FcεRl. The cellular allergic response and the activation of multiple signaling cascades are caused by the latter interaction. One of these leads to granule exocytosis and release of preformed or newly created inflammatory mediators (e.g., histamine, leukotrienes, prostaglandins, and platelet-activating factor).

There are two phases to a nasal allergic reaction: early and late. Early phase symptoms peak a few minutes after being exposed to the allergen in question, start almost immediately, and go away in a few hours. IgE-allergen interaction causes mast cell degranulation and the release of pro-inflammatory mediators like histamine, prostaglandins, cytokines, and leukotrienes within minutes of exposure. These molecules cause symptoms like nasal congestion, rhinorrhea, itching, and sneezing. Almost all of the early-phase symptoms are elicited by histamine, which binds to H1 receptors. Nasal congestion is the most common symptom in the late phase. Basophils, eosinophils, neutrophils, mast cells, and mononuclear cells infiltrate the nasal mucosa as a result of the mediators released during the early stage. It has been discovered that mast cells are important for both initiating and maintaining the allergic response over time. This is primarily due to the fact that Th2 lymphocyte recruitment to target organs is significantly aided by mediators generated by mast cell and histamine degranulation. Eosinophil activation is primarily caused by cysteinyl leukotrienes. Eosinophils are linked to the development of allergic symptoms and are the predominant cell type in the late-phase response. Eosinophils release proinflammatory mediators, cationic proteins, eosinophil peroxidase, and cysteinyl leukotrienes.

Allergy rhinitis may be suspected based on a comprehensive clinical examination and medical history. The diagnostic tests used to diagnose allergic rhinitis are divided into two categories: in vivo tests, which include skin prick tests; and radioallergosorbent tests, which include the immunoassay capture test (ImmunoCAP), multiple antigen simultaneous testing (MAST), fluoroallergosorbent test (FAST), and radioallergosorbent test (RAST). The most popular diagnostic procedures for allergic rhinitis are the allergen-specific immunoglobulin E (IgE) antibody test (RAST), which has been replaced recently by ImmunoCAP tests, and the percutaneous skin test, also known as the skin prick test. In skin prick testing, allergen and control substances are applied topically in predetermined concentrations. Skin testing elicits both early and late responses, but the primary objective is to identify the immediate allergic response brought on by the 15-minute wheal-and-flare reaction that is typically brought on by the release of mast cell or basophil IgE-specific mediators. A wheal with a diameter of at least 3 mm is considered positive. Allergen-specific IgE antibody testing (radioallergosorbent testing [RAST]) is useful in primary care if percutaneous testing is not practical (e.g., problems with reagent storage, expertise, frequency of use, staff training) or if it is contraindicated (e.g., medication such as tricyclic antidepressants, antihistamines). Although RAST has a high degree of specificity, it is less sensitive than skin testing and requires more expense and time to produce results. Even though the commercial RAST products that are currently on the market are usually trustworthy, they don't always offer repeatable, precise data.

The ImmunoCAP system is an in vitro test that uses a solid allergen phase made of three dimensions to identify particular IgE to allergen components. Comparing ImmunoCAP tests to skin prick tests, it has been discovered that the former is more sensitive to house dust and the latter to pollen, dog dander, and Candida. The MAST test permits the simultaneous analysis of several antigens and does not involve the use of radioactive materials. Comparable data is offered by the CAP and MAST systems. However, it appears that the CAP system is more sensitive. FAST is a chemical-radiating method that measures specific serum IgE; it was initially used as an inhibition assay to measure the activity of cross-reaction between aeroallergens. When compared to MAST, FAST analysis takes less time and requires using less serum.

Intranasal corticosteroids are a part of medical therapy; they are safer for adults and children to take, and they work better than oral antihistamines plus leukotriene receptor antagonists (LTRAs). Second-generation oral antihistamines have strong H1 receptor selectivity and weak anticholinergic action, while first-generation antihistamines are no longer advised due to their side effects. In comparison to intranasal antihistamines, intranasal corticosteroids are found to be more effective at controlling the symptoms of allergic rhinitis. It has been demonstrated that the combination of intranasal corticosteroids and intranasal antihistamines is even more effective than either medication used alone. Using isotonic or hypertonic saline, nasal irrigation is a common treatment for all forms of rhinitis. It aids in the removal of mucus and the clearance of anti-inflammatory drugs. Whether hypertonic saline is more effective than isotonic saline is still unknown. Because intranasal cromolyn and nedocromil stabilize mast cell membranes and inhibit mast cell degranulation, they are used prophylactically in AR. Despite the fact that their use is safe, it appears that they work less well than topical corticosteroids and antihistamines because they don't affect inflammatory factors that have already been released. The anti-IgE humanized monoclonal antibody omalizumab is licensed for the treatment of severe allergic asthma and chronic urticaria. Although it has been shown to lessen nasal and ocular symptoms in AR, it is not yet approved for use as a treatment for AR. In particular, omalizumab was shown to prevent and control nasal and ocular symptoms in moderate-to-severe seasonal allergic rhinitis to pollen in Japan through a randomized placebo control, double blinded trial. It is not yet authorized for the treatment of seasonal allergic rhinitis, though. Mepolizumab, reslizumab, and benralizumab are humanized monoclonal antibodies (mAbs) that target Il-5 and have been shown to alleviate eosinophilic asthma. These effects are also being studied in rheumatoid arthritis (AR).

People who have allergic rhinitis (AR) test positive for serum-specific (s)IgE/RAST or positive for the skin prick test. On the other hand, some individuals with seasonal or persistent rhinitis have positive nasal provocation tests (NAPT) for particular allergens and negative SPT and RAST results. This phenotype is not included in AR or NAR groups and is referred to as local allergic rhinitis (LAR). The presence of nasal-specific IgE (NsIgE) and nasal mucosa localized allergic response type 2 are characteristics of LAR. Young women, nonsmokers, moderate-to-severe rhinitis, persistent/perennial clinical behavior, conjunctivitis, and asthma are the most common characteristics of LAR patients. The most frequent allergen that causes LAR in people is house dust mites. In addition to mites, the mold Alternaria is a common allergen in LAR patients, whereas pollen and animal dander are more common in AR patients. Atopy/asthma in the family history, the clinical history, and the exclusion of CRS using a nasal endoscopy and/or CT scan are the first steps in the diagnosis of LAR. The diagnosis of AR is made if the results of the SPT and sIgE are positive. If these are negative, it is necessary to assess how the target organ reacts to an allergen challenge. The nasal allergy provocation test (NAPT) is the gold standard for diagnosing laryngitis (LAR); other options include sIgE detection in nasal secretions or a positive basophil activation test (BAT). It is important to note that some patients with chronic rhinitis only test positive for seasonal allergens on SPTs. Some of these patients have rhinitis phenotypes classified as dual allergic rhinitis (DAR), which refers to the simultaneous development of systemic and local sensitization in the same person, and are positive for NAPT to perennial allergens.

2.5.2. Non-Allergic Rhinitis (NAR)

Chronic rhinitis that lacks systemic allergic inflammation and endonasal infection symptoms (negative SPT, negative total blood IgE, and negative RAST tests) is known as non-allergic rhinitis. There are at least six subgroups that can be distinguished in the patients with non-allergic rhinitis:

- Drug-induced rhinitis
- Hormone-induced rhinitis
- Senile rhinitis or rhinitis of the elderly
- Gustatory rhinitis
- Occupational rhinitis
- Idiopathic rhinitis
- Atrophic rhinitis

A cellular inflammatory profile has been used to propose additional classifications for NAR. Non-allergic rhinitis with eosinophilia, or NARES, and neutrophilic NAR are the two most prevalent types. NARES is characterized by the presence of over 20%eosinophils in nasal smears without any indication of allergy or other nasal pathology. It is also linked to other comorbidities like asthma. The question of whether NARES is a unique phenotype or if its pathophysiologic mechanisms overlap with those of other conditions is not well-defined. When neutrophils account for 20% or more of the total cells on the nasal smear and other inflammatory organisms, like bacteria or fungi, are absent, the condition is known as neutrophilic NAR. NAR containing mast cells and mixed NAR (containing mast cells and eosinophils) are harder to diagnose, less common, and require more care.

2.5.2.1. Drug-Induced Rhinitis

Drug-induced rhinitis can be classified into three subgroups: (a) local inflammatory type, (b) neurogenic type, and (c) idiopathic type.

Local inflammatory reactions can be caused by medications such as aspirin and non-steroidal anti-inflammatory drugs (NSAIDs). These drugs inhibit the cyclooxygenase 1 (COX-1) mechanism, leading to an increase in arachidonic acid metabolism through the lipoxygenase pathway. This results in a decrease in prostaglandin 2 (PGE2), followed by an increase in cysteinyl leukotrienes such as LT4, D4, and E4. Of these, LTC4 is identified as the cysteinyl leukotriene responsible for aspirin-exacerbated asthma. Cysteinyl leukotrienes can cause bronchoconstriction, mucosal edema, hypersecretion, and vasoconstriction, as well as attract eosinophils to the airways. Activation of cysteinyl leukotrienes occurs through interaction with cysteinyl-LT receptors, with LTC4 synthase identified as the enzyme responsible for their activation, particularly in aspirin-induced rhinitis.

Neurogenic type: sympathetic, parasympathetic, and sensory fibers that are situated close to secretory glands and blood vessels in the nasal mucosa innervate the airways. The neurogenic type is brought on by sympatholytic medications like a and b adrenergic antagonists, which suppress the sympathetic nervous system and cause nasal congestion, vascular dilatation, and rhinorrhea. Because phosphodiesterase-5 selective inhibitors affect the erectile tissue of nasal turbinates and cause nasal obstruction, they can also cause neurogenic-type rhinitis due to their vasodilator effects. Examples of these inhibitors include sildenafil, tadalafil, and vardenafil. Rebound nasal congestion following overuse of nasal decongestants is a hallmark of medicamentosa rhinoritis. This condition is caused by two types of nasal decongestants: imidazolines (oxymetazoline, naphazoline, xylometazoline, and clonidine) and sympathomimetic amines (caffeine, Benzedrine, amphetamine, mescaline, phenylpropanolamine, pseudoephedrine, phenylephrine, and ephedrine). Norepinephrine is released presynaptically by sympathomimetic amines, and when it binds to postsynaptic a-receptors,

it causes vasoconstriction. Additionally, they stimulate vasodilation after the a-effect has ended and are b-receptor agonists. Imidazolines are postsynaptic a2 agonists that constrict blood vessels and, through a negative feedback mechanism, lower endogenous norepinephrine levels. Cocaine may also be the cause of medicamentosa rhinitis in addition to nasal decongestants. Long-term use of nasal decongestants can result in rebound nasal congestion as well as a number of histologic changes to the nasal mucosa, including goblet cell hyperplasia, squamous cell metaplasia, and more noticeable epithelial edema. When treating drug-induced rhinitis, one should stop taking the offending medication and start taking an intranasal corticosteroid, or if that doesn't work, a combination of intranasal corticosteroid and intranasal antihistamine.

Many medication classes, including b-blockers, angiotensin-converting enzyme inhibitors, calcium channel blockers, and antipsychotics, can induce idiopathic drug-induced rhinitis. Numerous of these lack comparable pathophysiological mechanisms.

2.5.2.2. Rhinitis of Elderly

Senile rhinitis, also known as elderly rhinitis, is characterized by clear, watery anterior rhinorrhea that is not brought on by a specific trigger and is thought to be impacted by cholinergic hyperreactivity as well as age-related anatomic nasal changes. These lead to weakening of the septal cartilage, degeneration of mucous glands and connective tissue, and atrophy of collagen. These alterations are thought to cause nasal congestion, drying, and reduced nasal flow, which can result in localized atrophy of the nasal mucosa, crusting, and atrophic rhinitis symptoms.

2.5.2.3. Hormone-Induced Rhinitis

Menstrual cycle-related rhinitis and pregnancy-related rhinitis are examples of hormone-induced rhinitis. Pregnancy-related rhinorrhea is most common in smokers and typically manifests in the final two months of pregnancy, clearing up two weeks after delivery. Premenstrual symptoms and premenstrual rhinitis are associated with recurrent cycles of symptoms. Although the precise mechanism is unknown, it is believed that hormone-induced rhinitis is caused by increased estrogen levels that cause vascular engorgement and nasal congestion. Other endotypes involve beta-estradiol, which causes eosinophilic migration and degranulation by increasing the expression of histamine H1 receptors on nasal epithelial and endothelial cells. Additional pathophysiologic mechanisms that have been proposed include increased levels of human growth factor that cause vasodilation by increasing the volume of blood in the circulation, progesterone, insulin-like growth factor-1, prolactin, a variant of placental growth hormone, and others. An additional sub-phenotype of hormone-induced rhinitis links nasal mucosal hypertrophy to elevated human growth hormone levels. Lastly, there is a possibility that thyroid issues and hormonal rhinitis are related, but this has not been proven scientifically.

2.5.2.4. Gustatory Rhinitis

Gustatory rhinitis is a non-inflammatory, non-allergic form of rhinitis that is triggered by eating hot, spicy food and is characterized by an abrupt onset of watery or mucoid rhinorrhea. Among the most frequent triggers are hot chili peppers, red cayenne, Tabasco sauce, onion, chili, vinegar, red pepper, and mustard. All of the aforementioned contain capsaicin, which stimulates afferent sensory nerves in the oropharyngeal mucosa, thereby initiating gustatory rhinorrhea. Four subtypes of gustatory rhinitis have been identified: gustatory rhinorrhea associated with cranial nerve neuropathy, post-traumatic, post-surgical, and idiopathic. Except for idiopathic, which is always bilateral, all of these types can be unilateral or bilateral.

Age, sex, or atopy are not linked to gustatory rhinitis. The age range for the peak prevalence is 20–60 years old. Debatable still are the pathophysiologic mechanisms underlying gustatory rhinitis. One theory states that gustatory rhinorrhea is caused by an offending food stimulating the trigeminal nerve endings, which in turn activates parasympathetic, cholinergic, muscarinic, and postganglionic fibers. Another prevalent pathophysiologic explanation involves a hyperactive neural system that is neither cholinergic nor adrenergic. TRPV1 (transient receptor potential vanilloid receptors subtype 1), which is found in neuronal and non-neuronal cells in the nasal mucosa and oral epithelium, is one of the receptors that capsaicin activates. Capsaicin activates TRPV1 on goblet cells and submucosal glands, which results in secretory hyperfunction. TRPV1 is also present on the fibers of sensory nerves C and Aδ. Capsaicin stimulates C fibers, which causes the local release of multiple neuropeptides, such as substance P (SP) and calcitonin gene-related peptide (CGRP). This increases vascular permeability, secretions, and vasodilation. Desensitization happens when there is a reduction in the quantity of secretory peptides that are available during and after prolonged exposure to capsaicin. Because of this, the mechanism underlying capsaicin's therapeutic effect in non-allergic rhinitis is desensitization.

Gulping rhinitis may also be caused by the interaction of the sympathetic and parasympathetic nervous systems. Noradrenaline and neuropeptide Y (NPY), which functions as a vasoconstrictor and neuromodulator for sensory and parasympathetic nerve function, are released in response to sympathetic nerve stimulation. The expression of gustatory rhinitis symptoms may be due to a decrease in neuropeptide Y on parasympathetic activity. Gustatory rhinitis is primarily diagnosed by exclusion and is based on medical history.

In addition, widely recognized stimulation tests are available for gustatory rhinorrhea. To prevent symptoms, it is essential to stay away from the offending agents. Treatment options include intranasal anticholinergics before consuming healthful foods, or, for best results, combining an anticholinergic agent with an intranasal corticosteroid. Despite their side effects, intranasal atropine and oxitropium bromide can also be used for gustatory rhinitis. Furthermore, the degeneration of C fibers and long-term relief from the symptoms of gustatory rhinitis may result from local capsaicin administration. Injecting botulinum toxin type A (BTXA) into the nasal septum and middle and inferior turbinate mucosa is an additional option. By attaching to peripheral cholinergic receptors, it is hypothesized to be effective in treating rhinorrhea by preventing the release of acetylcholine in cholinergic autonomic nerves and neuromuscular joints. Vidian nerve neurectomy or, less frequently, posterior nasal nerve resection, may be necessary as a last resort for the treatment of gustatory rhinitis.

2.5.2.5. Occupational Rhinitis

Occupational rhinitis is a condition where nasal symptoms like congestion, runny nose, nasal itching, and sneezing occur after exposure to specific substances in the workplace. It encompasses allergic, non-allergic, irritant-induced, and neurogenic types, making classification into subgroups challenging. Work-related rhinitis refers to symptoms developing in previously healthy individuals due to workplace exposure, while work-exacerbated rhinitis occurs in those with a history of rhinitis symptoms.

When an allergen is exposed to the immune system, it triggers an IgE-mediated Th2 response in allergic occupational rhinitis. On the other hand, certain allergenic triggers elicit IgG-mediated immunological reactions. Non-allergic occupational rhinitis lacks a distinct immunologic pathophysiologic foundation; however, it is associated with mechanisms that induce damage to or alteration of the epithelium as well as the release of neurokinin, both of which may have a role in the pathogenesis. Reactive upper airway dysfunction syndrome (RUDS) is the term used to describe rhinitis symptoms that occur after a single high-exposure to a particular agent. This type of rhinitis is unrelated to allergic occupational rhinitis. Occupational rhinitis is caused by a combination of low-molecular-weight (LMG) inorganic agents and high-molecular-weight (HMG) organic agents derived from plants, microorganisms, or animals. Exposure to HMW irritants has been shown to cause more reactions than LMW irritants. There is a strong correlation between occupational asthma and occupational rhinitis. The majority of individuals with occupational asthma also have occupational rhinitis, which is a condition that occurs before occupational asthma develops. Individuals who have occupational rhinitis are more likely to develop asthma. It is estimated that between 5% to 15% of people worldwide have occupational rhinitis and two out of every three people who have occupational asthma also have rhinitis. It is unclear, nevertheless, what proportion of patients with occupational rhinitis will go on to acquire occupational asthma.

The united airway model, which holds that the same inflammatory events in the upper and lower airways are the cause of both asthma and rhinitis, is still the most widely accepted theory explaining this relationship. With an emphasis on symptom type and duration, time of onset, factors that can improve or worsen the condition, and clinical examination, the medical history is crucial to the diagnosis process. The diagnostic strategy makes use of SPT or RAST testing to determine an agent's sensitivity. LMW irritants, however, usually do not cause an IgE-mediated reaction. In terms of diagnosis, nasal provocation tests are regarded as the gold standard. The diagnosis of occupational rhinitis is established by a combination of factors, including a comprehensive history and clinical examination consistent with the condition, and sensitization to a particular agent as demonstrated by a positive nasal provocation test. Using primary preventive techniques to minimize exposure to irritants appears to be crucial for managing occupational rhinitis. It may be necessary to employ secondary prevention techniques like symptom questionnaires and immunological assays for sensitization assessment. It is highly recommended to monitor patients with occupational rhinitis to prevent the development of occupational asthma. Intranasal corticosteroids are one medical treatment for occupational rhinitis that may help with nasal symptoms. Immunotherapy is typically not recommended as a therapeutic option.

2.5.2.6. Atrophic Rhinitis

Primary and secondary forms of atrophic rhinitis exist. The symptoms of both groups include dryness, epistaxis, halitosis, crusting, obstruction, and purulent discharge. Primary atrophic rhinitis primarily affects people who live in dry, warm climates and is characterized by glandular atrophy and nasal mucosa. Uncertainty surrounds the pathophysiological mechanisms. The most prevalent bacteria are Klebsiella ozaenae, Staphylococcus aureus, Proteus mirabilis, and Escherichia coli. Nasal dryness and a lack of mucosal secretions facilitate bacterial growth and mucosal colonization. The converse course could also be accurate. Fetor, crusting, and nasal congestion are the hallmarks of the secondary subtype, which is brought on by trauma, granulomatous diseases, or surgical removal of mucus-secreting tissue. Atrophic rhinitis is diagnosed by clinical suspicion and exclusion of autoimmune granulomatous diseases and other atrophic rhinitis-causing conditions, including scleroma, syphilis, leprosy, and tuberculosis.

The most common treatment for atrophic rhinitis is conservative, and it may involve paraffin nose drops to remove crusts and lubricate the nasal mucosa, nasal irrigations, or the use of glucose or glycerin to prevent infection by bacteria and other saprophytic organisms. Chloramphenicol-streptomycin drops, nemicetene antiozaena solution (containing propylene glycol, vitamin D2, and chloramphenicol estradiol diproprionate), acetylcholine with or without pilocarpine, vasodilators, and antibiotics after an infectious etiology evaluation are some other options for medical management. Antihistamines and decongestants should be avoided at all costs. Submucosal injections of placental extract are becoming more and more popular as a rather novel treatment option. For 24 weeks, the extract is injected weekly into each nasal cavity and possesses both angiogenic and mitogenic properties. Even if the symptoms of the nose are relieved, relapses may occur after the treatment is stopped.

2.5.2.7. Idiopathic Rhinitis

The most common type of non-allergic rhinitis is idiopathic or vasomotor rhinitis, making up approximately 71% of all cases. It affects 320 million people worldwide and is not linked to comorbid asthma. Idiopathic rhinitis is characterized by symptoms that are not triggered by allergies or infections and have no known cause. It is typically diagnosed after ruling out allergic rhinitis. The main underlying mechanism of idiopathic rhinitis appears to be related to abnormal neurogenic activity, as there is no association with other allergic conditions, structural issues, or specific inflammatory reactions in the body.

Idiopathic rhinitis is thought to be triggered by noxious odors, chemical irritants, cleaning products, and variations in environmental conditions like temperature, humidity, and barometric pressure. Numerous molecular pathways have been identified as being involved; one of these is typified by the release of tachykinin and the inhibition of sympathetic system mediators, which results in an increased parasympathetic response. There is not much evidence to support this mechanism. The idea that the non-adrenergic, non-cholinergic, or peptidergic neural systems are malfunctioning in at least some cases of idiopathic rhinitis is rather well-supported. Nasal peptidergic neurons, which affect blood vascularity and the secretory activity of mucous glands in the nasal cavity, are activated by inflammatory neuropeptides. Transparent response potential calcium ion channels (TRP) are responsible for activating the peptidergic and particularly C fibers. TRPs are triggered after the attachment to particular ligaments. Temperature variations, mechanical osmotic pressure, and chemical irritants all have an impact on those ligaments. The hot temperature activates the transient potential receptor vanilloid 1 (TPRV1), which is liganded by capsaicin. The TRPV1 receptor may become desensitized after repeated exposure to capsaicin, which is why it is regarded as a potentially useful medical treatment. Capsaicin is released when cold, dry air activates calcium channels that are similar to TRPV1, transient potential receptor ankyrin 1 (TRPA1), and transient potential receptor melastin 8 (TPRM8). The pathophysiological pathways associated with idiopathic or neurogenic rhinitis encompass a range of conditions, including gustatory rhinitis, occupational rhinitis, and others. Nasal hyperreactivity is the term used to describe increased nasal responsiveness to non-specific physical and chemical triggers in inspired air. Anticholinergic medications, aside from capsaicin, are widely recognized for their ability to improve the symptoms of idiopathic rhinitis patients.

2.5.3. Infectious Rhinitis

Because the sinuses and the nose have similar anatomical and vascular structures, sinusitis and rhinitis frequently coexist. Usually caused by viral agents rather than bacterial ones, acute viral rhinitis is the most prevalent type of upper respiratory infection. Adenovirus, influenza virus, respiratory syncytial virus, coronavirus, adenovirus, rhinovirus, and parainfluenza virus are among the common viruses that cause viral rhinitis. The viruses cause harm to the tight junctions between the epithelial cells, cause disruptions to their membranes, infiltrate the epithelial cells, and take control of the metabolic activity of the host cells. They use this control to further their growth and ultimately damage or kill the host cells. In most cases, medical treatment is not necessary as the disease progresses because the symptoms of infectious rhinitis are self-limiting. Unless there is a bacterial superinfection, antibiotic treatment is not recommended for viral rhinitis. Acute viral rhinitis has been shown to respond well to antiviral molecules like interferon alpha (INF-α), which reduces the length and intensity of symptoms.

Although the clinical phenotypes of rhinitis are well defined, the underlying pathophysiologic mechanisms of rhinitis are frequently not well understood. More research could lead to well-targeted treatments, which would then provide better symptom relief, manage related comorbidities, and lessen the financial burden associated with this extremely common illness.

2.6. Miscellaneous Disorders of Nasal Cavity

Air can be heated, cleansed, and humidified through the nasal passage and then enter the lungs and throat. The nasal septum, which divides this passage in half, can cause sinus issues and air flow obstructions when it is asymmetrical, or "deviated." The cilia on the nasal passage's outer walls, known as turbinates, expand and contract to control airflow via the nose. Usually, one side is more swollen and the other is shrinking to let air pass through the shrinking side and enable the swollen side to re-humidify itself. The swelling alternates to the other side roughly every two hours. Unless one takes deep breaths through their nose, this "nasal cycle" is usually invisible. Lying down causes the turbinates to swell more because the heart does not have to pump blood uphill to them as it does in a standing position. The turbinate swells more on the down side when one is on their side. The turbinates become enlarged or clogged due to allergies and colds.

Air pockets that drain into the nasal passage are called sinuses, and they are located in the face bones that surround the nose. They help to humidify the air and capture dust and debris by delivering pure mucus into the nose. In addition, because the sinuses absorb energy as they fracture, our head is lighter than it would be if it were made entirely of bone. The maxillary, sphenoid, ethmoid, and frontal sinuses are the four sinuses that lie on either side of the nose. Through the gap between the inferior and middle turbinates, the sinuses empty into the nasal cavity. The top of the nasal passage is where the sense of smell is produced. Here, chemical particles that produce odors activate special cells known as olfactory cells. Once activated, these cells communicate with the brain through nerve signals. The sense of smell may disappear temporarily or permanently if nasal disorders prevent smells from getting to the smell cells or if viruses infect these cells. A brain ailment may very seldom result in olfactory loss. It is interesting to note that scent accounts for 75% of the flavor that an object has. Flavor therefore suffers tremendously if scent is gone. This condition preserves the ability to distinguish between the four tastes—sweet, sour, bitter, and salt—and preserves the function of the taste buds.

2.6.1. Sinus and Nasal Disease

Numerous conditions can result in nasal obstruction or blockage of the nasal passage. A deviated septum is fairly common, and it only needs to be surgically corrected if it consistently causes bothersome nasal obstruction or if it is aggravating sinus disease. At times, it becomes imperative to decrease the turbinates' size through surgical procedures or radiofrequency reduction. Generally, the management of allergies involves avoiding the trigger if at all possible, in addition to using prescription drugs like decongestants, antihistamines, or nasal steroid sprays. In patients with more serious conditions or those who do not respond well to medication, allergy shots may also be helpful. The nose quickly becomes reliant on over-the-counter decongestant nasal sprays, so use them for no more than a few days at most. Regular use of saline (salt water) nasal spray is possible. Nasal obstruction may also result from enlarged adenoids. This is a common cause in children, but because the adenoids typically disappear in adolescence, it rarely happens in adults.

Although sinus illness and loss of smell are the most common side effects of *nasal polyps*, they can also cause nasal obstruction. Usually resulting from an allergic reaction, the lining tissue of the nose grows out of control to form polyps on both sides. The formation of polyps seems to be a genetic predisposition. Asthma and aspirin allergies are common in patients with polyps. Because polyps are so difficult to treat, steroid nasal sprays, oral or injectable steroid doses, and occasionally surgery are all necessary. A tumor or cancer may occasionally be the cause of polyps on one side of the nose, which are typically caused by inflammation or infection. Most of the time, these kinds of polyps require biopsies or surgical excision. See an expert in ear, nose, and throat care as soon as possible if you suspect that you have nasal polyps.

The common cause of sinusitis, also known as *sinus infection*, is obstruction of one or more sinuses' drainage channels. A deviated septum, polyps, changes in the shape of the nasal structures, or swelling of the nasal and sinus lining as a result of a cold or allergy can all be causes of this obstruction. A sinus infection is frequently the result of several of these variables working together. Because of this obstruction, bacteria from the nasal passage can enter the sinus and grow there in the stagnant mucus. Sinusitis can also occasionally be brought on by immune system abnormalities.

A presumptive diagnosis of sinusitis is frequently made based on symptoms commonly associated with sinus infection, even though a sinus infection can only be definitively diagnosed by X-ray or telescopic observation of pus draining into the nose from the sinus. Nasal blockage, fever, pain or pressure directly over the sinuses, colored mucous in the throat, coughing, and colored nasal drainage from the front of the nose are some of the symptoms that may accompany these conditions. Similar, but typically milder, symptoms can also indicate a chronic sinus infection. A sinus infection and a cold can present with many of the same symptoms, so it is important to distinguish between the two. The typical symptoms of a cold include body aches, less colorful discharge, and self-healing in 7 to 10 days. Seeking care or treatment for a "sinus infection" is generally discouraged unless the patient has had colored drainage for more than 7 to 10 days. Antibiotic resistance infections can arise later on and are expensive when antibiotics are misused.

An antibiotic, a decongestant tablet, and possibly the restricted use of a decongestant nasal spray (for no more than three days) are the usual treatments for acute sinusitis, which lasts for a few weeks. Consider getting some X-rays and/or seeing an ear, nose, and throat specialist if the symptoms don't go better after taking antibiotics for a few courses. Rarely, it might be required to clean the infected sinus in the workplace. Surgery is not always required. From time to time, an infection in the sinuses can spread to the eye socket, the skin around the eyes, or other structures. This frequently necessitates immediate surgery, IV antibiotics, and hospitalization.

Treatment for recurrent sinusitis (four or more episodes per year) or chronic sinusitis (lasting weeks to months) involves a precise diagnosis and a careful evaluation of the factors causing the sinusitis. This usually entails a detailed discussion of the patient's symptoms, an endoscopic (or telescopic) office examination of the nose, a CAT scan, and occasionally allergy testing. Next, a plan for treating these contributing factors is created. Surgery may be considered if medical therapy is ineffective or if it is evident that structural abnormalities play a significant role.

2.6.2. Sinus or Nasal Surgery

If other therapies are not working or don't seem to be helping, sinus or nasal surgery may be considered. The likelihood that the surgery would fix the issue or significantly improve it, along with the risks and discomforts associated with it, are all taken into consideration before making this decision. The Ear, Nose and Throat Center physician must thoroughly consult with you to determine which sinus or nasal procedures are necessary. Any given case will involve different factors, but the general principles listed below should help you get started.

Before Surgery

1. For two weeks before surgery, avoid taking any aspirin, Motrin, Advil, nuprin, ibuprofen, Aleve, naprosyn, Peptobismal, garlic pills, ginkgo, vitamin E, or similar products as they may increase bleeding. Also, stay away from these products and medications for two weeks following surgery. Take a Tylenol, please.
2. For preoperative blood work or tests, please make sure they are completed on time.
3. The day before surgery, avoid eating or drinking anything after midnight, not even water. If not, it might be necessary to postpone surgery.
4. Kindly contact the office as soon as possible if you have any questions concerning your surgical procedure.

The Day of Surgery

1. Avoid eating or drinking anything on the morning of the procedure.
2. If you take any prescription drugs regularly, please make sure to find

out which ones you should take the morning of surgery (with a small sip of water).

3. You must get to the surgical facility well in advance of the procedure's scheduled start time. You will receive a call from the doctor's nurse or a facility representative a day or two before surgery, with precise arrival time information.

After Surgery

1. Your operation will take between one and four hours, depending on what is being done. After surgery, a family member should stay in the waiting area until the doctor speaks with them.
2. Depending on the length and complexity of your procedure, you will typically return home one to four hours afterward. You won't be able to drive after surgery, so you should arrange for someone to drive you home.
3. After surgery, keep your head as high as you can. You could have a flat night's sleep.
4. Usually, one or both of your nose's sides will be packed. Two to five days following the procedure, this will be taken out in the office. You should have transportation to and from this initial appointment. You ought to after the packing is taken out.
   - Head straight home and spend the remainder of the day in silence.
   - For two weeks, refrain from blowing your nose; instead, open your mouth to sneeze.
   - avoid strenuous activity for two weeks.

2.6.3. Returning to Work

You might be able to go back to work the day after the packing is taken out, or you might have to wait up to two weeks, depending on the exact surgery that was done, how uncomfortable you are, and the requirements of your job.

2.6.4. Follow-Up Care

After surgery, you will need to come back to the office once or twice a week for a period of one to two months so that the nose can be cleaned and checked to make sure everything is healing properly. Adults can take their own cars to these appointments.

2.6.5. Risks of Surgery

Despite the generally low likelihood of surgical complications, no surgery is "risk-free.." The purpose of providing the following information is to inform patients rather than to scare them. The following is a list of common surgical procedures for the sinuses and nose. The majority of the potential risks associated with each procedure are listed along with the technical terms for each one. Any surgical procedure carries some general risks, such as those pertaining to anesthesia, infection, bleeding, and the formation of scar tissue. After surgery, there is always a chance of sinus or nasal problems returning due to allergies, scarring, or other reasons.

A Closer Look

Nasal Polyp

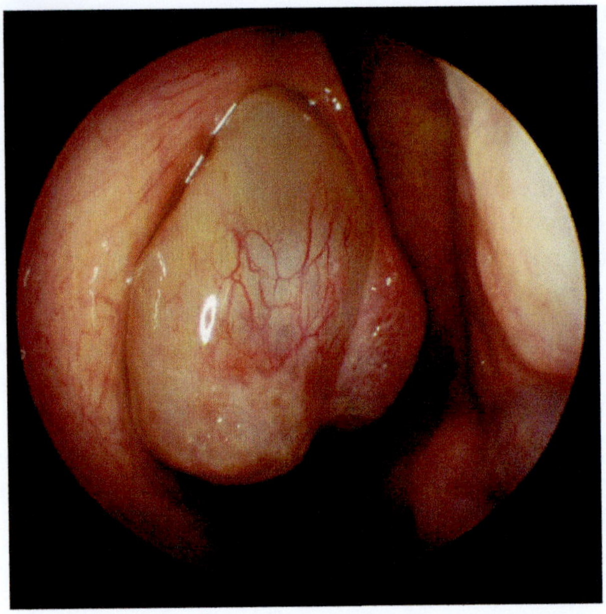

Source: By Mustafakapadiya – Own work, CC BY-SA 4.0, https://commons.wikimedia.org/w/index.php?curid=113507992.

A lump of tissue known as a nasal polyp protrudes into the nasal cavity and occasionally obstructs it. Allergies, inflammation, and infection can all lead to the formation of polyps. Because of their vast blood vessel network, allergic polyps are typically bright red in color. The nasal wall's upper and side walls are where these polyps are most frequently found. At times, they originate in the sinuses and then move into the nasal cavity. Although they can be surgically removed or treated with medication (injections or sprays), they typically return until the allergic source is removed. Both infections and nose injuries can lead to inflammatory polyps. Once removed, they do not return. These polyps are less fluid-filled than allergic polyps, but they are packed with white blood cells. Polyps can also occasionally develop from closely spaced blood vessels that enlarge due to high blood pressure or prior nose injuries.

Summary

- The nose, separated by the nasal septum, serves as the organ of smell and is divided into two parts. It filters out contaminants like pollen and dirt with tiny hairs in the nostrils, while also bringing humidified air to the lungs.
- The nose's typical duties include breathing, sinus drainage, conditioning inspired air, vocal resonance, smell, nasal resistance, and protection of the lower airway.
- One of the body's natural channels for breathing (perspiration) is the nose. Humans breathe through their noses most of the time for basic respiration. Breathing in causes the nose to function as an air conditioner.
- The nose is continually in contact with germs, viruses, and fungi that are inhaled. To fend off this attack, the respiratory system has evolved multiple defense mechanisms.
- A sinus infection (nasal vestibule) is referred to as nasal vestibulitis. Excessive blowing or picking of the nose is usually to blame. The area around your nose's opening may scab and crust over time. Antibiotic creams, tablets, or oral medications are used as treatments.
- The nasal septum divides the two nostrils and keeps the left and right airways of the nasal cavity apart. The depressor septi nasi muscle depresses it.
- A condition affecting the nasal septum where pus accumulates between the mucoperichondrium and septal cartilage is known as a nasal septal abscess.
- A reaction that results in a runny nose, itchy, and congested nasal passages is called rhinoitis. The majority of rhinitis types are brought on by inflammation and manifest as symptoms in the throat, ears, or eyes.
- Air can be heated, cleansed, and humidified through the nasal passage and then enter the lungs and throat. The nasal septum, which divides this passage in half, can cause sinus issues and air flow obstructions when it is asymmetrical, or "deviated."

References

1. Busse, W. W., & Holgate, S. T. (2000). *Asthma and Rhinitis*. Blackwell Science Ltd. http://dx.doi.org/10.1002/9780470694923.
2. Kaliner, M. A. (2006). *Current Review of Rhinitis* (2nd ed.). Current Medicine LLC.
3. Lasley, M. V., & Altman, L. C. (2000). *Rhinitis*. Saunders.

Chapter

DISEASES OF THE ORAL CAVITY AND SALIVARY GLANDS

3

Contents

Introduction

The oral mucosa, a mucous membrane that lines the oral cavity, is made up of the lamina propria, an underlying layer of connective tissue, and a stratified squamous epithelium that may or may not be keratinized. The major and several minor salivary glands produce mucus, which keeps the surface wet. The tongue's dorsal surface has unique sensory endings specifically for taste, and the oral mucosa is richly supplied with nerve endings. The submucosa of the oral cavity, which lies beneath the lamina propria, varies. The lamina propria and submucosa can occasionally blend invisibly due to their substantial similarity. The presence of small salivary glands in a loosely textured tissue will be the only way to distinguish the submucosa from the lamina propria microscopically.

The salivary glands are intricate organs. These could be exocrine, merocrine, or tubulo acinar glands that primarily secrete saliva. One of the primary soft tissue components in the maxillofacial region is the salivary gland. Saliva is a clear, mildly acidic mucosal fluid that coats the teeth and mucosa, contributing to the establishment and upkeep of a wholesome environment in the mouth. Numerous diseases, both systemic and local, can affect the salivary glands. The etiology of these diseases varies, as does their prevalence. Viral, bacterial, and infrequently fungal infections, as well as ductal blockage, can infect the glands and cause excruciating swelling or obstruction that impairs their ability to function. Numerous benign and malignant tumors can also impact the salivary gland.

Orientation and Directional Terms

Term	Definition	Illustration
Gingivitis	Gingivitis is the mildest and most common form of periodontitis. It is caused by the toxins in plaque and leads to periodontal disease. People at increased risk of developing gingivitis include pregnant women, women taking birth control pills, people with uncontrolled diabetes, steroid users, and people who control seizures and blood pressure using medication.	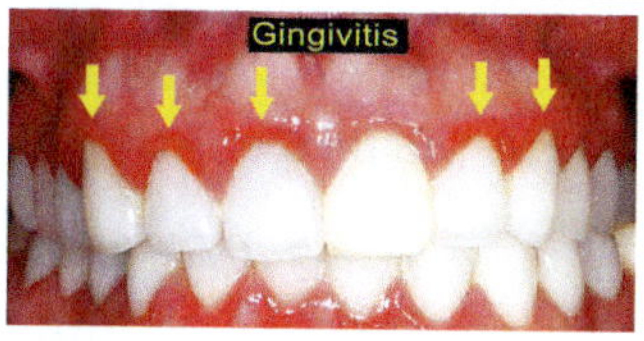
Chronic Periodontal Disease	Chronic periodontal disease is the most common form of the disease and occurs much more frequently in people over 45. Chronic periodontal disease is characterized by inflammation below the gum line and the progressive destruction of the gingival and bone tissue. It may appear that the teeth are gradually growing in length, but in actuality, the gums are gradually recessing.	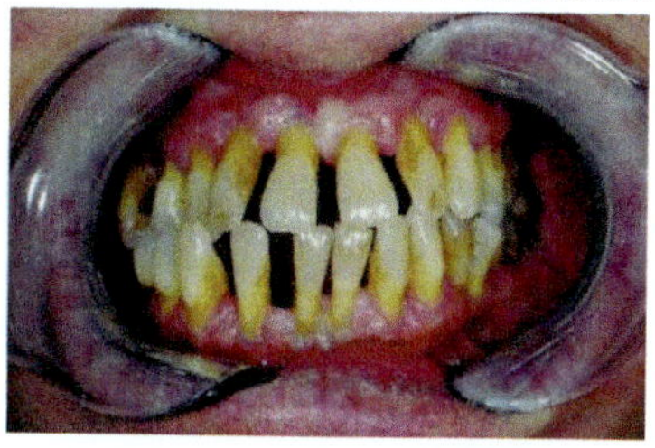
Erythroplakia	Erythroplakia is another symptom of smoking or chewing tobacco. People with erythroplakia have red patches that commonly appear behind their lower front teeth or under their tongue. Unlike leukoplakia lesions, erythroplakia patches are usually precancerous or cancerous.	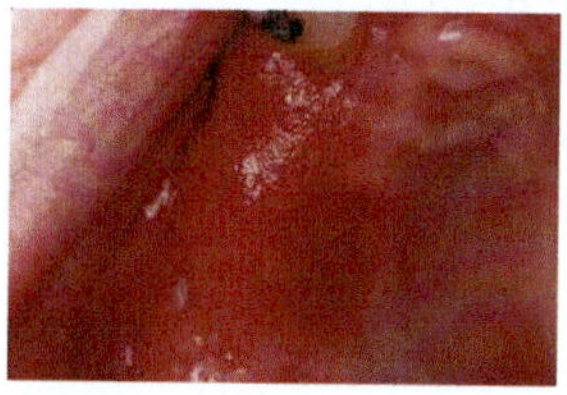
Bruxism	Bruxism is a common condition that refers to the voluntary or involuntary movement of the mandibular (bottom) jaw. This habitual movement results in clenching, grinding, or teeth clicking.	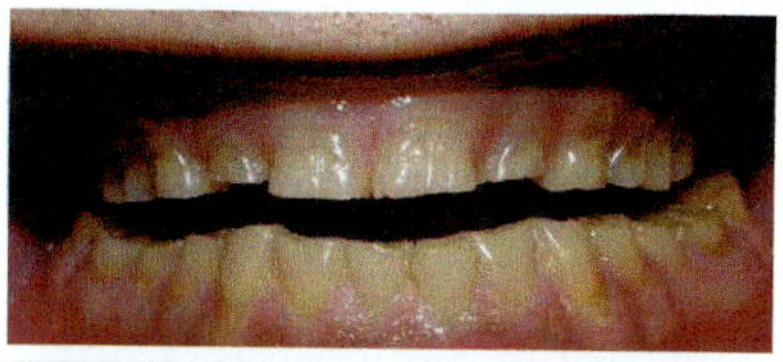
Dental caries	Dental caries results when plaque forms on the surface of a tooth and converts the free sugars (all sugars added to foods by the manufacturer, cook or consumer, plus sugars naturally present in honey, syrups and fruit juices) contained in foods and drinks into acids that destroy the tooth over time.	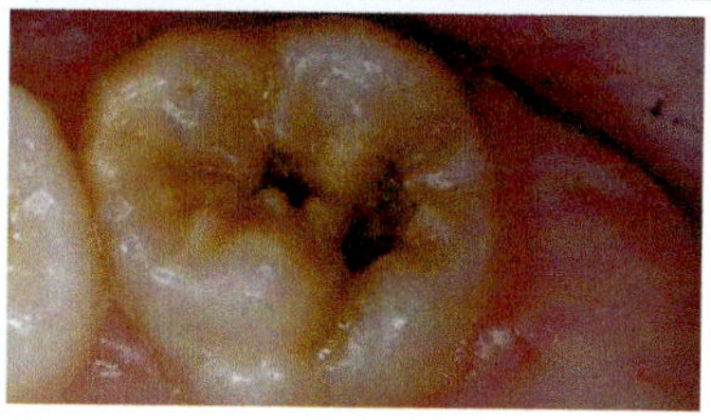
Leukoplakia	This condition causes white or gray patches inside your mouth. It develops because of excess cell growth. Chronic irritation from things like smoking or chewing tobacco can cause it. But sometimes it happens for no ap parent reason. Leukoplakia lesions usually are not cancerous.	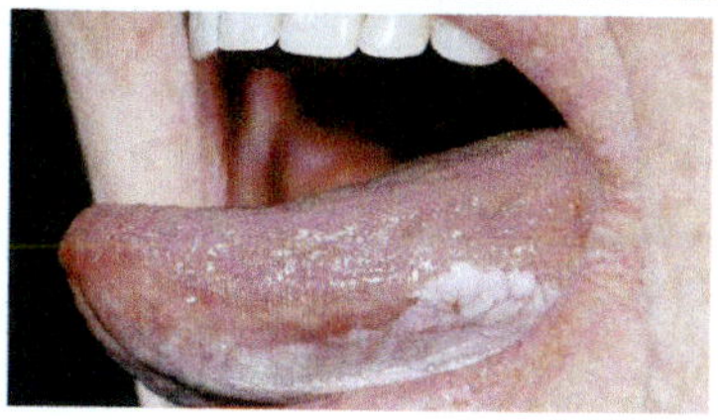

3.1. Anatomy of the Oral Cavity

The alimentary canal begins in the oral cavity, sometimes referred to as the mouth. It serves three main purposes.

- Digestion – is the act of breaking down food into molecules that can be absorbed; these processes occur in the stomach and small intestines.
- Communication – produces a variety of sounds by altering the sound made in the larynx.
- Breathing – serves as an air inlet in addition to the nasal cavity.

3.1.1. Divisions of the Oral Cavity

The oral cavity is located between the oropharyngeal isthmus, which is the opening of the oropharynx, and the oral fissure, which is the opening between the lips on the anterior side. The upper and lower dental arches—formed by the teeth and their bony scaffolding—separate it into two sections. The vestibule and the mouth cavity proper are the two sections that make up the oral cavity.

3.1.1.1. Vestibule

The vestibule, which has a horseshoe shape, is located in front. It is the area where the gums and teeth meet the lips and cheeks. Through the oral fissure and the space behind the third molar tooth, the vestibule is connected to both the interior and exterior of the mouth. The orbicularis oris, the primary facial expression muscle, regulates the diameter of the oral fissure. Salivary secretions are released into the vestibule through the opening of the parotid gland duct opposite the upper second molar tooth (Figure 3.1).

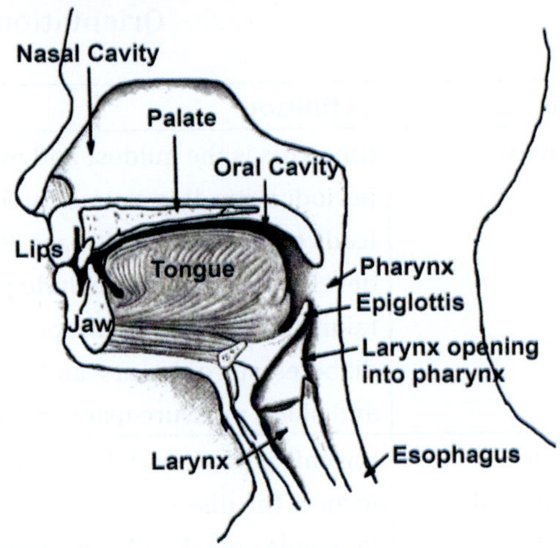

Figure 3.1. *Head and neck overview.*

Source: By Arcadian – http://training.seer.cancer.gov/head-neck/anatomy/overview.html, Public Domain, https://commons.wikimedia.org/w/index.php?curid=1678037.

3.1.1.2. Mouth Proper

The vestibule and the mouth proper are situated posteriorly. The cheeks, a floor, and a roof encircle it. A significant amount of the oral cavity is occupied by the tongue (Figure 3.2).

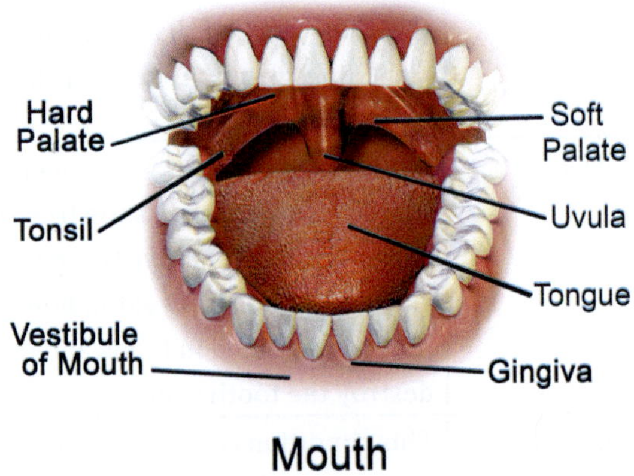

Figure 3.2. *Anatomy of the mouth.*

Source: By Bruce Blaus. Own work, CC BY 3.0, https://commons.wikimedia.org/w/index.php?curid=33041243.

3.1.1.2.1. Roof

The hard and soft palates make up the actual roof of the mouth. The hard palate is situated in front. The nasal cavity and the oral cavity are divided by this bony plate. It is covered by oral mucosa (stratified squamous epithelium) inferiorly and respiratory mucosa (ciliated pseudostratified columnar epithelium) superiorly. The hard palate continues posteriorly into the soft palate. It is a muscle structure as opposed to a hard palate. It functions as a valve that can be raised to divide the nasopharynx from the oropharynx and lowered to close the oropharyngeal isthmus.

3.1.1.2.2. Cheeks

The buccinator muscle, which has the oral mucous membrane lining it internally, forms the cheeks. The buccal branches of the facial nerve (CN VII) innervate the buccinator muscle, which contracts during chewing to keep food between the teeth.

3.1.1.2.3. Floor

The floor of the oral cavity consists of several structures (Figure 3.3):

- Muscular diaphragm: composed of the mylohyoid muscles on both sides. It pulls the larynx forward when swallowing and gives the floor of the mouth structural support.
- Geniohyoid muscles: Pull your larynx forward when you swallow.
- Tongue joined to the floor by the tongue's frenulum, an oral mucosal fold.
- Salivary glands and ducts.

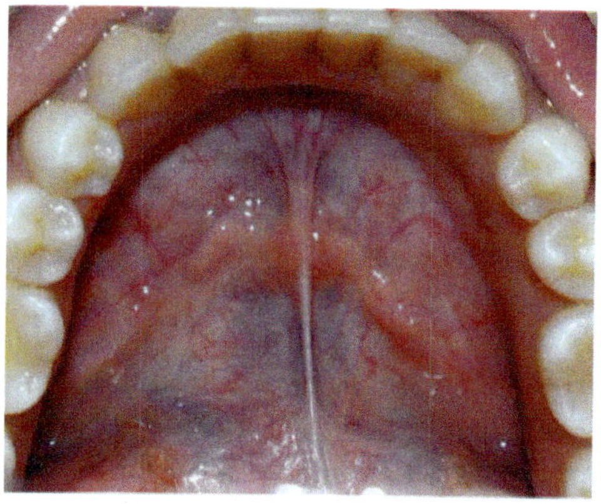

Figure 3.3. *Floor of the mouth with lingual frenum and sublingual fold.*

Source: By Shaimaa Abdellatif – Own work, CC BY-SA 4.0, https://commons.wikimedia.org/w/index.php?curid=68658680.

3.1.2. Innervation

The branches of the trigeminal nerve (CN V) supply sensory innervation to the oral cavity. The maxillary nerve (CN V2) gives rise to the greater palatine and nasopalatine nerves, which innervate the hard palate. The lesser palatine nerve, an additional branch of the maxillary nerve, innervates the soft palate. The lingual nerve, a branch of the mandibular (V3) division of the trigeminal nerve, provides sensory innervation to the floor of the oral cavity. Additionally, taste-related sensory fibers from the chorda tympani, a branch of the facial nerve (CN VII), innervate the tongue. The buccal nerve innervates the cheeks. Additionally, it is a branch of the trigeminal nerve's mandibular division (not to be confused with the buccal branches of the facial nerve).

3.2. Common Disorders of the Oral Cavity

Some of the more prevalent dental issues people are facing in today's world are referred to as oral diseases. Gum disease, oral cancers, dental cavities, infectious diseases, and trauma and injury are some of these issues. A bad diet, excessive alcohol consumption, smoking cigarettes, and neglecting oral hygiene are some of the more prevalent risk factors for receiving an oral health diagnosis. Dental diseases and oral conditions affect the state of your teeth, gums, and surrounding tissues. It is critical to prevent, diagnose, and treat oral health issues promptly because they are linked to overall health. Knowing the most typical oral health problems will help you decide when to see a physician.

3.2.1. Ulcers of the Oral Cavity

A common presenting symptom of a wide range of oral diseases with numerous etiologic factors is an ulcer. Because various types of ulcerated lesions share similar clinical and histologic characteristics, these lesions may present a special diagnostic challenge for medical professionals. The four types of ulcerative lesions of the oral mucosa are immune-related, traumatic, neoplastic, and infection-related (Figure 3.4).

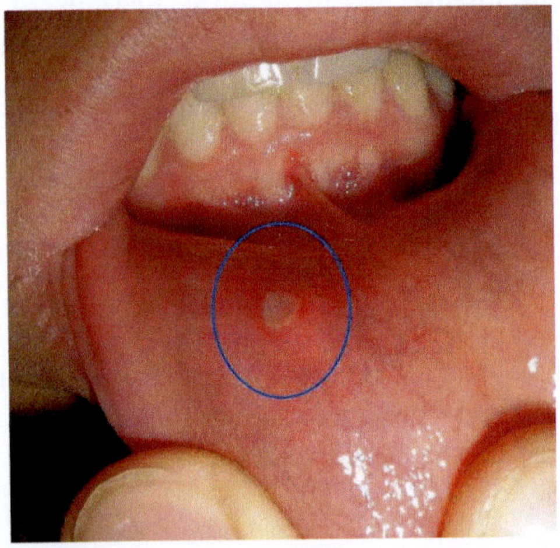

Figure 3.4. *A mouth ulcer (in this case associated with aphthous stomatitis) on the labial mucosa (lining of the lower lip).*

Source: CC BY-SA 3.0, https://commons.wikimedia.org/w/index.php?curid=513236.

3.2.1.1. Ulcerations of Infective Etiology

Because there is a large potential range of non-specific symptoms and health care providers are unfamiliar with the symptoms and presentations of these less common diseases, oral ulcerations caused by infections may present diagnostic challenges.

3.2.1.2. Bacterial: Syphilis and Tuberculosis

Treponema pallidum is the source of the sexually transmitted disease syphilis, which can manifest as primary, secondary, or tertiary disease or as a congenital condition. Syphilis is a non-specific, highly contagious ulceration that arises in cases of primary syphilis. The chancre usually appears as a painful, deep, solitary ulceration in the oral cavity. The lips are the most frequently involved site; the tongue, palate, or tonsillar region are less frequently involved. There's a chance the patient will exhibit related cervical lymphadenopathy. Usually, oral chancres involutrate within 3–8 weeks. Making a diagnosis can be difficult. particular assays for T-specific IgM or IgG antibodies. In the event that primary syphilis is suspected, pallidum should be given. Due to the non-specific nature of histopathology, special stains like Warthin-Starry may not yield positive results. Parenterally administered penicillin G is the recommended treatment for syphilis in all stages, and most patients only need one dose (Figure 3.5).

Mycobacterium tuberculosis is the cause of tuberculosis (TB), which affects more than 9,000 Americans annually. Up to 15% of these patients exhibit oral lesions, with ulcerations being the most frequent. When primary tuberculosis ulcerates, the lesion is not painful, and the patient may also have lymphadenopathy. Children are most likely to exhibit this presentation. Ulcerations are more common in adults and are painful with variable lymphadenopathy when secondary tuberculosis is present.

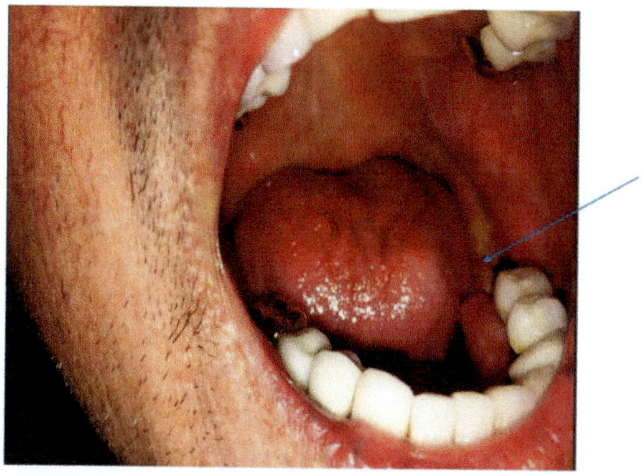

Figure 3.5. *Photograph of the open mouth with arrow pointed at exposed bone around teeth #18 and 19: bacterial culture grew alpha hemolytic streptococcus, Eikenella corrodens and Micrococcus spp.*

Source: *Ayoade F, Olayiwola A, Li A. (2018). "Holes" in the Jaw—A report of two cases of periapical actinomycosis. Diseases, 6(3), 79. https://doi.org/10.3390/diseases6030079.*

Although several lesions have been documented, tuberculosis ulcerations are typically solitary. The irregular ulcers can be deep or superficial, and necrotic tissue in the center may cover them. The ulcers do not go away on their own; instead, they gradually enlarge. Numerous laboratory tests, such as cultures, microscopic inspection, and molecular testing, are used to diagnose tuberculosis. The antimicrobial medications rifampin, isoniazid, pyrazinamide, and ethambutol are used in combination as treatment.

3.2.1.3. Viral: Human Herpesvirus: Herpes Simplex Virus, Varicella Zoster Virus, and Cytomegalovirus

Types 1 and 2 of the human simplex virus (HSV-1) are members of the human herpesvirus family. Although HSV-1 is more common in the oral mucosa, both viruses cause ulcerations that are comparable in nature. Patients with acute herpetic gingivostomatitis may develop oral ulcerations on the tongue, palate, gingiva, buccal mucosa, and labial mucosa, even though the primary infection is usually asymptomatic. Small vesicles that rupture and coalesce are the precursors of the ulcerations. Primary HSV infection symptoms can coexist with other acute oral ulcerative disorders, such as hand, foot, and mouth disease or herpangina, which are mainly observed in children. 40% of patients experience recurrent infection, which usually manifests as herpes labialis on the vermilion border. In healthy individuals, intraoral recurrences are ulcerations that are restricted to the hard palate and attached gingiva. Usually, these start out as several tiny, painless ulcerations that may come together and heal in 10 days. Recurrences on non-keratinized mucosa may occur in immunocompromised patients. The HSV-1 diagnosis is usually made in a clinical setting. Acyclovir rinses can be used to treat primary infections, and systemic acyclovir, valacyclovir, or famciclovir, as well as over-the-counter topical 10% n-docosanol cream, can be used to treat recurrences (Figure 3.6).

Varicella (chickenpox) is caused by a primary infection of the varicella-zoster virus (VZV); recurrences manifest as herpes zoster (shingles). Even though varicella typically affects the skin, severe cases can also result in oral ulcerations. They appear as tiny vesicles that burst quickly to produce shallow ulcers. The palate, buccal mucosa, and lips are where they are most frequently seen. Older or immunocompromised patients are susceptible to zoster. Usually, a few days before the acute phase's visible lesions, there is a prodromal stage of pain. The acute phase's oral symptoms begin as vesicles covering erythematous macules that ulcerate and crust over the course of 10 days. Both keratinized and non-keratinized mucosa are affected by these unilaterally distributed lesions. Postherpetic neuralgia may ensue, resulting in excruciating pain that could endure for up to a year. VZV is typically diagnosed clinically. For varicella, palliative care is appropriate; for zoster, patients benefit from systemic antiviral therapy if administered within 48 hours.

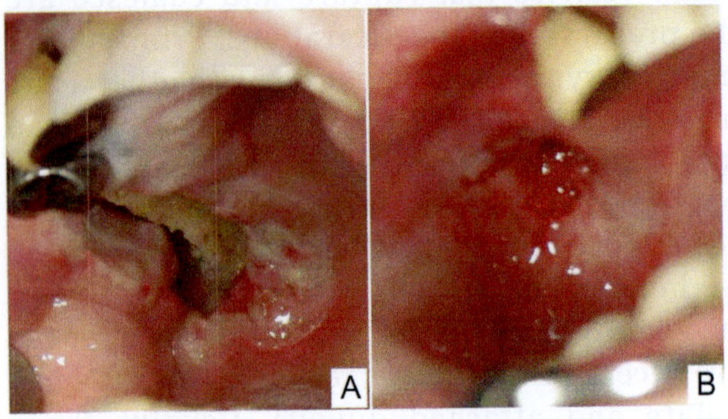

Figure 3.6. *Representative macroscopic findings for Epstein–Barr virus (EBV) in the gingival mucosa. The ulcer developed while the patient was on methotrexate (A). After the methotrexate dose was discontinued, the lesion spontaneously disappeared (B).*

Source: *Ikeda T, Gion Y, Nishimura Y, Nishimura MF, Yoshino T, Sato Y. (2021). Epstein–Barr Virus-Positive Mucocutaneous Ulcer: A Unique and Curious Disease Entity. International Journal of Molecular Sciences, 22(3), 1053. https://doi.org/10.3390/ijms22031053.*

Another member of the human herpesvirus family that sporadically causes oral ulcers is called cytomegalovirus (CMV). Immunosuppressed patients frequently develop these non-specific ulcerations, which typically affect the tongue, floor of the mouth, and hard or soft palate. When CMV-induced ulcerations are examined histopathologically, larger endothelial cells or salivary duct epithelium may be seen. Intranuclear inclusions will be highlighted by the use of periodic acid-Schiff (PAS) stain or Grocott-Gomori methenamine silver (GMS) stain. The afflicted cells also contain prominent nucleoli. Immunocompromised patients have historically been treated with ganciclovir.

3.2.1.4. Fungal: Deep Fungal Infections

Aspergillus fumigatus or *Aspergillus flavus* (aspergillosis), *Blastomyces dermatidis* (blastomycosis), *Histoplasma capsulatum* (histoplasmosis), *Cryptococcus neoformans* (cryptococcosis), *Coccidioides immitis* (coccidioidomycosis), and Paracoccidiodes brasiliensis (paracoccidiomycosis) are among the many fungal infections that can cause oral ulcerations. The majority of these infections manifest in immunocompromised individuals in a disseminated form. Aspergillosis ulcers are typically black or yellow necrotic lesions that affect the palate or tongue. It is possible for oral ulcerations caused by blastomycosis to resemble squamous cell carcinoma. These irregular, rolled-bordered, erythematous lesions can appear anywhere in the oral cavity. Histoplasmosis causes indurated, rolled-bordered ulcers that typically appear on the tongue, gingiva, or palate. Cryptococcosis can cause ulcerations on the tonsillar pillars, gingiva, or palate. Coccidioidomycosis can occasionally manifest as an oral ulcer. And last, the mucocutaneous form of paracoccidiomycosis can start off as tiny vesicles that ulcerate and grow over time, developing rolled borders and eventually becoming painful. The correct diagnosis is made by biopsies of the ulcerations using the proper special stains; intravenous amphotericin B is most frequently used for disseminated disease (Figure 3.7).

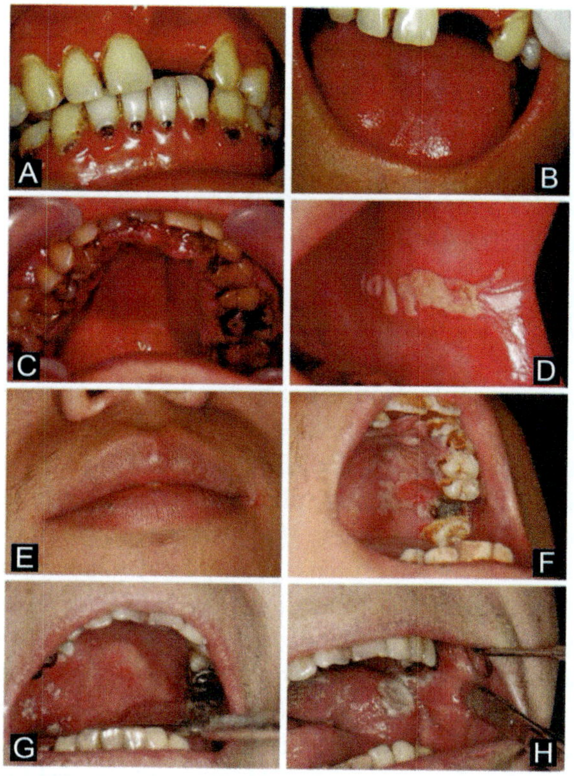

Figure 3.7. *Oral candidosis can be a mark of systemic disease.*

Note: (A,B) Erythematous candidosis, angular cheilitis, and rampant cervical caries led to the diagnosis of diabetes mellitus and iron deficiency anemia in a 30-year-old male who drank soda daily instead of water. (C,D) Pseudomembranous candidosis and diffuse gum hyperplasia with cyanotic change led to the diagnosis of acute myeloid leukemia in a 32-year-old man. (E,F) Cheilocandidosis and pseudomembranous candidosis around a necrotic ulcer over the palate led to the diagnosis of HIV infection in a 28-year-old man. (G,H) Pseudomembranous and erythematous candidosis with a necrotic tongue ulcer led to the diagnosis of severe leukopenia in a 33-year-old woman.

Source: Lu S-Y. (2021). Oral Candidosis: Pathophysiology and Best Practice for Diagnosis, Classification, and Successful Management. Journal of Fungi, 7(7), 555. https://doi.org/10.3390/jof7070555.

3.2.1.5. Ulcerations of Immune-Related Etiology

The majority of immune-mediated ulcerative diseases tend to persist, relapse, and occur frequently. Finding any potential trigger medications or coexisting symptoms that might point to a systemic illness is very important.

3.2.1.6. Recurrent Aphthous Stomatitis and Associated Conditions

Among younger patients, recurrent aphthous stomatitis (RAS) is one of the most prevalent oral mucosal lesions. The etiology is unknown and frequently complex, involving underlying genetic susceptibility as well as topical agents, foods, medications, hormones, stress, bacterial or viral microbiological agents, and systemic disease as potential contributing factors. There are three types of RAS: minor, major, and herpetiform.

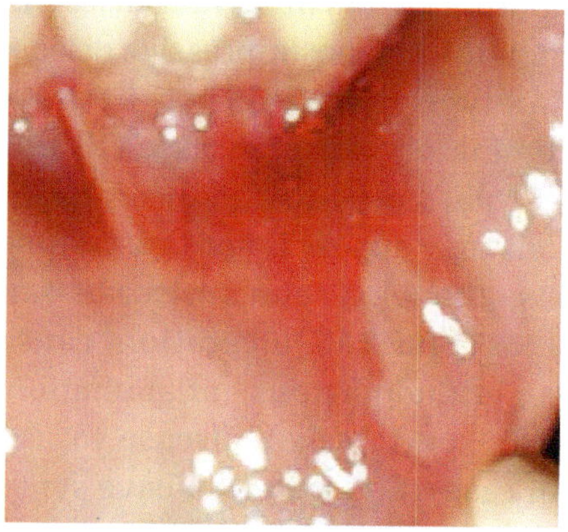

Figure 3.8. *An aphthous ulcer on the labial mucosa (note erythematous "halo" surrounding lesion).*

Source: *By The original uploader was Verslinykas711 at English Wikipedia. – Own work by the original uploader, Public Domain, https://commons.wikimedia.org/w/index.php?curid=9871404.*

These types differ in terms of the quantity of lesions, lesion recurrence frequency and duration, location of involvement, and severity.

In the absence of systemic illness, oral lesions that occur frequently or continuously and potential genital lesions are the hallmarks of complex RAS. All variations of the individual ulcerations are painful and have a central yellow necrotic area encircled by a characteristic red halo (Figure 3.8).

It is important to assess patients with RAS for potential correlations with foods, topical treatments or medications, underlying systemic diseases, and nutritional deficiencies. Sodium lauryl sulfate, an ingredient in toothpaste, is thought to have the potential to cause RAS. RAS-like lesions have been linked to a number of medications, including beta blockers, angiotensin-converting enzyme inhibitors, antibiotics, nonsteroidal anti-inflammatory drugs (NSAIDS), and antianginal drugs. Iron, B vitamin, vitamin C, or folate deficiencies may be contributing factors in certain cases. HIV and other systemic immunosuppressive diseases can lead to RAS-type ulcers. RAS may be associated with inflammatory bowel disease (IBD), which includes Crohn's disease and ulcerative colitis. Oral lesions may appear before gastrointestinal symptoms, though Crohn's disease can also manifest as non-RAS ulceration caused by persistent granulomatous inflammation. RAS has been linked to celiac disease in as many as 50% of cases. Children who have symmetric enamel defects and RAS should have a celiac disease evaluation. An evaluation for disorders like Behçet's disease, MAGIC, and Reiter's syndromes should be initiated if there has been a history of skin, genital, or ocular ulcerative lesions associated with arthritis. RAS is present in many illnesses, such as Sweet's syndrome, PFAPA syndrome, and cyclic neutropenia, along with recurrent fever and infection.

RAS is typically diagnosed clinically, and biopsy results, if taken to rule out other pathologies, typically reveal nonspecific ulceration. Topical corticosteroids are the first line of treatment for radiation-associated syndromes (RAS); however, systemic steroids or other immunosuppressive drugs may be necessary in complex or severe cases.

3.2.1.7. Erythema Multiforme and Medication-Related Ulcerations

The clinical severity of erythema multiforme (EM), an immune-mediated aberrant T-cell response, varies widely. Particularly in cases that recur, infectious agents are most frequently linked to EM. In between 61 and 100% of recurrent adult cases of EM and 35% of cases in children, the herpes simplex virus (HSV) has been linked. In certain cases, *Mycoplasma pneumoniae* and Epstein-Barr virus (EBV) have also been linked. 10 to 50% of adult cases of EM have been associated with medication, specifically NSAIDS, antibiotics, antifungals, and antivirals. Additional potential causative variables encompass cancer, radiation, vaccination, diet, and hormones. The majority of people with EM are in their early to middle years, and men are more likely to have the condition than women, especially in younger patients. Patients may experience self-limiting or recurrent episodes of oral, cutaneous, or genital lesions in addition to eye and genital lesions. Oral involvement is symptomatic and frequently manifests as lip ulcerations that crust over time, frequently affecting the buccal mucosa or other mucosal surfaces.

The results of a biopsy for certain conditions may show various symptoms such as ulceration, edema, acanthosis, and inflammation. Treatment focuses on identifying the cause of the condition. Recurrent erythema multiforme (EM) caused by herpes simplex virus (HSV) is often treated with antiviral medication. The use of corticosteroids for EM treatment is a topic of debate. Fixed-drug eruptions in the mouth, although different from EM, typically present as recurring or persistent ulcers in the same spot after using a specific medication. The condition may also affect the skin and genital mucosa. Medications that can cause this reaction include antihistamines, NSAIDs, acetaminophen, antifungal drugs, and antibiotics. Nicorandil, a medication for angina, has also been linked to oral ulcers. Like in EM cases, biopsy results are not specific and treatment involves identifying and eliminating the medication causing the issue.

3.2.1.8. Lichenoid Lesions and Related Conditions

Skin and the mucosa of the mouth, vagina, or eyes can be affected by oral lichen planus (OLP), an immune disorder mediated by T cells. Typically, middle-aged women experience symmetric and multifocal oral conditions, such as OLP, which often manifests in trauma-prone areas like the lateral tongue and buccal mucosa. From ulcerated, painful multifocal lesions to white, reticular, or lacy asymptomatic lesions, OLP and related conditions can present with a wide range of clinical appearances. Typically, ulcerated or atrophic forms of symptoms are reported by up to two-thirds of OLP patients. Patients who are asymptomatic may eventually develop ulcerations and exhibit symptoms.

Systemic illnesses, such as lupus erythematosus (LE) and graft-versus-host disease (GVHD), can resemble OLP. In patients with a history of bone marrow transplant, GVHD may present clinically and histologically like OLP. Moreover, oral lichenoid appearing lesions may also be present in patients with discoid lupus erythematosus (DLE) and systemic lupus erythematosus (SLE). OLP has been linked to hepatitis C in many populations. Oral lichenoid lesions (OLLs) may be linked to local irritants like amalgam, food additives, or dental materials. These should be looked into as potential triggers, particularly in cases of localized lesions. Although oral lichenoid drug reactions (OLDRs) have long been reported anecdotally, the complete understanding of this phenomenon is limited by the absence of credible studies. The list of drugs that are commonly linked to OLDRs is lengthy, but the most commonly implicated ones are NSAIDS, antihypertensives, antimalarials, and antiretroviral drugs. Less than one-third of cases in a recent systematic review of OLDRs showed resolution or improvement of the OLDR upon stopping the suspected medication. Unlike classic OLP, OLDRs are usually unilateral and erosive. The diagnosis and treatment of OLDRs can be complicated by the fact that they often show up weeks to months after starting medication and take several months to resolve after stopping it. Premalignant lesions, which need to be carefully distinguished from OLP, include epithelial dysplasia and proliferative verrucous leukoplakia (PVL), which have been linked to lichenoid features both clinically and histologically, as well as through DIF testing.

It has long been a challenge to establish trustworthy clinical and histopathologic diagnostic criteria for OLP. Variable surface thickness, "band-like" infiltration of primarily lymphocytes in the superficial lamina propria, basal layer degeneration, lymphocytic exocytosis, and the strict absence of epithelial dysplasia or verrucous surface change—which is common in PVL—are among the recently proposed updated criteria for the histologic diagnosis of OLP. Though these are nonspecific features, OLDRs and LE frequently exhibit a deeper and mixed inflammatory infiltrate with lymphocytes accompanied by plasma cells and eosinophils as well as a perivascular pattern of inflammation. Although nonspecific, direct immunofluorescence testing (DIF) is best used to differentiate OLP from clinical mimics like vesiculobullous disease and chronic ulcerative stomatitis. DIF testing may reveal fibrinogen or complement deposition at the basal layer. The diagnosis of OLP cannot be made with indirect immunofluorescence testing (IIF). Treatment for OLP is based on the severity of the condition; for the majority of symptomatic cases, topical corticosteroids continue to be the first line of treatment. Topical retinoids, topical calcineurin inhibitors, and low-level laser therapy are additional options. Due to a contentious correlation—estimated to be between 1–3%—between OLP and potential malignant transformation, long-term monitoring is crucial.

3.2.1.9. Vesiculobullous Lesions

The oral cavity can be affected by a number of immune-modulated vesiculobullous (VB) diseases, such as paraneoplastic pemphigus (PNP), mucous membrane pemphigoid (MMP), epidermolysis bullosa acquisita (EBA), and pemphigus vulgaris (PV). Furthermore, a number of drugs, including NSAIDS, penicillamine, antipsychotics, spironolactones, and sulfonamides, have also been linked to VB-appearing oral lesions.

Patients with oral VB disease typically exhibit recurrent transient ulceration and bullous formation in the oral cavity as well as other mucosal areas like the conjunctiva, larynx, oropharynx, and nasopharynx. Depending on the diagnosis and severity of the illness, the skin is affected differently. Although mucosal lesions may appear initially, cutaneous lesions are common in PV. MMP may cause scarring and affect the ocular mucosa. In contrast to PV, where gender distribution is roughly equal, the majority of MMP patients are middle-aged women. The oral cavity may or may not be involved; gingival involvement is the most common oral site where MMP presents. Oral PV primarily affects the gingiva and buccal mucosa. Similar to EM, PNP typically manifests abruptly and can cause extensive oral ulcers and lip crusting (Figure 3.9.

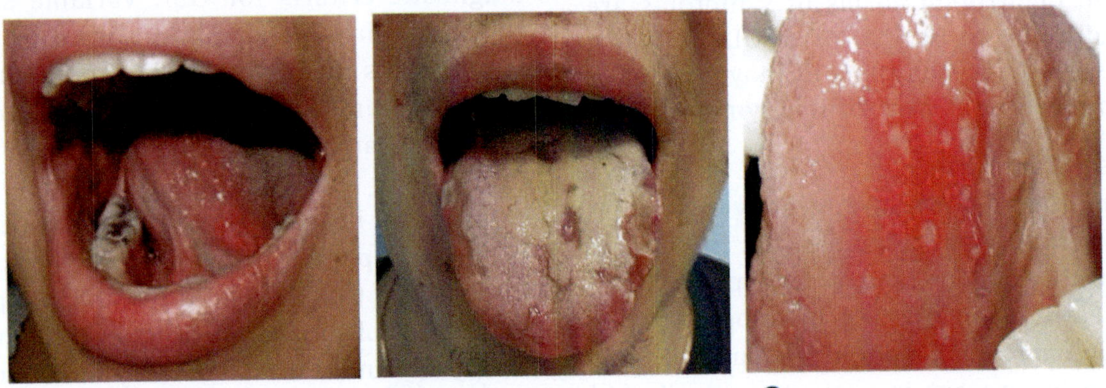

A B C

Figure 3.9. *Oral ulcers in patients with Behçet's disease.*

Note: (A) A centimetric aphthous lesion on the left ventral side of the tongue; (B) major deep aphthae on both sides of the tongue; and (C) aphthous lesions with a herpetiform distribution on the ventral side of the tongue. **Source:** *Gualtierotti R, Marzano AV, Spadari F, Cugno M., (2019). Main oral manifestations in immune-mediated and inflammatory rheumatic diseases. Journal of Clinical Medicine, 8(1), 21. https://doi.org/10.3390/jcm8010021.*

MMP biopsy results can indicate subepithelial separation related to suspected VB disease and EBA. In PV, intraepithelial separation has been observed (Both intraepithelial and subepithelial separation may be seen in PNP DIF is frequently required in order to differentiate between these entities and formulate a diagnosis. To differentiate PV, EBA, and PNP from MMP, IIF and ELISA testing may also be helpful. The diagnosis and degree of involvement are key factors in the treatment of oral VB diseases. Although systemic therapy is necessary for severe or widespread cases, topical corticosteroids are frequently effective in controlling MMP. Steroid sparing immunosuppressants or systemic corticosteroids are usually needed for PV treatment.

3.2.1.10. Ulcerations of Traumatic Etiology

Chemical, thermal, electrical, or mechanical trauma, whether acute or chronic, can cause oral ulcers. Proper classification of these lesions requires a thorough physical examination of the lesion in relation to dental restorations and appliances, as well as a thorough history of the lesion's onset and possible inciting events. Acute traumatized ulcers usually heal on their own without any complications in 14 days, but chronic ulcerations may not show a visible traumatizing source and may need to be biopsied to rule out neoplasia or other conditions.

3.2.1.11. Ulcerations Due to Chemical Trauma

Oral ulcerations have been linked to the use of illegal drugs, such as cocaine, amphetamines, and methylenedioxymethamphetamine (MDMA), as well as dental materials like formocresol, local anesthetics, sodium hypochlorite, hydrogen peroxide, and mouthwashes; finally, topical oral care products like hydrogen peroxide and denture cleaners have also been linked (Figure 3.10).

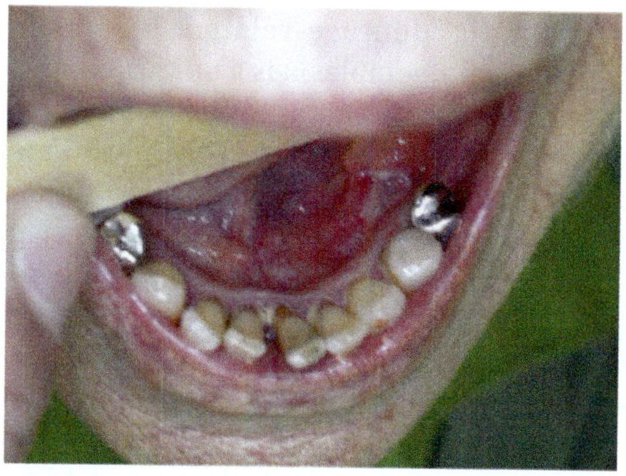

Figure 3.10. *Oral ulceration after using an antidepressant (sertraline hydrochloride).*

Source: Bertini, F., Costa, N.C.S., Brandão, A.A.H. et al. (2009). Ulceration of the oral mucosa induced by antidepressant medication: a case report. J Med Case Reports, 3, 98. https://doi.org/10.1186/1752-1947-3-98.

3.2.1.12. Ulcerations Due to Thermal or Electrical Trauma

Oral tissues can sustain thermal trauma from contact with hot materials most of the time, but it can also happen from extremely low temperatures (cryogenic burns), such as from contact with liquid nitrogen, dry ice, or frozen metal. The anterior third of the tongue and the palate are most frequently affected by thermal burns caused by intense heat, which are most frequently caused by hot food or beverages, especially those that have been microwaved. There have been more recent reports of oral burns brought on by electronic cigarettes that explode. Though they are uncommon, electric burns can be extremely painful and disabling, particularly in young people.

3.2.1.13. Ulcerations Due to Mechanical Trauma

Acute or chronic ulcerations can result from mechanical trauma. Roughly 20% of denture wearers with oral lesions in a recent study had traumatic denture-related ulcerations. Necrotizing sialometaplasia is a unique condition that can mimic cancer and arise from trauma resulting in deep ulcerations of the hard palate. Traumatic ulcerative granuloma with stromal eosinophilia (TUGSE) is a unique and concerning non-resolving chronic ulceration with elevated margins that is one type of chronic traumatic ulcer in the oral cavity. Although a similar lesion is seen in infants in tissues resembling natal teeth (Riga-Fede disease), TUGSE primarily affects middle-aged patients (Figure 3.11a–c). The tongue is the most frequently affected area by TUGSE, followed by the buccal mucosa, and infrequently the retromolar region, the floor of the mouth, or the lip.

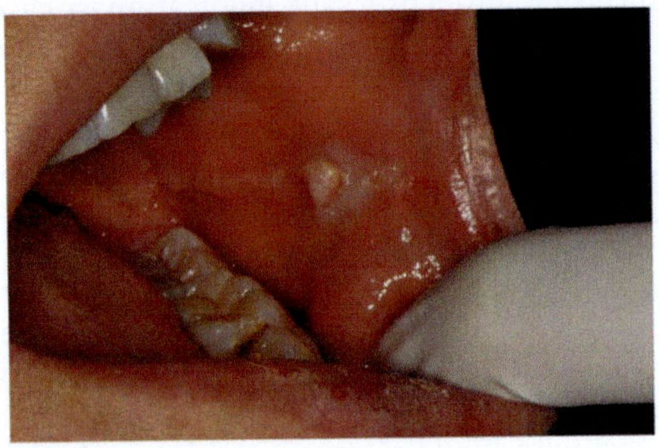

Figure 3.11. *Fibroma caused by mechanical irritation and parafunctional biting of buccal mucosa.*

Source: Radwan-Oczko M, Sokół I, Babuśka K, Owczarek-Drabińska JE. (2022). Prevalence and characteristic of oral mucosa lesions. Symmetry, 14(2), 307. https://doi.org/10.3390/sym14020307.

TUGSE is characterized by distinct deep-seated ulceration with a mixed inflammatory infiltrate consisting of lymphocytes, macrophages, numerous eosinophils, and proliferating blood vessels, even though the majority of traumatic lesions have nonspecific histologic findings. Even though TUGSE is a benign entity, large CD30+ cells may be present; however, in certain cases, resolution may require at least partial surgical excision. The goal of treating trauma-related ulcerations is to eliminate the trauma's etiologic source, though supportive care may also be required.

3.2.1.14. Ulcerations of Neoplastic Etiology

The accurate diagnosis of ulcerated malignant lesions imitating benign ulcerations is a major concern with regard to oral ulcers.

3.2.1.15. Ulcerated Oral Dysplasia and Squamous Cell Carcinoma

The conventional model of oral malignant change progression starts with normal-appearing epithelium, which develops into a thick white lesion, an erythematous component, and frequently a surface ulceration. It is acknowledged that there may not be a linear and progressive nature to this transition, and that OSCC may develop without any clinically evident precursors. While alcohol and tobacco use have long been recognized as risk factors for OSCC, the complete impact of high-risk human papillomavirus infection—which is strongly associated with oropharyngeal SCC—on OSCC remains to be determined. Although a lot of work has gone into creating adjunct devices or predictive tests to identify lesions that are highly likely to transform, their clinical utility is currently limited, and biopsy is still the gold standard. Therefore, biopsy is necessary to rule out dysplasia or invasive OSCC in non-healing ulcerated lesions, especially asymmetric or unilateral ones (Figure 3.12a, b). Malignant transformation is more likely to occur in dysplastic lesions on the floor of the mouth and the lateral and ventral surfaces of the tongue. The outcome of a biopsy can vary depending on the stage of the disease and can include carcinoma-in-situ, frankly invasive carcinoma, or mild to severe dysplasia. Several treatment protocols have been proposed for oral premalignant lesions; however, surgical removal of dysplasia at moderate or higher levels, with or without laser therapy, and long-term monitoring for recurrence or progression to malignancy remain the most widely accepted treatments.

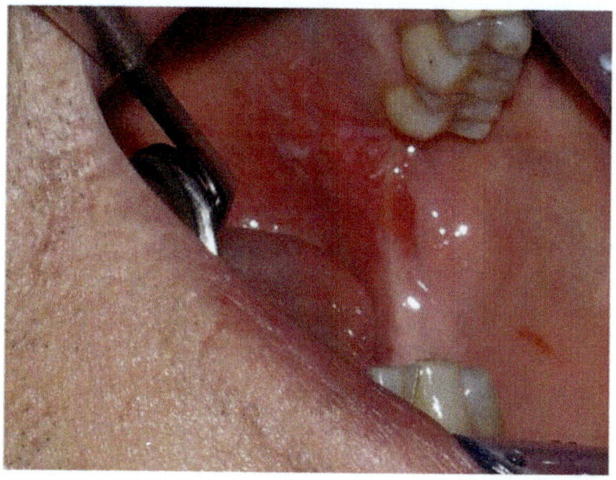

Figure 3.12. *Male, 61 years—erythroplasic area in the posterior hard palate, revealed severe dysplasia and in-situ carcinoma in the histopathologic examination.*

Source: Abati S, Bramati C, Bondi S, Lissoni A, Trimarchi M. (2020). Oral cancer and precancer: A narrative review on the relevance of early diagnosis. International Journal of Environmental Research and Public Health, 17(24), 9160. https://doi.org/10.3390/ijerph17249160.

3.2.1.16. Ulcerations Mediated by Underlying Hematologic Abnormalities

In the oral cavity, a broad range of hematologic abnormalities can appear, including tumors of B or T cell origin that are malignant or non-malignant. While diffuse submucosal swellings are the most common presentation of extranodal oral lymphomas, surface ulceration is a common symptom of certain hematologic disorders. In particular, leukemia frequently results in oral ulcers due to neutropenia and can also cause other oral symptoms like bleeding gingiva and/or inflamed, boggy gingiva.

Although they are uncommon in the mouth, cutaneous T-cell lymphomas (CTCL) frequently manifest as multiple ulcerations, and oral lesions may appear before skin lesions (Figures 3.12c, d). The most prevalent subtype of cutaneous T-cell lymphoma is mycosis fungoides (MF). Oral manifestations, which most frequently affect the tongue, palate, and gingiva, can include ulcers, erythematous plaques, or masses. Histologic features of MF include a diffuse infiltrate of atypical lymphocytes with an epidermotropic pattern and irregular cerebriform nuclei, which can cause a misdiagnosis by mimicking inflammatory conditions. Tests using immunohistochemistry (IHC) typically show positive results for CD3, CD4, and CD45. Because of the advanced stage, oral involvement in MF may be indicative of a poor prognosis. Seldom have reports of other CTCL subtypes in the oral cavity been made.

Extranodal NK/T-Cell Lymphoma (ENKTCL) is a unique and aggressive cancer that tends to involve the nasal cavity. It frequently results in ulcerative damage to the posterior third of the tongue, the uvula, the hard and soft palate, and the maxillary gingiva. The lesion is most common in Southeast Asia and populations in Central and South America, and it is strongly associated with EBV. Extensive necrosis that may mask malignancy features and a high inflammatory infiltrate combined with atypical lymphocytes that typically exhibit an angiocentric pattern are revealed by a biopsy of the lesions. It is typical to be positive for cytoplasmic CD3, CD56, and CD2. Radiation and/or chemotherapy are typically used to treat ENKTCL, but the results are not very good.

EBV is also linked to the EBV + mucocutaneous ulcer (EBVMCU), a newly identified lymphoproliferative disorder. Immunocompromised patients due to medication side effects or advanced age are most commonly affected by EBVMCU, a self-limiting indolent ulcerative lesion mediated by B-cells (Figure 3.12e, f). Additionally, EBVMCU has been reported in transplant recipients who fall under the post-transplant lymphoproliferative disorder (PTLD) spectrum. EBVMCU frequently manifests locally as lymphoid hyperplasia, but with ongoing immunosuppression, it may become more destructive or even develop into a lymphoid malignancy. Although it can also affect the skin or gastrointestinal tract, the oral cavity is the site of the ulceration most frequently. The palate, tonsillar region, tongue, and buccal mucosa are frequently affected by oral lesions. A necrotic ulcerated lesion with a mixed infiltrate of large atypical B-cells and small T-cells, along with Reed-Sternberg-like CD30+ cells, is revealed by the EBVMCU biopsy. IHC shows positive results for CD20 and CD30 along with positive results for EBV testing. Most lesions respond well to conservative treatment and a decrease in immunosuppression, and they frequently go away on their own.

A wide range of etiologic factors, such as infection, immunological dysregulation, trauma, and neoplasms, can result in oral cavity ulcerations. Even though a thorough clinical examination, medical history, and clinical assessment can often result in a strong presumptive clinical diagnosis, further testing, including a biopsy, may be required to confirm the diagnosis or rule out neoplastic sources.

3.2.2. Miscellaneous Lesions of Tongue and Oral Cavity

Both adults and children can get oral lesions, and the pharmacist may be the first person to see about treatment. Numerous oral lesions have varying prevalences depending on an individual's characteristics. Prevalence rates for a given lesion should therefore be stratified by risk factors and based on studies of general populations. These variables include age, racial or ethnic background, sex, use of removable dentures, and tobacco use. Pharmacists need to be aware of common oral lesions and the range of drugs used to treat them. From benign to malignant, there are many different diagnoses that can be made for oral lesions.

3.2.2.1. Lesions from Trauma or Irritation

White lesions are diagnosed based on whether they can be wiped off with gauze. A plaque-like white lesion in an irritated area could be an aspirin burn from sucking on a tablet or irritational keratosis from constant irritation from a dental appliance or biting. These lesions, although they don't rub off, are not cancerous. Treatment involves removing the source of irritation. If the lesion doesn't go away in a few months, a dental specialist should be consulted. Fibromas typically appear as smooth, pink nodules in areas of chronic irritation from biting or friction. They are harmless and usually require monitoring or surgical removal.

A mucocele occurs when secretions from a minor salivary gland duct in the inner part of the lip, usually the lower lip, leak into the surrounding tissues. In terms of clinical appearance, it manifests as a bluish swelling or as the mucosa's typical pink color. Throughout time, its size might grow or shrink. These lesions can be surgically removed and ought to be observed.

3.2.2.2. Candidiasis

A Candida species overgrowth—most commonly Candida albicans, which is a normal part of the flora—is the primary cause of oral candidiasis, which can present with a variety of clinical patterns. Age and certain risk factors—like HIV infection, smoking, dentures, chemotherapy, diabetes, corticosteroid therapy, xerostomia (dry mouth), and short- or long-term use of broad-spectrum antibiotics—affect the incidence differently. The most prevalent type of oral candidiasis is called acute pseudomembranous candidiasis, or thrush. It manifests as white, creamy, elevated plaques that are easily removed with gauze and leave an uncomfortable, raw, ulcerated surface behind. The palate, dorsal tongue, and buccal mucosa are the most frequently affected areas. Since there is no chairside test for oral candidiasis that can be performed in-office rather than in a lab, the diagnosis is typically made based on the patient's clinical presentation, either confirmed by a smear or culture of Candida.

Antifungals for the skin (e.g., clotrimazole or nystatin) are the recommended medications for individuals with normal immune function who have simple, localized thrush. In patients with compromised immune systems or in cases of widespread disease, systemic antifungals are typically recommended. Patients should keep taking the medication for at least two days after the lesions go away. Patients who use corticosteroid inhalers ought to be advised to rinse their mouths and brush their teeth after each use. It is advised to take acidophilus or yogurt along with broad-spectrum antibiotics to lower the risk of developing a candidiasis infection. Denture sore mouth, also known as chronic atrophic (erythematous) candidiasis, manifests as a velvet-textured plaque or red patch on the hard palate beneath a denture. The two most frequent causes are persistent denture wear and inadequate denture hygiene. It is important to advise the patient not to wear the denture while they sleep and to clean it every day. The inside of the denture can be treated with topical antifungal ointments or creams. Furthermore, troches of clotrimazole or pastilles of nystatin may be used.

Another form of candidiasis called angular cheilitis can present as mild erythema with superficial scaling fissures at the corners of the mouth, or it can present as intensely red and ulcerated lesions that hurt and burn. The multifactorial etiology involves infections with *Candida albicans* and *Staphylococcus aureus*, in addition to folic acid and vitamin B deficiencies. The recommended course of treatment is topical antifungal creams and ointments (Figure 3.13).

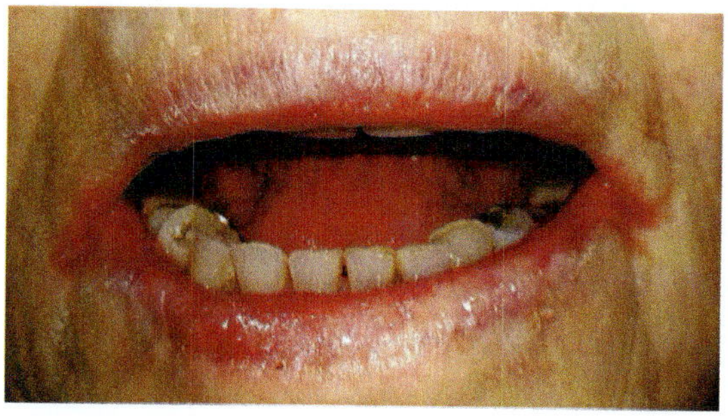

Figure 3.13. *Angular cheilitis.*

Source: By Matthew Ferguson 57 – Own work, CC BY-SA 3.0, https://commons.wikimedia.org/w/index.php?curid=45719116.

3.2.2.2.1. Leukoplakia and Erythroplakia

Benign or malignant neoplasms can arise in the oral cavity due to its diverse tissue composition. Leukoplakia is a white patch or plaque that defies clinical or pathological categorization as any other illness. With the exception of being a red patch, erythroplakia is defined similarly. A mixture of red and white lesions is called speckled leukoplakia. The use of tobacco products is the main risk factor for oral cancer. When heavy tobacco use is coupled with heavy alcohol consumption (four or more drinks per day), the synergistic risk factor increases. If a patient exhibits any red or white patches in their mouth, pharmacists should refer them right away to an otolaryngologist or oral surgeon.

3.2.2.3. Lichen Planus

A common dermatosis that affects the skin and oral mucosa is lichen planus. Skin lesions are present in about 50% of patients with oral lesions. The most common sites are the buccal mucosa and tongue. The reticular form of lichen planus is the most prevalent type and is characterized by fine, white lines that are slightly elevated and resemble lace, a feature known as Wickham's striae. Though its exact cause is unknown, lichen planus is known to be caused by an immunologically induced degeneration of the superficial epithelium. Lichen planus treatment options include topical corticosteroids (e.g., mouthwashes containing corticosteroids and/or fluocinonide are typically started if lesions exhibit symptoms.

3.2.2.4. Ulcerations

The most frequent recurrent oral lesion is recurrent minor aphthous stomatitis, also known as canker sores, and it is more common in women. Minor aphthous ulcers have an essentially unknown etiology, although streptococcal antigen hypersensitivity, stress, and hormonal changes have all been suggested. Although there may be a genetic predisposition, aphthous stomatitis is not a viral infection and is not contagious. Patients should also be assessed for folic acid or vitamin B12 deficiencies. Clinically, aphthous ulcers initially manifest as a papule on movable mucosa only, not as a vesicle (e.g., soft palate, lateral border of the tongue, and inner lower lip). Usually round in shape, the ulcerations have a red border and a depression in the middle. If more than one, they don't combine. They could hurt, particularly when eating and talking. Lesions typically heal in 7 to 10 days, but they frequently recur. Fever or lymphadenopathy linked to these lesions are uncommon.

The natural course of aphthous ulcers usually involves an eventual remission. When a patient experiences severe discomfort, palliative and supportive care are typically provided. The major objectives of therapy are pain relief and shortening the duration of ulcers. Topical corticosteroids, analgesics, and antibiotics are among the medications. On the skin, corticosteroids (e.g., The cornerstones of treatment, such as Kenalog in Orabase and Orabase HCA, only lessen pain; they don't increase the likelihood of recurrence. Pain relief is achieved by topical analgesics such as viscous lidocaine 2% and Orabase B (benzocaine). Applying Amlexanox (Aphthasol) 5% paste, which inhibits mast cell and neutrophil production of inflammatory mediators, up to four times a day may speed up healing and lessen pain, but it doesn't lessen the frequency of recurrent ulcer episodes.

Tetracycline use is supported by a small number of randomized, controlled trials. The patient was instructed to rinse four times a day for approximately five days after dissolving one 250 mg capsule in 180 mL of water. Rinsing four times a day for five days with 5 mL of tetracycline syrup (250 mg/5 mL) is an additional option. An antibacterial mouthwash such as chlorhexidine gluconate may lessen the intensity and discomfort of recurrences, but not their frequency. Furthermore, patients with HIV are treated for recurrent aphthous ulcers with immune modulators like thalidomide. Often, these ulcers take a long time to heal. Zinc lozenges (four to six lozenges per day), vitamin C (500 mg per day), and vitamin B complex (one tablet per day) are examples of alternative therapies that lack scientific backing.

3.2.2.5. Vesicular Lesions

3.2.2.5.1. Oral Herpes Simplex Virus Infection

The DNA virus known as herpes simplex virus (HSV) is typically categorized based on anatomical site. HSV-1 infections, also known as fever blisters, cold sores, or herpes labialis, are blisters that form above the chest and are usually connected to oral lesions. HSV-2 infections, also known as herpes genitalia, are typically associated with genital lesions and are found below the torso. But in roughly 30% of cases, oral-genital or genital-genital contact with an HSV-1-infected person can result in genital herpes.

3.2.2.5.2. Primary Herpetic Gingivostomatitis

The first HSV-1 outbreak typically affects children and is brought on by touching an infected person or sharing a cup with someone who has visible lesions. Primary HSV-1 is most commonly diagnosed in children between the ages of two and three, though it can also strike adults. The patient typically exhibits symptoms such as nausea, vomiting, malaise, headache, lymphadenopathy, and fever. Subsequently, tiny vesicles start to form in the mouth. When these rupture, tiny, painful ulcers are left behind, covered in membranes that are yellow-gray. Furthermore, there is acute gingivitis that is widespread.

Treatment for primary acute herpetic gingivostomatitis in adults and children in good health is still palliative and involves acetaminophen and fluids. Acyclovir treatment administered early on may reduce the length of time affected children remain contagious and exhibit all clinical symptoms. The only purpose of antibiotics is to stop secondary infections.

3.2.2.5.3. Recurrent Intraoral Herpes/ Herpes Labialis

This virus does not reactivate in the trigeminal ganglion following its initial exposure. It is believed that stress, sunlight, fever, HIV infection, specific foods, menstruation, trauma (e.g., after a dental procedure), or other allergens. Recurrent infections are not as serious as the initial infection. While not everyone experiences recurrent infections, some people may experience several recurrences annually. 12 to 36 hours before vesicle eruption, mild tingling, burning, or itching may be experienced as prodromal symptoms. The vesicles grow into ulcers that take 24 to 48 hours to crust over and heal. The course of spontaneous healing takes 7 to 10 days. Most ulcers occur on immobile mucosa (e.g., lateral border of the tongue and gingival, perioral, and vermillion border of the lips). These lesions are called fever blisters, cold sores, or herpes labialis (Figure 3.14).

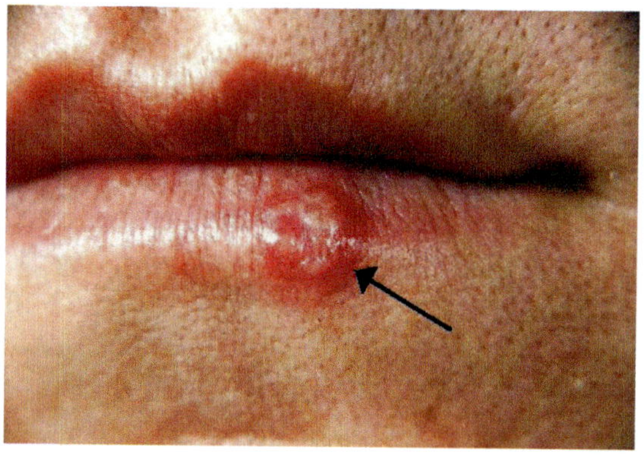

Figure 3.14. *Oral herpes of the lower lip. Note the blisters in a group marked by an arrow.*

Source: Public Domain, https://commons.wikimedia.org/w/index.php?curid=8011415.

Reducing the length of the active infection and managing symptoms are the two main goals of treatment. Most lesions are modest and self-limiting. Analgesics and topical antivirals can both speed up the healing process and reduce pain. Acyclovir 5% is a recognized standard topical treatment. Acyclovir, valacyclovir, and famciclovir are examples of systemic antiviral medications that can shorten the duration of symptoms, but they are only effective for prodromal symptoms. While these treatments do not cure infections, they may decrease their severity, duration, and recurrence rate. It is not recommended to use antibiotics as this is a viral infection. Herpes cannot be effectively treated with corticosteroids. Topical cream containing 10% docosanol (Abreva) prevents the virus from fusing with the human cell membrane, preventing entry and subsequent viral replication. It is intended to hasten the healing process of recurrent oral/facial herpes, and in approximately 34% of cases, applying it at the first sign of an outbreak (redness) prevented the condition from progressing to the blister stage. Until the infection heals, this over-the-counter drug should be used five times a day.

3.2.2.5.4. Xerostomia

Xerostomia can be due to medications (e.g., antipsychotics, anticholinergics, antihistamines, diuretics), illness (e.g., HIV or cancer), or aging. Innervation of the salivary glands is cholinergic and sympathetic. Either autonomic system can be activated to increase secretions, but the cholinergic system is the more significant. Anticholinergic medications cause dry mouth by attaching to cholinergic (muscarinic) receptors and preventing the salivary glands from secreting saliva.

The goal of treatment is to make the mouth more moisturizing or secretory. Artificial saliva, also known as saliva substitutes, contains the ions, lubricating mucins, and buffering qualities that are required. Oasis, Biotène, Optimoist, Xero-Lube, and Salivart are a few OTC products. Cholinergic medications, such as Salagen (pilocarpine) and Evoxac (cevimeline), may be prescribed by dentists or doctors.

3.2.2.5.5. Pharmacist's Advice to Patients

Any oral lesion that lasts longer than two weeks should be referred to an otolaryngologist or dentist. Oral lesions can be benign or malignant. In addition to going over the patient's medical history, the pharmacist should talk about the oral lesion's clinical appearance, including its color, location, appearance (flat or raised), and duration. Given that an innocuous lesion may have systemic causes, the pharmacist should carefully evaluate the patient's condition. Many over-the-counter (OTC) products can be recommended by the pharmacist to relieve pain in benign lesions like aphthous ulcers or herpes labialis.

3.2.3. Submucous Fibrosis

Juxtaepithelial deposition of fibrous tissue in the oral cavity and pharynx is a characteristic of the chronic, insidious process known as oral submucous fibrosis (OSMF). Joshi initially reported the ailment in India in 1953. Because of the habit of chewing betel nut, the disease is common in India, Pakistan, Taiwan, Sri Lanka, Nepal, and Thailand.

3.2.3.1. Symptoms

During the early stages of the illness, the mucosa has palpable fibrotic bands and feels leathery. In the advanced stage, the oral mucosa becomes blanched and stiff, losing its resiliency. Although mouth opening is thought to gradually decrease as a result of this blanched and stiff mucosa, this seems to be an oversimplification of the pathology. Many researchers overlook the fact that the degree of mouth opening is also influenced by the severity of oral symptoms, such as stomatitis and glossitis that is persistent or recurrent. The term "Reflectory Trismus" describes this phenomenon, in which the degree of mouth opening is determined by the activation of the 5th and 9th cranial nerves, as described above. Nonetheless, fibrosis and muscle injury are more significant contributors. It is thought that the illness started in the back of the mouth and moved outward over time. The idea that oral submucous fibrosis progresses posteriorly has recently been refuted in light of multiple reports suggesting that the disease may only affect the anterior portion of the oral cavity and not the posterior; the locations are determined by how the anterior and posterior parts of the oral cavity are used for spitting and swallowing, respectively.

Other features of the disease include:

- Xerostomia
- Recurrent ulceration
- Pain in the ear or deafness
- Nasal intonation of voice
- Restriction of the movement of the soft palate
- A budlike shrunken uvula
- Thinning and stiffening of the lips
- Pigmentation of the oral mucosa
- Dryness of the mouth and burning sensation (stomatopyrosis)
- Decreased tongue protrusion

3.2.3.2. Management

It is commonly known that OSMF is resistant and chronic. The main goal of treatment for OSMF is to stop the disease's progression into malignancy because it is a premalignant condition with the potential to become malignant. The patient should then receive symptomatic relief in order to enhance his nutritional status. This illness can be treated with a variety of methods, such as medication regimens, surgical procedures, and physical therapy. Teaching the patient about the harmful effects of areca nut and related chewing products is the first step in providing appropriate treatment and will help the patient break the habit. Then, there are three types of management approaches: surgical, medical, and conservative. Pharmacological and surgical treatment should be recommended in addition to physical therapy (Figure 3.15).

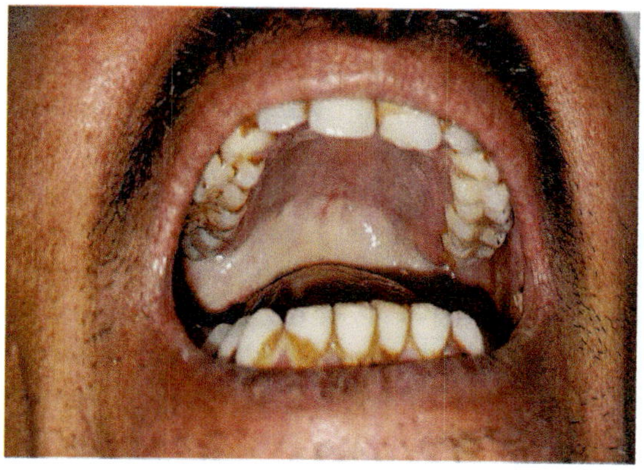

Figure 3.15. *Blanching and stiffness of soft palate and oropharynx.*

Source: *Chhabra A K, Sune R, Reche A (2023). Oral submucous fibrosis: A review of the current concepts in management. Cureus 15(10), e47259. doi:10.7759/cureus.47259.*

3.2.3.3. Conservative Treatment

Conservative treatment includes things like habit restriction, nutritional or supportive therapy, and oral physiotherapy.

3.2.3.3.1. Restriction of Habits

India is a country that consumes spices like chillies, areca nuts, gutkha, and paan masala. Encouragement of the patient to quit the habit at an early stage of OSMF is an important part of treatment, as it may help the illness progress more slowly.

3.2.3.3.2. Nutritional or Supportive Therapy

Free radical levels can be considerably reduced by micronutrients and minerals such as iron, copper, calcium, zinc, magnesium, and selenium, as well as vitamins A, B, C, D, and E. A lower intake of fruits and vegetables is linked to an increased risk of cancer and pre-malignancies. Fruits and vegetables should be included in a regular diet because they increase antioxidant levels and offer protection against the higher risk of cancer. Lycopene, a pigment present in tomatoes, has been shown to have a number of potent antioxidant and anti-carcinogenic qualities. Additionally, it has demonstrated noteworthy advantages in precancerous lesions such as leukoplakia. Green tea polyphenols have strong anti-free radical properties and can protect cells from DNA damage caused by reactive oxygen species. Moreover, it has the ability to start apoptosis and stop the growth of cancerous cells. As a result, the potent antioxidant activity of tea polyphenols has been linked to numerous potential benefits of tea. Numerous studies have established a causal and consequential connection between iron deficiency and the aetiopathogenesis of OSMF. As a result, regular measurements of hemoglobin levels and iron supplementation should be part of the treatment plan. Immune milk has strong anti-inflammatory properties and is a good source of vitamins A, B1, B2, B6, B12, C, pantothenic acid, nicotinic acid, folic acid, iron, copper, and zinc. Through modifying the cytokine assemblage and decreasing the inflammatory response, IgG antibody treatment has the potential to significantly reduce symptoms in patients with OSMF.

3.2.3.3.3. Oral Physiotherapy

Physiotherapy tools such as splints and exercise regimens can be employed to treat OSMF. Mouth-specific stretching exercises may help prevent future restrictions on mouth motions by applying pressure to the fibrous bands. It has been attempted to open the mouth violently while using acrylic surgical screws and mouth gags.

3.2.3.4. Medical Treatment

To enable improved mobility is the aim of symptomatic medical treatment. The following treatments are available as submucosal injections, oral medications, or topical applications.

3.2.3.4.1. Lycopene

Lycopene, an organic pigment found in plants, is a carotenoid known for its anti-carcinogenic and antioxidant properties. It has been proven to have significant benefits in treating precancerous lesions such as leukoplakia. In the case of Oral Submucous Fibrosis (OSMF), lycopene has been shown to effectively inhibit fibroblasts and control inflammation and lymphocyte stress response. It is often used as a first-line treatment for OSMF due to its high physical quenching rate constant for singlet oxygen.

3.2.3.4.2. Beta-Carotene

The precursor to vitamin A is beta-carotene. It has anti-oxidant and radical-scavenger properties. Beta-carotene lowers the damage caused by free radicals. The growth of cancer cells is slowed by the increased immune response. Beta-carotene stimulates T-cells and increases the mitogenic response. When beta-carotene is given, the concentration of the blood rises, boosting the patient's immune system and slowing the spread of cancer cells.

3.2.3.4.3. Alpha-Lipoic Acid (LA)

An example of a typical antioxidant is alpha LA. Free radicals from lipid and water-based media can be removed by it. Alpha LA diminishes solitary oxygen molecules and eliminates hypochlorous acid and hydroxyl radicals. The status of cellular antioxidants is indirectly maintained by alpha LA through stimulating the production of endogenous low molecular weight antioxidants or enzymes and encouraging their absorption. Alpha LA stimulates the production of glutathione (GSH), an endogenous antioxidant found in cells. Alpha LA is obtained through diet, where it is absorbed and stored in tissues.

3.2.3.4.4. Alpha-Tocopherol

Humans only contain alpha-tocopherol, which has antioxidant qualities, while plants contain eight different forms of vitamin E (delta-tocopherol/tocotrienols). Because of specific interactions with structural proteins, lipids, transcription factors, and enzymes, it inhibits platelet aggregation, monocyte adhesion, and cell growth.

3.2.3.4.5. Selenium

In order to avoid nutritional issues and degenerative diseases, selenium is essential. It is present in GSH peroxidase-active sites and has anticarcinogenic properties. This nutrient, which possesses antioxidant qualities, inhibits the development of aberrant cells by methylating selenium metabolites and selenoproteins.

3.2.3.4.6. Zinc

Zinc is essential for several cellular functions and enhanced immunity. By enhancing the activity of neutrophils and natural killer cells, which mediate innate immunity, zinc increases the efficacy of the immune system. The production of macrophages, cytokines, and intercellular killing caused by phagocytosis are all enhanced by zinc. Zinc is necessary for cell division, activation, and RNA transcription. It also enhances the functions and secretions of cytokines. It is an antioxidant and stabilizer of membranes.

3.2.3.4.7. Steroid, Placentrex and Fibrinolytic Drug Injections as Part of Medicinal Treatment

- **Steroids:** It is well known that steroids function as immunosuppressive medications, lowering the effects of this fibro-collagenous illness and preventing the inflammation seen in OSMF lesions. Steroids can also decrease collagen fiber count by preventing fibroblast proliferation. Topical steroids or weekly submucosal intralesional injections may help stop future damage in patients with moderate OSMF. Topically applied steroid ointments for ulcers and sore oral mucosa may be beneficial; local administration of 1 cc hydrocortisone has been shown to be efficacious.
- **Hyaluronidase:** In vitro studies suggest that hyaluronidase degrades collagen more quickly in OSMF patients than it does normal collagen. Hyaluronidase degrades the hyaluronic acid matrix, thins the intracellular cement, and initiates particular plasmatic processes. As a result, fibrous tissue becomes softer and smaller.
- **Collagenase:** The decreased amount of functional collagenase observed in OSMF patients is one of the elements causing the accumulation of collagen. Lin and Lin's finding—that intralesional collagenase injections significantly enhance mouth opening and lessen sensitivity to heat, cold, and spices—helps restore the ability to eat.
- **Placental extracts:** Vitamins, hormones, nucleotides, enzymes, and amino acids are all present in Placentrex, an aqueous extract of human placenta. It functions through a mechanism called biogenic stimulation. 1933 saw the introduction of tissue therapy.

Once the pathogenic elements have caused conflict in the body, these tissues or their extracts may be injected or implanted. This helps with healing by encouraging metabolic or regeneration processes.

- **Chymotrypsin:** Chymotrypsin is an endopeptidase that is capable of performing proteolysis.
- **Interferon (IFN)-gamma:** IFN-gamma plays a key role in the treatment of OSMF due to its immunoregulatory properties. It has been demonstrated that IFN-gamma has anti-fibrotic effects.
- **Aloe vera:** Aloe vera has antibacterial, anti-inflammatory, and medicinal properties in its resin, extract, and leaves. In all clinical-histopathological stages, aloe vera responds more favorably to every parameter assessed. This is especially true for patients with mild clinical stages and early histopathological stages of the disease. Aloe vera was used, and both the burning sensation and the mouth's and cheeks' flexibility improved. The aloe vera group helps patients feel better by healing their mouth opening and lessening the burning sensation.
- **Turmeric:** The yellow pigment curcumin, which is found in turmeric naturally, has anti-inflammatory, anti-cancer, and antioxidant qualities. Tight mucosa and limited mouth opening are two hallmarks of oral submucous fibrosis (OSMF), a potentially fatal condition. The oral mucosa and deeper tissues stiffen as a result of fibrosis, gradually reducing mouth opening and causing tongue protrusion. This makes it challenging to chew, swallow, and phonate.
- **Pentoxifylline therapy:** Depending on the dosage, the methylxanthine derivative pentoxifylline can have the following effects: (1) enhances microcirculation and reduces platelet aggregation and granulocyte adhesion; (2) increases leukocyte deformability and inhibits neutrophil adhesion and activation; additionally, it exhibits fibrinolytic, anti-thrombin, and anti-plasmin action; (3) can block T-cell and B-cell activation, boost the activity of natural killer cells, and cause neutrophils to degranulate; (4) can maintain cellular integrity and homeostasis after an acute injury; (5) improves vascularity and reduces OSMF patients' symptoms.

3.2.3.4.8. Surgery

In patients who have limited mouth opening, a biopsy is the preferred method if it reveals dysplastic or neoplastic alterations. It comprises:

- **Fibrotomy:** This surgical procedure involves the removal of fibrous bands and a forced mouth opening, leaving the wound surface raw. Relapse is a common side effect following surgical relief of the OSMF-caused oral trismus.
- **Fibrotomy with Grafts:** Surgeons originally intended to surgically remove the fibrotic bands, but in order to prevent additional scarring and trismus recurrence, they began using a variety of interposition

graft materials. The fundamental concept is that fibrous bands are cut (sometimes mislabeled "excised") or surgically released, the mouth is then forced open (by expanding the area or tissue that was incised), and any surgical deficiencies are covered with synthetic biological material or a variety of flaps.

- **Extra-Oral Flaps:** These include the platysma myocutaneous muscle flap, the superficial temporal fascia pedicled flap, the split-thickness skin graft, and the nasolabial flap.
- Intraoral flaps: These involve simple removal of fibrotic bands along with coronoidectomy, temporalis myotomy, split-thickness grafts, and other procedures used to treat patients with severe trismus. During the process, general anesthesia is administered. The mouth's small aperture makes intubation difficult. Using deep inhalational anesthesia or muscle relaxants with a regional block are the best techniques for tracheal intubation. Fiber optic guided intubation techniques have also been used.
- **Laser Therapy:** Oral surgeons now have a cutting-edge way to treat OSMF thanks to lasers. The yttrium scandium gallium garnet (Er Cr: YSGG) laser, which has a wavelength of 2780 nm and a high absorption by water, is used to treat soft tissue in the mouth without inflicting heat damage. Overall, the benefits of laser surgery include more visibility due to a mostly blood-free operating area, less need for local anesthetic, reduced risk of bacterial infection, less mechanical tissue stress, fewer sutures, faster healing, and a lower incidence of swelling, scarring, and tissue shrinkage following surgery. When discussing a follow-up attempt to treat a mild case of bilateral OSMF with Er Cr, the YSGG laser produced better results.
- **Microwave Diathermy:** The process of band fibrinolysis is how heat treatment operates. Microwave diathermy, which only heats juxta-epithelial connective tissue, limits the area that can be treated. As a result, applying it is easy and doesn't irritate the skin too much.

3.3. Tumors of the Oral Cavity

Any type of cancer that arises in any part of the mouth (oral cavity) is referred to as mouth cancer. One can develop mouth cancer on the:

- Lips
- Gums
- Tongue
- Inner lining of the cheeks
- Roof of the mouth
- Floor of the mouth (under the tongue)

Oral cancer, also known as oral cavity cancer, is the term used to describe cancer that develops inside the mouth. One of the several cancer types included in the head and neck cancers category is mouth cancer. Treatment for cancers of the mouth, neck, and other regions is frequently similar.

3.3.1. Signs and Symptoms

Depending on where the tumor is located, oral cancer may present with thin, uneven, white patches in the mouth as symptoms. They may also have a combination of red and white patches; when biopsied, mixed red and white patches have a significantly higher chance of being malignant. A raised, barely painful border and a persistent rough patch with ulceration are the classic warning signs. The ulcer is usually crusting and dry on the lip and more often a mass in the pharynx. A white patch, loose teeth, bleeding gums, a chronic earache, numbness in the lip and chin, or swelling can also be linked to it (Figure 3.16).

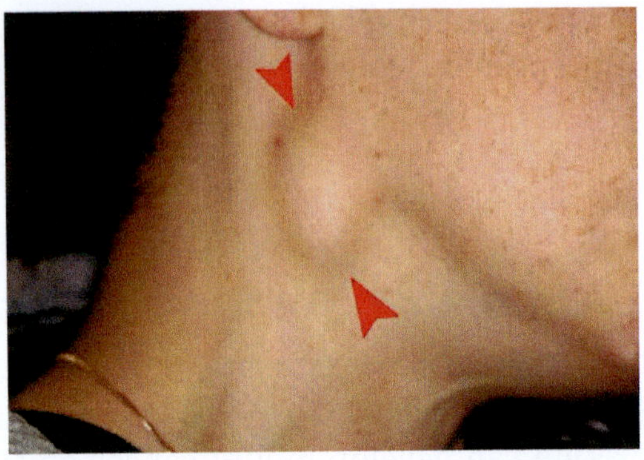

Figure 3.16. *Swelling of the right neck from the spread of oral cancer.*

Source: By Coronation Dental Specialty Group – Own work, CC BY-SA 4.0, https://commons.wikimedia.org/w/index.php?curid=77245466.

When a cancer spreads to the throat, symptoms may include pain when swallowing, a change in voice, and difficulty swallowing (typically caused by HPV16+ cancer at the base of the tongue) or a unilaterally noticeable enlarged tonsil. Until the lesions enlarge and are accompanied by a burning sensation, they usually cause very little pain. An insensitive hard lump will form as the lesion extends to the neck lymph nodes. General aches may arise if it spreads to other parts of the body; this is typically the result of bone metastasis.

3.3.2. Causes

Tobacco is the primary environmental factor that causes oral squamous cell carcinoma. The carcinogen's dosage, frequency, and mode of application all affect how quickly cancer develops, just like any other environmental factor (the substance that is causing the cancer). In addition to smoking cigarettes, other factors that can cause oral cancer include alcohol, radiation, viruses (especially HPV 16 and 18), and ultraviolet light.

3.3.2.1. Tobacco

The leading cause of oral and pharyngeal cancer is tobacco use. It is a recognized multi-organ carcinogen that, when combined with alcohol, works synergistically to cause cancers of the mouth and throat by causing direct damage to cellular DNA. It is estimated that smoking increases the risk of oral cancer by 3.4–6.8 points and accounts for about 40% of all cases of oral cancer.

3.3.2.2. Alcohol

According to epidemiological data, alcohol use is highly linked to oral cancer, which will account for 20.2% of cases worldwide in 2020. For light drinking, the relative risk is 1.13; for moderate drinking, it is 1.83; and for heavy drinking, it is 5.13. When alcohol and tobacco are combined, their combined effect is larger than multiplicative. Although the exact cause of the increased risk of cancer associated with alcohol use is still unknown, acetaldehyde is a significant contributor. Saliva contains higher amounts of acetaldehyde right after drinking, with a peak appearing in around two minutes. The oral microbiome, saliva glands, the liver, and the oral mucosa all produce acetaldehyde. Alcoholic drinks naturally contain it as well. At least half of the acetaldehyde present is attributed to the microbiome, making it the main contributor of these. Nicotine consumption, smoking, and excessive alcohol consumption raise the amount of acetaldehyde-producing bacteria in the mouth. The epidemiological significance of the numerous bacterial species that contribute to the production of acetaldehyde is unknown. When acetaldehyde interacts with oral epithelial cells, DNA alterations are produced that may result in mutations and the emergence of cancer. Because acetaldehyde cannot be completely metabolized in the mouth, it can linger in saliva for several hours. To reduce oral acetaldehyde exposure, L-cysteine tablets can be utilized.

Whether using mouthwashes with alcohol raises the risk of oral cancer has been a contentious issue. Though as of 2023 the evidence is still pending, it is suggestive. Like alcohol-based beverages, mouthwashes with alcohol do raise salivary acetaldehyde levels after usage. However, because mouthwashes are made to eradicate bacteria, they destroy the microorganisms that convert ethanol to acetaldehyde, which may lessen exposure to acetaldehyde overall and offer protection. Using alcohol-based mouthwash more than once a day was linked to a 4% increased risk of oral cancer in a 2021 meta-analysis, although the difference was not statistically significant. According to the same analysis, using mouthwash with alcohol once a day or less had a negligible and non-statistically significant impact on the risk of oral cancer.

3.3.2.3. Human Papillomavirus

Oral cancer is known to be independently caused by human papillomavirus (HPV) infection, specifically type 16 infection (of which there are over 180 types). Diagnoses that do not fit the historical stereotypes of the population are becoming more and more common. Those over 50, Blacks over Whites 2 to 1, Males over Females 3 to 1, and 75% of those who have used tobacco products or heavily drink alcohol have historically been the majority. Men slightly outnumber women in this newly formed and quickly expanding subpopulation of white individuals between the ages of 30 and 50 who mostly do not smoke.

3.3.2.4. Betel Nut

Chewing betel, paan, and areca leaves the mouth susceptible to oral cancer, even in the non-tobacco environment. Because of a number of genetic and associated factors, including local irritation of the mucous membrane cells from areca nut and slaked lime, it increases the risk of oral cancer by a factor of two and a half. Compared to just 4% in the UK, oral cancer accounts for up to 40% of all cancer cases in India, where these practices are widespread.

3.3.2.5. Stem Cell Transplantation

Following hematopoietic stem cell transplantation (HSCT), oral squamous cell carcinoma is more common. When compared to oral cancer in individuals who were not treated with HSCT, post-HSCT oral cancer may exhibit more aggressive behavior and a worse prognosis. This effect is thought to be caused by both chronic oral graft-versus-host disease and immune suppression that lasts a lifetime.

3.3.2.6. Premalignant Lesions

A benign, morphologically altered tissue with a higher than normal risk of malignant transformation is called a premalignant (or precancerous) lesion. Premalignant lesions can take many different forms, and they can happen in the mouth (Figure 3.17).

Leukoplakia (white patches), erythroplakia (red patches), or erythroleukoplakia (mixed red and white patches) are the initial stages of some oral cancers. Oral submucous fibrosis and actinic cheilitis are two other prevalent premalignant lesions. Chewing betel nut leads to a common condition in the Indian subcontinent called oral submucous fibrosis. This illness is typified by restricted mouth opening and a burning feeling when consuming spicy foods. This lesion progresses gradually, limiting the mouth's opening until eventually it becomes difficult to eat normally.

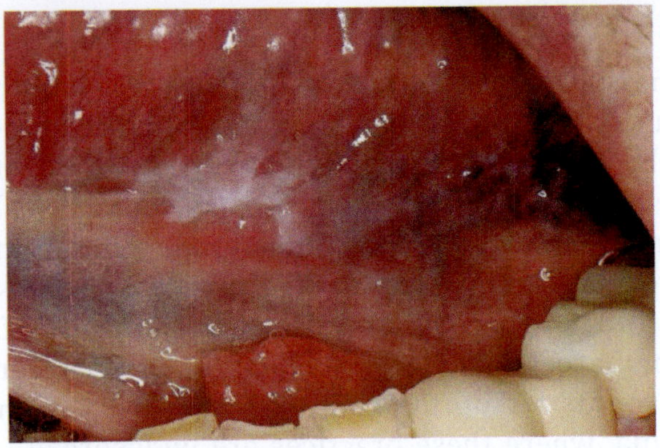

Figure 3.17. *Oral leukoplakia (white patch) on the left tongue. Proven to be severe dysplasia on biopsy.*

Source: By Coronation Dental Specialty Group – Own work, CC BY-SA 4.0, https://commons.wikimedia.org/w/index.php?curid=77923668.

3.3.3. Pathophysiology

Unchecked growth of mucous basal cells leads to the development of oral squamous cell carcinoma. An accumulation of mutated genes known as oncogenes causes a single precursor cell to divide into numerous daughter cells that make up the clone. An ability to metastasize is what distinguishes a malignant tumor from a benign one. This capacity is unaffected by the tumor's size or grade (adenoid cystic carcinoma, for example, can spread widely even though it often appears to grow slowly). A cancer is not only characterized by its fast growth; it can also spread due to its secretion of enzymes, angiogeneic factors, invasion factors, growth factors, and many other substances.

3.3.4. Diagnosis

Tests and procedures used to diagnose mouth cancer include:

- **Physical Exam:** Your lips and mouth will be examined by your physician or dentist to check for abnormalities, such as sores or white patches (leukoplakia), which are areas of irritation.
- **Removal of Tissue for Testing (Biopsy):** Your dentist or doctor may perform a biopsy, or sample of cells if they find a suspicious area for laboratory testing. A sample of tissue may be removed by the physician using a needle or a cutting instrument. The cells are examined in a lab to check for precancerous alterations that suggest a chance of developing cancer in the future or for cancer.

3.3.4.1. Determining the Extent of the Cancer

Following a diagnosis of mouth cancer, your doctor will try to ascertain the cancer's stage and extent. Tests for mouth cancer staging could involve:

- **Using a Small Camera to Inspect Your Throat:** Your doctor may insert a tiny, flexible camera with a light down your throat during an endoscopy procedure to check for evidence that cancer has spread outside of your mouth.
- **Imaging Tests:** Several imaging tests could be used to assess if cancer has progressed outside of your mouth. Imaging tests can involve, among other things, positron emission tomography (PET) scans, CT, MRIs, and X-rays. Not all people require every test. Which tests are appropriate will be decided by your doctor based on your condition.

Stages of mouth cancer are denoted by Roman numerals I through IV. A smaller cancer that is localized to one area is indicated by a lower stage, such as stage I. A higher stage, like stage IV, denotes a more advanced cancer or one that has spread to other parts of the body or to other parts of the head and neck. Your doctor can better assess your treatment options based on the stage of your cancer.

3.3.5. Treatment

The location and stage of your cancer, along with your general health and personal preferences, will all influence your treatment options for mouth cancer. It is possible for you to receive only one kind of treatment or to have several cancer treatments. Radiation, chemotherapy, and surgery are available treatment options. Talk to your doctor about your options.

3.3.5.1. Surgery

Surgery for mouth cancer may include:

- **Surgery to Remove the Tumor:** To be certain that all of the cancer cells have been eliminated, your surgeon may remove the tumor along with a margin of surrounding healthy tissue. Smaller cancers might be surgically removed. Larger tumors might necessitate more involved operations. For example, removing a larger tumor might require removing a portion of your tongue or jawbone.
- **Cancer that Has Spread to the Neck is Removed Surgically:** Your surgeon may suggest a neck dissection procedure to remove the lymph nodes and surrounding tissue if cancer cells have progressed to the lymph nodes in your neck, or if there is a strong likelihood that this has occurred given the size or depth of your cancer. Dissection of the neck eliminates any cancer cells that might have migrated to your lymph nodes. It can also help you determine if you will require further care following surgery.
- **Oral Reconstruction Surgery:** Following the removal of your cancer, your surgeon might suggest reconstructive surgery to rebuild your mouth and restore your ability to speak and eat. Your surgeon may reconstruct your mouth using skin, muscle, or bone grafts from other areas of your body. You can also use dental implants to replace your natural teeth.

There is a chance of bleeding and infection after surgery. Surgery for mouth cancer frequently impairs speech, eating, and swallowing abilities in addition to your outward look. To help you swallow, drink, and take medication, you might require a tube. The tube can be put into your stomach through your nose for short-term use. In the long run, you might have a tube put into your stomach through your skin. Your physician might suggest that you see experts who can assist you in adjusting to these changes.

3.3.5.2. Radiation Therapy

High-energy beams, like protons and X-rays, are used in radiation therapy to destroy cancer cells. Radiation therapy can be administered by radioactive seeds and wires positioned close to your cancer (brachytherapy), but it is typically administered by a machine outside of your body (external beam radiation). Following surgery, radiation therapy is frequently used. But in certain cases, if your mouth cancer is still in the early stages, it may be used alone. In other circumstances, chemotherapy and radiation therapy may be combined. Radiation therapy is more effective when this combination is used, but there is a higher chance of side effects. Radiation therapy may be used to treat advanced mouth cancer to relieve pain and other cancer-related symptoms.

Radiation therapy side effects to the mouth can include tooth decay, dry mouth, and jawbone damage. To ensure that your teeth are in the best possible condition before starting radiation therapy, your doctor will advise you to see a dentist. Any unhealthy teeth could require extraction or therapy. In order to lower your risk of complications, a dentist can also advise you on how to take the best possible care of your teeth both during and after radiation therapy.

3.3.5.3. Chemotherapy

Chemicals are used in chemotherapy to kill cancer cells. Chemotherapy medications can be administered as a single treatment, in combination with other cancer therapies, or with other chemotherapy medications. Radiation therapy and chemotherapy are frequently used in conjunction because of the potential for increased efficacy. The side effects vary depending on the medications you take. Hair loss, vomiting, and nausea are typical side effects. Inquire with your doctor about the possible side effects of the chemotherapy medications you will be taking.

3.3.5.4. Targeted Drug Therapy

Drugs that target specific characteristics of cancer cells that promote their growth are used to treat mouth cancer. Targeted medications can be taken on their own or in conjunction with radiation or chemotherapy. One targeted therapy used in some cases to treat mouth cancer is cetuximab (Erbitux). A protein that is present in many different kinds of healthy cells but is more common in some cancer cell types is inhibited by cetuximab. Skin rash, itching, headache, diarrhea, and infections are examples of side effects. If traditional therapies are not working, additional targeted medications may be an option.

3.3.5.5. Immunotherapy

Immunotherapy fights cancer by boosting your immune system. The immune system that fights disease may not be able to combat your cancer because cancer cells produce proteins that cause the immune system cells to become blind. Immunotherapy functions by obstructing that procedure. Immunotherapy is typically only used for patients with advanced oral cancer who are not improving with conventional care.

3.3.6. Risk Factors

Factors that can increase your risk of mouth cancer include:

- Usage of tobacco products of any kind, such as snuff, chewing tobacco, pipes, cigars, and cigarettes.
- Heavy alcohol use
- Excessive sun exposure to your lips
- A sexually transmitted virus called human papillomavirus (HPV)
- A weakened immune system

3.3.7. Prevention

There is currently no known method to stop mouth cancer. But you can lower your chance of developing mouth cancer if you:

- Give up smoking or avoid starting. Chewing or smoking tobacco exposes the cells in your mouth to chemicals that can cause cancer.
- If you consume alcohol at all, do so in moderation. or healthy adults, that translates to a maximum of one drink per day for men over 65 and women of all ages, and a maximum of two drinks per day for men under 65. Long-term, excessive alcohol consumption can irritate oral tissues, increasing your risk of developing mouth cancer. F

- Keep your lips from being exposed to too much sun. Stay in the shade whenever you can to avoid damaging the skin on your lips from the sun. Put on a wide-brimmed hat that will effectively block out the light on your whole face, including your mouth. As part of your regular sun protection routine, apply a sunscreen lip product.
- See your dentist on a regular basis. A routine dental exam should include an examination of your entire mouth by your dentist to look for abnormalities that could point to precancerous changes or mouth cancer.

3.4. Disorders of Salivary Glands

There are salivary glands in the mouth. The large salivary glands are located in three pairs. Each ear's parotid gland is located directly below and in front of it. There are submandibular glands beneath the jaw. The tongue has sublingual glands beneath it. Hundreds of smaller glands are also present. These glands produce spit, or saliva, which is then released into the mouth through duct openings. Food is moistened by saliva, which facilitates chewing, swallowing, and food digestion. Because saliva contains antibodies that destroy germs, it also helps to maintain a clean and healthy mouth. Damage to the salivary glands or insufficient saliva production can alter taste, complicate chewing and swallowing, and raise the risk of oral infections, cavities, and tooth loss (Figure 3.18).

In addition to these major glands, 600 to 1,000 very tiny, minor salivary glands are scattered throughout the mouth and throat. They are situated beneath the skin that is wet along the

- inner lips
- inner cheeks
- palate
- back of the throat
- back portion of the tongue
- pharynx
- sinuses

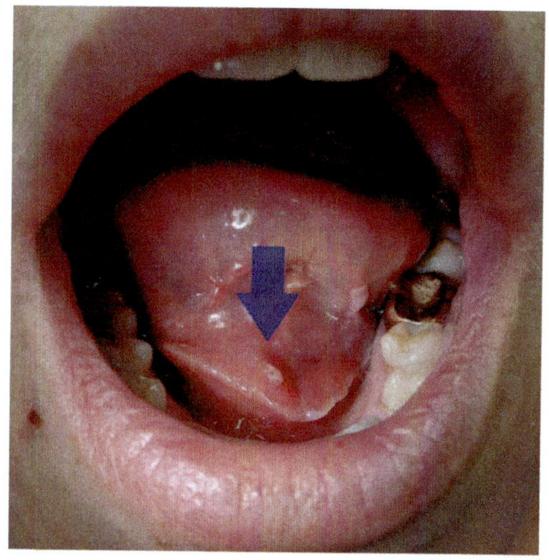

Figure 3.18. *Blockage of the submandibular gland by a salivary stone with subsequent infection. Arrow marks pus coming out of the opening of the submandibular gland.*

Source: By James Heilman, MD – Own work, CC BY-SA 4.0, https://commons.wikimedia.org/w/index.php?curid=69399533.

Some of the most common salivary gland disorders include:

- Sarcophagus (stones in the salivary glands). Inside the salivary glands, tiny stones rich in calcium can occasionally form. It is unclear what specifically causes these stones. Certain stones might be connected to the following:
  - dehydration, which thickens the saliva

- decreased food intake, which lowers the demand for saliva
- medications that decrease saliva production, including certain antihistamines, blood pressure drugs and psychiatric medications.

Sarcophagus (stones in the salivary glands). Inside the salivary glands, tiny stones rich in calcium can occasionally form. It is unclear what specifically causes these stones. Certain stones might be connected to the following:

- Sialadenitis (infection of a salivary gland). Sialadenitis is an excruciating infection that is typically brought on by bacteria. Older adults with salivary gland stones are more likely to experience it. Infants may also contract SIALDITIS in their first few weeks of life.

In the elderly or severely disabled, sialadenitis can worsen into a serious infection if left untreated.

- **Viral Infections:** Sometimes salivary gland infections are the result of systemic (whole-body) viral infections. This results in pain, edema, and trouble eating. The mumps is the most typical example.
- **Cysts (Tiny Fluid-Filled Sacs):** Sometimes issues with ear development prior to birth result in babies being born with parotid gland cysts. Different kinds of cysts may develop in the major or minor salivary glands later in life. They could be brought on by tumors or stones in the salivary glands, infections, or severe injuries.
- **Benign Tumors (Noncancerous Tumors):** The parotid gland is where most salivary gland tumors develop. Most of them are harmless. Benign parotid tumors are most commonly found as a slowly growing, painless lump located just below the earlobe at the back of the jaw. Radiation exposure and perhaps smoking are risk factors.
- **Malignant Tumors (Cancerous Tumors):** Cancers of the saliva glands are uncommon. They may or may not act aggressively. The two only known risk factors for salivary gland cancers are radiation exposure and Sjogren's syndrome. Smoking might also be a factor.
- **Sjogren's Syndrome:** It is a type of chronic autoimmune disease. The lacrimal glands (glands that produce tears), the salivary glands, and occasionally the sweat and oil glands on the skin are all targets of the body's immune system attacks. There is a chance that other body parts like the joints, lungs, and nervous system will be impacted.

Women make up the majority of those affected by this illness, and symptoms typically appear in middle age. Rheumatoid arthritis, polymyositis, scleroderma, and systemic lupus erythematosus (lupus) coexist with the illness in approximately half of cases.

- **Sialadenosis (Nonspecific Salivary Gland Enlargement):** The salivary glands can occasionally enlarge without showing signs of an infection, inflammation, or tumor. The term sialadenosis refers to this nonspecific enlargement. The parotid gland is typically affected, and its etiology is still unknown.

3.4.1. Symptoms

The specific type of salivary gland disorder will determine the symptoms.

- **Sialolithiasis:** The most typical sign is a sore lump in the gland that is impacted. Eating may make the pain worse.
- **Sialadenitis:** Symptoms may include:
    - a sore, tender lump beneath the chin or in the cheek.
    - a pus discharge from the duct into the mouth that has an unpleasant taste.
    - fever, chills, and overall weakness in extreme situations.
- Viral infections – The first symptoms often include:
    - fever
    - headache
    - muscle aches
    - joint pain
    - poor appetite
    - malaise.

Swelling of the parotid glands, usually on both sides of the face, occurs after these symptoms. It might not be easy to open the mouth completely.

- **Cysts:** A lump that hurts is caused by a cyst. It can occasionally get big enough to get in the way of eating.
- **Tumors:** The most typical sign of both malignant and noncancerous salivary gland tumors is a slow-growing lump. The lump hurts occasionally. There are four possible locations for this lump: the roof of the mouth, the tongue, the cheek, or beneath the chin.
- **Sjogren's Syndrome:** The primary symptoms of this syndrome are dry eyes, dry mouth, and enlargement of the salivary glands. Moreover, joint pain is typical.
- **Sialadenosis:** Usually, this disorder results in the parotid glands on both sides of the face swelling up painlessly.

3.4.2. Diagnosis

You will describe your symptoms. The doctor will review you're the following:

- medical history
- smoking history
- current medications
- diet

The doctor also may ask whether you

- were just admitted to the hospital for surgery. After surgery, cutting back on food and liquids can raise the risk of infections and stones in the salivary glands.
- have ever undergone radiation therapy for head or neck cancer?
- were ever given a mumps diagnosis or received a mumps vaccination.
- have come into contact with someone who has the flu or another virus recently.
- possess any kind of autoimmune disease, including rheumatoid arthritis.

Your head, neck, and oral cavity will then be examined by your physician. Your doctor will lightly press on certain cheek regions to check for parotid gland swelling. Additionally, he or she will feel for enlarged salivary glands beneath your jaw. If you feel any tenderness during the examination, let your doctor know. The doctor may request one or more of the following tests based on your symptoms, medical history, and physical examination results.

- **Tests on Blood:** To check for a high white blood cell count, which may indicate an infection with bacteria. Additional blood tests may be performed to check for viral infections, nutritional deficiencies, and Sjogren's syndrome.
- **X-rays:** To detect salivary gland stones.
- Computed tomography (CT) scans or magnetic resonance imaging (MRI). Tumors and stones that are not visible on X-rays can be found with these tests.
- **Fine-Needle Aspiration:** To ascertain whether a tumor is malignant, this procedure extracts cells from the salivary gland using a tiny needle.
- **Sialography:** To visualize the salivary flow pathways, a dye is injected into the gland's duct.
- A salivary gland biopsy involves removing a tiny sample of tissue in order to identify whether a cyst, tumor, or Sjogren's syndrome is present.
- **Test for Salivary Function:** To aid in the Sjogren's syndrome diagnosis.
- **Eye Tests:** To rule out Sjogren's syndrome or other possible causes of the symptoms of the eyes.

3.4.3. Expected Duration

The duration of a salivary gland issue varies depending on the particular condition.

- **Sialolithiasis:** On occasion, tiny stones come out of the duct by themselves. Larger stones, however, typically remain in the gland until they are extracted.
- **Sialadenitis:** After receiving antibiotic treatment, symptoms typically start to go away 48 hours later.
- **Viral infections:** With mumps, symptoms usually last about 10 days.
- **Cysts:** A small, superficial cyst may resolve on its own as it drains. Larger cysts typically continue to grow until they require surgical removal.
- Benign tumors typically do not spread until they are removed. Tumors that are cancerous persist until they are surgically removed, either with or without radiation therapy.
- Sjogren's syndrome is a chronic illness that is typically well controlled with medication.
- Sialadenosis associated with a medical issue typically continues for the duration of that issue.

3.4.4. Prevention

You can lessen your chance of salivary gland viral infections. Vaccinate against influenza and the mumps to achieve this. There are no particular precautions to guard against other kinds of disorders affecting the salivary glands. Still, it is beneficial to do the following:

- avoid smoking
- eat a healthy diet
- To prevent dehydration, consume six to eight glasses of water every day.

- Maintain proper oral hygiene by brushing and flossing your teeth on a regular basis

3.4.5. Treatment

The treatment varies, depending on the disorder:

- **Sialolithiasis:** Your doctor might be able to gently press out the stone if it is close to the duct's end. Surgery can be used to remove deeper stones.
- **Sialadenitis:** Treatment includes
    - drinking fluids or receiving fluids intravenously
    - antibiotics
    - compresses that are heated for the infected gland.
    - Chewing on sour, sugarless candies or consuming orange juice can stimulate saliva production.

Surgery can empty the gland if these treatments are ineffective in treating the infection.

- Infections caused by viruses typically resolve on their own. The goal of treatment is to reduce symptoms through the following:
    - rest
    - drinking fluids to prevent dehydration
    - taking acetaminophen (Tylenol) to relieve pain and fever
- **Cysts:** If left untreated, a small cyst may drain on its own. Larger cysts can be removed with laser surgery or conventional surgery.
- **Benign Tumors:** Surgical removal is typically used to remove noncancerous tumors. Radiation therapy is sometimes administered following surgery to stop the tumor from growing back.
- **Malignant Tumors:** Surgery alone is frequently sufficient to treat smaller, early-stage, low-grade tumors. Larger, high-grade tumors, however, typically need radiation therapy after surgery. Chemotherapy or radiation are used to treat tumors that are incurable.

Dry mouth is the primary salivary gland-related symptom of Sjogren's syndrome. Choices consist of:

- drugs that increase salivary flow, like cevimeline (Evoxac) and pilocarpine (Salagen).
- Eye drops like cyclosporine (brand name Restasis) that can decrease inflammation and boost tear production.
- tear duct plugs to increase lubrication in the eyes.
- Drugs like corticosteroids, hydroxychloroquine, and methotrexate are used to control or alter immune system activity.
- Candy and sugar-free gum to increase saliva production.
- staying away from drugs that exacerbate dry mouth.
- not smoking.

Dental hygiene is essential. Sjogren's syndrome patients experience gum and tooth issues due to reduced salivary flow.

- **Sialadenosis:** The goal of treatment is to address any underlying health issues. After the illness gets better, the salivary glands ought to return to their typical size.

3.4.6. Prognosis

The outlook depends on the disorder:

- **Sialolithiasis:** The prognosis is typically very good if a stone is removed as soon as possible. One in five people experience a return of stones.
- **Sialadenitis:** The prognosis is typically excellent if antibiotics are administered quickly. The elderly and those with incapacitating chronic illnesses are most at risk for complications.
- **Sialadenosis:** The salivary glands typically revert to their normal size after any underlying medical condition is treated.
- **Infections by Viruses:** Most patients recover completely and without any problems.
- **Cysts:** The prognosis is generally favorable. Some people develop cysts once more. However, these can typically be removed without any issues.
- **Benign Tumors:** Typically, there is a very good prognosis. Nonetheless, some people experience tumor recurrence up to 10 to 15 years after the initial tumor was removed.
- **Malignant Tumors:** Parotid tumors typically have the best prognosis. It is least fortunate for:
    - malignancies affecting the minor or sublingual salivary glands.
    - cancers that have invaded the nearby facial nerve
    - bulky cancers that have spread

The prognosis for Sjogren's syndrome varies. Some people only experience minor symptoms. Others suffer from more severe illnesses that have a negative impact on their quality of life.

A Closer Look

Salivary Duct Stones

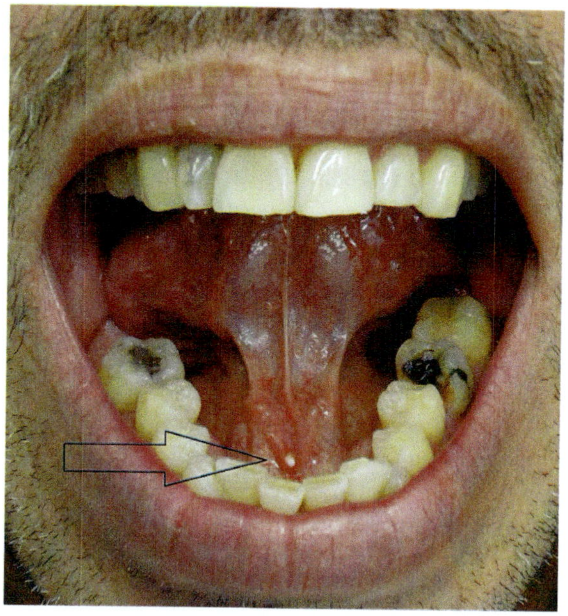

Source: By James Heilman, MD – Own work, CC BY-SA 3.0, https://commons.wikimedia.org/w/index.php?curid=24076829.

A calcified structure that can develop inside a salivary gland or duct is known as a salivary gland stone, also known as a salivary duct stone. It may stop saliva from entering the mouth. The submandibular glands at the base of the mouth are impacted by most stones. The sublingual glands, which are under the tongue, and the parotid glands, which are found inside the cheeks, are less frequently impacted by stones. Many patients with the illness have more than one stone.

Salivary Gland Stone Causes and Symptoms: When chemicals from the saliva build up in the gland or duct, salivary stones can develop. Most of them are made of calcium. The precise reason is unknown. However, conditions that cause saliva to thicken or produce less saliva may put people at risk for salivary stones. Dehydration, inadequate nutrition, and the use of specific medications, such as some antihistamines, blood pressure medications, psychiatric medications, and bladder control medications, are some of these risk factors. Salivary stones may also be more likely in cases of trauma to the salivary glands. When the stones get large enough to obstruct the duct, saliva backs up into the gland, causing pain and swelling. Initially, the stones don't cause any symptoms. The pain might come on and off, and it might get worse over time. The afflicted gland may then experience infection and inflammation. Salivary Gland Stones Diagnosis and Treatments: First, your doctor will perform a physical examination to rule out salivary gland stones if you are exhibiting symptoms. Occasionally, additional tests like an ultrasound, CT scan, or X-ray may be requested. The purpose of treatment is to remove any stones that are found. Sucking on a lemon or sour candy can stimulate saliva flow, which may help small stones pass on their own. When a stone is tiny, the physician or dentist may choose to massage it or force it out of the duct. To remove larger, more difficult-to-remove stones, doctors typically need to make a small oral incision. A less invasive procedure called sialendoscopy is being used by medical professionals more and more often to remove salivary gland stones. Sialendoscopy is a successful method that was developed and used for 10 years in Europe. It involves inserting small, lighted scopes into the mouth gland's opening to view the salivary duct system and find the stone. The surgeon can then relieve the obstruction by removing the stone with tiny instruments. Because the surgery is done under local anesthesia or light general anesthesia, the patient can return home the same day. In patients whose salivary gland damage is irreversible or whose stones are recurring, surgical excision of the gland may be required. In addition, if an infection has been brought on by salivary stones, antibiotics are recommended.

Summary

- The alimentary canal begins in the oral cavity, sometimes referred to as the mouth.
- The oral cavity is located between the oropharyngeal isthmus, which is the opening of the oropharynx, and the oral fissure, which is the opening between the lips on the anterior side. The upper and lower dental arches—formed by the teeth and their bony scaffolding—separate it into two sections. The vestibule and the mouth cavity proper are the two sections that make up the oral cavity.
- Some of the more prevalent dental issues people are facing in today's world are referred to as oral diseases. Gum disease, oral cancers, dental cavities, infectious diseases, and trauma and injury are some of these issues.
- Any type of cancer that arises in any part of the mouth (oral cavity) is referred to as mouth cancer.
- There are salivary glands in the mouth. The large salivary glands are located in three pairs. Each ear's parotid gland is located directly below and in front of it. There are submandibular glands beneath the jaw. The tongue has sublingual glands beneath it.

References

1. Berg, J. H., & Slayton, R. L. (2009). *Early Childhood Oral Health*. Wiley-Blackwell.
2. Jose, B. (2001). *Dental Caries and Oral Hygiene Practices of Children and Caregivers in Kerala, India* [Thesis, The University of Hong Kong]. http://hub.hku.hk/bib/B31954224 (accessed on 4 September 2024).
3. Myers, S. L. (2015). *General and Oral Pathology for Dental Hygiene Practice*. F. A. Davis Company.
4. Nestor, J. (2020). *Breath: The New Science of a Lost Art*. Riverhead Books.
5. Rantanen, I. (2003). *Betaine in Oral Hygiene with Special Attention to Dry and Sensitive Mucosa* [Doctoral dissertation, Turun Yliopisto]. http://books.google.com/books?id=qcJpAAAAMAAJ (accessed on 4 September 2024).
6. Studen-Pavlovich, D., & Ranalli, D. N. (2006). *Adolescent Oral Health*. Saunders.
7. Touger-Decker, R., & Sirois, D. (2011). *Nutrition and Oral Medicine* (2nd ed.). Humana Press.

Chapter

DISEASES OF THE PHARYNX

4

Contents

Introduction

The muscular tube in the middle of your neck is called the pharynx, or throat. It facilitates breathing and food digestion. A common cold to cancer are just a few of the medical conditions that can affect your throat. You can prevent infections and smoke to protect your pharynx.

Orientation and Directional Terms

Term	Definition	Illustration
Parotid Abscess	An acute infection of the parotid gland is characterized by a variety of symptoms such as the sudden onset of erythematous swelling in parotideal region, pain, fever, facial asymmetry, facial nerve palsy, and less frequently, pus/blood in the oral cavity and dysphagia.	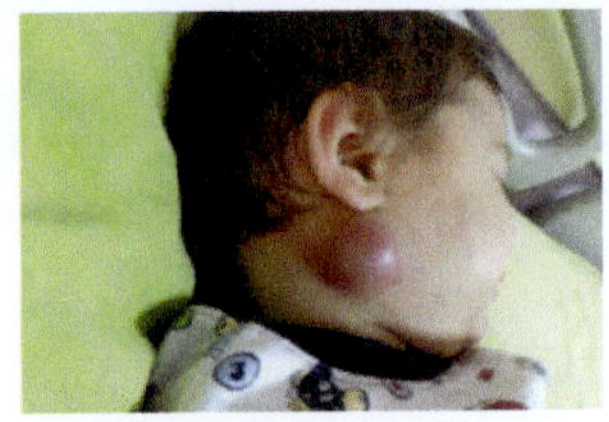
Ludwig's Angina	Ludwig angina is an infection of the floor of the mouth under the tongue. It is often due to a bacterial infection of the teeth or jaw.	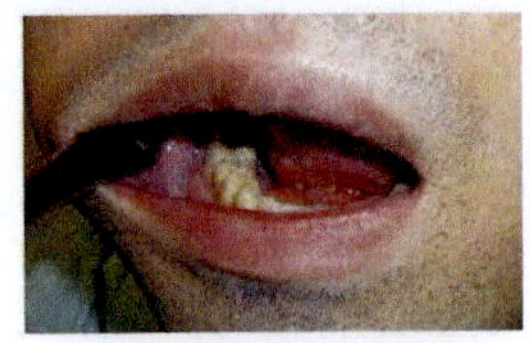
Peritonsillar Abscess	A peritonsillar abscess forms in the tissues of the throat next to one of the tonsils.	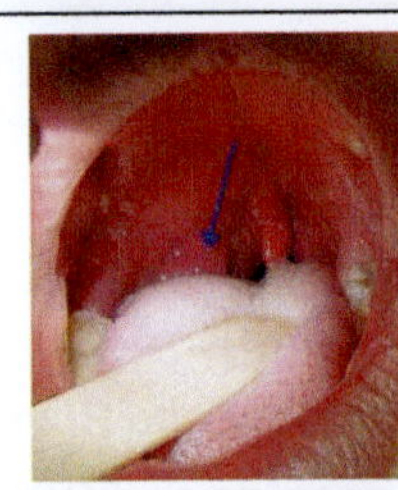
Retropharyngeal Abscess	A retropharyngeal abscess is pus deep in the back of your throat. It is caused by a bacterial infection affecting your throat's lymph nodes.	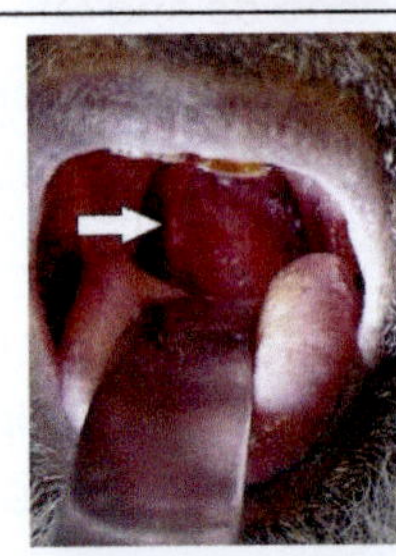
Parapharyngeal Abscess	Parapharyngeal abscesses are deep neck abscesses involving the parapharyngeal space.	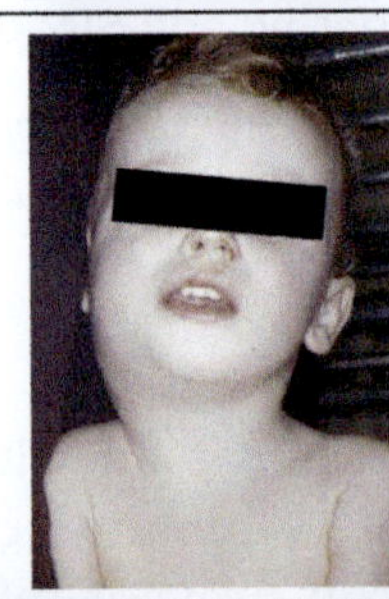
Masticator Space	The masticator space is the deep compartment of the head and neck that contains the muscles of mastication.	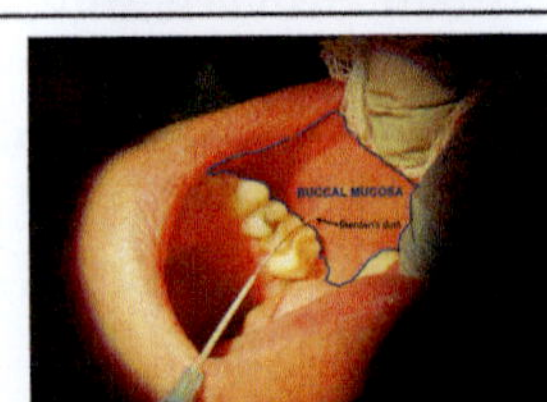

4.1. Anatomy and Physiology of Pharynx

The area of the throat that is directly behind the mouth and nasal cavity and above the esophagus and larynx in humans is called the pharynx. The pharyngeal plexus innervates the three sections that make up the human pharynx: the nasopharynx (epipharynx), the oropharynx (mesopharynx), and the laryngopharynx (hypopharynx) (Figure 4.1).

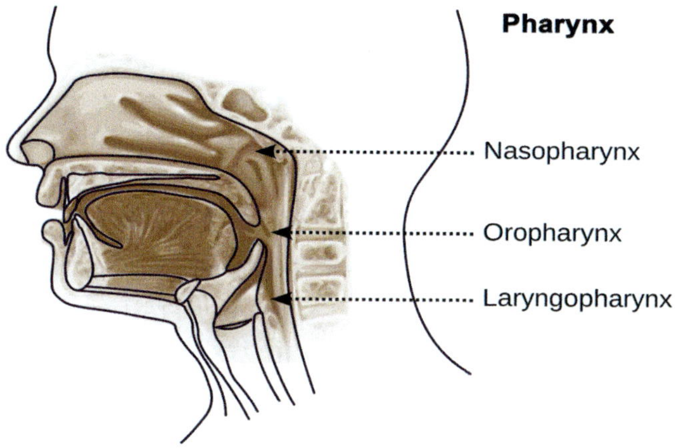

Figure 4.1. *The pharynx.*

Source: By Arcadian – http://www.cortexity.com:8080/nicksblog/images/pharynx.jpg, Public Domain, https://commons.wikimedia.org/w/index.php?curid=789690.

The respiratory system and the digestive system both include the pharynx. The pharynx is a part of the conducting zone for air entering the lungs because it is a part of the upper respiratory tract. As a result, one of its main jobs is to warm and humidify the air before the lungs receive it.

4.1.1. The Nasopharynx

The area above the throat is called the nasopharynx. It reaches from the base of the skull to the soft palate's upper surface, which is located above the oral cavity. The nasal cavity and throat are joined by the nasopharynx. The nasopharynx can assist in balancing the pressure inside the ear because of its connection to the middle ear's eustachian tubes. But it also facilitates the easy spread of infections from the nasopharynx to the ear. Psuedo-stratified squamous cell epithelia tissue, which is ciliated (covered in tiny hairs that move mucus), is found in the nasopharynx.

A mass of lymphatic tissue located in the roof of the nasopharynx is called the adenoids, also known as the pharyngeal tonsils. The adenoids have a small part in both the development of the embryo and the postnatal production of T lymphocytes for the immune system. Due to infection or hypertrophy (enlargement of the cells in its tissues), which can obstruct the passage of air from the nose to the lung if left untreated, the adenoids are frequently removed in children. Although the immune system's performance is not significantly affected by the removal of the adenoids, there are sometimes issues with the surgery. The torus tubarus, a mound of cartilage tissue from the auditory tube, supports the lateral walls of the nasopharynx, which are composed of the pharyngeal ostia (bone) of the auditory tube. The auditory tube's cartilaginous aperture gives rise to two folds. The salpingopharyngeus muscle makes up the salpingopharyngeal fold, a vertical fold of mucous membrane that extends from the inferior portion of the torus. The levator veli palatini muscle is located in the salpingopalatine fold, a smaller fold that runs from the superior part of the torus to the palate. There is a deep recess called the pharyngeal recess behind the auditory tube bone. The pharyngeal bursa is an irregular flask-shaped depression of the mucous membrane located in the midline, above the adenoid.

4.1.2. The Oropharynx

The middle section of the pharynx is called the oropharynx (mesopharynx). It has an opening to each of the following cavities: the laryngopharynx, below the nasopharynx, and between the oral cavity. The base of the tongue makes up the oropharynx's anterior wall, while the uvula and the soft palate's bottom surface make up the superior wall. Non-keratinized squamous stratified epithelium, which lines the oropharynx, is thicker than the epithelium in other respiratory tract regions to guard against food damage, but it is not as thick as skin because it does not contain keratin. The epiglottis is a flap of elastic cartilage that closes during swallowing to ensure that food enters the esophagus rather than the trachea. It is located between the oropharynx and the laryngopharynx.

The palatine tonsils, masses of lymphoid tissue on the lateral walls of the oropharynx, are located within the oropharynx. The palatine tonsils are not ciliated like the adenoids of the nasopharynx, and they have many folds, or crypts, in comparison. In some cases, individuals with infections or enlargements of the tonsils may also have these removed.

4.1.3. The Laryngopharynx

The part of the throat that joins the esophagus and trachea is called the laryngopharynx, also known as the hypopharynx. It is the caudal portion of the pharynx. It denotes the separation of the pathways leading to the digestive and respiratory systems and is located inferior to the epiglottis. The trachea's epiglottis closes during swallowing, causing a brief halt to airflow. The laryngopharynx, which is composed of a similar kind of stratified squamous epithelium tissue, naturally extends into the esophagus. There are several significant regions and demarcations within the laryngopharynx. At the level of the hyoid bone is the formal superior boundary that divides the laryngopharynx from the oropharynx.

The pyriform sinus, the postcricoid area, and the posterior pharyngeal wall are the three main regions that make up the laryngopharynx. These regions are divided by tiny cartilage folds. The laryngopharynx lacks tonsils, in contrast to the nasopharynx and oropharynx (Figure 4.2).

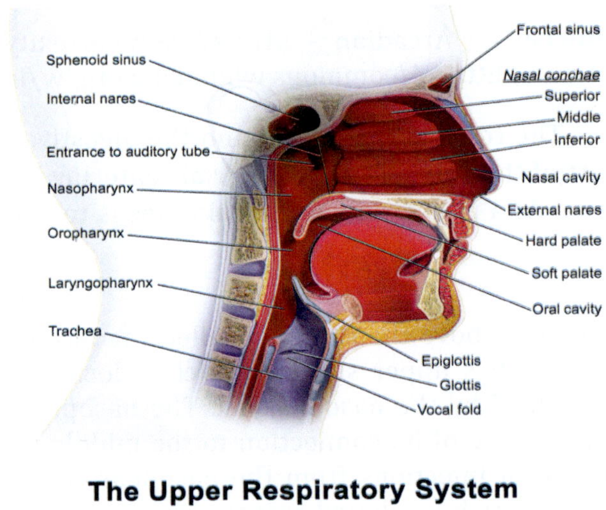

Figure 4.2. *Upper respiratory system, with the nasopharynx, oropharynx and laryngopharynx labeled at left.*

Source: By BruceBlaus – Own work, CC BY 3.0, https://commons.wikimedia.org/w/index.php?curid=27924400.

4.1.4. Muscles

The pharyngeal muscles are divided into two main groups: circular and longitudinal. With the exception of the stylopharyngeus (glossopharyngeal nerve), the majority of the pharyngeal muscles are innervated by the vagus nerve.

4.1.4.1. Circular

The superior, middle, and inferior circular pharyngeal constrictor muscles are the three types. They form an incomplete muscular circle around the pharynx, arranged like stacked glasses. The pharyngeal lumen is constricted by the circular muscles contracting successively from superior to inferior. and thus force the meal bolus into the esophagus inferiorly.

- Superior pharyngeal constrictor – the pharyngeal constrictor located highest. That can be found in the oropharynx.
    - originates from the sphenoid bone's pterygoid hamulus, the medial pterygoid plate, the alveolar process of the mandible, and the pterygomandibular ligament.
    - attaches posteriorly to the pharyngeal raphe and the pharyngeal tubercle of the occiput.
- Middle pharyngeal constrictor – located in the laryngopharynx.
    - originates from the horns of the hyoid bone and the stylohyoid ligament.
    - inserts into the pharyngeal raphe from the posterior.
- Inferior pharyngeal constrictor – situated in the throat and larynx. It is made up of two parts:
    - The thyroid cartilage is the source of thyroidopharyngeal fibers.
    - The cricoid cartilage serves as the source of cricophorangeal fibers.
    - The pharyngeal raphe is where all fibers insert posteriorly.

4.1.4.2. Longitudinal

The salpingopharyngeus, palatopharyngeus, and stylopharyngeus are the longitudinal muscles. During swallowing, they work to elevate the larynx and shorten and widen the pharynx.

- Stylopharyngeus –is inserted onto the pharyngeal wall from the styloid process of the temporal bone.
    - It is innervated by the glossopharyngeal nerve (CN IX), in contrast to the other pharyngeal muscles.
- Palatopharyngeus – comes from the oral cavity's hard palate and attaches to the pharyngeal wall.
    - Innervated by the vagus nerve (CN X).
- Salpingopharyngeus – comes from the Eustachian tube and attaches itself to the wall of the throat.
    - Innervated by the vagus nerve (CN X).
    - It aids in swallowing and releases air pressure in the middle ear by opening the Eustachian tube.

4.1.5. Innervation

The pharyngeal plexus provides motor and sensory innervation to most of the pharynx, with the exception of the nasopharynx.

The middle pharyngeal constrictor is topped by the pharyngeal plexus, which is formed by:

- The glossopharyngeal nerve (CN IX) gives rise to the pharyngeal branches.
- The vagus nerve's Pharyngeal Branch (CN X).
- branches coming from the laryngeal nerve externally.
- fibers of the superior cervical ganglion that are sympathetic.

i. **Sensory:** The glossopharyngeal nerve supplies sensory innervation to the pharynx. The maxillary nerve (CN V2) innervates the anterior and superior aspect of the nasopharynx. The internal branch of the vagus nerve innervates the inferior aspect of the laryngopharynx, which surrounds the larynx's origin.

ii. **Motor:** The vagus nerve (CN X) innervates every muscle in the pharynx, except for the stylopharyngeus, which is innervated by the glossopharyngeal nerve (CN IX).

4.1.6. Vasculature

The external carotid artery branches provide the pharynx with arterial supply.

- Ascending pharyngeal artery
- Branches of the facial artery
- Branches of the lingual and maxillary arteries.

The pharyngeal venous plexus, which empties into the internal jugular vein, facilitates venous drainage.

4.2. Adenoids and Other Inflammations of Nasopharynx

The adenoid, a structure in the immune system, is situated at the nose-throat junction (nasopharynx). Despite its advantages, problems with the adenoid may arise. The adenoid gland naturally grows larger between the ages of 2–4 years (though it can appear larger in infants younger than a year old), and this larger size can lead to complications. Your nose and respiratory system are connected by your nasopharynx, which is the top of your throat (pharynx). Adenoids, which are present in it, aid in preventing infection. Additionally, your eustachian tubes drain fluid and balance pressure by connecting your ears to your nasopharynx. Adenoids that are enlarged and the common cold can both affect your nasopharynx.

4.2.1. Adenoids

Similar to the palatine tonsils, the adenoids are a mass of lymphatic tissue that is attached to the rear wall of the nasal pharynx (i.e., the area where the throat's upper portion opens into the nasal cavity). One particular fold of this type of nasopharyngeal lymphatic tissue is referred to as an adenoid. The ciliated epithelial cells that make up the adenoidsal surface layer are mucus-thin. Microscopic hair-like projections from the surface cells called cilia move constantly in a wave-like pattern, pushing the mucus blanket down to the actual pharynx. The mucus is then transported to the stomach by the pharyngeal (throat) muscles as they swallow the material. In order to replenish the surface film, the adenoids also have glands that secrete mucus. The adenoids have a defensive purpose. The pharynx, where the epithelium is more resilient, is where infectious agents and dust particles that are inhaled through the nose tend to travel through the moving mucus film. It is believed that immune substances, or antibodies, are produced in the lymphatic tissue, which when paired with phagocytic activity, tends to halt and absorb infectious agents.

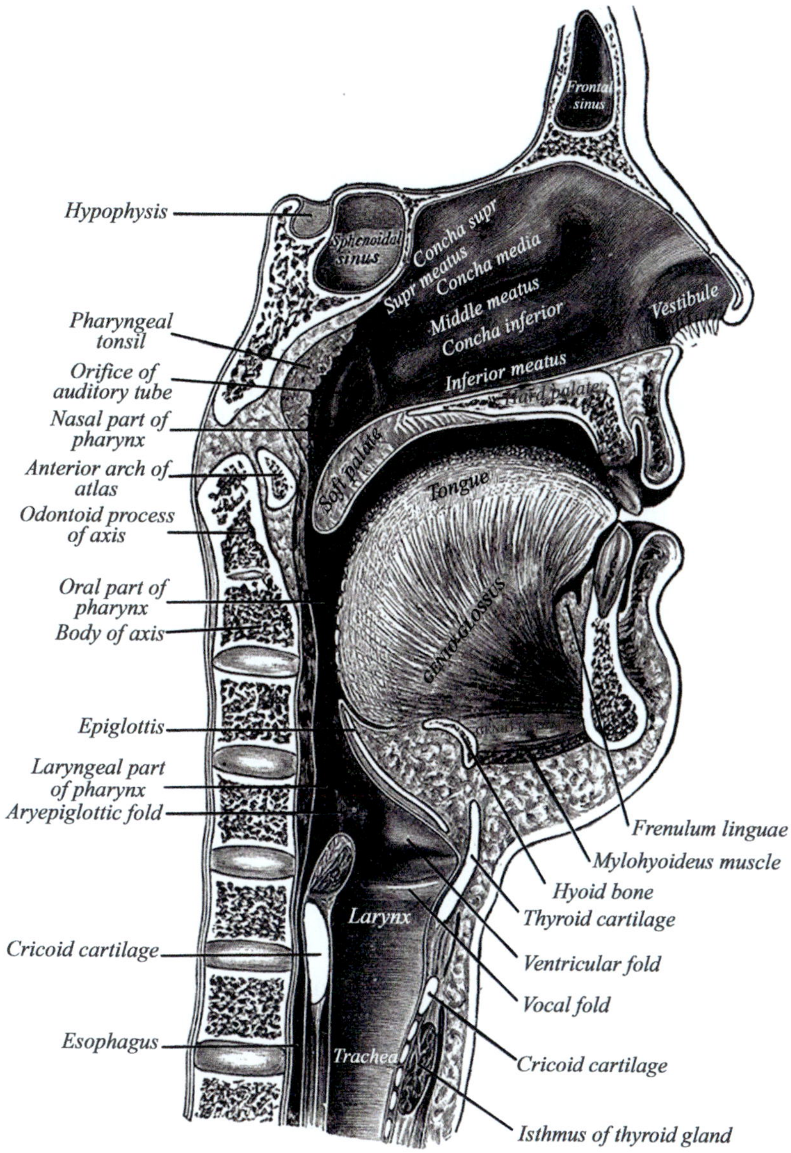

Figure 4.3. *Location of the adenoid.*

Source: By Henry Vandyke Carter – Henry Gray (1918) Anatomy of the Human Body Bartleby.com: Gray's Anatomy, Plate 994, Public Domain, https://commons.wikimedia.org/w/index.php?curid=698750.

Early childhood is typically when the adenoids enlarge. Childhood infections have the potential to permanently enlarge the adenoids by inducing swelling and inflammation. Big adenoids make it difficult to breathe through the nose and impede the drainage of the sinuses, which puts a person at risk for sinus infections. People with enlarged adenoids often have a vacant facial expression due to chronic respiratory obstruction and mouth breathing. The infection and enlargement of the adenoids also increase the risk of middle ear infections by blocking the eustachian tubes, which are the passageways that connect the nasal pharynx to the middle ear. For children with enlarged or infected adenoids, surgical removal is usually advised, frequently in conjunction with tonsillectomy. The size of adenoids typically decreases after childhood (Figure 4.3).

4.2.1.1. Adenoiditis

The nasopharyngeal tonsil, also known as the "adenoid pad" or "adenoids," is a collection of lymphoid tissue situated at the level of the soft palate on the posterior wall of the nasopharynx. Named for Heinrich Wilhelm Gottfried von Waldeyer-Hartz, a German anatomist at the turn of the 20th century, the adenoids, along with the faucial tonsils, lingual tonsils, and tubal tonsils of Gerlach, constitute what is known as Waldeyer's ring, a circumferential collection of lymphoid tissue that surrounds the upper aerodigestive tract. Collectively, these tissues play a crucial role in the early development of the human immune system. When antigens enter the nasal and oral cavities, they interact with Waldeyer's ring immune cells, which subsequently contribute to immunologic memory and the production of IgA antibodies. It is believed that during infancy, this process primes the immune system.

The adenoids are born and grow larger during childhood, reaching their maximum size by the time a child is seven years old. They typically experience a size regression during adolescence and may disappear entirely by adulthood. Adenoiditis is therefore frequently a concern in childhood and adolescence. When the adenoid tissue becomes inflamed due to an infection, an allergy, or irritation from stomach acid as a part of laryngopharyngeal reflux (LPR), the condition is known as adenoiditis. Seldom does adenotonsillitis, pharyngitis, rhinosinusitis, or other more widespread disease processes manifest alone as adenoidosillitis. Adenoid hypertrophy, which is the cause of many adenoid disease complications, such as Eustachian tube dysfunction and recurrent acute otitis media, can be brought on by ongoing irritation. There are two types of adenoiditis: acute and chronic.

4.2.1.1.1. Clinical Anatomy

The ascending pharyngeal artery, maxillary artery, and facial artery supply blood to the adenoids. Venous drainage happens via the veins in the throat. The vagus and glossopharyngeal nerves supply innervation. The size of an adenoid is rated from zero to four as follows:

- 0 absent
- 1+ <25% obstruction of the nasopharynx
- 2+ 25–50% obstruction
- 3+ 50–75% obstruction
- 4+ >75% obstruction

4.2.1.1.2. Etiology

The adenoid tissue can become inflamed due to a variety of substances and infections. Before acute adenoiditis, viral upper respiratory tract infections (URIs) are frequently observed. Bacterial pathogens have the ability to multiply and superinfect tissues in this condition.

The following are the most frequently isolated bacterial pathogens from adenoid specimens:

- Haemophilus influenza
- Streptococcus pneumoniae
- Streptococcus pyogenes
- Staphylococcus aureus

A polymicrobial infection, which may include anaerobic pathogens, is more common in cases of chronic adenoiditis. Children's recurrent upper respiratory tract infections may be exacerbated by chronic adenoiditis, which is often caused by biofilm development. Most of the time, adenoiditis coexists with pediatric rhinosinusitis. The pathogenesis of adenoiditis and the ensuing adenoid hypertrophy is thought to involve allergies. Adenoid tissue is exposed to allergens inhaled through the nose, which causes the tissue to multiply and produce IgA as a reaction to the allergens. Adenoiditis and adenoid hypertrophy may also be caused by gastric acid irritation over an extended period of time in patients with gastroesophageal reflux disease (GERD), especially young children and infants.

4.2.1.1.3. Epidemiology

Since adenoiditis is typically treated in conjunction with a regional disease process like rhinosinusitis and adenotonsillar disease, precise incidence and prevalence statistics for adenoiditis alone are difficult to ascertain. Adenoiditis usually affects children because adnoid tissue atrophies during puberty. Though there has been a positive correlation found between parental smoking and the disease, current research does not indicate that gender, race, region, or socioeconomic class are predisposing factors. In children, it can be difficult to distinguish bacterial sinusitis from adenoiditis. As a result, data on pediatric sinusitis may help us estimate the prevalence of adenoiditis. Children are thought to get six to eight viral URIs annually. 5–13% of these viral URIs are followed by a bacterial superinfection, which can cause sinusitis and possibly adenoiditis.

4.2.1.1.4. Pathophysiology

A viral upper respiratory tract infection (URI) is frequently followed by acute adenoiditis. Inflammation and an increase in exudate production are the outcomes of bacterial agents multiplying and infecting the adenoids and surrounding tissue. Post-nasal drip, snoring, fever, nasal blockage, rhinorrhea, and halitosis are among the symptoms. Many of the same symptoms are present in chronic adenoiditis, but they are persistent for at least 90 days and are frequently brought on by biofilm formation and polymicrobial infections. In cases of chronic adenoiditis, exudates are often absent. Environmental allergens or the caustic irritation caused by stomach acid when GERD/LPR is present are additional causes of adenoiditis.

Adenoid hypertrophy can result from lymphoid tissue proliferating due to chronic inflammation in any form. This hypertrophy can cause obstruction of the Eustachian tubes and nasal airways, which can result in otitis media and obstructive sleep apnea (OSA), among other issues. Other causes of adenoid hypertrophy include lymphoma, primary sinonasal malignancies, and HIV infection; however, these conditions do not always result in adenoid inflammation.

4.2.1.1.5. History and Physical

Since adenoid tissue usually regresses around puberty, prepubescent children with a recent history of URI are the typical patients with adenoiditis. Additionally, the patient may have a history of GERD/LPR, chronic nasal obstruction with mouth breathing, recurrent acute otitis media, sleep disordered breathing, or chronic otitis media. Purulent rhinorrhea, post-nasal drip, nasal obstruction, snoring, fever, mouth breathing, and halitosis are among the physical manifestations. A clinician may be able to see enlarged adenoids with exudates by using an indirect mirror exam, though this can be a very difficult exam to perform in children. A flexible nasal and laryngeal endoscopic examination can provide a more thorough evaluation of the adenoids, but its use may necessitate advanced training and parental and child cooperation. Rarely, the adenoid may be big enough to show through the edge of the soft palate and protrude downward. The patient's speech quality may be impacted if the adenoid is big enough to permanently or temporarily push out the soft palate.

Long-face syndrome, also called adenoid facies, can arise from chronic adenoiditis followed by adenoid hypertrophy in early childhood. A high-arched palate and a retrognathic mandible are two examples of craniofacial abnormalities that can arise from obligate mouth breathing caused by enlarged adenoids blocking the nasopharynx.

4.2.1.1.6. Evaluation

- **Clinical Evaluation:** The results of the following are used to make the clinical diagnosis of acute adenoiditis
  - Possible concurrent acute otitis media
  - Fever
  - Purulent rhinorrhea
  - Post-nasal drip
  - Nasal obstruction
  - Throat pain
  - Halitosis

A nasal endoscope or laryngeal mirror can be used to try visual inspection of the adenoids.

- Laboratory Testing:
  - Rapid Strep test
  - Cultures
  - Allergy testing

The doctor may run a quick Strep test if pharyngitis is present along with adenoiditis. There are two reasons to do this. First of all, this will provide a conclusive diagnosis of the patient's illness and aid in the management of antibiotic therapy. Second, a record of both positive and negative strep tests will be kept in the doctor's office. This information will be crucial in determining whether an adenoidectomy—with or without a tonsillectomy—is necessary. It is crucial to keep in mind that adenoiditis is still a clinical diagnosis, so if the Strep test comes back negative, the doctor can assume that another organism is causing the symptoms. Since direct cultures of the adenoids may be challenging in the office, the clinician may decide to perform throat cultures in cases of persistent infection despite antibiotic therapy in order to help identify the causative agent and guide treatment. HIV testing and a complete blood count are additional tests to think about.

Allergy skin testing may be used to help guide therapy if it is thought that the adenoiditis is caused by seasonal or environmental allergies.

- Radiology Testing:
  - Lateral neck X-ray
  - Computed tomography (CT) of the sinuses

If a sinus infection is clinically suspected, sinus CT scans or X-rays may be ordered to search for a sinus infection source. In most everyday situations, this is not necessary. An efficient method of evaluating specifically for adenoid hypertrophy is lateral neck X-rays. For patients who snore and have adenoid hypertrophy, a sleep study can be obtained to rule out obstructive sleep apnea.

4.2.1.1.7. Treatment / Management

Clinically, adenoiditis is frequently observed as a part of pharyngitis or rhinosinusitis. As a result, when treating adenoiditis, medical professionals frequently adhere to clinical management guidelines for rhinosinusitis and pharyngitis.

4.2.1.1.8. Medical Management

Observation: The doctor should avoid giving antibiotics if they think a common cold or another common viral infection is the cause of adenoiditis. Simple viral infections of the upper respiratory tract usually go away in five to seven days.

- **Antibiotic Treatment:** The first line of treatment is antibiotics that cover the most common pathogens if symptoms persist or if the clinical presentation suggests a bacterial etiology, such as a high fever or purulent discharge from the nose or throat. Amoxicillin has a low side-effect profile and good coverage, making it a popular first-line medication. Cefuroxime or cefdinir are other options that could be utilized, especially if the patient has not responded to amoxicillin. Alternatives such as clarithromycin or azithromycin are available if the patient is allergic to penicillins. In 48 to 72 hours, symptoms should improve with an effective antibiotic regimen. 10 days should be the length of the treatment, as shorter courses of action result in high rates of relapse and the development of antibiotic resistance. In order to eradicate possible beta-lactamase-producing organisms, amoxicillin-clavulanate should be recommended if the illness does not get better after a course of amoxicillin or other first-line medications. Saline sprays and nasal rinses may also reduce symptom duration by irrigating microorganisms and any stagnant mucous secretions.
- **Allergy Treatment:** If environmental allergies are thought to be the cause of the adenoiditis, the patient may be offered a trial of oral steroids, nasal steroid sprays, oral antihistamines, or a combination of these to see if any symptoms improve. If this works, official allergy testing and immune-modulating treatment may be beneficial for the patient to get long-lasting relief. In these situations, saline sprays and nasal rinses might also be helpful.
- **Reflux Treatment:** In cases where adenoiditis is thought to be a secondary symptom of LPR/GERD, treatment for this condition may be sufficient to relieve symptoms. This may involve dietary and lifestyle modifications, as well as raising the head of the bed with or without the use of H2 blockers or proton-pump inhibitors.

4.2.1.1.9. Surgical Management

Adenoidectomy: To receive additional evaluation and possibly surgical intervention, the patient should be referred to an otolaryngologist if there is no symptomatic improvement following treatment with amoxicillin-clavulanate or if the patient has repeated episodes of adenoiditis that require antibiotic treatment. Adenoidectomy with or without tonsillectomy, myringotomy with tympanostomy tube implantation, or endoscopic sinus surgery are among the surgical procedures that may be performed, depending on the situation. Adenoids are typically removed concurrently with tonsillectomy if the patient fulfills the Paradise criteria, which eliminates an additional potential cause of recurrent infections. Similarly, because adenoid hypertrophy may result in chronic Eustachian tube dysfunction, the majority of otolaryngologists will remove the adenoids if patients need repeat tympanostomies and pressure equalization tubes after the first set.

4.2.1.1.10. Differential Diagnosis

Differential diagnosis includes:

- Viral URI
- Sinusitis
- Rhinosinusitis
- Nasal polyposis
- Pharyngitis
- Tonsillitis
- Seasonal/environmental Allergies
- Nasopharyngeal neoplasm
- Laryngopharyngeal reflux
- Lymphoma
- HIV

4.2.1.1.11. Prognosis

The majority of patients responding well to the available medical treatment for adenoiditis. For patients with recurrent disease, adenoidectomy offers a permanent cure by excising the hypertrophic or infected adenoid tissue.

4.2.1.1.12. Complications

If the patient's adenoids become chronically infected due to untreated adenoiditis, a biofilm may form in certain situations. Rhinosinusitis, pharyngitis, tonsillitis, and otitis media may result from the adenoids acting as a nidus of infection for other structures that are closely related to them.

4.2.1.1.13. Adenoid Hypertrophy

Adenoid hypertrophy is the cause of several of the more prevalent side effects associated with adenoid disease. The tissues surrounding the enlarged adenoids may pose a serious barrier to airflow through the nasopharynx. OSA, snoring, and mouth breathing can all be brought on by this enlargement. If untreated, OSA can be fatal and impair a child's ability to develop cognitively, emotionally, and behaviorally. By increasing the amount of air passing through the nasopharynx, removing the adenoids can reduce the frequency of obstructive episodes, improve adherence to oral appliances and continuous positive airway pressure devices, or even completely resolve OSA.

Additionally, enlarged adenoids may block the Eustachian tubes of the nasopharynx from opening. When the Eustachian tube is not working properly, negative pressure in the middle ear can build up, causing the tympanic membrane to retract and an effusion to form in the middle ear and/or mastoid cavity. This can result in conductive hearing loss, difficulty speaking, and act as a breeding ground for bacterial infections. Adenoid facies, also referred to as long-face syndrome, can arise from chronic adenoiditis followed by adenoid hypertrophy. An obligate mouth breathing pattern brought on by enlarged adenoids can block the nasopharynx and cause craniofacial abnormalities such as a retrognathic mandible and high-arched palate.

4.2.1.1.14. Consultations

For additional assessment and care, patients with recurrent adenoiditis or issues related to adenoid hypertrophy should be referred to otolaryngology. Depending on the needs of the patient, additional specialties such as gastroenterology, allergy and immunology, and sleep medicine may need to be involved.

4.2.1.1.15. *Deterrence and Patient Education*

Since children are often exposed to common pathogens and allergens that cause inflammation of the upper aerodigestive tract, adenoiditis is a common problem that may not be preventable. However, as these can result in complications that could lower quality of life, treatment must be sought before chronic adenoiditis and adenoid hypertrophy develop.

4.2.2. Acute Nasopharyngitis

Acute nasopharyngitis, or the common cold, is a viral infection that primarily affects the upper respiratory tract, which includes the throat and nose. Acute nasopharyngitis is usually self-limiting, but it can still be uncomfortable and inconvenient. Symptomatic treatment and supportive care are the main goals of managing this condition.

4.2.2.1. *Signs and Symptoms*

Common cold symptoms include runny nose, sneezing, coughing, sore throat, and nasal congestion. Muscle aches, headaches, fatigue, and appetite loss can also occur. About 40% of cases include a sore throat, 50% involve a cough, and 50% also involve muscle aches. Fever is uncommon in newborns and early children but usually absent in adults. When compared to the cough that comes with influenza, the typical cough is mild. Adult influenza is more likely to manifest as a cough and fever, but these two symptoms share a lot of similarities. Asymptomatic infections can also be caused by several of the viruses that cause colds. The mucus or nasal secretion's color can range from clear to yellow to green, but it does not necessarily reflect the type of agent causing the infection.

4.2.2.2. *Progression*

A cold typically starts with headache, sneezing, exhaustion, and a feeling of being cold. A runny nose and cough usually follow a few days later. After exposure, symptoms can start as soon as 16 hours later and usually peak two to four days later. Though some symptoms can linger up to three weeks, they usually go away in 7 to 10 days. 18 days is the average duration of a cough, and occasionally people experience a post-viral cough that lasts long after the infection has cleared. In 35–40% of cases, a child's cough lasts longer than 10 days, and in 10% of cases, it lasts longer than 25 days (Figure 4.4).

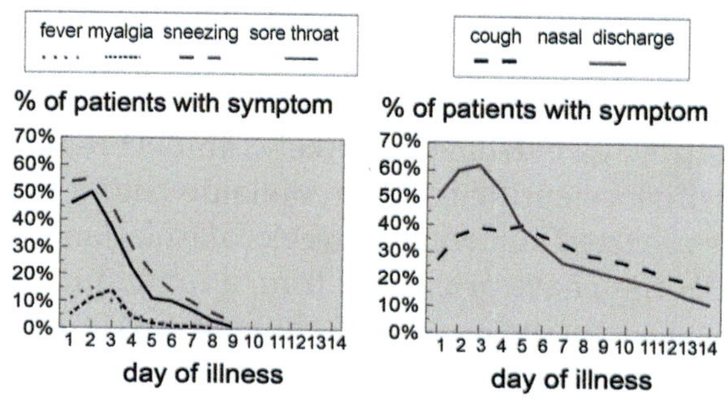

Figure 4.4. *Cold symptoms over time.*

Source: By US Government – The Centers for Disease Control and Prevention https://www.cdc.gov/getsmart/community/materials-references/print-materials/hcp/child-rhin-vs-sinus.pdf, Public Domain, https://commons.wikimedia.org/w/index.php?curid=54272465.

4.2.2.3. Causes

4.2.2.3.1. *Viruses*

A virus can cause an upper respiratory tract infection, which is what causes the common cold. The rhinovirus (30–80%), a kind of picornavirus with 99 known serotypes, is the most frequently implicated. RSV, parainfluenza, enteroviruses, and adenoviruses are among the other viruses that are frequently linked. There are usually multiple viruses present. More than 200 different viral types have been linked to colds overall. 20 to 30% of common colds have an unknown viral cause.

4.2.2.3.2. Transmission

Typically, direct contact with infected nasal secretions, airborne droplets (aerosols), or fomites (contaminated objects) are the ways that the common cold virus spreads. We do not yet know which of these routes is most important. The viruses can remain viable in the environment for extended periods of time (more than 18 hours in the case of rhinoviruses), and they can be transferred by people's hands to their eyes or noses, where they can cause infection. Animal-to-human transmission is regarded as extremely unlikely; an outbreak at a British scientific base on Adelaide Island that was reported following 17 weeks of isolation was believed to have originated from a contaminated object or an asymptomatic human carrier, not from the husky dogs that were also housed there.

The close proximity of numerous children with low immunity and often inadequate hygiene makes transmission common in daycare centers and schools. Other family members then get these infections at home. Evidence of recirculated air being used as a transmission method during commercial flights is nonexistent. It seems that the risk of infection is higher for those seated next to one another. In the initial three days of symptoms, rhinovirus-caused colds are highly contagious; subsequently, they become considerably less contagious.

4.2.2.3.3. Other

Herd immunity, which is a result of prior exposure to cold viruses, is crucial in preventing the spread of viruses, as evidenced by younger populations with higher rates of respiratory infections. One risk factor for disease is a weakened immune system. Malnutrition and insufficient sleep have been linked to an increased risk of infection after rhinovirus exposure; this is thought to be because of their effects on immune function. It is advised to breastfeed an infant who has a cold since it reduces the risk of lower respiratory tract infections and acute otitis media, among other illnesses. Breastfeeding may not be a sufficient defense against the common cold in the developed world.

4.2.2.4. Pathophysiology

It is thought that the immune system's reaction to the virus is largely responsible for the symptoms of the common cold.

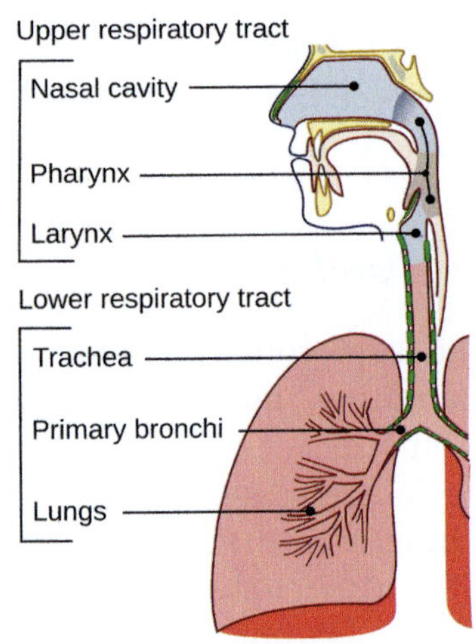

Figure 4.5. *The common cold is a disease of the upper respiratory tract.*

Source: By Lord Akryl, Jmarchn – Vectorized version of File:Illu conducting passages.jpg, which was in the public domain as a work of the US Government, Public Domain, https://commons.wikimedia.org/w/index.php?curid=112619332.

This immune response has a virus-specific mechanism. For instance, humans usually contract the rhinovirus through direct contact; it binds to ICAM-1 receptors on human bodies and, via unidentified mechanisms, the CDHR3 receptor, causing the release of inflammatory mediators. The symptoms are then brought on by these mediators of inflammation. The nasal epithelium is usually not harmed by it. In contrast, direct contact and airborne droplets are the means of contracting the respiratory syncytial virus (RSV). It then reproduces in the throat and nose, often moving on to the lower respiratory tract. RSV can harm epithelium. Usually, the human parainfluenza virus causes bronchial, throat, and nasal inflammation. Because of the small size of their airways, it can cause croup symptoms in young children when it affects the trachea (Figure 4.5).

4.2.2.5 Diagnosis

The common cold mainly affects the nose (rhinitis), throat (pharyngitis), and lungs (bronchitis). The location of symptoms is a loose indicator of which viral upper respiratory tract infection to differentiate. There may be a great deal of overlap, and the impact may extend to multiple areas. Self-diagnosis is commonplace. It is uncommon to isolate the virus agent in question, and symptoms typically do not allow for the type of virus to be identified.

4.2.2.6. Prevention

The most effective methods for reducing the transmission of cold viruses involve physical measures like proper hand washing and wearing face masks. Healthcare workers may also use gowns and disposable gloves in their workplaces. Isolation or quarantine is not typically used for the common cold due to its widespread nature and non-specific symptoms. Unfortunately, there is currently no vaccine available to prevent the common cold. The development of a universal vaccine is challenging due to the vast number of viruses that cause colds and their ability to mutate quickly. Therefore, creating a vaccine that effectively protects against all strains of the common cold is unlikely.

It seems that frequent hand washing can help stop the spread of cold viruses, especially in kids. It is unclear if adding antivirals or antibacterials to regular hand washing is more beneficial. There is not enough data to support keeping a larger social distance from infected individuals, but wearing face masks while around them may be advantageous. Whether taking zinc supplements influences the chance of getting a cold is unknown. Regular vitamin C supplements may shorten the duration of colds, but they do not lessen their likelihood or intensity.

4.2.2.7. Management

Medication and other therapies for symptomatic relief are the mainstays of treatment for the common cold. Reasonable precautions include getting plenty of rest, staying hydrated with fluids, and gargling with warm salt water. Still, a large portion of the advantages of symptomatic treatment are attributable to the placebo effect. There was no concrete evidence, as of 2010, that either herbal remedies or prescription drugs could shorten the course of an infection.

4.2.2.7.1. Symptomatic

Treatments for fevers such as acetaminophen (paracetamol) and ibuprofen, as well as basic painkillers, may help with symptoms. It is unclear, though, if acetaminophen reduces symptoms. The effectiveness of over-the-counter cough medicines in treating an acute cough is unknown. Children should not take cough medications because there is insufficient evidence to support their efficacy and there is a risk of injury. Due to worries about risks and unproven benefits, Canada restricted the use of over-the-counter medication for cough and cold in children aged six and under in 2009. A number of nations have banned dextromethorphan, an over-the-counter cough medication, due to misuse. It has not been discovered that intranasal corticosteroids are helpful. In adults, short-term use of nasal decongestants may provide some relief. Antihistamines can help with symptoms in the first day or two, but they do not offer long-term benefits and can cause drowsiness. Pseudoephedrine is an effective alternative for adults. Combined oral medications containing pain relievers, antihistamines, and decongestants are generally effective for older children and adults. Ipratropium nasal spray may help with a runny nose but may not be as effective for stuffiness. It can also assist with cough in adults. The use of nasal decongestants in children is uncertain. Some recommend avoiding exercise if there are severe symptoms like fever, muscle aches, or fatigue, but moderate exercise is generally safe if symptoms are limited to the head. While hot drinks are believed to help with cold symptoms, there is limited evidence to support this claim.

4.2.2.7.2. Antibiotics and Antivirals

Viral infections, such as the common cold, are immune system neutralizing agents. Antibiotics are generally harmful due to their side effects, but they are still prescribed a lot. People's expectations of antibiotics, doctors' willingness to assist, and the challenge of ruling out complications that might respond well to antibiotics are some of the factors contributing to the widespread prescription of antibiotics. Although some early research has demonstrated benefits, there are currently no effective antiviral medications for the common cold.

4.2.2.7.3. Zinc

When taken within 24 hours of the onset of symptoms, zinc supplements can shorten colds by as much as 33% and lessen their severity. There have been cases of smell loss following the direct application of zinc remedies to the nasal cavity.

4.2.2.7.4. Alternative Medicine

While there are numerous alternative and Chinese herbal medicines that claim to alleviate the common cold, there is currently a lack of scientific proof to back up these claims. Studies conducted up to 2015 show minimal support for the use of saline nasal irrigation. Furthermore, there is no concrete evidence that products containing Echinacea or garlic have any substantial effect on the treatment or prevention of colds.

4.2.2.7.5. Vitamins C and D

Supplementing with vitamin C may shorten the duration of the common cold, but it has no effect on its frequency. The effectiveness of vitamin D supplements in the prevention or treatment of respiratory tract infections is not well-established.

4.2.2.8. Prognosis

The majority of common cold symptoms usually go away after a week and are generally mild and self-limiting. In children, half of cases go away in 10 days and 90% in 15 days. If there are any severe side effects, they typically affect the very young, the very old, or immunocompromised people. It is possible for secondary bacterial infections to develop into sinusitis, pharyngitis, or ear infections 8% of cases are thought to involve sinusitis, and 30% involve ear infections.

4.2.2.9. Epidemiology

The most prevalent illness in humans, the common cold affects people everywhere in the world. Adults can expect two to three infections per year, while children can expect 6 to 10 colds (or up to 12 for school-age children). Because of their weakened immune systems, older people have higher rates of symptomatic infections.

4.2.2.9.1. Weather

There's a widespread misperception that being in cold weather for an extended period of time is enough to cause a cold. Even though it is now understood that colds are caused by viruses, many of these viruses do have a seasonal prevalence, appearing more frequently in colder months. It is unclear why there is seasonality in the first place. A lower immune response, changes in the respiratory system brought on by cold temperatures, and low humidity—possibly as a result of small viral droplets being able to travel farther and linger in the air longer—are some theories.

Social factors, such as people spending more time indoors, around infected people, and especially children at school, could also be the cause of the apparent seasonality. The majority of evidence suggests that severe exposure to cold, which results in a significant reduction of body temperature (hypothermia), may increase susceptibility to infection, even though it is controversial. Normal exposure to cold does not increase one's risk of infection.

4.2.3. Chronic Nasopharyngitis

Normal individuals have facial sinuses in their noses, which are in charge of exchanging nutrients and absorbing oxygen from the environment. Each sinus also has a vent and a mucosal layer covering it for protection. prevents the introduction of harmful bacteria. Bacteria have entered these areas in patients with chronic nasopharyngitis, resulting in mucosal edema in these sinuses, which has blocked the sinus openings, creating an environment that is conducive to bacterial growth. This growth, which may consist of both anaerobic and aerobic bacteria, eventually causes fluid and pus to drain down the throat, resulting in symptoms similar to chronic nasopharyngitis. Repeated symptoms following acute pharyngitis, lasting longer than one month and leading to chronic nasopharyngitis, are the signs of chronic nasopharyngitis. Chronic nasopharyngitis can be chronic tonsillitis, an inflammation of the tonsils brought on by bacterial or viral infections, dust and chemical pollution inhaled, reflux of the stomach, or chronic sinusitis.

Chronic tonsillitis-related nasopharyngitis frequently manifests after episodes of sore throat brought on by exposure to cold air, prolonged air conditioning use while sleeping, or consuming large amounts of cold water. Patients with a history of gastric illness are more likely to develop chronic nasopharyngitis caused by gastro-oesophageal reflux. Fluid from the inflamed sinuses running down the throat causes chronic nasopharyngitis, which results in dry coughing, burning and dry throat sensation, stuck in the neck, and possibly afternoon hoarseness.

4.2.3.1. Symptoms of Chronic Nasopharyngitis

The following are typical signs of chronic nasopharyngitis, which are frequently persistent and recurrent.

Long-lasting sore throat, pain that feels like it is burning, dry, and stuck in the throat. The aforementioned symptoms frequently manifest in the morning along with a lot of phlegm in the throat. Cough, protracted cough, frequent sputum production. A more severe case of hoarseness may result in voice loss. burning feeling behind the sternum, particularly in those who suffer from acid reflux. Systemic symptoms can include headaches, exhaustion, and fevers higher than 38°C.

4.2.3.2. Diagnosis of Chronic Nasopharyngitis

In addition to performing a clinical examination and taking a history, a number of paraclinical techniques, including endoscopy and CT scan, are now used to diagnose chronic nasopharyngitis caused by chronic sinusitis or other causes. During the examination, patients should collaborate with doctors to provide the most accurate information about their own medical condition and the most accurate symptoms in order to optimize the conditions for an accurate diagnosis. abnormal body symptoms in the nose, throat, respiratory system, and stomach that are frequently experienced to help physicians diagnose and treat patients more successfully.

4.2.3.3. Treatment of Chronic Nasopharyngitis Caused by Sinusitis

Following a thorough examination, history taking, and definitive diagnosis, the patient will receive appropriate regimens for the treatment of chronic nasopharyngitis. Currently, two treatment trajectories are being followed: treating the cause and treating the symptoms.

4.2.3.3.1. Treating the Cause

Chronic nasopharyngitis caused by conditions like tonsillitis and chronic sinusitis will typically be treated with antibiotics. Patients who also have a history of tobacco and alcohol use should be advised to quit these habits. In addition to medication, patients may be prescribed anti-edema and vasoconstrictor drugs to help open up the nasal passages and improve fluid drainage. Another effective method for treating chronic nasopharyngitis is the Proetz method, which involves washing the sinuses under negative pressure to remove fluid and pus. This method helps improve sinus function and reduce swelling over a period of about 2 weeks. It is a gentle and commonly used approach for treating this condition.

4.2.3.3.2. Symptomatic Treatment

In cases where the patient exhibits systemic symptoms like fever, headache, coughing or runny nose, and frequent sputum production, analgesics, anti-inflammatory medications, and cough suppressants must be administered. If the patient exhibits symptoms like foul breath or a dirty mouth, they should be advised to gargle with physiological saline solutions several times a day. Use physiological saline to clean the nose in order to reduce nasal secretions. In certain cases, such as polysinusitis, nasal polyps, and fungal-caused sinusitis, endoscopic sinus surgery is also necessary.

After treatment, the patient needs to be careful to heed the instructions. In order to stop the illness from coming again. Use physiological saline solution to rinse the throat and nose to avoid causing inflammation. Never consume food that is either too hot or too cold. In case you experience peculiar symptoms like stuffiness, sore nose, earache, etc., you must visit a medical facility to be examined and observed. If chronic sinusitis or other causes of chronic nasopharyngitis are not treated in a timely manner, they can result in severe complications like pneumonia, acute bronchitis, or even cancer. As a result, patients should visit a doctor right away for a prompt diagnosis and course of treatment if they exhibit any nasopharyngitis symptoms.

4.2.4. Tornwaldt's Disease (Pharyngeal Bursitis)

The inflammation or abscess of the embryonic cyst of the pharyngeal bursa is Tornwaldt's disease. It is situated in the middle of the nasopharynx's posterior wall. Mucosa in the adenoid mass covers it anteriorly. It is surrounded by the longus muscle on the back.

4.2.4.1. Signs and Symptoms

The signs typically show up when the pharyngeal bursa becomes inflamed, which results in a Tornwaldt cyst. This results from either spontaneous drainage in the nasopharyngeal cavity or from the nerve plexus becoming involved. The symptoms are occipital headache, cough, middle ear effusion, cervical myalgia, and halitosis, i.e., bad breath. The symptoms of a cyst enlargement include nasal obstruction, foul-smelling discharge discharged from the nose, blockage of the Eustachian tube resulting in otalgia and secretory otitis media, and pain just below the orbit.

4.2.4.2. Cause

Tornwaldt's disease can be triggered by various factors, including excessive alcohol and tobacco use, which weaken local immunity and allow pathogens to thrive, resulting in the disease. Other factors that can contribute to the development of Tornwaldt's disease include frequent exposure to high temperatures, malnutrition, chronic heart and kidney diseases, joint disorders, poor living and working conditions, and exposure to dust and harmful gases.

4.2.4.3. Pathogenesis

A rare benign disorder called Tornwaldt's disease is brought on by persistent notochord remnants. This illness essentially still has no symptoms. The pharyngeal ectoderm adheres to the cranial end of the notochord to form the pharyngeal pouch around the tenth week of embryonic development. This closes at the opening or crusts stick to the opening without shutting. The pharyngeal ectoderm comes into contact with these remnants, which causes the respiratory epithelium to grow. This creates Tornwaldt's bursa, which empties into the cavity behind the nose. This only develops into a cyst when the orifice is blocked by an infection, either totally or partially. Only after infection or inflammation takes place does a Tornwaldt's cyst develop into Tornwaldt's disease.

4.2.4.4. Diagnosis

A glass-shaped lesion with fluid on the upper portion of the posterior nasopharyngeal wall is visible on an MRI, and a solid mass of Tornwaldt's cyst is visible on a CT scan. On nasal endoscopy, there is also a cystic mass in the upper portion of the nasopharyngeal wall and mucopurulent discharge coming from the mass's upper portion. MRI is the most effective among them for identifying Tornwaldt's cyst.

4.2.4.5. Treatment

The infection is treated with antibiotics. Transnasal endoscopic marsupialization is the preferred surgical technique for treating large symptomatic lesions due to its safety, speed, and ability to provide clear visualization during the procedure. The endonasal approach is advised for small lesions.

4.3. Tumors of the Nasopharynx

A rare kind of cancer known as nasopharyngeal cancer affects the pharynx, the portion of the throat that connects the back of the nose to the back of the mouth.

4.3.1. Nasopharyngeal Angiofibroma

A benign vascular tumor called juvenile nasopharyngeal angiofibroma (JNA) develops in the nasal cavity. It can spread quickly and widely even though it is not cancerous. It can be extremely challenging to treat JNA because it can spread to many different parts of the head, such as the brain, the orbit (where the eye is located), and the sinuses.

- JNA primarily affects teenage boys; it very rarely manifests in younger children or males who have reached adolescence; it is rarely, if ever, observed in females.
- Patients with JNA usually experience an unexplained remission of the

illness once they are in their early 20s. Seldom will the illness worsen into a patient's 30s in certain cases.

- The main course of treatment is surgery. Patients may be prescribed medication to reduce tumor growth until the disease resolves in early adulthood if the entire tumor cannot be surgically removed.
- JNA is extremely rare, with only about 50 new cases per year in the U

4.3.1.1. Symptoms

Patients with juvenile nasopharyngeal angiofibroma may not exhibit any symptoms in the early stages of the condition. However, as the tumor grows, the following signs and symptoms could appear:

- difficulty breathing through the nose (due to airway obstruction)
- nosebleeds
- headaches
- If the tumor has grown considerably, you may experience double vision and other symptoms related to the cranial nerve

Patients rarely feel any significant pain.

4.3.1.2. Causes

The exact cause of JNA is unknown to scientists. JNA is not inherited, but it is slightly more common in children whose family members have familial adenomatous polyposis. Hormonal influences in JNA have been the subject of some research because the disease primarily affects teenage boys, although these investigations have yielded conflicting results.

4.3.1.3. Diagnosis

To find out if your child has JNA, several diagnostic techniques can be employed. Apart from a thorough medical history and physical assessment, these could consist of:

- **Endoscopic Evaluation:** To identify the presence of the JNA and the extent of nasal airway obstruction, doctors will use an endoscopic, which is a flexible or rigid telescope-like device that is inserted into the nose and frequently attached to a camera. Usually, this is done in the clinic for otolaryngology.
- Magnetic resonance imaging (MRI) is a diagnostic imaging procedure that creates two- and three-dimensional images of the body's soft tissue organs primarily using radio waves, a computer, and a large magnet.
- The computerized tomography scan, also known as a CT or CAT scan, is a diagnostic method that creates cross-sectional images, or slices, both horizontally and vertically by combining X-rays and computer technology. The skeletal structures of the body can be seen in more detail on CT scans.
- **Pathology:** To diagnose JNA, a combination of endoscopic examination, CT scan, and MRI is typically enough. Rarely, a biopsy may be required by your child's medical professionals in order to confirm the diagnosis.

Our experts convene following the completion of any required testing to go over and talk about what they have discovered about your child's condition. They then schedule a meeting with you to go over the findings and determine the best course of action for your child's care.

4.3.1.4. Treatments

Surgery is typically the first line of treatment, with the aim of removing the tumor as much as possible. It is ideal to remove the tumor completely. Depending on where the tumor has spread, it might not always be possible to remove it completely.

There are two parts to the first JNA treatment. Interventional radiologists performing angiographic embolization. In order to reduce blood loss during surgery, this is used right before the procedure to cut off the blood vessels supplying the tumor.

To remove the tumor, endoscopic surgery is the usual approach. This is a minimally invasive procedure that is typically performed through the nose. It is guided by pre-operative imaging studies and a special telescope called an endoscope. This can be completed in a single surgery if the tumor is localized and hasn't spread too far outside of the nasal cavity. Nevertheless, more than one operation might be needed if the tumor has grown considerably. Neurosurgeons will also be involved if it has affected the brain. Because of the location of the tumor, JNA surgery is extremely complicated, and it should only be performed by a surgeon with specialized training in this kind of procedure.

In certain cases, such as when the tumor has grown into the cranial cavity and is affecting the brain or carotid artery, surgeons may not be able to remove the entire growth. In these cases, there will still be fragments of tumor tissue. Your child's treatment team will talk with you and your child about additional therapies to treat this residual disease because it is possible for these tumor remnants to grow back. The supplementary treatment plan might involve the use of angiogenesis inhibitors, which are drugs that stop new blood vessels from growing. Occasionally, these drugs can reduce the size of the JNA tumor to the point where a surgical resection is necessary to remove the tumor. In other cases, the patient will have to keep taking the drugs until the illness clears up in their early adult years. Because radiation, especially so close to the brain, can have long-term side effects, radiation therapy is very rarely considered. Compared to radiation, medications frequently provide better disease control with fewer side effects.

4.3.1.4.1. Follow-Up Treatment

There is a chance that a new tumor could develop even if the patient's tumor is completely removed during surgery. Because of this, patients with JNA will require yearly follow-up appointments, where medical professionals will do endoscopic exams and obtain fresh imaging scans to keep an eye out for any potential recurrences. More frequent visits to a hematologist/oncologist will be necessary to monitor blood work, assess for side effects, and adjust medication dosages as needed if the tumor cannot be fully resected and adjuvant therapy is required. These visits will come in addition to the previously mentioned endoscopic exams and recurring imaging studies. Long-term results are typically quite favorable, despite the complexity of JNA. A skilled multidisciplinary team works to minimize any potential side effects from medication or surgery. Never is JNA is expected to be lethal.

4.3.2. Nasopharyngeal Carcinoma (NPC)

Cancer that develops in the nasopharynx, which is situated behind your nose and above the back of your throat, is known as nasopharyngeal carcinoma. In the US, nasopharyngeal carcinoma is uncommon. It happens in other parts of the world, particularly Southeast Asia, far more frequently.

Early detection of nasopharyngeal carcinoma is challenging. This is most likely due to the fact that the nasopharynx is difficult to examine and that nasopharyngeal carcinoma symptoms can be confused with those of other, more common illnesses. Treatment options for nasopharyngeal carcinoma typically include chemotherapy, radiation therapy, or a mix of the two. Depending on your unique circumstances, you can collaborate with your physician to decide on the best course of action.

4.3.2.1. Symptoms

Nasopharyngeal carcinoma may not exhibit any symptoms when it first appears. The following are some apparent signs of nasopharyngeal carcinoma:

- A lump in your neck caused by a swollen lymph node
- Blood in your saliva
- Bloody discharge from your nose
- Nasal congestion or ringing in your ears
- Hearing loss
- Frequent ear infections
- Sore throat
- Headaches

When to See a Doctor: It is possible that symptoms of early nasopharyngeal carcinoma won't always drive you to the doctor. See your doctor, though, if you experience any strange and persistent changes in your body that don't seem normal to you, like unusual nasal congestion.

4.3.2.2. Causes

Cancer starts when one or more genetic mutations allow healthy cells to proliferate uncontrollably, infiltrate nearby structures, and ultimately travel (metastasize) to different areas of the body. The squamous cells that border the nasopharynx's surface are where this process starts in nasopharyngeal carcinomas. Though elements that raise the risk of this cancer have been identified, such as the Epstein-Barr virus, the precise cause of the gene mutations that result in nasopharyngeal carcinoma remains unknown. The reason why some people who have all the risk factors never get cancer and others who don't seem to have any risk factors do is unknown, though.

4.3.2.3. Risk Factors

Certain factors have been identified by researchers as potentially elevating the risk of developing nasopharyngeal carcinoma. These factors include:

- **Sex:** In comparison to women, men are more likely to develop nasopharyngeal carcinoma.
- **Race:** More people in parts of China, Southeast Asia, and northern Africa are affected by this type of cancer. Asian immigrants in the US are more likely than Asian Americans to get this kind of cancer. In Alaska, there is also a higher chance of nasopharyngeal cancer among Inuit people.
- **Age:** Although nasopharyngeal cancer can strike anyone at any age, it typically manifests in adults between the ages of 30 and 50.
- **Salt-Cured Foods:** The cooking of salt-cured foods, like fish and preserved vegetables, releases chemicals into the steam that can enter the nasal cavity and increase the risk of nasopharyngeal carcinoma. Early childhood exposure to these substances may further raise the risk.

- **Epstein-Barr Virus:** Typically, this common virus causes mild symptoms similar to a cold. Infectious mononucleosis may occasionally result from it. Additionally, the Epstein-Barr virus has been connected to a number of uncommon cancers, such as nasopharyngeal carcinoma.
- **Family History:** Your risk of nasopharyngeal carcinoma is increased if you have a family member who has the condition.
- **Alcohol and Tobacco:** Smoking and excessive alcohol consumption can increase your risk of nasopharyngeal carcinoma.

4.3.2.4. Complications

Nasopharyngeal carcinoma complications can include:

- Cancer that spreads to infect adjacent buildings. If advanced nasopharyngeal carcinoma expands to the point where it invades surrounding structures, including the brain, bones, and throat, complications may result.
- Cancer that metastasizes to different bodily parts. Metastases, or the spread of nasopharyngeal carcinoma outside of the nasopharynx, are common.

Regional metastases are present in most cases of nasopharyngeal carcinoma patients. This indicates that cancer cells from the original tumor have spread to neighboring regions, like the neck lymph nodes. The most frequent destinations for distant metastases—cancer cells that spread to other parts of the body—are the liver, lungs, and bones.

4.3.2.5. Prevention

There is no foolproof method to stop nasopharyngeal cancer. However, you might think about giving up habits that have been linked to nasopharyngeal carcinoma if you're worried about your risk of developing the condition. For example, you could decide to limit your intake of foods that have been cured with salt or stay away from them completely.

4.3.2.5.1. Tests to Screen for Nasopharyngeal Carcinoma

The United States and other countries where nasopharyngeal carcinoma is uncommon don't routinely screen for the disease. However, in certain parts of the world, such as parts of China, where nasopharyngeal carcinoma is much more prevalent, physicians might recommend screenings to patients who are deemed to be at high risk of developing the illness. Blood tests may be used for screening in order to find the Epstein-Barr virus.

4.3.2.6. Diagnosis

4.3.2.6.1. Tests to Diagnose Nasopharyngeal Carcinoma

The following procedures and tests are used to diagnose nasopharyngeal carcinoma:

- **Physical Exam:** An examination in general is usually the first step in the diagnosis of nasopharyngeal carcinoma. Your physician will inquire about your symptoms. In order to check for lymph node swelling, he or she may apply pressure to your neck.
- Examine your nasopharynx with a camera to see inside. In case nasopharyngeal carcinoma is

suspected, a nasal endoscopy might be suggested by your physician.

The purpose of this test is to see inside your nasopharynx and look for abnormalities using a thin, flexible tube with a camera on the end. Either your nose or the orifice leading up into your nasopharynx at the back of your throat can be used to insert the camera.

Nasal endoscopy may require local anesthesia.

- Try to get rid of some suspicious cells from a sample. Your doctor may also perform a biopsy, or small tissue sample collection, using an endoscope or another device to check for cancer.

4.3.2.6.2. Tests to Determine the Extent of the Cancer

Following confirmation of the diagnosis, your doctor may prescribe additional tests, such as imaging studies, to ascertain the cancer's extent or stage.

Imaging tests may include:

- Computerized tomography (CT)
- Magnetic resonance imaging (MRI)
- Positron emission tomography (PET)
- X-ray

Your cancer is given a Roman numeral that represents its stage after your doctor has assessed the extent of the disease. There are four stages of nasopharyngeal cancer: I through IV. Your prognosis and treatment plan are based on the stage in addition to a number of other considerations. A lower number indicates that the nasopharyngeal cancer is localized and small. A greater number indicates that the cancer has progressed to the neck lymph nodes or other parts of the body from the nasopharynx.

4.3.2.7. Treatment

A treatment plan is developed in collaboration with your doctor and takes into account a number of variables, including the stage of your cancer, your desired course of treatment, your general health, and the side effects you can live with. Chemotherapy or radiation therapy alone are often the first lines of treatment for nasopharyngeal carcinoma.

4.3.2.7.1. Radiation Therapy

In radiation therapy, cancer cells are destroyed by powerful energy beams like protons or X-rays. External beam radiation therapy is the standard method used to deliver radiation therapy for nasopharyngeal carcinoma. Radiation is directed to the exact location where your cancer is located while you are lying on a table and a sizable machine is moved around you. Radiation therapy might be the only course of treatment required for small nasopharyngeal tumors. Chemotherapy and radiation therapy may be administered in other circumstances. Side effects from radiation therapy include hearing loss, dry mouth, and transient skin redness.

Brachytherapy, a form of internal radiation therapy, is occasionally utilized in cases of recurrent nasopharyngeal carcinoma. Radioactive seeds or wires are placed inside or near the tumor during this procedure. Radiation therapy to the head and neck, particularly when paired with chemotherapy, frequently results in painful sores in the throat and mouth. These sores can sometimes make it challenging to consume food or liquids. In such cases, the doctor may suggest inserting a tube into the throat or stomach for nourishment. This allows food and water to be provided through the tube until the mouth and throat have healed.

4.3.2.7.2. Chemotherapy

Chemotherapy is a pharmaceutical therapy that employs chemicals to eradicate cancer cells. Drugs used in chemotherapy can be injected intravenously, as pills, or both. There are three methods to treat nasopharyngeal carcinoma with chemotherapy:

- Concurrent use of radiation therapy and chemotherapy. Chemotherapy increases the efficacy of radiation therapy when the two are administered together. We refer to this combination of treatments as chemoradiation or concurrent therapy.

However, concurrent therapy is more difficult to tolerate because side effects from radiation therapy are compounded by side effects from chemotherapy.

- **Chemotherapy Following Radiotherapy:** Chemotherapy targets any cancer cells that are still present in your body, even if they may have separated from the original tumor and spread to other parts of your body. The question of whether giving nasopharyngeal carcinoma patients more chemotherapy genuinely increases their chances of survival is up for debate. Many patients who receive concurrent therapy and chemotherapy find they cannot handle the side effects and have to stop their treatment.
- **Chemotherapy Prior to Radiation Treatment:** Chemotherapy given either before radiation therapy alone or before concurrent therapy is known as neoadjuvant chemotherapy. To find out if neoadjuvant chemotherapy can increase survival rates in patients with nasopharyngeal carcinoma, more research is required.

4.3.2.7.3. Surgery

The most common treatment for nasopharyngeal carcinoma is not surgery. To remove cancerous lymph nodes in the neck, surgery may be required. A tumor in the nasopharynx may occasionally be removed surgically. To remove the cancerous tissue, surgeons typically need to make an incision in the roof of your mouth to gain access to the affected area.

4.3.3. Other Types of Nasopharyngeal Cancer

Though they are extremely uncommon, there are other cancers that can begin in the nasopharynx. Treatment for them differs frequently from that of the primary forms of nasopharyngeal cancer.

- **Adenocarcinoma and Adenoid Cystic Carcinomas:** These cancers may start in the nasopharyngeal minor salivary glands. However, the mouth and nose are more commonly affected by these cancer types.
- **Lymphoma:** Cancers known as lymphomas originate in the tissue of lymph glands, including the adenoids, or lymph nodes. The neck is full of lymph nodes. One of the most typical signs of lymphoma is painless lymph node swelling. Treatment for head and neck cancers, squamous cell nasopharyngeal carcinoma, and lymphoma differs.
- **Melanoma:** The pigment-producing cells that give skin its color are where melanoma begins to grow.

Melanomas of the head and neck can appear anywhere on the skin, in the oral cavity, or inside the nose or mouth. Seldom occurs nasopharyngeal melanoma.

- **Sarcoma:** Soft tissue sarcomas are cancers that arise in the body's supporting and connective tissues. Thus, soft tissue sarcomas can form and spread practically anywhere, though it is uncommon for them to do so in the nasopharynx.

4.4. Pharyngitis

Inflammation of the pharynx, the back of the throat, is known as pharyngitis. Most people just refer to it as "sore throat." Pharyngitis can also result in difficulty swallowing and a scratchy throat. One of the most frequent causes of doctor visits, according to the American Osteopathic Association (AOA), is a sore throat brought on by pharyngitis. Pharyngitis is more common in the winter months of the year. It is also among the most typical excuses given for missing work. Finding the source of a sore throat is crucial to treating it effectively. Infections caused by bacteria or viruses can result in pharyngitis.

4.4.1. Causes of Pharyngitis

There are numerous viral and bacterial agents that can cause pharyngitis. They include:

- measles
- adenovirus, which is one of the causes of the common cold
- chickenpox
- croup, which is a childhood illness distinguished by a barking cough
- whooping cough
- group A *Streptococcus*

The most common reason for sore throats is viruses. Viral infections like the common cold, the flu, or mononucleosis are the most common cause of pharyngitis. Antibiotics have no effect on viral infections, so the only purpose of treatment is to lessen symptoms. Bacterial infections are less common causes of pharyngitis. Medicines for bacterial infections are necessary. Group A Streptococcus is the culprit behind strep throat, the most prevalent bacterial infection of the throat. Gonorrhea, chlamydia, and corynebacterium are uncommon causes of bacterial pharyngitis.

Your chance of developing pharyngitis can rise if you get colds and/or flu frequently. This is particularly true for those who work in the medical field, have allergies, or get sinus infections frequently. Additionally, being around secondhand smoke may increase your risk (Figure 4.6).

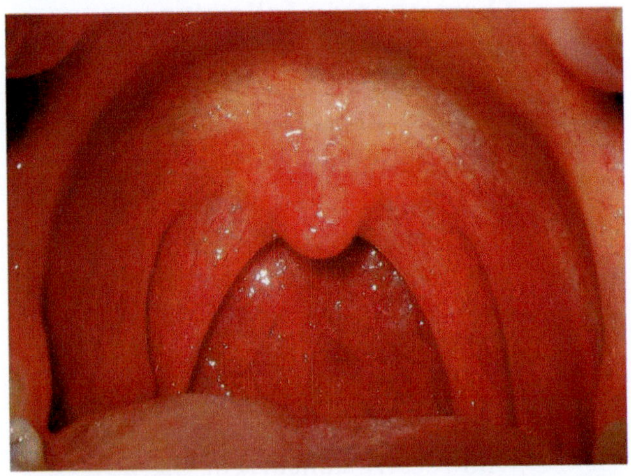

Figure 4.6. *Viral pharyngitis resulting in visible redness.*

Source: CC BY-SA 2.5, https://commons.wikimedia.org/w/index.php?curid=960953.

4.4.2. Symptoms of Pharyngitis

There is usually a two-to five-day incubation period. Depending on the underlying ailment, pharyngitis produces different symptoms. The symptoms of a cold or flu may include a scratchy, dry, or sore throat, such as:

- sneezing
- runny nose
- headache
- cough
- fatigue
- body aches
- chills
- fever (higher-grade fever from the flu and lower-grade fever from a cold).

In addition to a sore throat, the symptoms of mononucleosis include:

- swollen lymph nodes
- severe fatigue
- fever
- muscle aches
- general malaise
- loss of appetite
- rash

Strep throat, another type of pharyngitis, can also cause:

- difficulty in swallowing
- red throat with white or gray patches
- swollen lymph nodes
- fever
- chills
- loss of appetite
- nausea
- unusual taste in the mouth
- general malaise

The severity of your underlying illness will also affect how long the contagious period lasts. You will remain contagious if you have a viral infection until your fever subsides. You might not fully recover from strep throat until after taking antibiotics for a full day. Typically, a common cold passes after less than 10 days. The fever and other symptoms may peak in three to five days. This is how long you should expect your symptoms to last if you have pharyngitis linked to a cold virus.

4.4.3. Evaluation

To help with the diagnosis of Group A beta-hemolytic streptococcal pharyngitis and to direct testing and treatment, a number of clinical decision rules have been developed. Among the most popular is the Centor Score, especially for adult patients.

Centor Criteria (1 point for each) for Group A Beta-hemolytic Streptococci:

1. Tonsillar exudate
2. Tender anterior cervical left mentoanterior
3. History of fever
4. Absence of a cough

More likely in 5 to 15 years of age and not valid under 3 years old.

Point Totals and Recommended Actions:

- 0–1: No testing or antibiotics
- 2–3: Rapid antigen test
- 4: No testing, empiric antibiotics

To distinguish between bacterial and viral pharyngitis etiologies, white blood cell counts are not very useful. Higher than 50% lymphocytosis or more than 10% of atypical lymphocytes in the blood could be indicators of infectious mononucleosis. Though their sensitivity varies greatly, ranging from roughly 70% to 90%, rapid antigen detection tests (RADT) are very specific for Group A beta-hemolytic Streptococci. Treatment needs to start as soon as the test is positive. In the event of a negative result, especially in children, the course of treatment should be determined by obtaining a throat culture.

Although throat cultures have long been the gold standard for diagnosis, numerous variables can affect their sensitivity. The tonsillar surface is the ideal location for collection), the culture medium, the culture atmosphere, and the amount of bacteria present are some of these variables. The heterophile antibody, also known as the monospot test, has a sensitivity range of 70% to 92% and a specificity range of 96% to 100%. This test is widely accessible for infectious mononucleosis; however, Epstein-Barr virus serology is the recommended gold standard. Testing one to two weeks into the illness and the patient's age (less than 12 years) both reduce the test's sensitivity.

A culture must be obtained to detect gonococci. The most used type is Thayer-Martin agar. Use a potassium hydroxide preparation or Sabouraud agar to test for Candida.

In routine cases, a chest X-ray is not necessary. A lateral neck X-ray ought to be taken if airway compromise is thought to be present. A peritonsillar abscess (or quinsy) may be identified with the aid of a computed tomography (CT) scan.

4.4.4. Treatment / Management

Patients with Group A beta-hemolytic streptococcal pharyngitis typically receive antibiotic treatment for the condition. Antibiotics have the potential to reduce the duration of symptoms by 16 to 24 hours and avoid rheumatic fever, which is thought to occur in 1 in 400 untreated cases of strep pharyngitis, according to older data. Based on a positive culture or a rapid antigen detection test, antibiotics should only be administered to patients who test positive for Group A beta-hemolytic streptococci, especially if they are pediatric patients. To guarantee the elimination of bacterial carriage and avoid rheumatic fever, a 10-day oral penicillin course is advised.

For Group A beta-hemolytic streptococcal pharyngitis, oral amoxicillin or penicillin V therapy is available. Clindamycin, macrolides, and cephalosporins can also be employed. Another treatment option is intramuscular penicillin. Azithromycin and clarithromycin are not regarded as first-line antibiotics for this indication because resistance may arise during treatment. Cephalosporins can be used in patients with mild penicillin allergies. Patients who have previously experienced penicillin anaphylaxis may benefit from using azithromycin or clindamycin. After taking antibiotics for 24 hours, the disease is no longer contagious.

The evidence supporting the use of single-dose corticosteroids, such as dexamethasone, to lessen symptom severity is scant. It is advised to treat symptoms with gargles, acetaminophen, or nonsteroidal anti-inflammatory medications. When there is extreme dehydration, proceed with caution. Due to the possibility of splenic rupture, patients with infectious mononucleosis should refrain from participating in contact sports for six to eight weeks.

4.4.5. Differential Diagnosis

- Airway obstruction from any cause
- Allergic rhinitis
- Cancer of the head and neck
- Gastroesophageal reflux disease
- Peritonsillar abscess
- Diphtheria
- Epiglottitis
- Herpes simplex virus
- Mononucleosis

4.4.6. Prognosis

Since bacterial and viral infections usually self-limit to 5 to 7 days, the prognosis for pharyngitis is generally favorable. More than 20 million people in developing nations get acute rheumatic fever from group A Streptococci. In young people, this disorder is the primary cause of death. Pharyngitis rarely results in death, but it can if the airway is compromised. Pharyngitis usually goes away in 7 to 10 days. Poor compliance, untreated close contacts, and antibiotic resistance are the main causes of treatment failures.

4.4.7. Complications

Complications of bacterial pharyngitis include:

- Epiglottitis
- Otitis media
- Mastoiditis
- Sinusitis
- Acute rheumatic fever
- Post-streptococcal glomerulonephritis
- Toxic shock syndrome

4.4.8. Postoperative and Rehabilitation Care

If a patient has group A streptococci and their household members show symptoms, they should receive a full 10-day course of antibiotics without any prior testing. People who are asymptomatic don't need medical attention.

4.4.9. Deterrence and Patient Education

It is important to inform patients and their parents about the distinctions between viral and bacterial pharyngitis. To reduce their risk of developing rheumatic heart disease, patients with a diagnosis of group A streptococcus infection should be encouraged to finish the entire course of antibiotics. Antibiotics are not necessary for treating viral pharyngitis; instead, patients should be advised to treat their symptoms with over-the-counter pain relievers. This will lessen the overprescription of antibiotics and the development of bacterial drug resistance. It is important to emphasize the value of rest, fluids, and handwashing to all pharyngitis patients.

4.5. Tonsillitis

The inflammation of the tonsils, which are two oval-shaped tissue pads at the back of the throat, one on each side, is known as tonsillitis. Swollen tonsils, sore throats, trouble swallowing, and tender lymph nodes on the sides of the neck are all indications of tonsillitis. Although bacterial infections can also result in tonsillitis, common viral infections account for the majority of cases. It is critical to receive a timely and precise diagnosis because the best course of treatment for tonsillitis depends on the underlying cause. Once a common procedure to treat tonsillitis, tonsillitis removal surgery is typically reserved for cases where the illness is severe, doesn't respond to medication, or causes significant complications.

4.5.1. Symptoms

The majority of children with tonsillitis are in preschool through mid-teenage years. The following are typical tonsillitis signs and symptoms.

- Red, swollen tonsils
- White or yellow coating or patches on the tonsils
- Sore throat
- Difficult or painful swallowing
- Fever
- Enlarged, tender glands (lymph nodes) in the neck

- A scratchy, muffled or throaty voice
- Bad breath
- Stomachache
- Neck pain or stiff neck
- Headache

Tonsillitis symptoms in young children who are unable to express their feelings include:

- Drooling due to difficult or painful swallowing
- Refusal to eat
- Unusual fussiness

When to See a Doctor: If your child exhibits symptoms that could point to tonsillitis, it is critical to obtain a precise diagnosis.

If any of the following apply to your child, contact a doctor.

- A sore throat with fever
- A sore throat that doesn't go away within 24 to 48 hours
- Painful or difficult swallowing
- Extreme weakness, fatigue or fussiness

Get immediate care if your child has any of these signs:

- Difficulty breathing
- Extreme difficulty swallowing
- Excessive drooling

4.5.2. Causes

Common viruses are the most common cause of tonsillitis, but bacterial infections can also be to blame. The most frequent cause of tonsillitis is the same bacterium that causes strep throat, Streptococcus pyogenes (group A streptococcus). Tonsillitis can sometimes be brought on by other strep strains and other bacteria.

The first line of defense for the immune system against oral bacteria and viruses is the tonsils. The tonsils may be especially prone to inflammation and infection because of this function. But after puberty, the tonsils' immune system begins to deteriorate, which could be the reason for the uncommon cases of tonsillitis in adults (Figure 4.7).

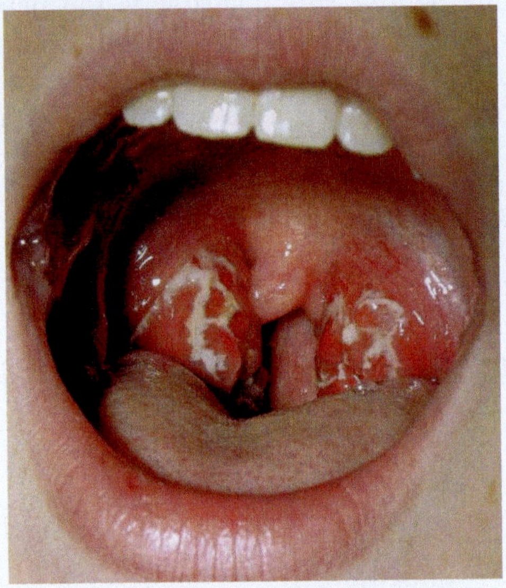

Figure 4.7. *A culture-positive case of streptococcal pharyngitis with typical tonsillar exudate in a 16-year-old.*

Source: By James Heilman, MD – Own work, CC BY-SA 3.0, https://commons.wikimedia.org/w/index.php?curid=11596322.

4.5.3. Diagnosis

The physician for your child will begin with a physical examination, which will consist of:

- Examine your child's throat with a lighted instrument, as well as likely the ears and nose, as these areas could also be infected.
- looking for the scarlatina rash, which has been linked to strep throat in certain cases.
- Gently palpate your child's neck to look for enlarged lymph nodes or glands.

- Listening to his or her breathing with a stethoscope
- looking for signs of splenic enlargement (to rule out mononucleosis, which also irritates the tonsils).

4.5.3.1. Throat Swab

Using a sterile swab, the doctor performs a quick test to obtain a sample of secretions from your child's throat. The sample will be examined for streptococcal bacteria in a lab or in the clinic. Numerous clinics are outfitted with a lab capable of obtaining test results in a matter of minutes. But a second, more trustworthy test is typically sent to a lab, which can usually return results in a few days or several hours. Your child most likely has a bacterial infection if the fast in-clinic test results are positive. In the unlikely event that the test is negative, your child most likely has a viral infection. To identify the infection's source, your doctor will, however, hold off until after the more trustworthy out-of-clinic lab test.

4.5.3.2. Complete Blood Cell Count (CBC)

A small sample of your child's blood may be requested by your doctor for a complete blood cell count (CBC). This test, which is frequently performed in a clinic, yields a count of the various blood cell types. It is possible to determine whether an infection is more likely to be caused by a bacterial or viral agent by looking at the profile of what is elevated, normal, or below normal. In most cases, a CBC is not required to diagnose strep throat. To help identify the cause of tonsillitis, the CBC may be required if the strep throat lab test comes back negative.

4.5.4. Treatment

The cause of tonsillitis determines how to treat it. Although bacterial and viral tonsillitis can have similar symptoms, there are differences in how they are treated. The course of treatment could involve:

4.5.4.1. At-Home Care

Whether a bacterial or viral infection is the cause of your child's tonsillitis, at-home care techniques can help them feel more comfortable and heal more quickly. These tactics are the only ones available for treating tonsillitis if a virus is the likely culprit. Antibiotics are not prescribed by your doctor. It is expected that your child will recover in 7 to 10 days.

At-home care strategies to use during the recovery time include the following:

- **Encourage Rest:** Encourage your youngster to sleep well.
- **Provide Adequate Fluids:** In order to keep your child's throat moist and avoid dehydration, give them lots of water.
- Provide comforting foods and beverages. Cold treats like ice pops and warm liquids like broth, caffeine-free tea, or warm water with honey can help relieve sore throats.
- **Prepare a Saltwater Gargle:** A sore throat can be relieved by your child gargling a solution of 1/2 teaspoon (2.25 milliliters) table salt mixed with 8 ounces (237 milliliters) of warm water, if they are able to do so. After gargling the solution, have your child spit it out.
- **Humidify the Air.** To avoid adding to the irritation of a sore throat, use a cool-air humidifier or spend some time in a steamy bathroom with your child.
- **Offer Lozenges:** Children older

than age 4 can suck on lozenges to relieve a sore throat.

- **Avoid Irritants:** Keep throat-irritating cleaning supplies and cigarette smoke out of your house.
- **Treat Pain and Fever:** To reduce throat pain and manage a fever, discuss with your doctor the use of ibuprofen (Advil, Children's Motrin, and other brands) or acetaminophen (Tylenol, and other brands). Treatment is not necessary for low fevers that are painless.

Unless aspirin is prescribed by a doctor to treat a particular disease, children and teenagers should not take aspirin. Aspirin use by children to treat symptoms of cold or flu-like illnesses has been linked to Reye's syndrome, a rare but potentially life-threatening condition.

4.5.4.2. Antibiotics

In case a bacterial infection is the reason for tonsillitis, your physician will recommend a course of treatment. The most popular antibiotic prescribed for group A streptococcus-induced tonsillitis is penicillin, which is taken orally for 10 days. Your child's doctor will recommend an alternate antibiotic if they have a penicillin allergy. Although the symptoms may completely disappear, your child still needs to take the entire course of antibiotics as directed. Infections can get worse or spread to other parts of the body if medication is not taken exactly as prescribed. In particular, your child's risk of developing rheumatic fever and severe kidney inflammation may increase if the antibiotic course is not finished. Discuss what to do if you forget to give your child's medication with your doctor or pharmacist.

4.5.4.3. Surgery

Tonsillitis that doesn't go away after treatment with antibiotics, chronic tonsillitis, or bacterial tonsillitis can all be treated with tonsillectomy surgery. The general definition of frequent tonsillitis is:

- seven or more episodes in the year before.
- In the previous two years, at least five episodes per year.
- In the previous three years, at least three episodes per year.

If tonsillitis causes hard-to-manage complications like these, a tonsillectomy may also be necessary

- Obstructive sleep apnea
- Breathing difficulty
- Swallowing difficulty, especially meats and other chunky foods
- An abscess that doesn't improve with antibiotic treatment

Unless your child is extremely young, has a complicated medical condition, or if complications arise during surgery, a tonsillectomy is typically performed as an outpatient procedure. In other words, on the day of the procedure, your child ought to be able to return home. Typically, a full recuperation takes seven to 14 days.

4.5.5. Risk Factors

Risk factors for tonsillitis include:

- **Young Age:** Tonsillitis most often affects children, and tonsillitis caused by bacteria is most common in children ages 5 to 15.
- **Frequent Exposure to Germs:** School-age children are in close contact with their peers and are frequently exposed to viruses or bacteria that can cause tonsillitis.

4.5.6. Complications

Complications from recurrent or persistent (chronic) tonsillitis can include tonsil swelling or inflammation. Others include:

- breathing problems that occur when you sleep (obstructive sleep apnea).
- infection (tonsillar cellulitis) that permeates the surrounding tissue deeply.
- infection that causes a peritonsillar abscess, or collection of pus behind the tonsil.

4.5.6.1. Strep Infection

Your child is more likely to develop rare disorders like the following if the tonsillitis brought on by group A Streptococcus or another strain of streptococcal bacteria is left untreated or if antibiotic treatment is not given in full such as:

- dangerous inflammatory disease that can harm the skin, joints, heart, and nervous system is rheumatic fever.
- consequences of streptococcal scarlet fever, an infection marked by a noticeable rash.
- glomerulonephritis, or kidney inflammation, caused by streptococcal infection.
- joint inflammation is the result of post-streptococcal reactive arthritis.

4.5.7. Prevention

It is communicable to contract bacterial and viral tonsillitis from the same germs. Thus, maintaining proper hygiene is the best form of prevention. Instruct your youngster to:

- In particular, after using the restroom and before eating, wash his or her hands thoroughly and often.
- Refrain from sharing cutlery, water bottles, drinking glasses, or food.
- After receiving a tonsillitis diagnosis, change their brush.

To help your child prevent the spread of a bacterial or viral infection to others:

- When your child is sick, keep them at home.
- Find out from your doctor when it is safe for your child to go back to school.
- Instruct your youngster to sneeze or cough into a tissue or, if required, their elbow.
- Instruct your youngster to wash their hands after coughing or sneezing.

4.6. Deep Neck Space Infect

Deep neck space infections (DNSIs) are a dangerous subtype of ENT presentations that carry a high risk of airway compromise and a quick patient decline. The mortality rate ranges from 1% to 2%.

Usually, the infection moves into the fascial planes from the oropharyngeal area. These are the primary DNSI types:

- Parapharyngeal abscess – is formed when an infection moves to the nasopharynx's posterolateral potential space (the most common subtype).
- Retropharyngeal abscess – The potential space anterior to the prevertebral fascia (often observed from necrotizing lymph nodes in children) is where infection spreads.
- Submandibular space abscess is most frequently caused by a dental infection that spreads to possible

submandibular, submental, or sublingual spaces (also known as Ludwig's angina); infection in these areas results in significant tongue swelling, which can quickly obstruct airway passage.

Given that their typical source is the upper respiratory tract and oral cavity, DNSIs are typically polymicrobial. The most frequent offender is *Streptococcus viridans*, although other common culprits include *Staphylococcus*, anaerobes, and Gram-negative bacilli.

4.6.1. Anatomy

Anatomically, there are two types of cervical fascia: superficial fascia and deep fascia. Skin, subcutaneous tissue, and the platysma make up the superficial fascia, whereas the superficial, middle, and deep layers comprise the deep fascia. The submaxillary and parotid glands, as well as the muscles deep to the platysma (the trapezius, sternocleidomastoid, and strap muscles), are covered by the superficial layer, also known as the investing layer, of the deep fascia. The masticator and submandibular spaces, which can serve as a focal point for dental or submandibular infections, are enclosed by this layer. The visceral organs of the neck, namely the parathyroid and thyroid glands, the pharynx, the esophagus, the larynx, and the trachea, are enclosed by the middle layer, also known as the pretracheal layer.

The paravertebral muscles and the vertebral column are covered by the deep layer, also known as the prevertebral layer. A thin membrane known as the alar fascia divides the retropharyngeal space, a potential space between the middle and deep layers anteriorly. The "danger space" is located posterior to the retropharyngeal space and stretches from the inferior oropharyngeal region into the posterior mediastinum up to the diaphragm. The parapharyngeal space is a potential area on both sides of the neck that is bounded inferiorly by the hyoid bone and superiorly by the base of the skull. It resembles an inverted cone. The superficial fascia borders it laterally, and the pretracheal fascia borders it medially. It is separated into anterior and posterior compartments by the muscles that attach to the styloid process.

4.6.2. Clinical Features

A wide range of symptoms can be present in patients, such as hoarseness or voice loss, neck stiffness, drooling, breathing difficulties, severe sore throat, and new-onset dysphagia or odynophagia. Upon examination, the patient will appear sick, exhibiting systemic infection symptoms such as pyrexia. Stridor, trismus, cervical lymphadenopathy, and pharyngeal swelling—which is frequently discrete—are among the clinical indicators of DNSI. Because there may not be any localized symptoms of erythema, oedema, or fluctuance, a low degree of suspicion is needed. Make sure to check for oral salivary gland openings, dental infections, and peritonsillar abscesses. Check for any parotitis that is suppurative. This is due to the fact that these are the most frequent infection sources that can lead to abscesses in the deep neck space.

In order to evaluate the patency of the airway and the supraglottic structures, a fiberoptic nasal endoscopy is a crucial addition to the examination. Since these structures are typically oedematous and inflammatory in a DNSI, take care not to upset the patient any more while doing this examination. To detect any parapharyngeal swelling, it is crucial to examine the pharyngeal wall in addition to supraglottic structures. Any pharyngeal wall enlargement or asymmetry should raise questions about DNSI.

4.6.3. Differential Diagnosis

There are numerous differentials for patients presenting with some or all of the characteristics of DNSIs because these infections have a variety of etiologies. Meningitis or encephalitis, tonsillitis or peritonsillar abscess, Ludwig's angina, epiglottitis, and foreign bodies are a few of these.

4.6.4. Investigations

Initial blood work will reveal elevated (sometimes very high) inflammatory markers, and if the patient is septic, there may be indications of end-organ dysfunction. In suspected cases, blood cultures ought to be obtained as well. The cornerstone of the investigation is a CT neck with intravenous contrast, which should be carried out as soon as possible in any suspected cases. This test will determine the location and extent of the infection. Plain film lateral view neck radiographs lack the sensitivity and specificity to be routinely used for investigation in modern practice, even though they can demonstrate widening of retropharyngeal tissue (>7 mm at C2, >22 mm at C7).

4.6.5. Management

Given the polymicrobial nature of DNSIs, patients should begin on broad-spectrum antibiotics with adequate aerobic and anaerobic cover, in accordance with local guidelines. One option to help reduce any airway swelling is to administer intravenous dexamethasone.

Maintain sufficient fluid resuscitation and use saline nebulizers to provide humidified oxygen (adrenaline nebulizers can be trialed as well); if there are any indications of airway compromise, a low threshold for intubation should be used. When feasible, maintain the patient's temperature at 45 degrees and make sure senior support is provided promptly.

4.6.5.1. Surgical Management

Surgical drainage and washout of the DNSI, sometimes with radiological guidance, constitute the cornerstone of management. Depending on the type of abscess, drainage can be done through the neck or mouth, and drains must be left in. On rare occasions, cardiothoracic involvement may be necessary due to the DNSI's potential to have spread inferiorly to the mediastinum. Patients should be closely monitored for clinical and biochemical improvement following surgery. There may be times when DNSIs re-accumulate and spread, necessitating repeated infection washouts and explorations.

4.7. Tumors of the Oropharynx

The most prevalent type of cancer in the throat is oropharyngeal cancer. It develops in an organ known as the oropharynx. Where the back of the mouth ends is where the oropharynx begins. It consists of the tonsils, the base of the tongue, the soft palate, the back and side walls of the throat behind the tonsils, and the soft part of the roof of the mouth. The pharynx includes the oropharynx. A tube called the pharynx extends from the rear of the nasal cavity. It attaches to the mouth, esophagus, and trachea in order of connection. Swallowing and breathing both require the pharynx. Almost all oropharyngeal cancers begin in the mucosa, the lining that covers the tonsils and base of the tongue. The majority of cases of oropharyngeal cancer are squamous cell carcinoma because this lining is composed of thin, flat cells called squamous cells.

4.7.1. Symptoms of Oropharyngeal Cancer

Oropharyngeal cancers frequently have no symptoms. A lump in the neck is usually the initial symptom. Some symptoms could be:

- Neck mass
- Difficulty or pain with swallowing
- Muffled voice

- Ear pain
- Throat pain or sore throat
- Lump or mass in the back of the throat

4.7.2. Diagnosis

Many oropharyngeal cancer patients first exhibit a neck mass. An evaluation, which entails a thorough head and neck examination to ascertain whether there is a tumor from which the cancer has migrated to the neck, should be scheduled for any adult who has had a neck mass for longer than two weeks. This could involve the doctor passing a tiny scope through the nose and looking into the throat to check for any suspicious masses. Oropharyngeal tumors ought to undergo biopsies. Some tumors that are accessible in the clinic may be the subject of local anesthesia during biopsies. Biopsies for other tumors are frequently done in the operating room with the patient asleep. This allows for a comprehensive assessment of the tumor's extent and offers diagnostic as well as treatment planning information. Under local anesthesia, a fine needle aspiration biopsy is performed in a clinic. This procedure involves inserting a small needle into the neck mass in order to extract cells. This makes it possible for a pathologist to examine the cells under a microscope and determine whether the neck mass is connected to HPV or is malignant. Imaging is a necessary part of a full work-up, and this can involve an MRI, CT scan, or PET scan.

4.7.3. Oropharyngeal Cancer Treatment

Treatment for oropharyngeal cancer is contingent upon a number of factors, such as the nature of the cancer, the size and location of the tumor, lymph nodes, swallowing and speech abilities, and the patient's general health. Chemotherapy, radiation therapy, and minimally invasive robotic surgery are among the available treatments. Sometimes, radiation is required following surgery. Treatment for these tumors usually entails a combination of chemotherapy and radiation when surgery is not an option. A multidisciplinary group contributes to creating the best possible plan for every patient. Researchers are looking into methods for treatment de-intensification that can lessen side effects while preserving survival rates. This could mean shorter treatment schedules for radiation, chemotherapy, or immunotherapy.

4.8. Hypopharyngeal Cancer

One uncommon type of throat cancer is hypopharyngeal cancer. Physicians also refer to it as head and neck cancer. It forms directly behind your voicebox, in the hypopharynx, the lowest region of the throat (larynx). Most cancers of the hypopharynx are squamous cell carcinomas. This kind of cancer develops in the cells that line the throat. A small percentage of cases of head and neck cancer are hypopharyngeal cancer. In total, roughly 65,000 individuals in the U.S. each year are diagnosed with head and neck cancer. Less than 3,000 of those cases are related to hypopharyngeal cancer. The incidence of hypopharyngeal cancer has generally decreased recently. The hypopharyngeal cancer can strike anyone. However, it usually affects men more than women, especially after 50.

4.8.1. Symptoms

Typically, hypopharyngeal cancer doesn't show obvious symptoms. Early-stage patients might not even exhibit any symptoms of throat cancer. Many of the symptoms of hypopharyngeal cancer can mimic common, easily treated ailments. Your medical professional can help you diagnose the issue and direct you toward the best course of action.

Hypopharyngeal cancer may cause:

- alterations to your voice, which could come out as harsh or raspy.

- Feel a lump along your neck.
- Sore throat that lasts for a long time.
- difficulty swallowing (which can make eating difficult or uncomfortable).
- Pain, ringing, or fullness in one or both ears that is not explained.

4.8.2. Causes

When something causes a particular type of mutation (change) in the DNA of healthy cells, cancer results. Cells grow uncontrollably as a result of this alteration. Cancer cells can grow into a mass or tumor if they are not treated. Certain cancer cells metastasize to different bodily parts. There is still much to learn about the reasons behind healthy cells developing into cancer. According to current research, alcohol and tobacco use are major contributors to the development of many head and neck cancers. The same holds true for cancer of the hypopharynx. Over time, tobacco products and alcohol harm the cells in the mouth and throat. At least 3 out of 4 head and neck cancers are caused by them. It is obvious that using tobacco products or drinking alcohol increases your risk of developing hypopharyngeal cancer.

4.8.3. Risk Factors

There are certain risk factors that increase your chance of developing hypopharyngeal cancer. The presence of one or more risk factors does not ensure that you will contract the illness. However, cancer can sometimes develop in the absence of risk factors. However, cancer may be avoided by adopting healthy decisions (such as giving up smoking).

Hypopharyngeal cancer risk factors include:

- Using any kind of tobacco (like smoking or chewing).
- too much alcohol consumed on a regular basis.
- Any head and neck cancer, including cancer of the salivary glands, that was previously diagnosed.
- getting radiation therapy close to the head or neck (to treat cancer or another issue).
- suffering from Plummer-Vinson syndrome, a condition associated with severe, chronic iron deficiency anemia and dysphagia.

4.8.4. Diagnosis and Tests

The first thing your healthcare provider will do is assess your symptoms. You might be asked by your doctor about the duration of your symptoms and whether or not you use tobacco or alcohol. Your provider can use this information to determine if you require additional testing. Your doctor will likely feel your neck during a physical examination to look for enlarged lymph nodes. They might use a tiny mirror to peer down your throat in search of anything strange.

To diagnose hypopharyngeal cancer, medical professionals may employ one or more of the following tests:

- **Endoscopy:** This scoped procedure is usually carried out in the office by an ENT specialist to examine further down your throat. A long, flexible tube that slides down the throat and into the mouth or nose is equipped with a camera.
- **Biopsy:** To remove abnormal cells, your specialist might do a separate biopsy procedure in the operating room. Subsequently, a pathologist—a physician in a lab—examines tissue cells carefully under a microscope to

search for indications of cancer. A biopsy can identify hypopharyngeal cancer or rule it out.

- **Imaging Tests:** To find out more about how cancer affects you, your provider may order imaging tests if a biopsy confirms the disease. Advanced computer technologies are used in imaging tests (such as a PET/CT scan, MRI, or CT scan) to obtain detailed images of internal organs.

4.8.5. Management and Treatment

A treatment plan tailored to your needs will be created by your care team. Surgery, radiation therapy, chemotherapy, and immunotherapy are among the treatments that are employed. Your recommended course of treatment may involve more than one type of treatment and will be based on several factors.

- **Chemotherapy:** Strong drugs are used to treat cancer cells all over the body. Chemotherapy may be used to reduce a tumor. Or, after surgery, it might aid in the destruction of any cancer cells that are still present in the body. In order to treat hypopharyngeal cancer, providers typically advise chemotherapy in addition to radiation therapy.
- **Radiation Therapy:** With the use of sophisticated machinery, specific radiation beams are directed to kill cancer cells while sparing healthy tissues. Based on the particulars of your case, your provider will suggest a type of radiation therapy as well as the length of time you'll need treatment.
- **Immunotherapy:** These more recent medications strengthen your body's defenses naturally. Immunotherapy improves the ability of your immune system to identify and eliminate cancer cells.

4.8.5.1. Surgery

Your doctor will take into account a number of factors, including the location and size of a tumor. Some patients require multiple surgeries.

Initially, your surgeon will take out as much of the tumor as they can. They might also remove neck structures or lymph nodes, among other tissues where cancer might have spread.

Surgery options include:

- **Pharyngectomy:** The pharynx is removed entirely or in part by the surgeon.
- **Laryngopharyngectomy:** The pharynx and larynx are removed entirely or in part by the surgeon.

4.8.5.2. Recovery after Surgery

The complexity of your surgery will determine how long it takes you to recover. Your surgeon will give you an expectation sheet. Surgery may have minor or major effects on your ability to breathe, eat, and speak. Certain modifications, such as a laryngectomy, might be irreversible. Prior to surgery, you might wish to inquire with your surgeon about:

- **Reconstructive Surgery:** In more complex cases, doctors may perform a second or simultaneous procedure to rebuild structures (like the pharynx or create a voice prosthesis). You may benefit from reconstructive surgery to maximize your overall functionality.
- **Speech or Swallowing Therapy:** Following surgery, your physician

might advise you to see a rehabilitative specialist, like a speech therapist. This qualified expert can assist you in adjusting to any difficulties you may have swallowing or speaking.

4.9. Snoring and Sleep Apnea

Others find snoring annoying, but it can also be an indication of obstructive sleep apnea (OSA), a more serious disorder that affects 3% of the population. Multiple breathing pauses lasting longer than 10 seconds at a time, caused by upper airway narrowing or collapse, are the hallmark of OSA. As a result, the blood's oxygen content decreases, making the heart work harder. The snorer may perform worse during the day because they don't get enough sleep, which makes them drowsy. Untreated OSA increases the risk of high blood pressure, stroke, heart attacks, car accidents, and other conditions (Figure 4.8).

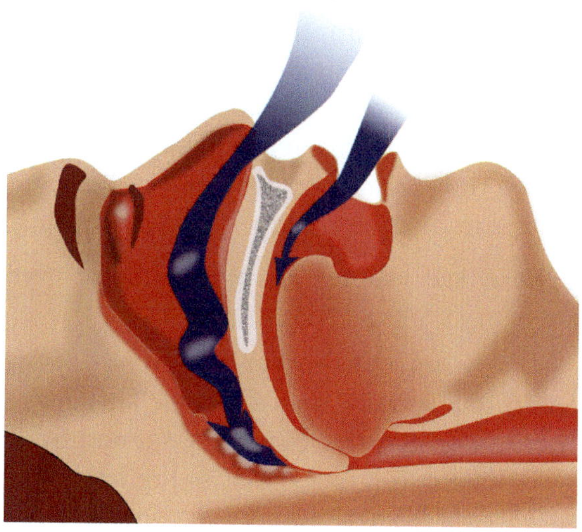

Figure 4.8. *Obstructive sleep apnea.*

Source: By Credits to Habib M'henni / Wikimedia Commons – Own work based on: http://topnews.in/health/files/sleep-apnea_0.jpg, Public Domain, https://commons.wikimedia.org/w/index.php?curid=10961498.

4.9.1. Symptoms of OSA

Symptoms associated with OSA can include:

- Loud snoring
- Pauses in breathing during sleep
- Waking up gasping or choking
- Waking up with a dry mouth or sore throat
- Daytime sleepiness or fatigue
- Frequent nighttime urination
- Morning headache
- irritability, fluctuations in mood, depression, and trouble focusing.
- Heart disease, stroke, hypertension, or other cardiac problems.

4.9.2. Causes

When there is a partial blockage to the airflow through the passages at the back of the mouth and nose, it can produce the loud sounds of snoring. This is the portion of the airway that collapses where the uvula and soft palate meet the tongue and upper throat. When these structures collide and vibrate while breathing, snoring results. When there is a more significant air flow obstruction, breathing becomes difficult or impossible altogether, resulting in apnea. Snoring in kids could indicate issues with the tonsils and adenoids. Adults may have more difficulty locating the obstruction. Adult obstruction can result from a variety of factors in several locations, making diagnosis and treatment more difficult.

Other factors that contribute to snoring and sleep apnea are:

- **Poor Muscle Tone in the Tongue and Throat**: The tongue can fall backward into the airway or the throat muscles can draw in from the sides into the airway when the muscles are overly relaxed. Sleep-inducing substances like alcohol can exacerbate muscle relaxation and blockage.

- **Excessive Bulkiness of Throat Tissue:** Youngsters who have big adenoids and tonsils frequently snore. People who are overweight may have an abundance of soft tissue in their necks, which can narrow their airways. Large tongues can make a person more prone to OSA and snoring. Tumors or cysts are uncommon reasons for airway narrowing.
- **Long Soft Palate and/or Uvula:** The opening from the nose into the throat is made narrower by a long palate. When breathing in a relaxed manner, the long soft palate and/or uvula function as a noisy flutter valve.
- **Obstructed Nasal Airways**: It takes more work to get air through a stuffy nose. This pulls the loose tissues of the throat together by producing an excessive vacuum in the throat. Sometimes the only times someone snores are during allergy season, when they have a cold or sinus infection. Snoring and OSA can also be brought on by abnormalities of the nose or nasal septum, such as a deviated septum, which is an abnormality of the wall dividing one nostril from the other.

4.9.3. Treatment

To make sure that sleep apnea is not the cause of their snoring, heavy snorers—those who snore continuously in any position or who interfere with their bed partner's sleep—should consult a doctor. An otolaryngologist, also known as an ENT (ear, nose, and throat) specialist, will perform a comprehensive examination of the nose, mouth, throat, palate, and neck, frequently with the use of a fiberoptic scope. A physical examination can determine whether snoring is due to tonsil and adenoidal enlargement, nasal allergies, infections, or nasal obstructions. If snoring is caused by OSA, a sleep study at home or in a lab may be required.

The most common treatment for OSA is using a device that slightly opens the airway under positive pressure. An appliance worn during sleep delivers this pressure through the mouth, nose, or both. For patients with OSA, continuous positive airway pressure, or CPAP, is the first treatment option that is currently recommended. The fact that obstruction of the airway can happen at several different levels presents a challenge in treating OSA. Though some wearers cannot tolerate CPAP and must look for other options, CPAP can be very effective in stabilizing pressure at all points in the upper airway.

For some patients with snoring or OSA, a custom-fit oral appliance that moves the lower jaw forward may also be taken into consideration. An ENT specialist, dentist, or oral surgeon with experience in sleep dentistry should fit this. Significant weight loss in certain patients can also help with OSA and snoring.

There are numerous surgical treatments for snoring/OSA, including:

- Uvulopalatopharyngoplasty (UPPP) is a type of throat plastic surgery in which the airway is opened by removing or repositioning excess soft tissue. Tissue vibration is also reduced because, as it heals, the remaining tissue becomes more rigid. Expanding the airway can also be aided by a tonsillectomy.
- The tissue bulk in the tongue base, soft palate, and/or nasal

turbinates—structures on the inside wall of the nose—is reduced by thermal ablation techniques. Both snoring and OSA are treated with these procedures, and multiple treatments might be necessary.

- Stiffening rods can be inserted into the soft palate or an irritating substance can be injected near the uvula to stiffen the soft palate.
- "Hypoglossal nerve stimulator" technology implants a tongue pacemaker, which stiffens and projects the tongue forward during sleep. Other procedures may be used to surgically target tongue muscles or the boney configuration of the midface. During sleep, a tongue pacemaker implanted with "hypoglossal nerve stimulator" technology causes the tongue to stiffen and protrude forward. The bone structure of the midface or the tongue muscles may be surgically targeted using alternative techniques.

A Closer Look

Peritonsillar Abscess (Quinsy)

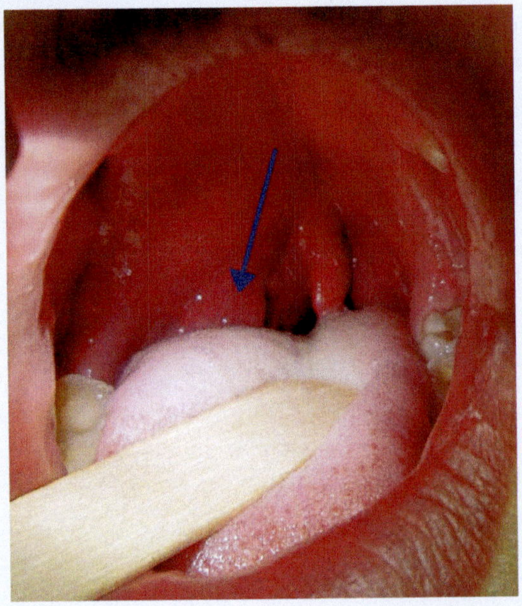

Source: By James Heilman, MD – Own work, CC BY-SA 3.0, https://commons.wikimedia.org/w/index.php?curid=15307040.

Quinsy, also known as a peritonsillar abscess, is one of the most prevalent deep head and neck infections in adults. It seems to be a distinct illness rather than a tardy consequence of tonsillitis because it affects adults and is caused by a different type of bacteria.

The effects are felt equally by men and women. The most frequently implicated bacteria are Fusobacterium and Group B beta-hemolytic streptococci (*Streptococcus pyogenes*). In the US, there are roughly 45,000 cases annually.

- **Causes:** A quinsy is believed to be caused by tonsillar tissue suppuration, or if the patient has already had a tonsillectomy, residual tissue at the upper tonsillar pole extending into the loose surrounding areolar tissue.

  Another explanation for the development of a quinsy following tonsillectomy is that an embryological remnant of the second internal pharyngeal pouch may form a congenital fistula. This is because the scar formation following the surgical procedure may block off this tract and prevent the free drainage of any infection occurring therein.

  Its etiology might also involve dental infection. Once more, quinsy formation can result from lesions caused by syphilis, tuberculosis, injury to this region, or the presence of foreign bodies. Additionally, it has been proposed that tonsillectomy itself lowers the risk of infection in this area by impairing the local immune response.

- **Symptoms:** Quinsy typically manifests as a fever, sore throat, and difficulty opening the mouth due to pain. The patient has pain over the same side of the ear, their voice sounds muffled, and they find it difficult to even swallow saliva.
- **Diagnosis and Management:** Both the physical examination and the history are highly suggestive. The soft palate is inflamed, the uvula is pushed to the side opposite the swelling, and the peritonsillar area on the affected side is swollen and reddened. Up to 95% of cases using an intraoral ultrasound scan result in a correct diagnosis, and its specificity is between 80 and 100%. If there is severe trismus in the patient, it may also be removed externally.

Antibiotics for both aerobic and anaerobic bacteria are the first line of treatment. Steroids can be used to shorten the healing time and to relieve pain and swelling. They do, however, also impede the immune response.

While aspiration of the peritonsillar abscess is generally regarded as the gold standard in management, incision and drainage may also be thought to be equally effective in confirming the diagnosis and relieving the condition.

When tonsillectomy is performed as part of the management at the time of presentation, it is a safe procedure that leads to a quicker recovery than interval tonsillectomy, which is performed three to six months after the initial management of quinsy.

It is more practical, lessens the need for follow-up, prevents a repeat admission, and offers instant relief.

However, since most patients recover fully from a needle aspiration under skilled hands, it might be deemed excessive treatment. 92% of patients may experience a quinsy recurrence; therefore, after the abscess has successfully cleared up initially, a group at high risk of recurrence may be chosen for interval tonsillectomy.

These signify the existence of congenital fistulae, recurrent tonsillitis, and dental disease or interventions.

Summary

- The area of the throat that is directly behind the mouth and nasal cavity and above the esophagus and larynx in humans is called the pharynx. The pharyngeal plexus innervates the three sections that make up the human pharynx: the nasopharynx (epipharynx), the oropharynx (mesopharynx), and the laryngopharynx (hypopharynx).
- The adenoid, a structure in the immune system, is situated at the nose-throat junction (nasopharynx).
- Acute nasopharyngitis, or the common cold, is a viral infection that primarily affects the upper respiratory tract, which includes the throat and nose.
- The inflammation or abscess of the embryonic cyst of the pharyngeal bursa is Tornwaldt's disease. It is situated in the middle of the nasopharynx's posterior wall. Mucosa in the adenoid mass covers it anteriorly. It is surrounded by the longus muscle on the back.
- A rare kind of cancer known as nasopharyngeal cancer affects the pharynx, the portion of the throat that connects the back of the nose to the back of the mouth.
- Cancer that develops in the nasopharynx, which is situated behind your nose and above the back of your throat, is known as nasopharyngeal carcinoma.
- Inflammation of the pharynx, the back of the throat, is known as pharyngitis. Most people just refer to it as "sore throat." Pharyngitis can also result in difficulty swallowing and a scratchy throat.
- The inflammation of the tonsils, which are two oval-shaped tissue pads at the back of the throat, one on each side, is known as tonsillitis. Swollen tonsils, sore throats, trouble swallowing, and tender lymph nodes on the sides of the neck are all indications of tonsillitis.
- Deep neck space infections (DNSIs) are a dangerous subtype of ENT presentations that carry a high risk of airway compromise and a quick patient decline.
- The most prevalent type of cancer in the throat is oropharyngeal cancer. It develops in an organ known as the oropharynx.
- One uncommon type of throat cancer is hypopharyngeal cancer. Physicians also refer to it as head and neck cancer. It forms directly behind your voicebox, in the hypopharynx, the lowest region of the throat (larynx). Most cancers of the hypopharynx are squamous cell carcinomas.
- When there is a partial blockage to the airflow through the passages at the back of the mouth and nose, it can produce the loud sounds of snoring. This is the portion of the airway that collapses where the uvula and soft palate meet the tongue and upper throat.

References

1. Albahout, K. S., & Lopez, R. A. (2023). Anatomy, head and neck, pharynx. In *StatPearls* [Internet]. StatPearls Publishing. Retrieved from: https://www.ncbi.nlm.nih.gov/books/NBK544271/ (accessed on 4 September 2024).
2. Fasick, J. (2006). *Respiratory System* (PDF). Benjamin Cummings (Pearson Education, Inc).
3. Snell, R. S. (2004). *Clinical Anatomy by Regions* (8th ed.). Lippincott Williams & Wilkins. ISBN 978-0-7817-6404-9.

Chapter 5

DISEASES OF THE LARYNX AND TRACHEA

Contents

Introduction

The voice box, or larynx, is located above the windpipe (trachea), at the back of the throat. The cartilage rings that make up the bump on the Adam's apple provide support for it. Stretchy bands of tissue connected to the inside of the larynx are called the vocal cords. These cords force the air that enters and exits the lungs. The vocal cords can contract or relax due to cartilage movements, altering the pitch of sounds. The nose, mouth, tongue, jaw, and throat are additional body parts that affect a person's voice quality. The epiglottis, a crucial flap or valve located in the larynx, covers the trachea when we swallow in order to keep liquids or food from going into our lungs. The larynx can be impacted by a number of illnesses and conditions, including cancer. Hoarseness is the typical symptom.

Depending on the suspected cause, different tests may be performed, such as:

- blood tests or throat cultures to look for infections.
- imaging tests such as computed tomography (CT), positron emission tomography (PET), or magnetic resonance imaging (MRI).
- To see your vocal cords while they are vibrating, use videostroboscopy.
- To examine your larynx, get a laryngoscopy.
- A biopsy involves removing tissue to be examined under a microscope.

The tube that begins beneath the larynx, or voice box, and ends behind the breastbone is called the trachea, also referred to as the airway or windpipe. The bronchi, which lead to the lungs, are formed when it splits into two smaller tubes. A healthy trachea expands and contracts with each breath. The trachea may become scarred and narrowed due to inflammation, or it may become soft and floppy as a result of birth defects or injury. Blockage of the main bronchi or the trachea can also be caused by tumors. Breathing can be adversely affected by any of these conditions.

Orientation and Directional Terms

Term	Definition	Illustration
Throat culture	A throat culture is a quick, painless test to look for infections. Your provider may do a throat culture if you have a sore throat.	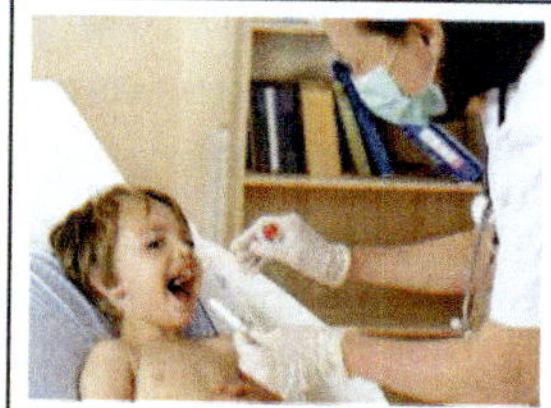
Magnetic Resonance Imaging (MRI)	Magnetic Resonance Imaging (MRI) is a non-invasive imaging technology that produces three-dimensional detailed anatomical images.	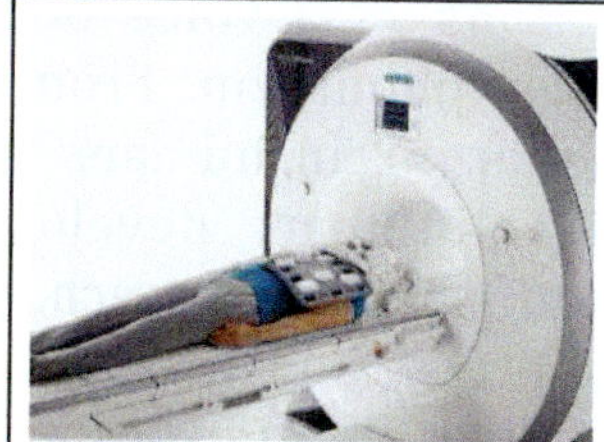
Videostroboscopy	A videostroboscopy is a test that can diagnose certain conditions that affect your vocal cords or swallowing.	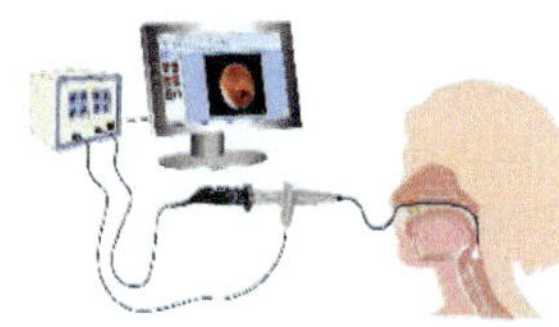
Laryngoscopy	Laryngoscopy is when a doctor uses a special camera to look down the throat to see the voice box (larynx) and vocal cords.	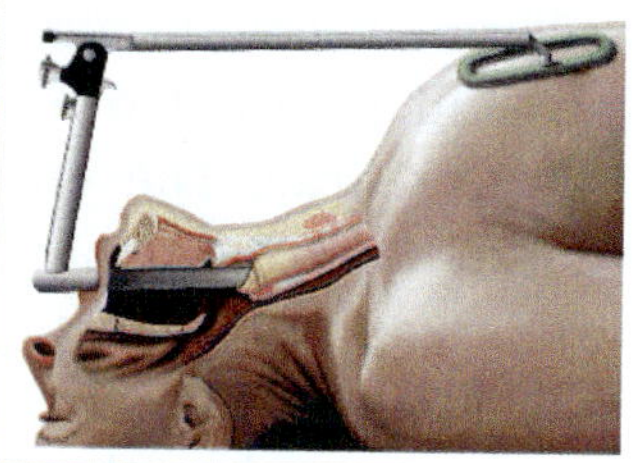
Biopsy	A biopsy is a procedure to remove a piece of tissue or a sample of cells from your body so that it can be tested in a laboratory.	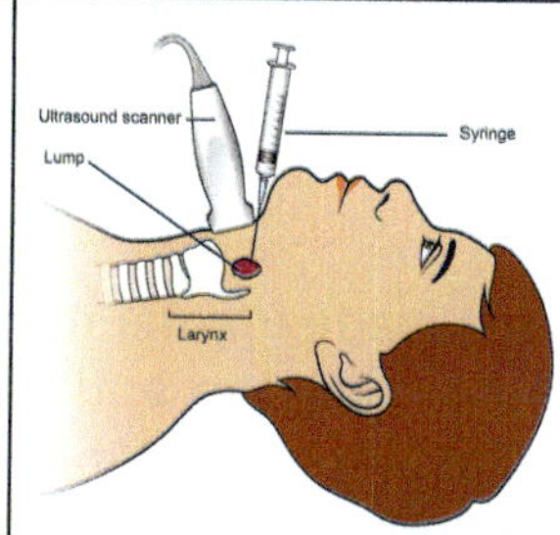

5.1. Anatomy and Physiology of the Larynx

The cartilaginous larynx of the respiratory tract is situated in the anterior aspect of the neck. In humans and other vertebrates, the larynx's main job is to keep the lower respiratory tract safe from food particles that might enter the trachea during breathing. It also contains the vocal cords and functions as a voice box for producing sounds, i.e., phonation. From a phylogenetic view, the larynx in humans has achieved its highest evolutionary development with the capacity to articulate speech, which is absent in invertebrates and fishes. The larynx has a slightly shorter anterior-posterior diameter and measures between 4 and 5 cm in length and width. Its size changes with puberty; it is larger in men than in women and larger in adults than in children. A larger larynx is associated with a lower voice pitch.

The larynx is held in place by muscles and ligaments and is situated at the level of the C3 to C7 vertebrae. The epiglottis, which is connected to the hyoid bone that is part of the inferior pharynx, is the area of the larynx that is the highest point. The superior region of the trachea is connected to the inferior aspect of the larynx.

5.1.1. Structure and Function

The larynx is made up of a mucous membrane, a cartilaginous skeleton, and a few muscles and ligaments that move and stabilize it. The thyroid, cricoid, epiglottis, arytenoid, corniculate, and cuneiform cartilages are the nine cartilages that make up the laryngeal skeleton. The cartilages in the last three are paired, while the first three are unpaired.

Thyroid cartilage extends vertically from the superior to inferior regions of the larynx, serving as a shield of defense around its anterior portion. The laryngeal prominence, also referred to as Adam's apple, is the largest of the six cartilages. It resembles a half-opened book with the back facing the front and the two halves meeting in the center to form the protrusion. Since it is the only cartilage that completely encircles the trachea, the cricoid cartilage is also referred to as the cricoid ring or signet ring. It consists of two parts: the anterior part, also known as the arch, and the posterior part, which is much wider than the anterior and is called the lamina. It is located at the level of the C6 vertebra in the inferior part of the larynx.

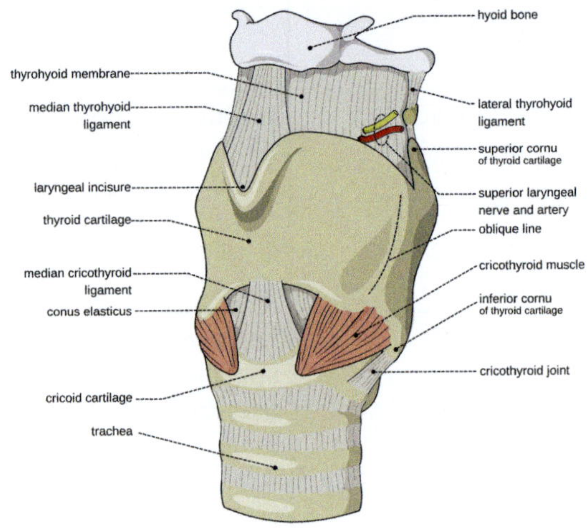

Figure 5.1. *Anatomy of the larynx, anterolateral view.*

Source: By Olek Remesz (wiki-pl: Orem, commons: Orem) – Own work based on: Gray951.png, CC BY-SA 2.5, https://commons.wikimedia.org/w/index.php?curid=3492701.

The epiglottis is a leaf-shaped flap made of elastic cartilaginous tissue that covers the larynx's opening. It protrudes over the pharynx and is attached to the inside surface of the thyroid cartilage, which permits air to enter the trachea, lungs, and larynx. When swallowing, the hyoid bone raises the larynx, allowing food or liquids to pass through the esophagus and keeping food from going into the trachea. There are three paired cartilages in the second set of cartilages. Two small, flexible, hard, pyramid-shaped cartilages called arytenoid cartilages cover the posterior region of the cricoid cartilage. Every cartilage base has two processes: the vocal process is located at the anterior angle, and the muscular process is located at the lateral angle. The apices of the arytenoid cartilages articulate with the small, elastic, cone-shaped corniculate cartilages, also known as the Santorini cartilages (Figure 5.1).

The two long, fibrous segments of yellow cartilage on either side of the aryepiglottic fold are called the cuneiform cartilages, or Wrisberg cartilages. They support the vocal folds and the lateral aspects of the epiglottis but do not directly attach to other cartilages. There are multiple joints that allow the laryngeal cartilages to move. The thyroid cartilage and the cricoid arch are joined by the cricothyroid joint. Each arytenoid cartilage is connected to the cricoid cartilage by the cricoarytenoid joints, and the Santorini cartilage is connected to the arytenoid cartilage by the arycorniculate joint.

5.1.1.1. Larynx Ligaments

There are two different kinds of ligaments: intrinsic ligaments, which link the larynx cartilages together, and extrinsic ligaments, which attach the larynx to other structures like the trachea or hyoid. The cricothyroid, cricocorniculate, thyroepiglottic, thyroarytenoid, and arytenoidepiglottic ligaments are the intrinsic ligaments. With its base in the superior border of the cricoid cartilage and its apex in the center of the thyroid cartilage, the cricothyroid membrane, also known as the cricothyroid ligament, is shaped like a pyramid. The Santorini cartilage and the cricoid cartilage are connected by two fibrous bands called the cricocorniculate ligaments. The thyroid ligament and the epiglottis are joined by the thyroepiglottic ligament. The thyroarytenoid ligaments split into the superior ligament, which rests next to the superior vocal cords, and the inferior ligament, which rests on the inferior vocal cords. They run from the outer portion of the arytenoid cartilages to the middle portion of the thyroid cartilage. The arytenoid cartilages are joined to the epiglottis by the arytenoidepiglottic ligaments.

The cricotracheal, hyoepiglottic, and thyrohyoid ligaments are the extrinsic ligaments. The upper border of the thyroid cartilage and the posterior surface of the hyoid bone are joined by the thyrohyoid ligament, also known as the membrane. The surface of the epiglottis and the upper border of the hyoid bone are joined by the hyoepiglottic ligament. The cricoid ligament and the first ring of the trachea are joined by the cricotracheal ligament.

5.1.1.2. Laryngeal Cavity

The larynx's internal space reaches the lower edge of the cricoid cartilage by way of the laryngeal inlet. It has a pyramidal form, with the trachea at the apex and the tongue at the superior base. It is composed of one posterior and two lateral parts, as well as a base and an apex. The anterior wall of the pharynx forms the posterior portion of the internal space of the larynx, which contains two vertical recesses known as the piriform sinus. The larynx cartilage, which is divided into three parts—a superior part that resembles the thyroid cartilage, an inferior part that resembles the cricoid cartilage, and a middle part known as the cricothyroid space—determines the shape of the lateral aspects. The trachea is joined to the larynx by a hole formed by its apex. The pharynx and larynx communicate through the oval-shaped base of the larynx.

The larynx's internal space is divided into three sections: supraglottic, glottis, and infraglottic. The internal space is broad in the superior and inferior regions but becomes narrow in the middle, forming a section known as the glottis. The glottic space is made up of the larynx ventricles, the glottis, and the vocal cords. The vocal cords consist of two superior and two inferior folds of fibro-elastic tissue that are inserted anteriorly into the thyroid cartilage and posteriorly into the arytenoid cartilage. The inferior vocal cords are wider and have a muscular fascicle running the length of them, whereas the superior vocal cords are narrow, ribbon-shaped, and devoid of muscle elements. When looking at the larynx from above, one can see that there are four vocal cords because the space between the superior and inferior vocal cords is greater. Since only the inferior vocal cords can approach one another, the inferior vocal cords are referred to as true vocal folds, and the superior vocal cords are referred to as false vocal cords or folds.

The area of the larynx that is made up of the four vocal folds and the space between them is called the glottis. The inferior (actual vocal folds) and superior vocal cords (vestibular folds) are separated by a fusiform fossa, which is known as the laryngeal ventricles or Morgagni sinus. The vocal cords and trachea define the boundaries of the subglottic section, which is the region beneath the glottis and has the shape of an inverted bottleneck. The hyoepiglottic ligament is typically thought of as the roof of the supraglottic cavity, which is formed by the supraglottic section and extends along the free edge of the epiglottis and the aryepiglottic folds down to the arytenoid cartilages.

5.1.2. Embryology

The laryngotracheal groove, a longitudinal notch, marks the location of the earliest human larynx, which originated in the first four weeks of intrauterine life on the primitive pharyngeal floor. Around the fifth week of embryonic life, this groove will eventually form the esophagotracheal septum, with the respiratory system located anteriorly and the esophagus on the dorsal side.

Splanchnic mesenchyme, which is situated ventral to the foregut, is the source of the cartilage, smooth muscles, and connective tissue that will make up the larynx. The third, fourth, and sixth pharyngeal arches give rise to the larynx cartilages.

Because of some paired arytenoid swellings brought on by the mesenchyme's proliferation, the primitive glottis has a T-shaped form during this time, resulting in a small opening for the larynx. The laryngeal epithelium grows rapidly, momentarily obliterating the laryngeal lumen before breaking apart and re-canalizing in the tenth week. Two lateral depressions connected to the mucous membrane's anterioposterior folds give rise to the future vocal cords.

5.1.3. Blood Supply and Lymphatics

The superior and inferior laryngeal arteries provide blood to the larynx. The epiglottis, supraglottic area, and superior vocal cords are supplied by the superior laryngeal artery, a branch of the superior thyroid artery. The subglottic area and the inferior vocal cords are supplied by the inferior laryngeal artery, which is a branch of the superior thyroid artery. The posterior cricoarytenoid and arytenoid muscles are supplied by a small branch of the superior thyroid artery that occasionally branches off of the inferior laryngeal artery.

The laryngeal veins bear the same names as the arteries, i.e., the laryngeal veins, superior and inferior. These veins empty into the internal jugular and subclavian veins, respectively, after emptying into the superior and inferior thyroid veins. The lymph drainage of the larynx is separated into the infraglottic and supraglottic lymphatics. The deep cervical lymphatics receive the output of the dense supraglottic lymphatic nodes. Pre and paratracheal nodes, as well as prelaryngeal nodes, are where the less dense subglottic lymphatics drain into the lower deep cervical nodes. There are no lymphatics in the glottic area or the vocal folds.

5.1.4. Nerves

The inferior laryngeal nerve, recurrent laryngeal nerve, and superior laryngeal nerve innervate the larynx. The inferior ganglion of the vagus nerve gives rise to the superior laryngeal nerve, which is a branch of the vagus nerve (X cranial nerve). It also receives branches from the sympathetic nervous system's superior cervical ganglion. It descends between the pharynx and carotid vessels before arriving at the larynx, which is located just below the hyoid bone. There, it splits into the internal and external branches. The cricothyroid muscle is supplied by the external laryngeal nerve. Together with the superior laryngeal artery, the internal laryngeal nerve descends to the thyrohyoid membrane, extending across the epiglottis and supplying the mucous membrane that envelops the laryngeal opening.

With the exception of the cricothyroid muscle, all of the intrinsic laryngeal muscles are innervated by the inferior laryngeal nerve, also known as the recurrent nerve. The recurrent nerves on the left and right are asymmetrical. The right recurrent nerve loops around the subclavian artery, while the left recurrent nerve originates from the vagus nerve bellow into the thorax, loops around the aortic arch, passes upward to the trachea and esophagus, and then enters the larynx just posterior to the cricothyroid joint beneath the inferior constrictor muscle. At the base of the neck, the right recurrent nerves split off from the vagus, looping around the subclavian artery before ascending lateral to the trachea and entering the larynx between the thyroid and cricoid cartilages. The Galen anastomosis is where the inferior and internal laryngeal nerves normally join.

5.1.5. Muscles

The two main types of laryngeal muscles are extrinsic muscles, which move the larynx, and intrinsic muscles, which produce voice. We'll look at the former first before the latter.

5.1.5.1. Intrinsic Muscles

The cricothyroid muscle attaches to the cricoid arch, the thyroid's lower lamina to the superior belly, and the inferior cornu to the inferior belly. It has two concave surfaces: the superior and inferior. Higher pitch phonation is produced by these muscles by elongating the vocal folds. The arytenoid cartilage and the posterior cricoid cartilage are where the posterior cricoarytenoid muscle is attached. Unlike the lateral cricoarytenoid muscles, these muscles abduct, or open, the vocal cords. From the lateral cricoid cartilage to the muscular process of the arytenoid cartilage, the lateral or anterior cricoarytenoid muscles extend. These muscles do the opposite action of the posterior cricoarytenoid muscles, which is to adduct the vocal folds.

The middle cricothyroid ligaments and the thyroid cartilage are the sources of the thyroarytenoid muscles, which insert into the arytenoid cartilage. As they loosen up, these muscles resemble the vocal folds. The aryepiglottic muscles reach the epiglottis from the arytenoid cartilages. The aryepiglottic folds are adducted by these muscles. The transverse and oblique regions between the arytenoid cartilages are covered by the arytenoid muscles. The only laryngeal intrinsic muscle that is compromised is the transverse arytenoid muscle. The vocal folds are adducted by these muscles.

5.1.5.2. Extrinsic Muscles

The larynx can move because of the paired extrinsic larynx muscles. The body of the hyoid bone and the thyroid cartilage are where the thyrohyoid muscle inserts. The hypoglossal nerve as well as the first cervical nerve innervate the. Its main purpose is to elevate the larynx by depressing the hyoid bone. The sternothyroid muscles originate from the sternum and first rib, travel to the lamina of the thyroid cartilage, and are innervated by the Ansa cervicalis. They are located beneath the sternohyoideus muscle. The larynx is depressed by these muscles.

The cricoid and thyroid cartilages to the pharyngeal raphe are the locations of the inferior pharyngeal constrictor muscles. These muscles narrow the pharynx diameter to aid in swallowing and are innervated by the vagus nerve through branches of the pharyngeal plexus and recurrent laryngeal nerve. The muscles of the stylopharyngeus extend from the thyroid cartilage to the styloid process located in the temporal bone. The pharynx and larynx are elevated by these muscles, which derive their nerve supply from the glossopharyngeal nerve. The palatine aponeurosis and pterygoid processes give rise to the palatopharyngeus muscles, which insert into the thyroid cartilage. They elevate the larynx and pharynx and are a component of the soft palate. The pharyngeal branch innervates them.

The geniohyoid, mylohyoid, digastric, or stylohyoid muscles, which elevate the larynx, and the omohyoid and sternohyoid muscles, which cause laryngeal depression, are examples of other muscles that may also contribute to the movement of the larynx but are not strictly considered laryngeal because they do not insert in the larynx or any of its parts.

5.1.6. Physiologic Variants

The fundamental reason why male and female voices differ is because of the larynx, a structure that can display multiple gender-specific differences. The larynx of males is typically more pronounced than that of females. Similar variations between the sexes can also be seen in the thyroid, which is thicker and has a different angle in men (95 degrees versus approximately 115 degrees in women). Individual differences may also exist in laryngeal innervation. As a result, numerous variants of the recurrent laryngeal nerve have been identified through extensive research. The recurrent laryngeal nerve, for instance, can split into two or more branches. It has been observed that the anterior branch enters the larynx either anteriorly or posteriorly to the cricothyroid joint. Because the left recurrent nerve loops around the aortic arch, aortic aneurysms or even individual variations in the aortic arch may cause variations in the nerve's course. Studies have also been conducted on "non-recurrent" inferior laryngeal nerve cases, in which the recurrent laryngeal nerve travels straight from the vagus in the neck to the larynx without circumnavigating the subclavian artery.

The relationship between the inferior thyroid artery and the recurrent laryngeal nerve has also drawn a lot of attention. Generally, the nerve ascends posterior to the artery (about 60%), but on rare occasions, it may ascend anteriorly (about 32.5%) or even between the artery's branches (roughly 60.5%). The risk of surgical injury makes the position of the recurrent nerve crucial.

5.2. Laryngotracheal Trauma

Trauma to the larynx is rare but may prove to be fatal. There are two types of laryngeal trauma: penetrating and blunt. Even with a minor injury, a fibrous union, a deformity, and impaired laryngeal function, laryngeal injuries can heal. These wounds can occur in the supraglottic, glottic, or infraglottic regions and can be blunt or penetrating. It is important to understand laryngeal damage in detail because blunt trauma, as opposed to penetrating laryngeal trauma, can cause different sequences and levels of wound severity. Before undergoing further testing, patients with a history of anterior neck trauma should have their larynx carefully examined for damage symptoms and have a secure airway confirmed.

Acute, subacute, penetrating, or blunt trauma can all occur in the trachea. Even though there may be subacute injuries, a blow to the neck can result in a crush injury to the upper chest, a knife wound, or an acute traumatic disruption of the trachea. After a blunt neck injury, the trachea can become disrupted, usually within 3 cm of the carina. Based on the etiology, tracheal trauma may be followed by involvement of the digestive system or vascular damage to nearby structures, such as the main arteries, carotids, or jugulars. However, to avoid complications and the loss of respiratory function, early detection and surgical treatment are required.

5.2.1. Etiology

Although motor vehicle accidents remain the primary cause of laryngeal injuries, advancements in car safety measures such as seat belts and airbags have significantly reduced the occurrence of such injuries. Other causes, such as attacks, strangulation, and penetrating wounds, also contribute to laryngeal damage. Additionally, iatrogenic injuries can occur during medical procedures like bronchoscopy, intubation, or tracheostomy.

The larynx is frequently shielded from blunt trauma by the sternum and jaw. A clothesline injury occurs when the exposed neck is struck by a hard object, like a tree branch or wall wire, or when an attack is meant to harm the larynx. Stress and damage to the neck can result in injuries. A rear-end collision that causes whiplash-like injuries or intentional harm to the larynx can also result in injuries. When there are penetrating neck injuries, the larynx can get injured. If a patient has had a traumatic or penetrating neck injury, it is typically clear from the vital trauma assessment or the patient's history. On the other hand, it is advised to use minimal force to establish a surgical airway and to be on the lookout for anterior neck injuries in general.

5.2.2. Epidemiology

Less than 1% of all traumatic injuries are laryngeal injuries. They may be quite severe even though they are uncommon. Laryngeal injuries are the second most common cause of death for patients with head and neck injuries, after intracranial injuries. In certain academic investigations, the Schaefer classification system is used to rate the degree of laryngeal injury (Table 5.1).

Table 5.1. Schaefer Classification System for Laryngeal Injuries

Type of Injury	Classification System of Schaefer for Laryngeal Injuries
1	Minor hematoma of endolarynx or fracture less laceration
2	Extreme edema, hematoma, a fracture that is not dislocated or a break in the mucosa in which cartilage is not exposed
3	Extensive edema, extensive break in the mucosa, dislocated fractures or immobility of vocal cord, exposed cartilage
4	Serious interruption of the anterior larynx, unsteady fractures, fracture lines, and severe trauma of mucosa
5	Total isolation of trachea and larynx

Source: Malvi A, Jain S (2022) Laryngeal trauma, its types, and management. Cureus 14(10): e29877. doi:10.7759/cureus.29877.

This might give the medical practitioner a useful starting point. In clinical practice, the majority of medical professionals divide patients' airways into stable and unstable groups because this directly affects the ensuing workup and assessment. In order to secure a stable airway in unstable patients before undergoing additional testing, an emergency tracheostomy or cricothyrotomy is typically performed. Patients who are stable might undergo further fiberoptic inspection testing.

5.2.3. Laryngeal Trauma: Pathophysiology

5.2.3.1. Blunt Trauma of the Larynx

The force applied and the area it covers often determine the severity of the situation. Due to high-velocity traumas that fracture the cartilage lining the larynx and trachea, the organs may develop structural malformations. The most serious injury, known as a clothesline injury, happens when a motorcyclist runs into a small, stationary object, such as a tree branch or fencing net, and it hits the rider's neck below the helmet line. Its forceful impact across restricted space may seriously damage the larynx and trachea's cartilage, crumbling and disintegrating it and restricting airway movement. Laryngotracheal separation could occur as a result of the shearing pressures. Minor blunt laryngeal injuries can happen in sports or fights. They may result in submucosal endolaryngeal injuries or hyoid fractures, which may not always be visible upon inspection due to shearing pressures. Owing to anatomical flaws, patients may experience symptoms of delayed airway obstruction right away or gradually develop airway blockage.

5.2.3.2. Penetrating Laryngeal Injury

The mechanism will once more decide the severity. For instance, knife wounds may initially exhibit mild symptoms of a lower-velocity penetrating injury, but the airway may become blocked by edema or hematoma that develops after the injury. Weapon-related high-velocity injuries, such as those from hunting or military rifles, can be extremely severe, shattering and destroying the tissues and supporting systems of the larynx. A relative devascularization and scarring of these tissues may cause severe long-term constriction in addition to any acute airway difficulties caused by tissue disturbance or post-injury edema.

5.2.4. History and Physical

Knowing the history is crucial to figuring out whether a laryngeal injury is possible. Individuals with anterior cervical trauma should be closely monitored for laryngeal trauma. This includes the type of injury (penetrating or blunt), how long it has been since the injury, and any additional injuries that might have happened. When a patient has experienced multiple traumas, such as a car accident, it is important to consider the possibility of laryngeal damage because the patient might not be cooperative or coherent. A history of anterior neck injury, a husky voice or altered voice, anterior neck pain, dyspnea, difficulty swallowing, and subcutaneous emphysema are concerning clinical features of laryngeal trauma.

Estimating the patient's breathing condition is the first step in the actual assessment. Take note of the emergency trauma assessment's breathing, circulation, and airway. Depending on the degree of damage, stridor may be inspiratory, expiratory, or biphasic, and vocal abnormalities may or may not accompany it. Every patient who has had neck trauma should have their cervical spines checked for any accompanying injuries. When examining the neck, one should look for any soreness, ecchymoses over the anterior neck, subcutaneous emphysema, or loss of the characteristic prominence of the thyroid cartilage. If at all possible, one should also listen for hoarseness in the voice.

5.2.5. Assessment

In an emergency situation, establishing a secure airway should come first; this may require tracheostomy or orotracheal intubation. A computed tomography (CT) scan is advised to check for and evaluate any laryngeal damage after the patient has been stabilized and the airway and cervical spine have been secured.

5.2.5.1. Flexible Laryngoscopy

The most critical assessment occurs when a patient's airway is determined to be intact. If there is any doubt about the airway, tracheostomy and cricothyrotomy procedures should be considered. After primary and secondary trauma evaluations are completed, flexible laryngoscopy is used to examine the interior mucosal tissues of the larynx and upper aerodigestive tracts. This examination can identify common issues such as edema and potential problems like laryngeal lacerations, hematomas, mucosal tears, or other structural abnormalities that could lead to complications. It can also determine the severity of any mucosal wounds, check for exposed vocalis muscle or cartilage, and assess the range of motion of the vocal cords. If there is suspicion of hidden laryngotracheal damage or vocal fold paresis, further investigation is necessary. In some cases, it may be challenging to see the subglottis during the exam. While a routine flexible laryngeal exam is a positive sign, additional testing such as bronchoscopy in the operating room may be required if there are concerns about potential hidden injuries based on the patient's symptoms and the nature of the damage. An asymptomatic patient who has undergone a standard flexible laryngeal exam before further evaluation or imaging may not need intubation or tracheostomy.

5.2.5.2. Computed Tomography (CT)

Imaging ought to be utilized only in situations where it is secure and informs the management plan. Patients with a positive history, clinical picture, routine review, and laryngoscopy are probably not good candidates for imaging. In a similar vein, those who have an obvious injury are unlikely to benefit because surgery will be required. A CT scan may be beneficial for patients who have a stable airway, a positive assessment, and a strong clinical suspicion of undiscovered harm. A non-contrasted CT scan of the neck can show the bony and cartilaginous parts of the hyoid and larynx, as well as any small or nondisplaced fractures that may require stabilization.

5.2.5.3. Esophagram

An additional 4–6% of laryngeal fractures will cause damage to the esophagus. Esophagrams are rarely used for acute conditions, but they can be useful if chronic damage is suspected. If there is any doubt about esophageal damage in relation to laryngeal injury, the best course of action is a thorough evaluation under anesthesia after securing the airway. In the operating room, procedures may include an open neck evaluation, esophagoscopy, and direct laryngoscopy.

5.2.5.4. Chest X-Ray

In the event of a polytrauma patient with questionable neck trauma, this data may usually be obtained using a portable roentgenogram when the patient is in a stable state and has a secured airway. Subcutaneous emphysema may indicate chest wall damage and a laryngotracheal injury on a clinical examination.

5.2.6. Treatment/Management

Recognizing and opening an airway is the first step in treating laryngeal injuries. Having a stable airway is the first criterion to be considered when making a decision. The airway is at least patent if the patient is speaking normally, though it might not be steady. Laryngeal fracture symptoms have been reported to include coughing, hemoptysis, anterior neck discomfort, stridor, dyspnea, and hoarseness. Clinical manifestations include pain, hematoma, ecchymosis, cracking when palpated, and surgical emphysema. The following conditions increase the need for intubation, cricothyroidotomy, or tracheotomy: breathlessness, neck hematoma, severe hemorrhage, subcutaneous neck emphysema, stridor, sore throat, expectoration of blood, thrill or bruit, and altered throat architecture. For anyone with an obvious larynx fracture, stridor with elevated breathing labor, or an impending airway blockage, tracheostomy or cricothyrotomy should be performed immediately. Approaching blockage of the airway: Skilled airway care results in a tracheostomy, cricothyrotomy, or intubation. Following that, each patient has an oesophageal scoping and direct laryngoscopy. The following actions should be taken after esophagogoscopy and laryngoscopy (Table 5.2).

Table 5.2. Treatment Modality/Management for the Type of Injury

Type of Injury	Treatment modality/ Management
Normal endolarynx or fracture, less trauma of mucosa.	Monitoring
Fracture of the thyroid or cricoid with an uninjured endolarynx.	Examination of the throat, open reduction, and internal fixation (ORIF) of skeletal fractures of the larynx with plating without thyrotomy.
Unsteady fractures or anterior commissure interruption, or major mucosal lacerations.	ORIF of fractures, correction of laceration of the mucosa, and stent of endolarynx or keeper of the lumen.
Steady fractures of the larynx, uninterrupted anterior commissure, change of mucosa which is less severe.	Examination of the throat, ORIF of skeletal fractures of the larynx with plating thyrotomy, primary closure of lacerations.

Source: Malvi A, Jain S (2022) Laryngeal trauma, its types, and management. Cureus 14(10), e29877. doi: 10.7759/cureus.29877.

Neck computed tomography and laryngoscopy with flexible fiber optics are used to treat stable airways. Videostroboscopy and laryngeal electromyography may also be used, based on availability and local knowledge. The course of treatment is determined by the findings of many studies (Table 5.3).

Table 5.3. Treatment for the Type of Injury

Type of Injury	Treatment Modality/Management
Normal endolarynx in which reversible trauma to mucosa may or may not be present without fracture	Monitoring
Interruption of cartilage or endolarynx	Tracheostomy or intubation, direct laryngoscopy and esophagoscopy, throat examination, and correction of findings like "impending airway obstruction."

Source: Malvi A, Jain S (2022) Laryngeal trauma, its types, and management. Cureus 14(10), e29877. doi: 10.7759/cureus.29877.

When airway injuries are treated within 24 hours, the best results are achieved. Medical management/close observation: For cases involving Schaefer type 1 and type 2 injuries, close observation may be adequate. In addition to inhalational (nebulized) steroids, intravenous dexamethasone is used to treat edema. Pulse oximetry airway monitoring and serial flexible laryngoscopy should be carried out for the first 24 hours at the very least. In such cases, where there is a normal or nearly normal mucosal layer and a small risk of unfavorable laryngeal scarring, this may be all that is required.

Treatment by surgery: In all other cases, comprehensive anesthetic examinations of the larynx and esophagus using direct endoscopy and laryngoscopy are required. If mucosal lacerations are mild to moderate, endoscopic repair may be attempted to cover all muscle and cartilage and avoid scarring. A thyrotomy is likely required for treatment in cases of significant mucosal lacerations, unstable fractures, or displaced fractures, which will require an open neck examination. In order to provide a covering and avoid scarring or webbing, the mucosa should be repaired first. Finally, any laryngeal fractures should be reduced and corrected. Any oesophageal injuries should be attended to. Soft tissue and skin repairs ought to come first. If the intralaryngeal lesions are mild, there may be no need for a formal thyrotomy; however, this procedure should be tailored to the particular injuries that are present. If there are large lesions of the intralaryngeal mucosa, a stent might be necessary. However, these devices should only be used sparingly, as they can leave scars. Following surgery, these patients ought to stay under close supervision for the first night in the critical care unit. Until their larynx heals completely and they can have a formal evaluation with the assistance of a speech therapist, many patients will require tracheostomy. Patients should be fed through nasogastric or gastrostomy tubes until their larynx heals, as there is a serious risk of aspiration.

5.2.7. Prognosis

It is imperative to manage the airway as soon as possible because laryngotracheal injuries can be fatal. If a severe laryngeal injury is missed, it may lead to airway blockage and death. Patients receiving conservative care, including frequent scopes, steroids, and continuous monitoring, are treated for minor tears or abrasions of the larynx or trachea. Since early airway treatment speeds up healing, laryngeal fracture patients benefit from it. Early diagnosis and treatment help patients' voice and airway outcomes.

5.2.8. Complications

Complications could be extremely minor or catastrophic in severity. Any lesion to the intralaryngeal mucosa is likely to have some granulation tissue as it heals. This can very rarely become an obstructive tumor, but it can occasionally be pretty serious and leave scars. The best defense against the horrifying complication of cicatrix development is prompt mucosal healing and avoiding laryngeal muscle or exposed cartilage. If scarring is severe or persistent, it may lead to a long-term reliance on tracheostomy. Although they are rare, wound healing complications like recurrent tracheo- or laryngo-cutaneous fistulae can still occur. Undiagnosed gastric injury is a potentially lethal adverse consequence. After trauma, vocal fold paresis, or paralysis that is visible at presentation, usually gets better, but it can take up to a year. Furthermore, this kind of injury might not go away and require more attention. During the healing process, damage to the superior or recurrent laryngeal nerves may also occur, which could result in dysphonia or aspiration and require further medical attention.

5.2.9. Postoperative and Rehabilitation Care

For observation, all traumatic laryngeal injuries need to be admitted to the hospital.

Laryngotracheal injuries that can be treated conservatively with head elevation, humidified air, analgesics, steroids, vocal rest, and a clean diet include minor mucosal injuries, nondisplaced fractures, and hematomas. Restoring these people's voices and swallowing systems is the long-term therapy goal. More severe injuries might require prolonged speech and swallowing therapy in addition to the potential for longer-term tracheostomy or gastrostomy reliance.

5.2.10. Consultations

In cases of suspected laryngeal injuries, head and neck surgeons should be consulted to aid in the diagnosis and treatment of laryngeal trauma. A surgeon and anesthesiologist with experience in managing complex airways are essential if such information is not available. In an emergency, if there is any doubt about the stability of the airway, the physician with the greatest experience performing such treatments should perform an elective surgical airway (often through an awake tracheostomy).

5.2.11. Deterrence and Patient Education

Individuals who have sustained a neck injury—from a car accident, a gunshot, a neck knife, an attempted hanging, or an attack—should visit the emergency room for a check-up because tracheal or laryngeal injuries are serious and sometimes fatal. Even in cases where the patient is asymptomatic at the moment, serious delayed complications may occur. For those who have respiratory problems, a tracheostomy is usually required. Until a more thorough image of the patient's upper airway is obtained, intubation attempts must be delayed; if this is not possible, a tracheostomy must be performed. Patients may need imaging, hospitalization, or monitoring if they are stable and have not experienced any severe trauma.

5.3. Acute and Chronic Inflammations of the Larynx

The sudden inflammation of the larynx brought on by a viral infection, like the common cold, is known as acute laryngitis. The larynx may swell and redden due to irritation from cigarette smoke or overuse of the voice, such as yelling or singing. Voice abuse, like shouting a lot, or irritation from cigarette smoke are the two main causes of persistent hoarseness. Chronic laryngitis can also be brought on by prolonged exposure to air pollutants like dust, which can irritate your larynx.

5.3.1. Laryngitis

Inflammation of the larynx, or voice box, is known as laryngitis. In addition to a hoarse voice, other symptoms might include fever, coughing, frontal neck pain, and difficulty swallowing. These usually don't last more than two weeks. If the symptoms of laryngitis disappear after three weeks, the condition is classified as chronic; otherwise, it is classified as acute. The most common cause of acute cases is a viral upper respiratory tract infection, although other infections and trauma from coughing can also be factors. Chronic cases can be brought on by sarcoidosis, rheumatoid arthritis, allergies, acid reflux, smoking, or tuberculosis. The vocal cord irritation is the fundamental mechanism.

Symptoms that might necessitate additional research include stridor, a history of neck radiation therapy, difficulty swallowing, longer than three weeks, and a smoking history. If there are any alarming symptoms, a laryngoscopy should be performed to examine the vocal cords. Similar symptoms can also be caused by croup, epiglottitis, inhaling a foreign body, and laryngeal cancer. The acute form usually goes away on its own without special care. Drinking enough water and resting the voice could be beneficial. In general, antibiotics don't seem to be helpful when used acutely. The chronic form is uncommon, but the acute form is frequently seen. Men are more likely than women to experience the chronic form, which typically manifests in middle age (Figure 5.2).

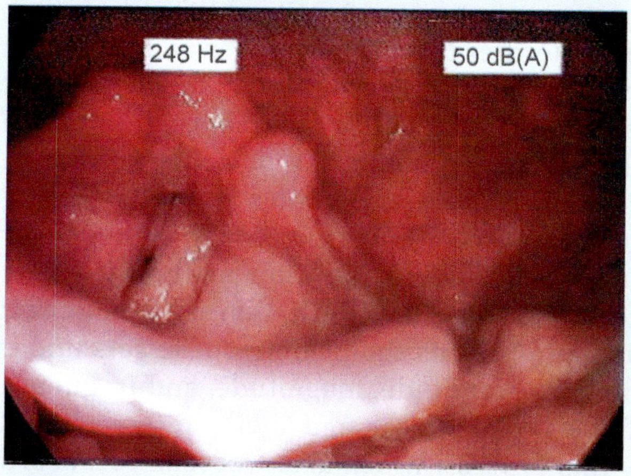

Figure 5.2. *Endoscopic image of an inflamed larynx caused by acid reflux.*

Source: By Phoni – Own work, CC BY-SA 3.0, https://commons.wikimedia.org/w/index.php?curid=12218422.

5.3.1.1. Etiology

There are two categories for the etiology of acute laryngitis: infectious and non-infectious. The more prevalent infectious form typically develops after an upper respiratory tract infection. Potential etiologic agents are viral agents, which are listed in approximately decreasing order of frequency: rhinovirus, parainfluenza virus, respiratory syncytial virus, coronavirus, adenovirus, influenza, and so on. When viral laryngitis is present, bacterial superinfection can happen; this usually happens seven days after the onset of symptoms.

In that order, *Streptococcus pneumoniae, Haemophilus influenzae*, and *Moraxella catarrhalis* are the most frequently encountered bacterial species. Accurate immunization history is important because exanthematous febrile illnesses like whooping cough, chickenpox, and measles can also cause acute laryngitis symptoms. Fungal-induced laryngitis is extremely uncommon in immunocompetent people; instead, it typically manifests as chronic laryngitis in immunocompromised people or in patients on inhaled steroids.

The viral organisms mentioned above are the most common cause of adult acute infectious laryngitis. These same medications are frequently used to treat pediatric acute laryngitis, but it is also vital to keep in mind that the parainfluenza virus, most frequently parainfluenza-1, can also cause croup (laryngotracheobronchitis) in children. Isolated vocal symptoms are possible, but the typical presentation is a distinctive barking cough that can develop into inspiratory or biphasic stridor. Acute non-infectious laryngitis may result from inhalational injuries, allergies, asthma, gastric reflux disease, abuse, misuse, or trauma to the voice, as well as functional or conversion disorders and environmental pollution. As can be observed after several days of shouting or yelling, vocal misuse or abuse can have an abrupt onset. After an event, coaches, spectators, and athletes frequently act like this. This is also evident in vocalists who have never received official voice or singing coaching, especially those whose frequency or intensity of performance has increased recently.

The extremely common cause of voice symptoms and laryngitis is gastroesophageal reflux disease (GERD), more precisely extra-esophageal GERD, also known as laryngopharyngeal reflux (LPR). Both chronic and episodic forms of these symptoms are possible. While one-third of GERD patients will only have laryngeal/voice symptoms, they may not follow or accompany the traditional GERD symptoms. Signs and symptoms include globus pharyngeus sensation, recurrent coughing or throat clearing, and coarseness in speech. Skilled vocalists may experience a decrease in performance. Chronic use of steroid inhalers can increase the risk of fungal laryngitis, especially if patients do not drink plain water after using the inhaler as directed. Asthma can also increase the risk of laryngitis due to chemical irritation from the inhaler. Another asthma condition that can result in voice abnormalities similar to acute laryngitis is cough-variant asthma, which can harm the vocal cords repeatedly.

Seasonal and environmental allergies, as well as intermittent or continuous air pollution, are examples of environmental factors that can irritate the vocal cords and result in acute laryngeal symptoms. Inhaling harmful substances can cause irritation to the larynx, edema of the vocal folds, and voice problems. This can happen accidentally or as a result of smoking or using other drugs. Certain patients might be allergic to detergents, colognes, perfumes, or other aromatics that are frequently used in daily life. A collection of real conversion disorders collectively referred to as functional dysphonia include a broad spectrum of voice symptoms and physical examination findings. This is an exclusion diagnosis, but well-known triggers include recent significant life stressors like losing a loved one or a job.

5.3.1.2. Epidemiology

Although it can strike patients at any age, acute laryngitis is more common in adults, typically affecting those between the ages of 18 and 40, though it can strike children as young as three. In children under three years old, isolated voice symptoms should initiate a more comprehensive workup for additional pathology such as vocal cord paralysis, GERD, and neurodevelopmental disorders. Because acute laryngitis is still underreported and many patients appropriately choose not to seek medical attention for this frequently self-limited condition, it is still difficult to determine the accurate incidence of this condition.

5.3.1.3. Pathophysiology

Acute laryngitis is caused by localized inflammation of the vocal folds and surrounding tissues in response to a trigger, which can be either infectious or non-infectious. It usually goes away in two weeks. Should the symptoms continue after this period, they may indicate the onset of chronic laryngitis or superinfection. Early on, inflammation and congestion of the larynx are the hallmarks of acute laryngitis. This can include, depending on the triggering organism, the supraglottic, glottic, or subglottic larynx (or any combination of these). White blood cells travel to the infection site to eliminate the pathogens as the healing phase gets under way. The amplitude, magnitude, and frequency of the typical vocal fold dynamic are altered by this process, which also worsens vocal cord edema and negatively impacts vibration. The pressure threshold for phonation can rise as the edema deepens. It gets harder to generate enough phonation pressure, and the patient experiences phonatory changes as a result of altered tissue dynamics brought on by both conscious and unconscious adaptation as well as changes in the fluid-wave dynamics of the edematous and inflamed tissue. Sometimes the edema is so severe that it is hard to produce enough phonation pressure. The patient might experience frank aphonia in this circumstance. These maladaptations can cause vocal symptoms from an acute laryngitis episode to last longer than expected after the triggering event has passed. Referrals to otolaryngologists and/or speech-language pathologists are appropriate in these circumstances.

5.3.1.4. History and Physical

A complete history and physical examination are always the first steps in the evaluation of a patient with acute laryngitis. Recent URIs or other illnesses, sick contacts, or any other indications of systemic illness should all receive extra care. The doctor should also look into the patient's past medical history, including any allergies, vaccinations, confounding pathologies like GERD, immune status, and immunization history. The beginning and duration of the symptoms, as well as whether they have occurred previously, should all be carefully considered. The effectiveness and type of any prior treatment must also be investigated if the patient has received it.

Acute laryngitis usually presents with sudden onset of symptoms that worsen over two or three days. If treatment is not received, symptoms may last up to a week. These might consist of:

- Alteration in voice quality; in advanced stages, total voice loss (aphonia) is possible.
- ache and discomfort in the throat, especially after speaking.
- Dysphagia and odynophagia (be cautious if they exist as they may indicate underlying pathology).
- Dry cough
- Fever, malaise, and dry throat are common symptoms.
- Frequent throat-clearing
- vocal range loss or early voice fatigue.

The diagnosis can be verified by a laryngeal examination. It is necessary to perform an indirect examination of the airway using a flexible laryngoscope or mirror. Variations in laryngeal appearance can be attributed to disease severity. The vocal cords, aryepiglottic folds, arytenoids, and epiglottis all exhibit erythema and edema in the early stages. The vocal cords may become erythematous and edematous as the illness worsens. Though less common, the subglottic area may become involved depending on the triggering agent. Additionally, there may be ropy, sticky secretions in the inter-arytenoid space or between the vocal cords. The vocal folds can exhibit a number of changes when vocal abuse or misuse occurs. Reinke's edema is frequently observed in cases of laryngitis, both acute and chronic. Acute vocal trauma may cause submucosal hemorrhage, or there may be nodules or pseudo-nodules that have not been identified before. All of these have the potential to develop into chronic voice pathology if untreated.

5.3.1.5. Evaluation

Usually, a very detailed history and physical examination are used to make the diagnosis. For cases that are complicated or resistant to treatment, formal voice analysis and fiberoptic laryngoscopy can be used to confirm the diagnosis. Stroboscopy may show reduced mucosal wave patterns, asymmetry, and aperiodicity, or it may be relatively normal. Unless an unusual infection or tumor is suspected, no additional imaging or lab tests are necessary. In rare cases, a culture may be necessary if the patient has exudate in their vocal cords or oropharynx.

5.3.1.6. Treatment / Management

Depending on the severity of the laryngitis, the course of treatment is typically supportive.

- **Voice Rest:** This is the most crucial element. When laryngitis is present, using one's voice causes a partial or delayed recovery. While nearly impossible to attain, complete voice rest is advised. When speaking, the patient should be told to speak in a confidential voice, which is to say, speak in a normal phonatory voice at a low volume without projecting or whispering.
- **Steam Inhalation:** Breathing in humidified air improves upper airway moisture and aids in secretion and exudate removal.

- **Avoidance of Irritants:** Alcohol and smoking ought to be avoided. Smoking prevents the disease process from ending quickly.
- **Dietary Modification:** It is advised that patients with gastroesophageal reflux disease restrict their diet. This entails staying away from chocolate, peppermint, spicy and fatty foods, and beverages with added caffeine. Avoiding late meals is a significant lifestyle change as well. Meals should be consumed by the patient no later than three hours before bed. The patient needs to hydrate well. The effectiveness of these dietary interventions for classic GERD has been demonstrated, and while their applicability in LPR is debatable, they are frequently still used.
- **Medication:** At this time, there is no evidence to support the prescription of antibiotics for an otherwise healthy patient with acute laryngitis; however, high-risk patients and those with severe symptoms may receive antibiotics. Some writers advise against using narrow-spectrum antibiotics unless a gram stain and culture are visible.

Oral antifungal medications like fluconazole can be used to treat fungal laryngitis. Typically, treatment lasts for three weeks, though it can be extended if necessary. This should only be administered to patients whose laryngeal examination and/or culture have confirmed a fungal infection. Secretions can be removed with the help of mucolytics like guaifenesin. Anti-reflux drugs are used in the treatment of LPR-related laryngitis in addition to dietary and lifestyle changes. Proton pump inhibitors have been found to be the most effective medication for LPR, but H2 receptor and proton pump blocking agents are also effective in treating gastroesophageal reflux. For these to work in this situation, higher dosages or a twice-daily dosing schedule might be necessary. The current body of evidence does not support the use of oral corticosteroids or antihistaminics to treat acute laryngitis.

5.3.1.7. Differential Diagnosis

This includes:

- Spasmodic dysphonia
- Reflux laryngitis
- Chronic allergic laryngitis
- Epiglottitis
- Neoplasm

5.3.1.8. Prognosis

Because this condition tends to improve on its own, the outlook is positive. Completing the suggested treatment can lead to a full recovery of normal voice function. In cases where voice issues persist, speech therapy can help address any maladaptive behaviors.

5.3.2. Acute Epiglottitis (Syn. Supraglottic Laryngitis)

Epiglottitis is an inflammatory disease of the epiglottis and surrounding structures, such as the vallecula, arytenoids, and aryepiglottic folds. It is typically caused by an infection. Asphyxia and respiratory arrest can result from the severe swelling of the upper airways caused by epiglottitis, a potentially fatal condition. Prior to the creation of the *Haemophilus influenzae* type B vaccine, *H.influenzae* was the primary cause of cases and the illness was much more prevalent. The pathogens causing illnesses in the post-vaccine era are more diverse and sometimes multimicrobial. Because the infections may affect the supraglottic structures more broadly, the term supraglottitis is frequently preferred. When an infection of the epiglottis and supraglottic structures causes edema, the condition can worsen quickly, resulting in respiratory distress, airway obstruction, and even death. The edema can progress gradually until a critical mass is reached. Any patient diagnosed with true supraglottitis should have their airway secured under the most controlled circumstances possible, and every effort should be made to keep the patient as calm and comfortable as possible until an airway is secured. This is because symptoms can be made worse by patient discomfort and agitation, especially in children. No patient with a possibly unstable airway should be sent to the radiology department for imaging, nor should the airway be instrumented for oral exams or endoscopy in the clinic or emergency room.

5.3.2.1. Etiology

Whether bacterial, viral, or fungal in origin, infectious agents are the most frequent cause of epiglottitis. *Haemophilus influenzae* type B (HIB) remains the most common cause in children. But since vaccinations have become widely accessible, this has significantly declined. Other pathogens that have been linked include *Streptococcus pyogenes, S. pneumoniae*, and *S. aureus. Candida* and *Pseudomonas* aeruginosa have been identified in immunocompromised patients. Traumatic non-infectious causes include heat, caustic substances, and foreign body ingestion.

Although viruses do not cause epiglottitis, bacterial superinfection may arise as a result of a previous viral infection. Herpes simplex, Epstein Barr virus, and varicella-zoster are among the viruses that can lead to a superinfection.

5.3.2.2. Epidemiology

In many parts of the world, the annual incidence of childhood epiglottitis has declined since the HIB vaccine was added to the infant immunization schedule. On the other hand, the incidence in adults has not changed. Furthermore, in the post-vaccine era, the age range of children who have experienced epiglottitis has increased from three to 6 to 12 years old. Although epiglottitis was once thought to be primarily an illness of young children, practitioners are now much more likely to find adults with epiglottitis/supraglottitis.

5.3.2.3. Pathophysiology

In comparison to an adult, a child's airway is significantly different. An adult's epiglottis is positioned more anteriorly and superiorly than that of a small child. Along with the trachea, there is an even more oblique angle. It is the glottis in adults and the subglottis in infants and children that is the narrowest part of the airway. Moreover, compared to an adult, whose epiglottis is more rigid, an infant's cartilage is far more flexible. This is due to the normal maturation process of cartilage, which explains why laryngomalacia is more common in very young children. Since the cartilage is pliable, a ball-valve effect can occur whereby each inspiration pulls an edematous epiglottis over the laryngeal airway, resulting in symptoms. This means that an infectious process that causes edema and increases the weight and mass of the epiglottis is more likely to cause symptoms in a child. However, an infection that affects more of the supraglottis's tissues and causes edema can cause symptoms and an unstable airway. In adults, whose cartilages are stiffer, an isolated epiglottic infection and the ensuing increase in epiglottic mass may be resisted by the more rigid laryngeal/epiglottic cartilage.

H. influenzae and other, infections of the epiglottis can lead to marked edema and swelling of the epiglottis and supraglottis of patients of any age. The symptoms of an airway blockage may appear quickly as a result of this edema's quick spread to surrounding structures. While *H. influenzae* remains the most common pathogen in both adults and children, other organisms such as *S. Pneumoniae, S. aureus,* and beta-hemolytic *Streptococcus sp.* are important pathogens also in both adults and children. Mycobacterium tuberculosis must be on the long list of possible causes in immunocompromised patients, along with a long list of other possible causes, all of which have the same relative frequencies.

5.3.2.4. Toxicokinetics

Other complications of epiglottitis include:

- Cervical adenitis
- Empyema
- Epiglottic abscess
- Meningitis
- Pneumonia
- Pneumothorax
- Sepsis
- Septic arthritis
- Septic shock
- Vocal cord granuloma
- Ludwig angina-type submental infection

5.3.2.5. History and Physical

Though not always, the history will frequently show an antecedent URI. For a few hours or days, symptoms might be extremely mild before sharply worsening to resemble a sudden onset. The majority of the time, this will have happened in the last 12 or 24 hours. The patient will seem extremely uncomfortable and perhaps even aggressively toxic. Most kids don't exhibit prodromal symptoms. The child in the emergency room will probably be sitting up straight, with their mouth open in a tripod position, and may even have a muffled voice. Although adults may be downplaying their symptoms, they will probably not want to lie down or find it uncomfortable. There may be signs of drooling, dysphagia, discomfort, or anxiety (particularly in children, but also in adults). These are commonly known as the 3 Ds. Because they cause turbulent airflow during inspiration or stridor, swelling of the upper airway causes this. Tachypnea, cyanosis, and intercostal or suprasternal retractions are signs of severe upper airway obstruction that should alert the healthcare provider to the possibility of respiratory failure. Avoid performing a throat exam using a flexible laryngoscope or tongue blade as this could cause the airway to become trapped. Anterior neck examination may show lymphadenopathy. A poor prognosis and advanced infection are indicated by the presence of cyanosis.

5.3.2.6. Evaluation

When evaluating a suspected case of epiglottitis, an oropharyngeal exam is typically not conducted because oral cavity manipulation could result in catastrophic consequences, such as respiratory arrest. The main basis for this diagnosis is clinical suspicion. Thumb sign, or swelling of the epiglottis, can be seen on a lateral neck radiograph. Although it can be used to focus the provider's differential diagnosis, it is not required to make the diagnosis. Only the most stable, comfortable, and cooperative patients should have this procedure done on them. Theoretically, a flexible fiberoptic laryngoscopy is possible, but only under strict control—in the operating room, for example—because there is a chance of causing laryngospasm. This is nearly never finished. The patient should be taken as soon as possible to the operating room for an airway examination under the best circumstances if there is a clinical suspicion of acute epiglottitis.

Another method of assessing these patients has been suggested: ultrasound, which shows an alphabet P sign in a longitudinal view. This may not be the best course of action for children and needs to be considered against the clinical condition. Patients who have an endotracheal tube that is securely fastened should only have an epiglottal culture, blood culture, and complete blood count with differential. A CT scan of the neck is rarely necessary, but it can be disastrous. Restrictions on breathing can occur when a patient is placed in a supine position. Should a CT scan reveal this diagnosis unexpectedly, the child or adult should not be left unaccompanied in the radiology suite; instead, they should be taken immediately to the operating room for intubation and airway assessment.

In 10–15% of cases, the chest X-ray may reveal concurrent pneumonia. In certain cooperative patients, a lateral neck X-ray can be obtained as previously described (with great caution). The diagnosis may also be suggested by a standard portable P-A X-ray, which can be confused with the steeple sign of laryngotracheal bronchitis (croup) due to the narrowing of the laryngotracheal area. As a result, this diagnosis is still solely clinical.

5.3.2.7. Treatment / Management

Securing the airway is the one and only, most crucial part of the treatment plan. These patients are considered to have difficult airways, so experienced healthcare professionals should perform intubation. Should the need arise, someone qualified to perform a tracheotomy ought to be on hand. Though this varies from patient to patient, this probably entails an inhalation induction of general anesthesia and subsequent intubation. After the airway is secured, the patient should be admitted to the intensive care unit, and culture swabs should be sent at the time of intubation once the tube is inserted. It has been reported that patients who receive corticosteroids for edema reduction stay in the intensive care unit for a shorter period of time overall. The use of empirical antimicrobials ought to begin. The regimen needs to be modified as soon as the results of the culture and sensitivity tests are known. Extubation can be considered if a leak around the endotracheal tube can be shown with the cuff deflated.

Every non-intubated patient needs to be admitted for observation, and by the patient's bedside, a tracheostomy tray needs to be available. In the event that an emergency airway is needed, the admission must be reported to the anesthesiologist and the ENT surgeon. It is important to advise nurses not to put a child in a supine position. Although this is uncommon, patients who have a strong suspicion of epiglottitis ought to be intubated right away. In the best case scenario, an emergency airway can be obtained in the operating room. A laryngoscope should be used to first visualize the airway. A tracheostomy should be done if endotracheal intubation is not an option. Typically, cefuroxime, ceftriaxone, and cefotaxime are prescribed as antibiotics to treat common respiratory and oral flora.

5.3.2.8. Differential Diagnosis

The HIB vaccine and its accessibility have made acute epiglottitis caused by *H. influenzae* as the most common pathogen responsible for the condition in both adults and children, despite being less common (though this is occasionally increasing due to public misconception regarding vaccination). As a result, most medical professionals might be less knowledgeable about the illness. Antibiotic initiation is frequently delayed as a result of this deficiency. Acute epiglottitis may cause an abrupt blockage of the airway. If this diagnosis is even slightly suspected, it is never a good idea to send the patient somewhere without adequate monitoring and resuscitation equipment. A foreign object blockage in the airway, acute angioedema, airway compromise from caustic ingestion, diphtheria, or peritonsillar and retropharyngeal abscesses are some other conditions that can resemble the presentation.

5.3.2.9. Prognosis

When epiglottitis is diagnosed and treated promptly, the prognosis is good for the majority of patients. Even those who need intubation are typically free of any lasting effects after being extubated within a few days. However, in children, delayed diagnosis can lead to airway compromise and even death. The patient's sudden upper airway obstruction, difficulty intubating them, and significant laryngeal swelling are typically the cause of death. A tracheostomy tray must therefore be placed at the patient's bedside, and any patient admitted with a diagnosis of acute epiglottitis must see an ear, nose, and throat surgeon or anesthesiologist. Patients with unstable airways have been reported to have a 3–7% mortality rate worldwide.

5.3.3. Acute Laryngo-Tracheo-Bronchitis

Acute laryngotracheobronchitis, also known as croup, is a contagious respiratory illness that affects infants and children.

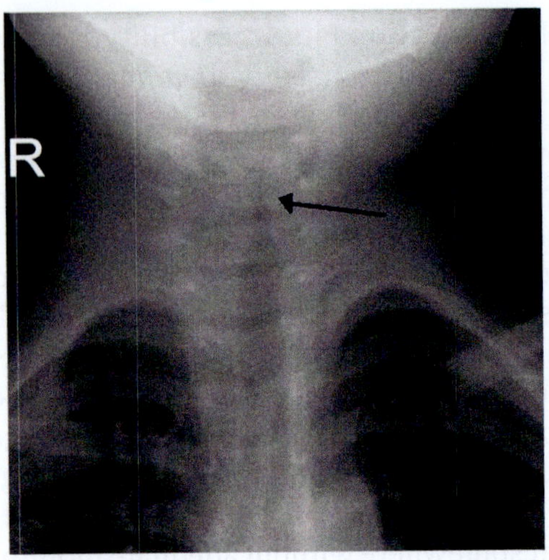

Figure 5.3. *The steeple sign as seen on an AP neck X-ray of a child with croup.*

Source: By Frank Gaillard – Own work, CC BY-SA 3.0, https://commons.wikimedia.org/w/index.php?curid=6792682.

It can be brought on by an infection of either the trachea or the larynx. It may result in a partial or severe blockage of the airway, which makes coughing and breathing difficult. It may even be fatal for certain kids (Figure 5.3).

5.3.3.1. Cause

Though it can also result from infection with the measles virus, adenoviruses, or respiratory syncytial virus (RSV), parainfluenza virus is the most common cause of croup. It is also known that croup can result from allergic reactions, acid reflux, or foreign body irritation of the airway. Children are more susceptible to croup than adults due to their narrower airways, which increases the risk of swelling and increases the likelihood that it will obstruct breathing.

5.3.3.2. Symptoms

The afflicted child's age range is typically 3 months to 5 years, with a peak incidence occurring around 24 months of age. Typically, croup begins as a regular cold but gets worse over a few days. The most striking characteristic is the barking cough, which is sometimes compared to a seal barking. Other characteristics include noisy breathing and a hoarse voice. Breathing problems could also occur, particularly at night. Most of the time, the symptoms only begin mildly. They are particularly bad on the first and second nights and can last up to a week.

5.3.3.3. Diagnosis and Management

The symptoms and cough are used to diagnose croup. A physical examination will reveal a number of symptoms associated with inflammation of the larynx and respiratory difficulties. Most of the time, croup responds to home care when prescribed by a physician. It is important to comfort the child because fear and anxiety exacerbate the obstruction and quicken breathing. Steam, or moist air, is frequently used to remove the obstruction. Vaporizers with cool air could be useful. But science has no support for this age-old method of healing. Acetaminophen is used to treat fever in children, with dosages determined by the child's age and body weight. On a doctor's prescription, antibiotics or steroid inhalers may be necessary in specific situations. When taken systemically, steroids help to relieve the obstruction of the airway but take time to start working. Steroids inhaled work far more quickly. When a child is in critical distress, exhausted from breathing, or cyanosed due to insufficient oxygen reaching the body, medical attention is imperative. Of the children with croup, about 5% require admission. In severe cases, nebulization with epinephrine may be part of the hospital treatment to rapidly reduce inflammation. Additional actions consist of:

- The child is relieved by using an oxygen tent to increase oxygenation and thereby decrease breathing effort.
- Glucocorticoids, which can be administered orally, intravenously, or by inhalation, have been shown to be very effective in reducing the need for hospital admission for children with inflammatory swelling.
- Liquids for dehydration, administered intravenously or orally is more common.
- Antibiotic treatment in the event that a secondary infection is present or likely.

5.3.4. Laryngeal Diphtheria

Diphtheria is a dangerous bacterial infection that primarily affects the throat and nose mucous membranes. Because of widespread vaccination against the disease, diphtheria is incredibly rare in the United States and other developed nations. Still, there are still a lot of nations with poor access to healthcare and immunization programs that have high diphtheria rates. Medication is a treatment option for diphtheria. However, when diphtheria progresses, it can harm the kidneys, heart, and nervous system. Diphtheria can be fatal even with treatment, particularly in young children.

5.3.4.1. Symptoms

Signs and symptoms of diphtheria typically appear two to five days after infection. Symptoms and indicators could be:

- A thick, gray membrane covering the throat and tonsils
- A sore throat and hoarseness
- Swollen glands (enlarged lymph nodes) in the neck
- Difficulty breathing or rapid breathing
- Nasal discharge
- Fever and chills
- Tiredness

Some people only experience a mild illness or no symptoms at all from a diphtheria-causing bacterial infection. Those who carry the infection but remain oblivious to it are called carriers of diphtheria. Because they can spread the infection without getting sick themselves, they are known as carriers.

- **Skin (Cutaneous) Diphtheria:** Similar to other bacterial skin infections, a second type of diphtheria can affect the skin and cause pain, redness, and swelling. Gray membrane-covered ulcers may also indicate skin diphtheria. Skin infections from diphtheria are not limited to tropical regions; they can also occur in the United States. People who live in crowded environments and have poor hygiene are particularly susceptible to it.

- **When to See a Doctor:** If you or your child have come into contact with someone who has diphtheria, call your family doctor right away. Make an appointment if you're unsure if your child has received the diphtheria vaccination. Verify the status of your own vaccinations.

5.3.4.2. Causes

The bacteria *Corynebacterium diphtheriae* is the cause of diphtheria. Usually, the bacteria grows on or close to the skin's or throat's surface. *C. diphtheriae* propagates via:

- **Airborne Droplets:** When an infected person's sneeze or cough releases a mist of contaminated droplets, people nearby may inhale *C. diphtheriae*. Diphtheria spreads easily this way, especially in crowded conditions.
- Personal or household items tainted with contaminants. Handling contaminated items, such as used tissues or hand towels, that have been handled by an infected person can occasionally expose a person to diphtheria.

Bacteria causing diphtheria can also be transmitted by touching an infected wound. Even if they don't exhibit any symptoms, people who have been infected with the diphtheria bacteria and have not received treatment can still infect others who have not received the vaccine.

5.3.4.3. Diagnosis

Physicians may suspect diphtheria in a sick child if the child has a sore throat and a gray membrane covering their tonsils and throat. Growth of *C. diphtheriae* in a lab culture of material from the throat membrane confirms the diagnosis. In order to determine whether a patient has cutaneous diphtheria, doctors can also remove tissue from an infected wound and have it tested in a lab.

Treatment starts as soon as a doctor suspects diphtheria, even before the findings of bacterial tests are known.

5.3.4.4. Treatment

A dangerous disease is diphtheria. Physicians take quick action and treat it vigorously. First, doctors make sure there is no obstruction or reduction of the airway. To keep the airway open until inflammation subsides, a breathing tube may occasionally need to be inserted into the throat.

Treatments include:

- **Antibiotics:** Antibiotics, like erythromycin and penicillin, assist in killing bacteria in the body to treat infections. The duration of a diphtheria patient's contagious period is reduced by antibiotics.
- **An Antitoxin:** When a doctor suspects diphtheria, they will prescribe a medication that blocks the body's production of the diphtheria toxin. The Centers for Disease Control and Prevention is the source of this medication. This medication, known as an antitoxin, is injected into a muscle or vein.

Doctors might do skin allergy testing prior to administering an antitoxin. In order to ensure that the infected individual is not allergic to the antitoxin, these steps are taken. A person's doctor will probably advise against taking the antitoxin if they have an allergy. Diphtheria frequently requires hospitalization for treatment in both children and adults. Given that diphtheria can spread quickly to those who have not received the vaccination, they might be kept apart in an intensive care unit.

5.3.4.4.1. Preventive Treatments

Seek medical attention from a physician for testing and potential treatment if you have come into contact with an infected person. To help stop you from getting the illness, your doctor might prescribe antibiotics to you. A booster dose of the diphtheria vaccine might also be necessary. Antibiotics are given to those who are discovered to be carriers of diphtheria in order to eradicate the bacteria from their bodies.

5.3.4.4.2. Self Care

It takes a lot of bed rest to recover from diphtheria. If you have heart problems, it is especially crucial to avoid physical activity. Pain and difficulties swallowing may mean that you have to take your nutrition in the form of liquids and soft foods for a while. Maintaining complete seclusion while you are infectious aids in stopping the infection from spreading. Limiting the spread of the infection requires everyone in your home to wash their hands carefully. To avoid contracting the disease again after recovering from diphtheria, you must receive the entire course of vaccinations. It is not a lifetime immunity to diphtheria, unlike some other infections. In the event that you are not fully vaccinated against diphtheria, you may contract it more than once.

5.3.4.5. Risk Factors

The following individuals have a higher chance of contracting diphtheria.

- Adults and children without current vaccination records.
- People who reside in filthy or congested environments.
- Anyone visiting a region where cases of diphtheria are more prevalent.

In Western Europe and the United States, where children have been immunized against diphtheria for decades, the illness rarely occurs. Nonetheless, in developing nations with low vaccination rates, diphtheria is still widespread. In regions where vaccination against diphtheria is mandatory, the illness primarily poses a risk to individuals who are not vaccinated or who have not received enough vaccinations and who travel abroad or interact with individuals from developing nations.

5.3.4.6. Complications

Left untreated, diphtheria can lead to:

- **Breathing Problems:** Bacteria that cause diphtheria could create a toxin. This toxin usually affects the nose and throat, causing tissue damage in the immediate area of infection. The infection creates a hard, gray membrane there that is composed of bacteria, dead cells, and other materials. Breathing may be hindered by this membrane.
- **Heart Damage:** It is possible for the diphtheria toxin to enter the bloodstream and harm other bodily tissues. For instance, it may harm the heart muscle, leading to issues like myocarditis, or inflammation of the heart muscle. Myocarditis may cause mild or severe heart damage. Myocarditis can, in the worst case scenario, result in heart failure and abrupt death.
- **Nerve Damage:** There's a chance that the toxin damages nerves. Usually, the nerves leading to the throat are the target, as inadequate

nerve conduction can lead to swallowing difficulties. Muscle weakness may also result from inflammation of the nerves that supply the arms and legs.

Breathing muscles may become paralyzed if the diphtheria toxin damages the nerves that aid in controlling these muscles. By then, breathing might require mechanical assistance. Most diphtheria patients recover from these complications with treatment, though recovery is frequently sluggish. About 5–10% of cases of diphtheria result in death. Children under five or adults over 40 have higher death rates.

5.3.4.7. Prevention

Before the discovery of antibiotics, diphtheria was a common childhood illness. These days, there is a vaccine that can prevent the illness in addition to treating it. Usually, the whooping cough (pertussis) and tetanus vaccinations are given in addition to the diphtheria vaccine. The diphtheria, tetanus, and pertussis vaccine is the name of the three-in-one vaccination. The most recent iteration of this vaccination is referred to as the Tdap vaccine for adults and adolescents and the DTaP vaccine for children.

During infancy, doctors in the United States advise children to receive the vaccine against pertussis, tetanus, and diphtheria. Children at these ages receive vaccinations in the form of a series of five shots, usually given in the arm or thigh.

- 2 months
- 4 months
- 6 months
- 15 to 18 months
- 4 to 6 years

Diphtheria can be prevented with the help of the vaccine. However, there might be adverse effects. During receiving a diphtheria, tetanus, and pertussis (DTaP) shot, some children may experience a mild fever, fussiness, drowsiness, or tenderness at the injection site. Consult your physician about ways to lessen or alleviate these effects for your child. Problems don't happen very often. Rarely, a child may experience major but manageable side effects from the DTaP vaccination, such as an allergic reaction (rash or hives appear minutes after injection). Certain children might not be able to receive the DTaP vaccine, such as those who have epilepsy or another disorder affecting the nervous system.

5.3.4.7.1. Booster Shots

To help you maintain your immunity, you need booster shots of the diphtheria vaccine after the initial series of vaccinations in childhood. This is due to the fact that immunity to diphtheria waned with age. Around age 11 or 12, children who completed all recommended vaccinations before the age of 7 should get their first booster shot. It is advised to have another booster shot 10 years later, and then every 10 years after that. Getting booster shots is especially crucial if you are visiting a region where diphtheria is prevalent. The booster is administered as the tetanus-diphtheria (Td) vaccine, which combines the tetanus and diphtheria boosters, or as the tetanus, diphtheria, and pertussis (Tdap) booster. Injections of this combination vaccine are administered, typically into the arm or thigh. For adults who have never received a booster shot and adolescents aged 11 to 18, the Tdap vaccine is an alternate vaccination option. It is also advised to have it once while pregnant, regardless of prior immunization history. If you're not sure whether you've had all the shots you need, ask your doctor about vaccinations and booster shots. For children aged 7 to 10 who are not up to date with the vaccination schedule, a Tdap vaccination may also be advised as part of the tetanus-diphtheria (Td) series.

5.3.5. Edema of the Larynx

It affects the supraglottic and subglottic regions, where the laryngeal mucosa is loose. It was formerly known as oedema glottidis. Due to the sparse subepithelial connective tissue, oedema of the vocal cords is rare.

5.3.5.1. Aetiology

1. Infections (a) Tuberculosis, syphilis of the larynx, acute epiglottitis, and laryngo-tracheo-bronchitis. (b) Neighbor-wide infection, e.g., Ludwig's angina, retropharyngeal abscess, and peritonsillar abscess.
2. Trauma. The procedures include tongue surgery, floor of mouth surgery, laryngectomy, foreign body removal, endoscopy, particularly in pediatric patients, intubation, burns from heat or caustic chemicals, or inhalation of irritating gases or fumes.
3. Neoplasms. Laryngopharyngeal or laryngeal cancer is frequently linked to deep ulcers.
4. Allergy. Anaphylactic shock or angioneurotic oedema.
5. Radiation. For pharyngeal or laryngeal cancer.
6. Systemic diseases. Heart failure, myxoedema, or arthritis.

5.3.5.2. Symptoms and Signs

1. Obstruction of the airway. Respiratory distress varies in intensity. Tracheostomy might end up being necessary.
2. Inspiratory stridor.
3. Indirect laryngoscopy. It displays subglottic or supraglottic oedema. Direct laryngoscopy may be necessary for children.

5.3.5.3. Treatment

If there is an obstruction to the airway, tracheostomy or laryngeal intubation will need to be done right away. Treatment for less serious cases is conservative and is based on the underlying cause. A 0:3–0:5 ml injection of adrenaline (1:1,000) is useful in cases of allergic or angioneurotic edema; if necessary, repeat every 15 minutes. When traumatic allergies or radiation exposure cause oedema, laryngo-tracheo-bronchitis, or epiglottitis, steroids can be helpful.

5.3.6. Polypoid Degeneration of Vocal Cords (Reinke's Oedema)

Reinke's edema, also called polypoid corditis, is a condition in which swelling or polyps impair the superficial lamina propria, a structure necessary for regular voice function. The edema does suggest significant damage to the vocal cords, even though it is not thought to be precancerous. To make sure they do not have any precancerous lesions, patients with the condition should have a thorough examination of their mouth, nose, and throat performed (Figure 5.4).

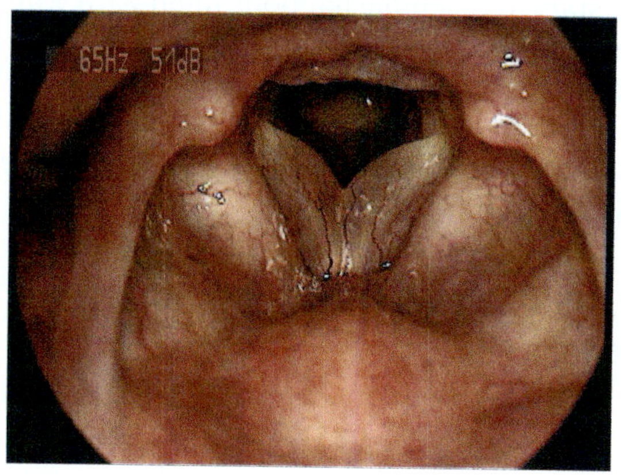

Figure 5.4. *Reinke's edema.*

Source: By Phoni – Own work, CC BY-SA 4.0, https://commons.wikimedia.org/w/index.php?curid=47558409.

Usually affecting smokers, Reinke's edema is brought on by the vocal cords' constant exposure to cigarette smoke. Reinke's edema is less common, but it can also happen to people who have severe acid reflux or who talk a lot.

5.3.6.1. Symptoms of Reinke's Edema

The superficial lamina propria becomes boggy and less vibrates as it swells and gains mass. The voice may consequently grow much deeper and more gravelly. Due to the greater noticeable nature of the vocal changes, women are typically diagnosed with the condition at a higher rate than men. Women with Reinke's edema frequently experience voice changes so severe that people mistake them for men. Sometimes the swelling gets so bad that breathing becomes difficult. At first, this might only be felt during physically demanding activities, but over time, it can worsen to the point where it affects breathing during rest and even aggravates sleep apnea.

5.3.6.2. Diagnosing Reinke's Edema

Swelling all the way down the vocal folds is a hallmark of Reinke's edema. The vocal folds may even start to resemble balloons filled with water. One vocal fold may be affected more than the other, or it may affect both vocal folds equally and move when breathing. It is also possible that the patient's swelling is only apparent when they inhale deeply.

5.3.6.3. Treatments for Reinke's Edema

The first step is to stop smoking because smoking-related damage is the cause of Reinke's edema in the majority of cases. Giving up smoking may be sufficient to allow for some voice improvement and halt the condition's further progression, depending on the severity of the damage. Quitting smoking can greatly lower the chance of recurrence, even if additional treatment is needed. Surgery may be required in severe cases of Reinke's edema in order to reduce the superficial lamina propria. Reinke's edema was traditionally treated with a direct laryngoscopy, which involved making incisions in the vocal folds to remove extra tissue. Using a laser, microlaryngoscopy is a much more common technique for minimally invasive surgery nowadays. Through this procedure, normal vocal fold vibration can be preserved while removing excess tissue. After surgery, the majority of patients report a noticeable improvement in voice quality.

5.3.7. Pachydermia Laryngitis

It is a type of chronic hypertrophic laryngitis that affects the posterior portion of the vocal cords as well as the posterior part of the larynx in the interarytenoid region. Clinically, the patient exhibits throat irritation and hoarseness or husky voice. When an indirect laryngoscopy is performed, it can reveal accumulations of red or grey granulation tissue in the interarytenoid region and the posterior thirds of the vocal cords. The vocal cords can also exhibit ulceration from continuous vocal process hammering during speech, a condition known as a "contact ulcer." The ailment is symmetrical and bilateral. It doesn't experience harmful alterations. To distinguish the lesion from tuberculosis and carcinoma, a biopsy of the lesion is necessary. The cause is unknown. It is most common in men who smoke and drink excessively. Extra-forceful speech and gastro-oesophageal reflux disease, which causes the posterior part of the larynx to be continuously drenched in stomach acid, are additional contributing factors. Treatment involves removing granulation tissue under an operating microscope, which may involve speech therapy, reflux control, and repetition.

5.3.8. Atrophic Laryngitis (Laryngitis Sicca)

Laryngitis sicca is characterized by extreme dryness of the larynx, nearly invariably accompanied by mucus crusting. It frequently causes voice hoarseness.

5.3.8.1. Causes of Laryngitis Sicca

Radiation treatment for laryngeal cancer is one of the causes. Radiation therapy may harm or even destroy the glands that produce mucus in the larynx in addition to killing the tumor it is intended to target. The result of this damage to the glands may be a decrease in mucus production as well as a rise in proteinaceous mucus, which makes it thicker and stickier. This thick mucus is also susceptible to bacterial colonization and crusting, particularly in the winter when indoor humidity is lower. Apart from any use of radiation therapy, a second kind of laryngitis sicca appears to accompany bacterial infection alone. The mucosa reddens with inflammation, and the mucus crusts turn yellow or green.

5.3.8.2. Treatment for Laryngitis Sicca

Although some cases appear steadfastly resistant to such treatment, even after multiple courses of broad-spectrum antibiotics, antibiotic therapy may help to improve or solve the issue. Enhancing the larynx's hydration and teaching the patient how to "gargle" in the larynx may both be of some assistance.

5.3.9. Tuberculosis of the Larynx

The most prevalent granulomatous disease of the larynx, laryngeal tuberculosis (LT), has historically been linked to pulmonary tuberculosis (PT), though it can also occur locally as a primary lesion in the larynx without pulmonary involvement. LT may result in odynophagia, dysphagia, and hoarseness. Because of the mycobacteria's hemogenic and lymphatic dissemination, the granulomatous lesions associated with Lymphoma Trauma (LT) may affect the entire larynx. The non-pathognomonic complaints and physical findings, particularly in patients without pulmonary disease, can make the diagnosis of lung cancer (LT) challenging. Furthermore, it may be more challenging to diagnose LT in patients with HIV infection due to changes in tuberculosis manifestations. The infection starts in the subepithelial space with exudation, moves on to the round cell infiltration stage, and ends with fibrosis in the lung tissue. Vibrations may be adversely affected and the voice quality may be irreversibly altered by fibrotic alterations in the layers of the lamina propria of the vocal folds. Treatment is similar to that for tuberculosis in the lungs. It is crucial to take breaks for your voice.

5.3.10. Lupus of the Larynx

It is an indolent TB infection linked to pharyngeal and nasal lupus. Lupus affects the anterior part of the larynx, in contrast to tuberculosis of the larynx, which primarily affects the posterior parts. First affected is the epiglottis, which may be totally destroyed by the illness. Aryepiglottic folds and occasionally ventricular bands are affected by the lesion. When lupus of the nose is present, a routine laryngeal examination may reveal the presence of lupus of the larynx, which is a painless and frequently asymptomatic condition. Pulmonary tuberculosis does not exist. Antitubercular medications are the treatment. The prognosis is favorable.

5.3.11. Syphilis of the Larynx

It is a rare condition these days. Sometimes, only tertiary stage gumma is visible. It can start as a smooth swelling that spreads to any part of the larynx and eventually becomes an ulcer. Only serological testing and biopsies are used for diagnosis. Laryngeal stenosis is a common side effect.

5.3.12. Leprosy of the Larynx

It is an uncommon ailment that is frequently linked to leprosy of the nose and skin. It manifests as arytenoids, aryepiglottic folds, and diffuse nodular infiltration of the epiglottis. Ulcers may form on lesions. It is linked to leprosy of the nose. After a biopsy of the lesion, a diagnosis is made. After healing, this disease leaves behind stenosis and a deformity of the laryngeal inlet.

5.3.13. Scleroma of the Larynx

The cause of this persistent inflammatory ailment is *Klebsiella rhinoscleromatis*. In India, nasal involvement is highly prevalent. Occasional cases of laryngeal involvement can occur with or without a nasal lesion. It usually manifests as a red, smooth swelling in the subglottic area. In addition to the nasal lesion, other symptoms that may be present include dyspnea, wheezing, and hoarseness of voice. On biopsy, a diagnosis is made. Steroids are frequently used in conjunction with streptomycin or tetracycline as a treatment to avoid fibrosis. Subglottic stenosis is a common side effect that needs to be treated with reconstructive surgery later on.

5.3.14. Laryngeal Mycosis

The larynx can infrequently be affected by fungi that cause infections like blastomycosis, histoplasmosis, and candidiasis. The diagnosis is typically made after a biopsy and the discovery of a lesion that is similar in other body parts.

5.4. Congenital Lesions of the Larynx and Stridor

Congenital anomalies can result from intrauterine events that impact fetal and embryonic growth, or they can be the outcome of errors in embryogenesis, known as malformations. There are more chances for deformity the more intricately a structure is formed. Many malformations result from defects in the development and growth of the larynx.

5.4.1. Laryngomalacia

The most common cause of stridor in newborns is laryngomalacia, and the majority of these abnormalities manifest symptoms at birth or in the first few days of life. Supine positions, feeding, and crying can aggravate mild cases of stridor. Almost all children with laryngomalacia experience a resolution of symptoms by the time they turn one year old, with 50% of cases experiencing worsening symptoms during the first six months of life. Surgery is necessary for children (10%) who have severe laryngomalacia; symptoms in these children can include apnea, cyanosis, severe retractions, and failure to thrive. Cor pulmonale is seen in cases that are very severe.

Flexible transnasal fiberoptic laryngoscopy confirms the diagnosis. Short aryepiglottic folds with cuneiform cartilage prolapse are characteristic findings. A tightly curled (Ω-shaped) epiglottis is also observed in certain cases. The supraglottic structures exhibit a characteristic collapse upon inspiration due to the Bernoulli effect. Additionally common is inflammation suggestive of reflux laryngitis. The infant's symptoms dictate whether or not intervention is necessary, not the larynx's appearance during an endoscopy. Acute airway compromise is a rare presentation for children with laryngomalacia. Within one to two weeks of presentation, operative management for the 10% of children who need it can be scheduled in a semi-elective manner. It is wise to treat gastroesophageal reflux disease (GER) before surgery. The preferred intervention is now supraglottoplasty, also known as epiglottoplasty, instead of tracheotomy. This quick and efficient endoscopic treatment targets the infant's unique laryngeal pathology. Usually, one or both aryepiglottic folds are divided. Furthermore, it is possible to remove one or both cuneiform cartilages. In most cases, postoperative intubation is not necessary if the aryepiglottic folds are divided; however, if more extensive surgery has been done, it may be necessary to consider overnight intubation.

After supraglottoplasty, it is preferable to stay overnight in the intensive care unit due to the possibility of laryngeal edema impairing the airway and requiring reintubation. Extubation can typically be performed 24 hours after surgery. Some children experience postoperative obstruction. Laryngeal edema and persistent laryngomalacia can be distinguished by bedside fiberoptic laryngoscopy. Controlling reflux aids in the reduction of laryngeal edema. Sometimes the larynx looks good after surgery, but the baby is still having trouble breathing. In these situations, laryngomalacia may have an underlying neurological cause. Even though the neurological issues might be incredibly subtle at first, they might eventually become much more noticeable. This group of kids is far more likely to need to have a tracheotomy placed.

5.4.2. Bilateral Vocal Fold Paralysis

Bilateral paralysis, in contrast to unilateral vocal fold paralysis, is typically congenital. Despite being primarily idiopathic, this condition can also be associated with pathologies of the central nervous system, such as hydrocephalus and brainstem Chiari malformation. A tracheotomy is recommended for a baby with bilateral paralysis-related stridor and retractions. Similar to laryngomalacia, awake flexible transnasal fiberoptic laryngoscopy is used to make the diagnosis. As an alternate temporizing strategy, intubation, CPAP, or a high-flow nasal cannula can all be used to achieve stabilization. By the time a child is a year old, up to 50% of cases of paralysis spontaneously resolve. As a result, surgical intervention to accomplish decannulation is typically delayed until after this time. Achieving a sufficient decannulated airway while preserving voice and avoiding worsening aspiration are the goals of surgery. Laser cordotomy, endoscopic or open partial or full arytenoidectomy, endoscopically guided or open vocal process lateralization, and posterior cricoid cartilage grafting are among the surgical options available. There is no one solution that works perfectly. Before decannulation, it is frequently preferable to keep a child's tracheotomy in place to guarantee a sufficient airway. Compared to idiopathic cord paralysis, acquired bilateral vocal cord paralysis is typically more resistant to treatment, and decannulation may need multiple procedures. Post-extubation stridor in patients who have had any of these procedures may improve with CPAP therapy or a high-flow nasal cannula. Before returning to a regular diet, a video swallow study should be used to determine the child's postoperative risk of aspiration. Certain textures, especially thin fluids, can occasionally increase the risk of aspiration during the first few weeks after surgery.

5.4.3. Subglottic Stenosis

A failure of the laryngeal lumen to recanalize is thought to be the cause of congenital SGS, which is defined as a lumen 4.0 mm in diameter or less at the level of the cricoid in a term newborn. It belongs to a spectrum of embryologic failures that also includes webs, stenosis, and laryngeal atresia. Congenital SGS manifests as a typical cricoid with a smaller diameter than average, typically elliptical in shape, in its mildest form. Recurrent upper respiratory infections can cause mild SGS, wherein airway obstruction is caused by minimal subglottic swelling. The biggest obstruction in a young child is typically located 1–3 mm below the actual vocal folds. Acute airway compromise may be present at delivery in more severe cases. In the event that endotracheal intubation is successful, the patient might need medical attention prior to being removed. Placing a tracheotomy at the time of delivery may be lifesaving if intubation is not possible. It is crucial to remember that babies usually exhibit surprisingly few symptoms. Even people with grade 3 SGS (occlusion of 71–99%) might not exhibit any symptoms for several weeks or months.

One common association between congenital SGS and other head and neck syndromes and lesions (e.g., a patient with Down syndrome's tiny larynx). The larynx will develop with the patient following the first management of SGS and might not need additional surgery. On the other hand, there is a significant chance of developing an acquired SGS in addition to the underlying congenital SGS if initial management calls for tracheal intubation. The location and duration of the stenosis may be revealed to the clinician through radiologic evaluation of an unintubated patient's airway. Three imaging modalities are useful: (1) chest X-ray; (2) inspiratory and expiratory lateral soft-tissue neck films; and (3) fluoroscopy to show the dynamics of the trachea and larynx. High-kilovoltage airway film, however, is the one and only most crucial study. These films are able to distinguish between potential tracheal stenosis and the classic steepling seen in SGS patients. Complete tracheal rings are typically the cause of the latter condition, which puts the patient at risk for a potentially fatal outcome during rigid endoscopy.

Assessment of subglottic stenosis (SGS) necessitates endoscopic evaluation. Flexible fiberoptic endoscopy provides insight into vocal fold dynamics, while rigid endoscopy with Hopkins telescopes offers the most thorough examination. A detailed assessment of the endolarynx, including grading of the SGS, is essential. In cases of mild SGS in children with minor symptoms, endoscopic treatments like radial incisions with steroid injections and laryngeal dilatation may be effective. Severe SGS typically requires open airway reconstruction, with laryngotracheal reconstruction using costal cartilage grafts being a reliable option. These procedures can be performed in one or two stages, with careful post-operative management to ensure successful recovery. Cricotracheal resection is preferred over laryngotracheal reconstruction for severe SGS cases, although it is a complex procedure with potential complications. Patients must be thoroughly evaluated and optimized before undergoing subglottic airway reconstruction, including managing conditions like GER, EE, and tracheal infections.

5.4.4. Saccular Cysts

At the anterior end of the laryngeal ventricle, the laryngeal saccule is a small diverticulum that extends superiorly between the vestibular fold and the inner surface of the thyroid cartilage. It is home to a large number of mucous glands. Mucus-filled congenital saccular cysts typically extend posterosuperiorly into the aryepiglottic fold and false vocal fold (the lateral saccular cyst). In the first few days of life, these cysts usually cause dysphagia, a muffled cry, and respiratory obstruction. One of the biggest risks for children with saccular cysts is the induction of general anesthesia, which can result in the loss of the airway and total obstruction because low muscle tone predisposes to obstruction. Preoperative awake transnasal flexible laryngoscopy is therefore required to assess the airway, as this will alert the patient to potential issues with the subsequent anesthesia. An appropriate ventilating bronchoscope, a styleted endotracheal tube, or an endotracheal tube covered by a small Hopkins rod telescope can all be used to secure the airway during anesthesia. The use of anesthesia carries risks, so this should only be tried in the presence of people and equipment that can secure the airway. It could be extremely dangerous to send a baby for a radiologic evaluation that calls for sedation or anesthesia. As a result, it is best to assess and stabilize the airway in the operating room and then to consider doing a radiologic evaluation.

Saccular cysts have traditionally been treated endoscopically through needle aspiration, marsupialization, or endoscopic excision; however, the outcomes have not been good, frequently necessitating repeated procedures and the placement of a tracheotomy. The author prefers to employ an anterior cervical approach, in which the thyrohyoid membrane is incised along its superior border after identifying the thyroid alar cartilage's superior border. By using this method, the cyst can be gently dissected free and removed whole. After the cyst is removed, part of the thyroid cartilage may be removed to allow for better access and replacement.

5.4.5. Posterior Laryngeal Clefts

The inability of the laryngotracheal groove to fuse during embryogenesis leads to posterior laryngeal clefts. Anomalies that impact the respiratory system or other organ systems are frequently present in patients. Tracheomalacia (>80%) and tracheoesophageal fistula (TEF) formation (20%) are associated airway anomalies. Anogenital anomalies and GER are examples of non-airway associations. Opitz-Frias syndrome, which is characterized by hypertelorism, anogenital anomalies, and posterior laryngeal clefting, is the most prevalent syndrome linked to posterior laryngeal clefting.

Benjamin and Inglis proposed a useful anatomic classification that splits posterior laryngeal clefts into four subtypes.

- Type 1: The supraglottic interarytenoid cleft is located at the level of the true vocal folds, not below them. An alternative name for this cleft would be a deep interarytenoid notch.
- Type 2: partial cricoid cleft that penetrates the posterior cricoid cartilage but does not go through it.
- Type 3: complete cricoid cleft, either closed or open to the cervical trachea.
- Type 4: the thoracic trachea is reached by the cleft.

A cleft that reaches into or past the carina is an uncommon variation of type 4 (also known as type 4 long). Clinicians should be aware that symptoms do not always indicate the severity of a cleft; in fact, there is a lot of overlap in symptoms between the different types of clefts. The primary clinical characteristic of this anomaly is aspiration. Microaspiration, choking episodes, transient cyanosis, and recurrent chest infections are common symptoms of gross aspiration, though it can also be accompanied by apnea, cyanosis, and even pneumonia. The airway may be seriously compromised by severe tracheomalacia, particularly in children who also have a tracheoesophageal fistula.

The gold standard for diagnosis is rigid bronchoscopy and esophagoscopy, despite the availability of diagnostic tools such as flexible nasopharyngoscopy, fiberoptic endoscopic evaluation of swallowing, video fluoroscopy-barium swallow, and flexible bronchoscopy. Because the cleft in the posterior glottis is frequently obscured by superfluous mucosa, it frequently goes misdiagnosed or unnoticed during the initial evaluation using flexible or rigid bronchoscopy. The goal of management is to reduce the chance of aspiration while maintaining a suitable airway. Determining whether the infant needs a Nissen fundoplication, tracheotomy, or gastrostomy tube insertion should be the first step in managing the patient. All of these improve the chances of a successful cleft repair, even though none of them are necessary. Additionally important is protection against aspiration; nasojejunal feeding can help stabilize a baby. Most type 1 and some type 2 clefts can be repaired surgically endoscopically; longer clefts that extend into the cervical or thoracic trachea, however, need to be repaired openly. The transtracheal technique preserves the recurrent laryngeal nerves while offering the cleft an unmatched level of exposure. It is advised to use a two-layer closure, but if necessary, an interposition graft can be done. A free transfer of the sternal periosteum is a helpful interposition graft.

The uncommon type 4 long cleft is the hardest to repair. These clefts are prone to anastomotic breakdown, and the baby frequently has a variety of non-airway and airway abnormalities. Microgastria, polysplenia, and annular pancreas are examples of the latter. Microgastria is resistant to fundoplications and can cause uncontrollable reflux of the stomach. Prior to attempting cleft repair through surgery, the surgeon must determine whether the child is still viable. Depending on a variety of factors, posterior laryngeal cleft success rates can range from 50% to 90%. A congenital tracheoesophageal fistula present at birth is the most important factor compromising successful cleft repair. The degree of the cleft, the surgeon's procedure of choice, and whether a single- or double-layer closure is used are additional variables. Compared to primary surgery, revision surgery has lower success rates.

5.4.6. Laryngeal Webs

A failure of glottic airway recanalization in the early weeks of embryogenesis is represented by laryngeal webs. The majority of glottic webs, or 95% of them, are anterior; nevertheless, these webs are uncommon, making up only 5% of congenital laryngeal abnormalities. Congenital glottic webbing is not currently associated with any known gene; however, a noteworthy correlation has been observed between this abnormality and chromosome 22q11.2 deletion syndrome, also known as velocardiofacial syndrome. It is wise to refer all patients with congenital anterior glottic webs for genetic evaluation, as more than half of patients with anterior glottic webs have chromosome 22q11.2 deletion syndrome. While some webs are extremely thin, the majority are thick and typically connected to a subglottic "sail" that threatens the subglottic lumen. They could thus be categorized as a particular type of partial laryngeal atresia. At birth, newborns typically exhibit an unusual cry or respiratory distress. An emergency airway intervention is necessary if a newborn with an anterior glottic web exhibits severe airway compromise during the first few hours or days of life. However, the infant is remarkably tolerant of airway compromise, and even infants with a moderate to severe glottic web may initially present with mild airway symptoms, which the clinician should be aware of. The first few months of life are usually when these symptoms get worse. Biphasic stridor and retractions become more noticeable in infants with moderate to severe webs, especially when these babies are agitated or feeding.

Rigid or flexible bronchoscopy is necessary for a conclusive assessment. Evaluations are made of the web's severity as well as its subglottic extension. Rigid bronchoscopy is better for assessing the degree of associated SGS, but flexible bronchoscopy offers a great view of the anterior commissure. When a child has a severe web, it is important to avoid making their already compromised airway worse. Intubation or an emergent tracheotomy is not preferred over spontaneous ventilation where the infant maintains his or her own airway. Compared to the far more common thick web with subglottic extension, the management of an infant with a gossamer-thin anterior glottic web is different. Since it is believed that intubation for airway stabilization may actually lyse the web and completely resolve the issue in a child with neonatal airway compromise due to such a web, the infant with a thin glottic web may never be diagnosed. When an infant is suspended on a small Lindholm laryngoscope and presents with a thin anterior web during bronchoscopy, dividing the web with a sickle knife can be therapeutic.

When a thick glottic web is present in an infant, the first decision to be made is whether to repair it later in life or early in the neonatal period. Since late repair is technically easier in a larger larynx, it is preferred in children with mild to moderate webs and no clinical airway compromise. To enhance a child's voice before they reach school age, late repair is typically completed by the time they are 4 years old. Early repair may be necessary for children whose glottic compromise is more severe. As an alternative, a tracheotomy might be performed and a delayed repair might be arranged. Approximately 40% of patients with thick webs require this approach. Open keel placement and open anterior commissure reconstruction are two options for treating a congenital anterior glottic web. It is not recommended to perform endoscopic procedures like laser division of the web or endoscopic keel placement. Laser division does not sufficiently address the inherent SGS that is typically present and is likely to cause web reformation. Similarly, SGS is not addressed by endoscopic keel placement. Furthermore, it is technically demanding for an infant, even though it might be a suitable option for an older child.

5.4.7. Subglottic Hemangioma

Hemangiomas can develop in any anatomic location, despite the fact that they typically manifest cutaneously. The most typical airway presentation site is the larynx, specifically the subglottis. A synchronous subglottic lesion may be present because cutaneous hemangiomas are present in over 50% of patients with subglottic hemangiomas. Individuals whose hemangioma is distributed throughout their beard (i.e., the chin, jawline, and preauricular areas) are most vulnerable to subglottic hemangioma. Subglottic hemangiomas grow and involute more quickly than cutaneous lesions, but their natural history is similar to that of cutaneous lesions in that it begins with proliferation and ends with involution. The airway typically deteriorates over time as the hemangioma grows larger. Biphasic stridor with retractions is one of the symptoms, particularly when the child is distressed or feeding. There could also be a barking cough, which is comparable to the croup. Severe airway obstruction can cause cyanosis, apnea, and "dying spells."

The best method for doing a preliminary assessment is using awake transnasal flexible laryngoscopy. This could make the compromised subglottis visible, but more importantly, it should rule out other possible causes of stridor in newborns, like vocal fold paralysis and laryngomalacia. When a child has both a normal glottic and supraglottic examination and progressive stridor, they need to have a laryngoscopy and bronchoscopy done in the operating room while under general anesthesia. As previously discussed in this section, by the time the child arrives for a rigid bronchoscopy, the subglottic lumen may have already been compromised to an extent of 80–90% because infants are so remarkably tolerant of progressive subglottic airway compromise. In infants in whom extralaryngeal involvement is suspected (e.g., those with cutaneous hemangiomas occurring in a beard distribution), magnetic resonance imaging (MRI) with T2-weighted gadolinium contrast is performed. Biopsies are not recommended due to the potential for bleeding.

5.5. Laryngeal Paralysis

A condition known as vocal cord paralysis causes you to lose control over the movement of the muscles that produce your voice. It occurs when your voice box's (larynx) nerve impulses are interfered with. The muscles of the vocal cord become paralyzed as a result. Breathing and speaking can be difficult in cases of vocal cord paralysis. This is so that your vocal cords, also known as vocal folds, can do more than just generate sound. Additionally, they shield your airway by keeping food, liquids, and even saliva from choking you in the trachea, your windpipe. Viral infections, certain malignancies, and nerve damage sustained during surgery are all potential causes of vocal cord paralysis. Surgery and occasionally voice therapy are used as treatments for vocal cord paralysis.

5.5.1. Symptoms

The two pliable bands of muscle tissue that are located at the windpipe's opening are called your vocal cords (trachea). The bands come together and vibrate to produce sound when you speak. The vocal cords are kept loose and open during the remainder of the speech to allow for breathing. Typically, vocal cord paralysis affects just one paralyzed vocal cord. It is an uncommon but dangerous condition to have paralysis of both vocal cords. This may result in serious issues with breathing and swallowing, as well as trouble speaking. Vocal cord paralysis symptoms and indicators could be as follows.

- A breathy quality to the voice
- Hoarseness
- Noisy breathing
- Shortness of breath
- Loss of vocal pitch
- choking or hacking up food particles, liquids, or saliva.
- the requirement to inhale deeply while speaking
- Inability to speak loudly
- Loss of your gag reflex
- Ineffective coughing
- Frequent throat clearing

When to See a Doctor: If you experience persistent hoarseness for over 2 to 4 weeks, or if you observe any unexplained alterations in your voice or discomfort, please get in touch with your healthcare provider.

5.5.2. Causes

The nerve impulses that supply the larynx, or voice box, are interfered with in vocal cord paralysis, resulting in muscle paralysis. Many times, medical professionals are unable to pinpoint the precise cause of vocal cord paralysis. However, a few recognized causes could be:

- **Vocal Cord Damage Resulting from Surgery:** The nerves supplying the voice box may sustain damage from surgery performed on or near the neck or upper chest. Surgery on the thyroid or parathyroid glands, esophagus, neck, and chest are among the procedures that have a potential for harm.
- **Neck or Chest Injury:** The nerves supplying the vocal cords or the voice box itself may be damaged by trauma to the neck or chest.
- **Stroke:** A stroke damages the area of the brain that communicates with the voice box and stops blood flow to that area.
- **Tumors:** Vocal cord paralysis can result from tumors, both malignant and noncancerous, growing in or near the muscles, cartilage, or nerves that control the voice box's function.
- **Infections:** Certain infections, like Epstein-Barr virus, herpes, and Lyme disease, can inflame the voice

box's nerves and cause direct harm to them. There is some evidence that a COVID-19 infection can result in vocal cord paralysis.

- **Neurological Conditions:** Vocal cord paralysis can result from a number of neurological disorders, including Parkinson's disease and multiple sclerosis.

5.5.3. Risk Factors

There are several factors that could raise your chance of vocal cord paralysis.

- **Undergoing Throat or Chest Surgery:** Individuals undergoing surgery for thyroid, throat, or upper chest conditions are more susceptible to damage to their vocal cords. Vocal cord nerve damage can occasionally result from breathing tubes used during surgery or to assist breathing if you are experiencing severe respiratory problems.
- **Having a Neurological Condition:** Individuals with specific neurological disorders, like multiple sclerosis or Parkinson's disease, are more susceptible to vocal cord paralysis or weakness.

5.5.4. Complications

Vocal cord paralysis-related breathing issues can range from being so minor as to only cause hoarseness to being so severe as to be life-threatening. As a result of vocal cord paralysis, the airway's aperture cannot fully open or close, which can lead to additional complications like choking or aspirating food or liquids. Although rare, aspiration that results in severe pneumonia is dangerous and needs to be treated right away.

5.5.4.1. Diagnosis

Your doctor will probably listen to your voice, ask you about your symptoms and lifestyle, and inquire about the duration of your voice issues. Your voice issues may be further assessed by doing the following tests:

- **Laryngoscopy:** Your physician uses either a mirror, a thin, flexible tube (called a laryngoscope or endoscope), or both to examine your vocal cords. Another test that you might have is a videostrobolaryngoscopy. It makes use of a specialized scope with either a larger camera attached to the scope's viewing piece or a tiny camera at its tip.

  In order to ascertain the movement and position of your vocal cords as well as whether one or both of them are affected, your care provider can view your vocal cords directly through these specialized high-magnification endoscopes or on a video monitor.
- **Laryngeal Electromyography:** The electrical currents in your voice box muscles are measured by this test. In order to accomplish this, the medical professional usually uses tiny needles that are inserted through the neck skin into the vocal cord muscles.

  Although this test is not meant to direct treatment, it might provide your doctor with insights into your potential for recovery. When this test is conducted between six weeks and six months after the onset of your symptoms, it is most beneficial.
- **Blood Tests and Scans:** To determine the underlying cause of the paralysis, you might require

more testing as several illnesses can result in nerve damage. Tests could involve MRIs, CT scans, X-rays, or blood work.

5.5.5. Treatment

The cause, the intensity of the symptoms, and the length of time since the onset of symptoms all affect how vocal cord paralysis is treated. Surgery, injections given in large quantities, voice therapy, or a mix of these therapies may be used as treatments. You might occasionally recover without undergoing surgery. Because of this, your surgeon may decide to postpone major surgery for a minimum of a year after your vocal cord paralysis first manifests. Nonetheless, within the first three months of voice loss, surgical treatment using different bulk injections is frequently administered. In order to prevent you from using your voice incorrectly while the nerves heal, your doctor might recommend voice therapy while you wait for surgery.

5.5.5.1. Voice Therapy

Exercises and other activities are performed during voice therapy sessions to strengthen your vocal cords, enhance breath control during speech, avoid tense other surrounding muscles of the paralyzed vocal cord or cords, and safeguard your airway when swallowing. If your paralyzed vocal cords are in a place where you don't need to add bulk or realign, voice therapy might be all you need to treat them.

5.5.5.2. Surgery

Your ability to swallow and speak may be improved by surgical treatments if the symptoms of your vocal cord paralysis don't go away on their own. Options for surgery include:

- **Bulk Injection:** Your vocal cord's muscle will most likely become weak and thin if the nerve that supplies it is paralyzed. A laryngologist, a physician who specializes in disorders of the larynx, may inject body fat, collagen, or another approved filler material into your paralyzed vocal cord to give it more volume. When you speak, swallow, or cough, the extra bulk pushes the affected vocal cord toward the center of your voice box, where it can make closer contact with the other, functioning, moving vocal cord.
- **Structural Implants:** This procedure, also called laryngeal framework surgery, medialization laryngoplasty, or thyroplasty, uses an implant in the larynx to realign the vocal cord in place of a bulk injection. In rare cases, patients may require a second procedure to realign the implant.
- **Vocal Cord Repositioning:** The paralyzed vocal cord is pushed toward the center of your voice box by the surgeon during this procedure, which involves moving a window of your own tissue from the outside inward. Your unimpaired vocal cord can now vibrate more effectively against its paralyzed partner as a result.
- **Replacing the Damaged Nerve (Reinnervation):** In order to replace the damaged vocal cord during this surgery, a healthy nerve is transferred from another part of the neck. Your voice may not get better for up to six or nine months. Some medical professionals pair this procedure with a bulk injection.
- **Tracheotomy:** Your airflow will be

reduced if both of your vocal cords are paralyzed and positioned near to each other. This makes breathing extremely difficult and necessitates tracheotomy surgery.

A tracheotomy involves making an incision in the front of the neck to expose the trachea, or windpipe. By inserting a breathing tube, air is able to pass through the vocal cords.

5.5.5.3. Emerging Treatments

The inoperable vocal cords may be able to open and close again by connecting them to another electrical stimulation source, such as a cardiac pacemaker or a nerve from another area of the body.

5.5.5.4. Coping and Support

Disabling vocal cord paralysis can interfere with day-to-day activities. Interpersonal communication can be challenging. You can acquire the communication skills you need with the assistance of a speech therapist. Voice therapy can assist you in learning useful strategies to compensate for the loss of your former voice, even if it is not possible to restore it. Furthermore, you can learn how to use your voice from a speech-language pathologist without endangering your vocal cords.

5.6. Benign Tumors of the Larynx

Male and female individuals can develop benign laryngeal tumors at any age. The most typical sign is a person's voice changing. The prognosis for this kind of tumor is typically favorable because it is not malignant. Recurrent respiratory papillomas are the most prevalent kind of benign laryngeal tumor (RRP). About 4.6 out of 100,000 children and 1.8 out of 100,000 adults experience it. Experts surmise that human papillomavirus exposure during childbirth is the cause of childhood RRPs. Papillomas account for about 85% of benign tumors of the larynx.

Types of benign laryngeal tumors include:

- papillomas
- fibromas
- hemangiomas
- leiomyomas
- rhabdomyomas
- schwannomas
- myxomas
- chondromas
- neurofibromas

Benign tumors are caused by alterations in the larynx, and they differ from cancer in that they usually do not spread.

5.6.1. Symptoms of Benign Laryngeal Tumors

Harshness, breathy voice, dyspnea, aspiration, dysphagia, otalgia (ear pain), and hemoptysis are among the signs and symptoms of benign laryngeal tumors. The most common cause of otalgia, which is pain that is referred to the ear due to vagus nerve irritation or distension, is a malignant tumor that is growing quickly.

5.6.2. Diagnosis

A physician may carry out or prescribe the following procedures in order to diagnose a benign laryngeal tumor.

- a physical examination that includes a vocal cord examination.
- a CT scan to ascertain the tumor's exact location, size, and form.
- a biopsy to take tissue samples for examination in a lab.
- a throat examination by

laryngoscopic, which is usually performed in conjunction with a biopsy

The process of diagnosing involves excluding other potential conditions. To exclude alternative reasons for the symptoms, a physician might inquire about:

- a person's history of allergies
- episodes of reflux
- instances of vocal overuse
- previous intubations
- symptom onset and progression
- trauma history

A tissue biopsy can rule out malignancy even though a visual examination or imaging results may indicate that a tumor is benign.

5.6.3. Treatment for Benign Laryngeal Tumors

Surgical excision is typically the first step in the treatment of a benign laryngeal tumor. Tumors have the potential to grow and obstruct a person's airway, so removal is a crucial component of treatment. A few tumors, like neurofibromas and papillomas, have the potential to develop into cancer. Physicians use laser surgery or conventional surgical methods to remove benign laryngeal tumors. Due to the tendency of laryngeal papillomas to recur, repeat surgeries may be necessary. Physicians may think about extra therapeutic alternatives, such as drugs and photodynamic therapy, if:

- An individual needs more than four surgeries in a calendar year.
- Papillomas regrow quickly.
- The person's airway is compromised by the tumor.
- The papillomas dispersed to different locations.

5.6.4. Outlook

The majority of patients with benign laryngeal tumors have good prognoses. Even benign tumors, though, can result in side effects like airway obstruction. Tumors can occasionally develop into malignant growths. Around 1% and 4% of benign papillomas progress to squamous cell carcinoma. Furthermore, there are hazards associated with laryngeal tumor removal surgery, just like with any other surgery.

5.7. Cancer of the Larynx

One-third of all head and neck cancers are laryngeal cancers, which can also be a major cause of morbidity and death. Patients with a history of heavy smoking are most likely to be diagnosed with them, as they are also more susceptible to cancers in the remaining portions of the aerodigestive tract. They may affect various laryngeal subsites, which may have an impact on symptom presentation, dissemination patterns, and treatment approaches. With either surgical or radiation monotherapy, often with larynx preservation, early-stage disease is highly curable. On the other hand, late-stage disease is less frequently larynx-preserving, has a worse prognosis, and necessitates multimodal therapy. In the present era, speech rehabilitation techniques for individuals in need of laryngectomy have improved.

About 13,000 laryngeal cancers, mostly squamous cell cancers, are diagnosed in the United States each year. Unlike laryngeal cancer, which was treated primarily surgically in the past, organ preservation is now the focus of the treatment strategy, which involves chemoradiation. Numerous investigations demonstrate that this method yields outcomes comparable to a total laryngectomy. Furthermore, endoscopic techniques are now available for the treatment of laryngeal cancer.

5.7.1. Etiology

With smoking being linked to between 70 and 95% of cases, smoking is the single biggest risk factor for laryngeal cancer. Any smoking history is associated with increased risk; smokers who are currently smoking have higher relative risks overall compared to non-smokers as well as higher relative risks for supraglottic cancers compared to glottic cancers. A correlation with excessive alcohol intake has also been identified; however, since alcohol is typically used in conjunction with tobacco, the effect of alcohol alone is unclear. For younger patients, smoking marijuana may have an impact. Unlike other head and neck cancers, there is no proof that the human papillomavirus (HPV) is the cause of this one.

The following are additional risk factors for laryngeal cancer:

- Advanced age
- A diet low in green leafy vegetables
- Infection with HPV
- A high-fat, salt-preserved meat diet.
- Exposure to radiation, paint, asbestos, and fuel fumes.

5.7.2. Epidemiology

In 2017, there were 13,150 new cases of laryngeal cancer, or approximately one-third of all head and neck cancers. 3,710 deaths were linked to this disease. Patients are 65 years old on average, and there is a greater percentage of males than females and blacks than whites. Age-adjusted incidence rates have dropped by roughly 2% per year in recent years, which has been linked to a decline in tobacco use. Around 2% of all cases of laryngeal cancer are glottic cancers, which are three times more common than supraglottic and subglottic cancers. Approximately 98% of laryngeal cancers originate in the supraglottic or glottic regions. Early-stage cancers are very treatable; local control rates for T1 glottic cancers range from 90 to 95%, and for early-stage supraglottic cancers, they range from 80 to 90%. Moreover, surgical therapy that spares the vocal cords is typically an option for these early-stage cancers. On the other hand, control rates for locally advanced cancers range from 40 to 70%; laryngectomy is frequently necessary for bulky and/or T4 disease. But improvements in laryngectomy patients' speech rehabilitation and increased laryngeal preservation have been made possible by advancements over the years.

5.7.3. Pathophysiology

Squamous cell carcinomas that are well-differentiated account for the majority of laryngeal cancers. Verrucous, sarcomatoid, and neuroendocrine carcinomas are among the squamous cell variants that account for a small percentage of cases. In the past, verrucous and sarcomatoid carcinomas were thought to be radioresistant; however, more recent research has shown otherwise. The location of the primary mass and the natural lymphatic supply determine the patterns of spread. There are three subsites for laryngeal cancers: supraglottic, glottic, and subglottic. The pathophysiology and course of treatment vary depending on the subsite.

5.7.3.1. Supraglottic

False vocal cords, aryepiglottic folds, arytenoids, suprahyoid epiglottis, and infrahyoid epiglottis are the divisions of the supraglottis. Before exhibiting symptoms, suprahyoid epiglottic tumors may expand superiorly and exophytically, occasionally to greater sizes. In other situations, they might encroach inferiorly into the epiglottis' tip and obliterate the surrounding cartilage. On the other hand, infrahyoid epiglottic tumors typically grow circumferentially, involving the aryepiglottic folds before potentially infiltrating the false vocal cords inferiorly. Additionally, they encroach anteriorly into the pre-epiglottic fat space, the base of the tongue, and the vallecula.

Unlike glottic or subglottic cancers, supraglottic cancers are characterized by lymphatic involvement; at presentation, 55% of patients show clinical evidence of nodal metastasis, and 16% show contralateral involvement. Cancer primarily spreads to cervical nodal chain levels II, II, and IV in order to reduce the risk of involvement. Locally advanced tumors are more likely to metastasize to nodes, either by superior extension and invasion into the base of the tongue, vallecula, and pyriform sinus, or by bilateral tumor involvement, which also raises the risk of lymphatic spread in the bilateral neck.

5.7.3.2. Glottic

The transition from the supraglottic to the glottic larynx is represented by the ventricle's apex. The vocal cords end posteriorly at a commissure with the vocal process and vary in thickness from 3 to 5 mm. They do not pose a risk of lymphatic involvement unless there is a supraglottic or glottic extension because they have a sparse lymphatic supply. Usually, glottic cancers only show up in the front part of one vocal cord's upper free margin. They may cause vocal cord fixation through sheer muscle mass, intrinsic muscle and ligament involvement, or, in rarer cases, recurrent laryngeal nerve involvement.

5.7.3.3. Subglottic

The subglottis begins 5 mm below the vocal cord and ends at the lower border of the cricoid cartilage (or 10 mm below the ventricle apex). It has limited lymphatic drainage, which collects into cervical nodal chain levels IV and VI.

5.7.4. Histopathology

Squamous cell cancers account for the majority of laryngeal cancers. On the other hand, adenocarcinomas, sarcomas, lymphomas, and neuroendocrine tumors are uncommon forms of cancer. Squamous cell carcinoma's histopathology ranges widely, from hyperplasia and dysplasia carcinoma in situ to an invasive cancer.

5.7.5. History and Physical

Most patients are men who have smoked tobacco in the past or present. Due to vocal cord immobility or fixation, hoarseness is frequently the first symptom of glottic cancers to manifest, with swallowing difficulties and referred ear pain signifying more advanced disease. On the other hand, the most typical early sign of supraglottic cancer is difficulty swallowing, and hoarseness signals that the disease has progressed and is now affecting the glottis. Nodal metastases appear in the neck as hard, stable, painless masses. All subsites experience late symptoms such as dysphagia, airway compromise, aspiration and its aftereffects, and weight loss.

An invasive assessment of the primary lesion, which often involves fiberoptic endoscopy, mirror examination, and indirect laryngoscopy, is the most important physical examination component. The aim is to evaluate the local extent of the tumor by observing the size and involvement of surrounding structures and evaluating the mobility of the vocal cord. Direct laryngoscopy provides improved capacity for obtaining tissue specimens and for defining the extent of disease. It is essential to perform a complete neck examination to check for the extension of the primary lesion as well as nodal metastases. Thyroid cartilage tenderness signifies direct tumor extension, while firm fullness felt just above the thyroid notch traditionally denotes pre-epiglottic space invasion.

5.7.6. Diagnosis

Your medical history and symptoms will be inquired about by a healthcare professional.

They will examine your neck and throat during a physical examination. You will most likely require additional testing to confirm a diagnosis after the initial examination.

Diagnostic tests include:

- **Imaging Scans:** A CT or MRI scan can produce finely detailed internal body images. They are able to display the location and size of a tumor. An X-ray of the chest can reveal whether cancer has spread to the lungs.
- **Laryngoscopy:** An endoscope is a thin, lighted tube that a healthcare professional uses to examine your larynx during a laryngoscopy.
- **PET Scan:** A tiny, safe dose of a radioactive material is injected into your vein by the healthcare professional during a PET scan. The material draws attention to cancerous cell growths.
- **Biopsy:** A biopsy involves the removal of a tiny piece of abnormal tissue from your larynx for microscopic examination. A pathologist, who is an expert in this field, will assess the cells and search for specific protein markers. Certain cancer treatments are limited to targeting cancer cells that possess particular protein markers.

5.7.7. Treatment / Management

Treatment for laryngeal cancer is decided by the:

- Type of cancer
- Extent or stage of the tumor
- Precise portions of the larynx involved with the tumor.

5.7.7.1. Early-Stage Laryngeal Cancer

T1-2N0 disease and other early-stage laryngeal cancers can be effectively treated with one locally-directed treatment modality, such as surgery or local radiation therapy.

5.7.7.2. T1-2N0 Glottic Cancer

It is advised to undergo local radiation therapy or surgery; the choice of modality will largely depend on the patient's preferences and the experience of the provider. These treatment approaches have one thing in common: they only treat the main tumor due to the true glottis's sparse lymphatic drainage. Although there are no Level I data comparing the two methods, previous experience indicates that the local control rates of respiratory therapy (RT) and surgical methods are similar. For a number of these cancers, voice-sparing surgery is an option, but not always. In one case, 10% of T1 and 55% of T2 tumors required a total laryngectomy as the surgical procedure of choice. Laryngofissure, partial laryngectomy, and transoral laser excision are further methods. Although there is insufficient data to compare surgery and RT, randomized studies show that definitive RT results in better voice preservation than transoral laser excision.

5.7.7.3. T1-2N0, Selected T1-2N1/ T3N0-1 Supraglottic Cancer

Supraglottic cancers can be treated with either larynx-sparing surgery or radiation therapy alone, with comparable overall efficacy to early-stage glottic cancers. The treatment of the neck in light of the possibility of nodal metastases is the primary distinction amongst glottic cancers. For T1-2 and low-volume T3 disease, surgical techniques include endoscopic resection or partial supraglottic laryngectomy; neck dissection frequently reveals T2 or T3 lesions. Many patients receive adjuvant radiation therapy (RT), with common indications being extracapsular extension, positive margins, and positive nodal disease. Usually levels II to IV, at-risk cervical nodal stations are included in definitive radiotherapy.

5.7.7.4. Locally Advanced Laryngeal Cancers

Treatment for locally advanced cancers, such as T3-4N1-3 disease, is more complex and usually entails combination therapy. Even if these tumors could be surgically removed, laryngeal preservation surgery is not an option. However, conclusive radiation therapy combined with cisplatin chemotherapy is still a viable option for laryngeal preservation. When it comes to treating locally advanced disease, as opposed to early-stage disease, level I evidence is used. The combination of radiation and chemotherapy has been shown to improve locoregional control and preserve the larynx. Comparing laryngectomy and adjuvant radiotherapy to chemotherapy and salvage surgery, similar locoregional control rates have been shown in T4 disease. Larynx-preserving chemotherapy and radiation is linked to a lower prognosis in patients with T4 disease.

When a tumor is morbidly invaded and has advanced to a nodal stage on surgical pathology (pT3-4, pN2-3), along with other high-risk pathologic features like close margins (less than 5 mm), perineural invasion, lymphovascular space invasion, and extracapsular extension, post-operative radiation therapy (RT) is indicated. Furthermore, extracapsular extension, numerous positive nodes, and close or involved margins require the addition of chemotherapy in addition to RT. It is important for the reader to understand that while the morbidity of surgery has decreased, survival rates for laryngeal cancer have not increased significantly as a result of novel treatment approaches. Transoral laser microsurgery has gained popularity recently as a treatment for supraglottic and early glottic cancers. Experience as a surgeon is crucial, though. The cancer is removed piecemeal during the procedure, and the margins are assessed.

5.7.8. Differential Diagnosis

The following differential diagnoses should be taken into account and ruled out in relation to laryngeal cancer.

- Acute sialadenitis
- Bacterial lymphadenopathy
- Benign tumors (rare)
- Branchial cleft cyst
- Chronic laryngitis
- Chronic sialadenitis
- Contact granuloma
- Hemangioma
- HPV papillomas
- Laryngocele
- Polyps on the vocal cord(s)
- Reinkes edema
- Thyroglossal duct cyst

5.7.9. Staging

The next step after being diagnosed with cancer is staging. The stage indicates the extent of the cancer's spread. The TNM system is typically used by oncologists to stage laryngeal cancer.

- T stands for the primary tumor's size and whether or not it has spread to nearby tissue.
- The number N indicates the extent to which the cancer has spread to lymph nodes.
- M denotes the presence of metastases, or the spread of the cancer to distant lymph nodes or other organs.

The American Cancer Society states that lung metastases are the most typical for laryngeal cancer. The least dangerous cancers are small tumors that haven't spread to your lymph nodes or metastasized. Tumors become more dangerous as they enlarge. The likelihood of survival significantly reduces if cancer spreads to your lymph nodes or metastasizes. These cancers are later-stage or more advanced.

5.7.10. Enhancing Healthcare Team Outcomes

An interprofessional team comprising an ENT surgeon, oncologist, dietitian, pulmonologist, speech therapist, intensivist, and radiation therapists manages laryngeal cancer. Most patients initially visit their primary care physician complaining of weight loss, dysphagia, otalgia, and hoarseness. Most patients are men who have smoked tobacco in the past or present. If the hoarseness persists and is accompanied by other symptoms suggestive of a cancer, a referral to an ENT surgeon should be made. Evaluation and follow-up therapy require an interprofessional approach involving an ENT or oncologic surgeon, oncologist, respiratory therapist, speech therapist, and other clinicians due to the complexity of the treatment. To achieve the best results, the patient and family need coordinated education regarding procedures and aftercare.

An invasive assessment of the primary lesion, which often involves fiberoptic endoscopy, mirror examination, and indirect laryngoscopy, is the most important physical examination component. Complex and technically demanding surgery is the treatment for laryngeal cancer. Patients require close monitoring to ensure airway patency because postoperative complications are common. While there is hope for those with early-stage laryngeal cancer, the prognosis for those with advanced cancer is not good.

5.8. Voice and Speech Disorders

There are numerous causes for voice disorders in humans. A shift in voice quality is known as a voice disorder. Speech-language pathologists and medical professionals with training in ear, nose, and throat disorders diagnose and treat voice problems. The cause of the voice change determines the course of treatment. Interventions may involve medication, injections, surgery, or voice therapy.

5.8.1. Causes

The larynx, another name for the voice box, is composed of soft, moist areas, muscle, and a smooth covering. The voice box is located at the base of the tongue and the top of the windpipe, also called the trachea. Tone is produced by the vocal cords vibrating. The vocal cords vibrate as air passes through the voice box, drawing them closer together. In order to prevent you from breathing in food or liquid when swallowing, the vocal cords also assist in closing the voice box. Vocal cords cannot function normally if they swell or become inflamed, grow, or become immobile. Any of these could be the source of a voice issue.

Some common voice disorders include:

- Laryngitis
- Spasmodic dysphonia is the term for abnormalities in voice that are linked to the brain and nervous system.
- Growths on the vocal cords that are not cancerous include polyps, nodules, or cysts.
- Precancerous and cancerous growths
- Vocal cord paralysis or weakness
- White patches, also known as leukoplakia

5.8.2. Risk Factors

A voice disorder can result from numerous factors, including.

- Aging
- Alcohol use
- Allergies
- Disorders affecting the nervous system and brain, like stroke or Parkinson's disease.
- Gastroesophageal reflux disease (GERD)
- Illnesses like upper respiratory infections or colds.
- Scarring resulting from neck surgery or injuries to the front of the neck.
- Screaming
- Smoking
- Throat cancer
- Throat dehydration
- Thyroid problems
- Voice misuse or overuse

5.8.3. Diagnosis

Your physician will examine you and inquire about any issues you may be having with your voice. Before the exam, you may be given a numbing medication by your provider. One or more of the following tools may be used by your provider.

- **Mirror:** A dental mirror or other tool may be inserted into your mouth by your healthcare provider. It has an angled mirror and is long.
- **Flexible Laryngoscope:** This flexible tube is equipped with a light and camera. It is inserted by a provider using their nose.
- **Rigid Laryngoscope:** Using the mouth, a healthcare professional inserts this rigid viewing tube.
- **Video Stroboscope:** The vocal cords can be seen moving in slow motion thanks to a camera and flashing light.

A care provider may use other tests such as:

- **Sound Analysis:** This test uses a computer to measure any abnormalities in the vocal cords' sound.
- **Laryngeal Electromyography:** The electric currents in the voice box muscles are measured by tiny needles inserted through the skin.

5.8.4. Treatment

The treatment(s) that your healthcare provider recommends may vary depending on your diagnosis.

- **Rest, Liquids and Voice Therapy:** The vocal cords require regular rest and hydration just like any other part of the body. Speech-pathology experts instruct on proper voice usage, throat clearing techniques, and fluid consumption.
- **Allergy Treatments:** A medical professional can identify the cause of an allergy and treat it if it is producing excessive amounts of mucus in the throat.
- **Stopping Smoking:** The voice, among many other aspects of health, can be enhanced by stopping smoking. For instance, it can reduce the risk of cancer and improve heart health.
- **Medicine:** Voice disorders can be treated with a variety of medications. Medication can treat

gastroesophageal reflux, prevent blood vessel regrowth, or lessen swelling or inflammation, depending on the underlying cause of the voice disorder. During surgery, medication may be injected into the vocal cords, administered orally, or applied topically to the vocal cords.

Procedures:

- **Removal of Growths:** Surgery may be required to remove growths on the vocal cords, even if they are not cancerous. Microsurgery, carbon dioxide laser surgery, and other laser treatments, such as potassium titanyl phosphate (KTP) laser treatment, can all be used by a surgeon to remove growths.

  Modern therapy known as KTP laser treatment involves severing the blood supply to vocal cord lesions in order to treat them. This enables the growth to be removed while the majority of the underlying tissue is left intact.

- **Injections:** Small doses of pure botulinum toxin injected under the skin of the neck can help prevent spasms in the muscles and abnormal movements. This medication addresses a neurological and/or brain-related movement problem. This disorder, known as spasmodic dysphonia, affects the larynx's vocal muscles.

  Sometimes the vocal cords become immobile. Hoarseness may result from a single paralyzed vocal cord. When consuming liquids, it can also result in choking. However, it rarely creates issues with solid food swallowing. Sometimes the issue goes away on its own. In the event that the issue persists, the paralyzed vocal cord may be moved toward the center of the windpipe using one of two techniques. The vocal cords can meet and vibrate closer together with either procedure. As a result, the voice is better and the larynx can close during swallowing. Among the treatments are:

- **Fat or Collagen Injection:** The paralyzed vocal cord is made larger by injecting human-made collagen or body fat through the neck or mouth skin. Vocal cord weakness is also treated by it.
- **Thyroplasty:** A tiny hole made from the outside of the voice box by the tissue, also known as cartilage. An implant is inserted into the opening by the surgeon, who then presses it up against the paralyzed vocal cord.

5.9. Tracheostomy and Other Procedures for Airway Management

A tracheostomy, also known as a tracheotomy, is a surgically made opening in the neck that allows air to enter the trachea, or windpipe, and fill the lungs. Surgeons create the tracheostomy opening in the neck and then insert a tube through it to remove secretions from the lungs and to provide an airway. Instead of breathing through their mouth and nose, a person who has a tracheotomy breathes through a tracheostomy tube, also known as a trach tube. A tracheostomy can be either long-term or short-term.

5.9.1. Anatomy and Physiology

The trachea starts at the subglottic larynx and ends at the carina and mainstem bronchi. It is made up of incomplete cartilaginous rings, with the exception of the first ring, which is complete. The anterior wall of the esophagus and the posterior wall of the trachea are shared. The cricoid cartilage, a complete ring that includes the larynx's cricothyroid joint, is the first ring that joins the trachea to the larynx. The thyroid gland normally sits on top of the second or fourth tracheal rings in the neck, and the trachea is situated deep between the sternohyoid and sternothyroid muscles. The peritracheal lympho-fatty tissue and the recurrent laryngeal nerves are located directly lateral to the cervical trachea. The middle layer of the deep cervical fascia, also known as the pretracheal layer, encircles these structures. The common carotid arteries are located lateral to these structures. They are covered by the carotid sheath, which is a part of the deep layer of the deep cervical fascia. The thoracic trachea runs posterior to the heart, covered by the thymus and anterior mediastinal contents. As the innominate artery emerges from the aorta, it passes over the trachea.

Anatomic Landmarks for Tracheostomy:

- **Thyroid Notch**: a palpable landmark that can be used to locate the midline superior aspect of the larynx.
- **Cricothyroid Membrane**: a discernible dip between the thyroid and cricoid cartilages. This is where an emergency cricothyrotomy is to be performed.
- **Cricoid Cartilage**: a palpable landmark that indicates where the trachea and larynx meet. Usually, the skin incision is made 1 to 2 cm below the cricoid.
- **Sternal Notch**: a detectable marker to locate the thoracic inlet. In order to rule out the possibility of a high-riding innominate artery during tracheostomy, it is crucial to palpate this area.

5.9.2. Indications

It is possible to categorize the indications for tracheostomy into two groups: elective and emergent.

Indications for emergent tracheostomy include:

- Acute upper airway obstruction with failed endotracheal intubation (foreign body, angioedema, infection, anaphylaxis, etc.)
- Post-cricothyrotomy: After an airway is secured, a cricothyrotomy should be promptly formalized into a tracheostomy if one has been placed.
- Penetrating laryngeal trauma
- LeFort III fracture

The most common circumstances for performing an emergent tracheostomy are acute airway obstructions, such as aspirating a foreign body into the upper airway, having Ludwig's angina, or experiencing penetrating trauma to the airway that makes endotracheal intubation unfeasible. Emergency tracheostomy may also be required in cases of severe facial or cervical trauma, especially in cases of pan-facial fractures where nasal intubation is contraindicated due to craniofacial dislocation. Most of the time, less invasive airway management techniques can be tried before attempting an awake emergent tracheostomy (with the exception of penetrating laryngeal trauma and LeFort III fractures). However, before any airway manipulation takes place, all necessary instruments must be prepared and available to proceed with an emergent tracheostomy.

Indications for elective tracheostomy include:

- Prolonged ventilator dependence
- Preventive tracheostomy before head and neck cancer surgery.

- Obstructive sleep apnea that is unresponsive to other therapies.
- Chronic aspiration
- Neuromuscular disease
- Subglottic stenosis

There has been much discussion about when to undergo an elective tracheostomy in cases of prolonged intubation (i.e., failure to wean off of mechanical ventilation). According to conventional wisdom, tracheostomy should be performed five to seven days following endotracheal intubation to reduce the possibility of long-term intubation complications, such as subglottic stenosis. This time may be extended if there is a chance of extubation thanks to the development of low-pressure cuffs on endotracheal tubes, which have a maximum pressure of 20 cm H_2O. As an alternative, early tracheostomy has been recommended to improve patient comfort, lessen sedation, and possibly shorten the duration of hospitalization or ventilator days.

Early tracheostomy (3–7 days after intubation) is advised by the Eastern Association of Surgical Trauma (EAST) guidelines for patients who have severe closed-head injuries or who need continuous ventilatory support. Similar to this, tracheostomy at post-intubation days 5–7 has been advised by multiple professional organizations for non-trauma patients who have failed to wean off of their ventilator. In cases where extensive head and neck procedures are required because of trauma or upper aerodigestive tumors, a preventive tracheostomy may be required. An elective tracheostomy is necessary prior to the start of treatment because anticipated edema from the surgery or the radiation therapy that follows could foreshadow upper airway obstruction. When treating refractory obstructive sleep apnea, tracheostomy may be helpful, particularly in patients who are morbidly obese and cannot receive continuous positive airway pressure treatment. Long-term neurologically compromised patients may not be able to control their oral secretions, increasing their risk of repeated aspiration. Therefore, in order to prevent aspiration pneumonia in such a pulmonary toilet, an elective tracheostomy may be necessary. In conclusion, individuals suffering from neuromuscular disorders like amyotrophic lateral sclerosis might not possess the necessary muscle strength for autonomous breathing, necessitating the use of a tracheostomy to enable mechanical ventilation.

5.9.3. Contraindications

The only complete contraindication to tracheostomy is active cellulitis of the skin on the anterior neck. Before a tracheostomy or other invasive procedure is performed on a terminally ill patient, end-of-life issues should be discussed and goals for continued care should be established.

5.9.4. Equipment

Personal protective equipment and a tracheostomy tray are necessary pieces of equipment in the operating room. Additionally needed for percutaneous tracheostomy is a bronchoscope. In challenging cases, fiberoptic bronchoscopy or laryngoscopy may be useful.

5.9.5. Personnel

Anesthesiologist, scrub tech, nurse, surgeon, and surgical assistant are required for an open tracheostomy performed in the operating room. Two doctors are needed for a percutaneous tracheostomy, whether it is done in the operating room or at the patient's bedside. One does the percutaneous part at the neck, and the other looks through a bronchoscope to see how the wire and tube are passing through the trachea. A critical care physician or pulmonologist, for example, is a non-surgeon who may perform a bedside percutaneous tracheostomy.

5.9.6. Preparation

As mentioned above, an open tracheostomy is typically performed in the operating room by a surgeon and support personnel. A local anesthetic can be used in cases like Ludwig angina, and the tracheostomy can be done while the patient is awake instead of the usual general anesthesia and intubation. A non-fenestrated, cuffed tracheostomy tube is first utilized. When there is a risk of aerosolization of respiratory secretions, the team must wear specialized PPE, and the procedure needs to be carried out in a negative pressure room (Figure 5.5).

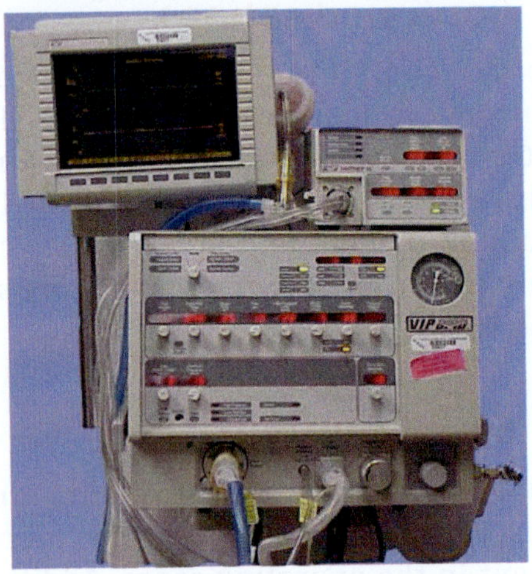

Figure 5.5. *Tracheotomy tubes and endotracheal tubes are often attached to ventilators to assist in breathing.*

Source: *By Brian Hall – Own work, Public Domain, https://commons.wikimedia.org/w/index.php?curid=1786487.*

5.9.7. Technique or Treatment

5.9.7.1. Open Tracheostomy

Anatomic landmarks that are palpable and marked include the sternal notch, thyroid notch, and cricoid cartilage. To identify a high-riding innominate artery, the surgeon should feel the sternal notch closely. Next, a skin incision is made 1 to 2 cm inferior to the cricoid cartilage in the midline anterior neck. One may use a vertical or horizontal incision. The median raphe is identified by extending the incision through the platysma muscle to reveal the strap muscles, sternohyoid and sternothyroid. The thyroid gland and cricoid cartilage are visible when the strap muscles are pulled laterally. Based on where the thyroid isthmus is located in the trachea, it is located and, if necessary, ligated. Hemostats can be used to cross-clamp the isthmus. To guarantee thyroid tissue hemostasis, each stump can then be oversewn with a silk suture. The trachea and larynx are then elevated into the operating field by a cricoid hook that is positioned beneath the cricoid cartilage. It is determined which are the second and third tracheal rings.

Lateral stay ligatures may be used to help with tube placement traction on the trachea and tube security during the recovery phase. A tracheostomy tube is inserted following the creation of an incision between the second and third rings. A number of changes have been suggested: the removal of an anterior window of cartilage (typically involving the removal of a segment of one to two rings); the use of a vertical anterior incision across one or two rings (used in pediatric tracheostomy); or the development of a Bjork flap, which entails the creation and attachment of an inferiorly-based cartilage flap to the subcutaneous tissues. To lower the chance of developing stenosis later on, the first ring is omitted. After the tube is positioned, the end-tidal CO_2 is verified and it is connected to the anesthesia circuit. The cricoid hook is only released at that point. Up until the first tracheostomy tube change on postoperative day five, the tracheostomy tube is sutured to the anterior neck skin and fastened with a soft trans-cervical tie.

5.9.7.2. Percutaneous Tracheostomy

Under bronchoscopic guidance, this technique

uses a modified Seldinger technique to dilate the tissue. Several studies that have compared the two methods have indicated various possible benefits that each method may have over the other. The percutaneous approach eliminates the need to take potentially seriously ill patients to the operating room, making it more suitable for bedside use. In comparison to the open technique, the percutaneous technique has also been linked to reduced rates of infection and blood loss. After the open procedure, the percutaneous technique has been linked to a number of extremely rare but devastating complications, including esophageal perforation, aortic injury, and tracheal laceration (Figure 5.6).

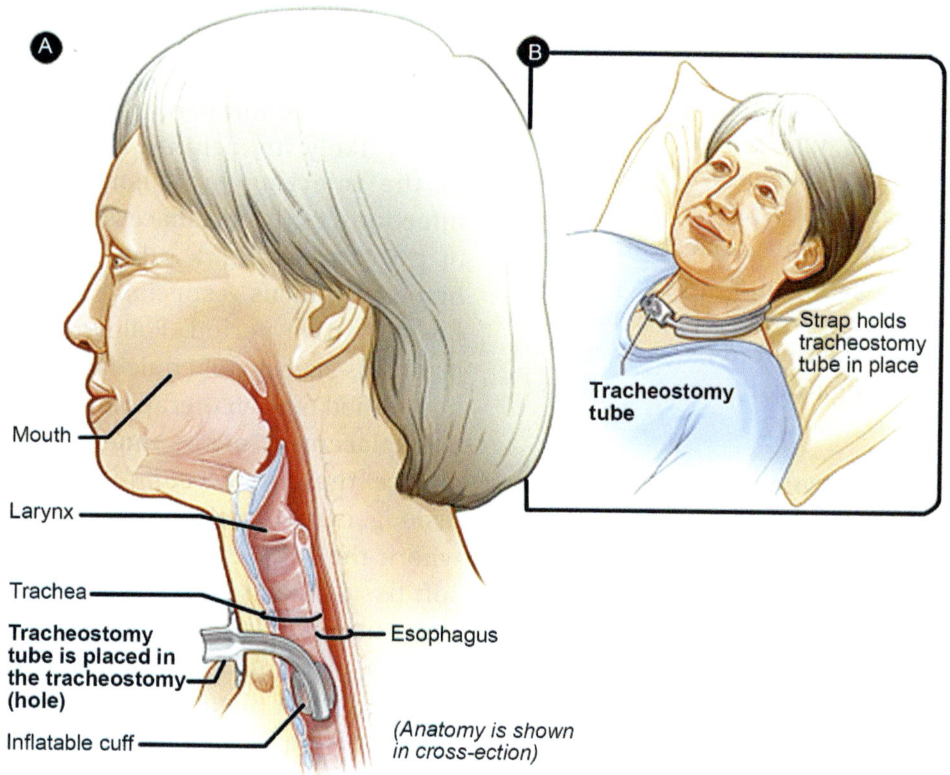

Figure 5.6. *(A) shows a side view of the neck and the correct placement of a tracheostomy tube in the trachea, or windpipe. (B) shows an external view of a patient who has a tracheostomy.*

Source: *By National Heart Lung and Blood Institute (NIH) – National Heart Lung and Blood Institute (NIH), Public Domain, https://commons.wikimedia.org/w/index.php?curid=29588234.*

5.9.8. Complications

The best times to think about complications following tracheostomy are during the operative, early, and late postoperative phases.

5.9.8.1. Operative Period

Bleeding is the most frequent intraoperative complication. A coagulopathy that is present in many critically ill patients requiring tracheostomy should ideally be treated prior to surgery. Before undergoing any airway surgery, a thrombocytopenic patient might need a platelet transfusion to reach a platelet count of more than 50,000. Although the anterior jugular veins can typically be retracted laterally anatomically, they may occasionally be aberrant or bridging, in which case they need to be ligated. The thyroidea ima artery, which runs along the anterior surface of the trachea, will be present in about 5% of patients. When it is divided, it can retract inferiorly and cause continuous bleeding, so when ligating it, extreme caution must be used. As was previously mentioned, the risk of bleeding from the thyroid isthmus can be reduced by carefully ligating it with transfixing ligatures.

Airway fire is an uncommon but extremely dangerous intraoperative complication. High oxygen concentrations in the anesthetic tubing and the ignition source of the electrocautery unit are the causes of this. Accurate communication between the anesthetic and surgical teams can prevent this. In the event of a fire, the patient should have the entire circuit removed and be mask-bagged until the tracheostomy is implanted. Then, using laryngoscopy, bronchoscopy, and esophagoscopy, the aerodigestive tract should be examined for any possible thermal injury. Pneumothorax or pneumomediastinum is the last surgical complication. This can happen if the tracheostomy tube is positioned in front of the trachea, unintentionally creating a false passage. A pneumothorax can also be caused by an injury to the lung's apex or by a ruptured blcb. In most cases, pneumomediastinum is self-limited. A chest radiograph should be taken after surgery if the pneumothorax is a concern, and a chest tube should be inserted if necessary. Although some surgeons get postoperative chest X-rays on every tracheostomy patient, this is also incredibly uncommon following a standard tracheostomy.

5.9.8.2. Early Complications

It is extremely uncommon for infections following tracheostomy to require antibiotics. Since most infections are just secretions leaking into the field from the new stoma, they can usually be treated with local wound care. The immunocompromised patient is more likely to require antibiotics specific to the infecting organism for certain deep infections or frank abscesses. Acute blockage of the tracheostomy tube may be caused by blood or mucus, especially in the immediate postoperative period. Following postoperative protocols such as scheduled tracheal suctioning, humidified oxygen therapy, and regular cleaning or replacement of the inner cannula can help reduce the risk of complete blockage. Tube dislodgement can also lead to acute obstruction, where the tube exits the trachea and rests in soft tissue. Stay sutures during the surgery and skin sutures post-surgery can help secure the tube in place. Reintubation may be necessary to establish a clear airway, and can be done visually using flexible laryngoscopy through the tracheostomy tube.

5.9.8.3. Late Complications

Pressure necrosis brought on by the tracheostomy tube's cuff being overinflated is one of the most feared late complications. Because of developments in low-pressure cuffs and increased awareness of cuff pressure as a risk factor, these are less common than in the past. To avoid this, tracheostomy cuff pressure should be checked frequently, ideally at a maximum of 20 cm H_2O. Because of ischemia, high tracheal pressure can cause the wall to necrotize. Later healing leads to stenosis and scanning.

5.9.8.4. Persistent Tracheocutaneous Fistula

Following the removal of the tracheostomy tube, the stoma typically heals on its own in 24 to 48 hours. Granulation tissue can occasionally remain at the site and cause problems. Topical silver nitrate is typically effective in treating this. Debridement and closure in layers, which support the repair by using the strap muscles, are usually successful if surgical closure is needed.

5.9.8.5. Tracheoesophageal Fistula

A very rare complication of tracheostomies—less than 5% of cases—is tracheoesophageal fistula. Usually, they start when the posterior membranous trachea—the party wall that the trachea and esophagus share—experiences excessive pressure. The tracheostomy tube's cuff over-inflating may be the cause of this. In cases where ventilatory pressures are higher than anticipated, a flexible scope should be passed via the tracheostomy tube to ensure proper intra-lumenal orientation. It is possible for the tracheostomy tube to be oriented posteriorly, which would put excessive pressure on the posterior tracheal wall. Such a problem could be resolved by resizing the tube or replacing it with a proximal or distal XLT tube.

For patients who require tracheostomy, alternate enteral feeding (via a gastrostomy tube) is recommended as the risk of this complication is increased when an indwelling nasogastric tube is present in addition to the rigid tracheostomy tube. Individuals who have a tracheoesophageal fistula may exhibit symptoms of severe or recurrent pneumonia, bronchopulmonary suppuration, or tracheobronchial contamination with food or gastric contents. The fistula, which typically measures 1 to 4 cm in length, needs to be treated with care for both the esophagus and the trachea. Resection of the fistula with primary esophageal closure, primary tracheal anastomosis, and insertion of a viable muscle flap are the procedures involved in definitive repair.

5.9.8.6. Tracheoinnominate Fistula

Less than 1% of tracheostomies result in tracheoinnominate fistulas, a very rare but potentially fatal complication with an estimated 80% mortality rate. A sentinel bleed, or pulsatile bleed from the stoma that ceases on its own, may occur before the event. A few days later, the bleeding might resume, followed by exsanguinating hemorrhage. There are several known risk factors that could put a patient at risk for developing a tracheoinnominate fistula. These include the tracheostomy being positioned below the third tracheal ring, the innominate artery being more cephalad (high-riding), and the use of an incorrectly sized tube (either too large in diameter or too long), which puts undue pressure on the anterior tracheal wall behind the sternum.

The pressure necrosis of the anterior wall of the trachea between the relatively rigid, high-pressure wall of the innominate artery and the tracheostomy tube or its cuff is the primary cause of tracheoinnominate fistula. Another factor that has been identified as causative is the innominate artery's abnormal cephalad location. To lower the risk of tracheal necrosis, tube cuff pressure should also be monitored and kept below 20 cm H_2O.

As soon as it is determined that there may be a tracheoinnominate fistula, surgical intervention is required. The tracheostomy tube should be removed, and oral tracheal intubation with the cuff inflated distal to the bleeding source are the immediate measures. The innominate artery can then be blocked by applying digital pressure by pinching it against the posterior surface of the manubrium with a finger that has been inserted through the tracheostomy stoma. The occluding finger and hand should be prepared for surgery in the operating room as soon as possible after the patient is stabilized. In order to facilitate tracheal healing, the open repair entails a median sternotomy combined with ligation of the innominate artery and an interpositional flap. Additionally, case studies have shown the possibility of both embolization and endovascular stenting.

5.9.9. Clinical Significance

For patients requiring prolonged mechanical ventilatory support, a tracheostomy offers a stable, long-lasting airway. It can also give people who are unable to expel secretions a way to use the pulmonary toilet. Prior to surgery, quality of life and end-of-life concerns should be discussed with the patient or their proxy. This is especially important for elderly and terminally ill patients. Compared to many other surgeries, tracheostomy aerosolizes respiratory particles from the patient more, and in cases of virulent airborne pathogens (tuberculosis, COVID-19, etc.), extra care should be given to safeguard operating room personnel.

5.9.10. Enhancing Healthcare Team Outcomes

5.9.10.1. Post-Tracheostomy Care

It is important to keep an eye on tube cuff pressure in the range of 20 to 25 mm Hg. Humidification of gases is crucial because it helps avoid thick or parched secretions, which are more likely to obstruct. To reduce the chance of aspiration, the head of the bed should be raised, and a speech pathologist should examine oral feeding first. The lumen should be suctioned hourly for the first 24 hours. Up until the first tracheostomy tube change, which occurs five to seven days after surgery, this can be increased to once every four hours. At this point, all stay sutures and skin sutures are taken out. The tracheostomy tube's caliber may be reduced at this time if the patients are cooperative, awake, and alert. Since the cutaneous-tracheal tract is still developing and prone to loss, changing the tracheostomy tube during the first five days of implantation is not advised as it may cause the airway to become trapped. If tube replacements are required during this time, emergency supplies and sufficient lighting akin to that found in the operating room or operating suite should be taken into account. The provision of exchange catheters, endotracheal tubes, trach tubes in smaller sizes, and perhaps bronchoscopic guidance are further precautions.

5.10. Foreign Bodies of Air Passages

A foreign body in the air can pose a serious risk to one's life. Both the diagnosis and treatment of patients with suspected airway foreign bodies—which are most frequently observed in patients with foreign body aspiration (FBA)—now revolve around flexible and rigid bronchoscopy. The development of smaller diameter flexible bronchoscopes has increased the role of pulmonary physicians in the diagnosis and treatment of patients who present with FBA, even though FBA was traditionally managed by otolaryngologists and thoracic surgeons. We will go over the assessment and management of FBA in adults in this section. Separate topics covered include rigid bronchoscopy technical aspects, central airway obstruction, and FBA in children.

5.10.1. Etiology

There is always a chance of respiratory compromise or subsequent inhalation into the distal airways, which could result in subacute symptoms like coughing, wheezing, or shortness of breath after aspirating a foreign body into the larynx or proximal trachea. Anything that can fit in the mouth has the potential to cause aspiration. Parents must exercise extreme caution when it comes to letting their unsupervised child have access to certain objects. This is especially concerning when it comes to newborns and early children who explore and interact with their surroundings by putting things in their mouths. Similarly, there is a tendency for babies and young children to aspirate or inhale food when eating, and their coordination for swallowing has not fully developed. In the West, peanuts are the most commonly consumed food item, with hotdogs being the most deadly. Compared to female children, male children are more likely to aspirate. Aspiration is most common in foods and other objects with smooth, round shapes, such as nuts, beans, grapes, hotdogs, sausages, etc. Preparing these foods in a way that makes them more angular and easier to chew and swallow is one way to prevent aspiration (quartering grapes, for example).

5.10.2. Epidemiology

Though the elderly are also at risk, aspirating foreign bodies is more common in children, who are more likely to be male than female, and in people who have developmental delays. The most frequently aspirated food item in the west is peanuts, which are followed in frequency by hotdogs and hard candies. In addition to food, aspiration occurs frequently with other round, smooth objects like rubber balls and marbles. Another factor that contributes in children is the absence of molars for food chewing. Most statistical data comes from research conducted at a single location. It has only been recently that larger cohorts and a national analysis have been assembled to examine more data. According to these studies, there are 0.66 cases of foreign-body airway obstruction (FBAO) for every 100,000 people. In the United States, inhaling foreign bodies was the cause of 17,000 emergency room visits in children under the age of 14. The leading cause of unintentional infantile deaths and the fourth most frequent cause of death for preschoolers under five is foreign body aspiration.

5.10.3. Pathophysiology

If the glottic or tracheal airway is completely blocked, there will be immediate respiratory distress, cyanosis, audible and visible choking, and death if treatment is not received quickly. In the event of a mainstem bronchial obstruction, total obstruction of the bronchus or intermediate bronchus may be surprisingly asymptomatic, but over time, it may result in distal infection. Depending on the airway structure involved, partial obstruction may result in inflammation of local tissue and varying degrees of dyspnea, SOB, wheezing, coughing, or other symptoms. Generally speaking, symptoms will be more severe, noticeable, and fast the closer the airway is to the body. Compared to metal or plastic objects, food may cause more inflammation because it is an organic material that can swell and cause a more severe obstruction that persists over time. Severe airway inflammation and distal airway stenosis have been linked to medications like iron tablets.

5.10.4. History and Physical

A history of aspiration or suspected aspiration is frequently enough to justify a thorough examination that includes a rigid bronchoscopy. Aspiration can manifest itself in various ways. Acute large airway obstruction is characterized by drooling, stridor, choking signs, and acute, obvious clinical distress. Doctors and other staff members should not overly agitate these patients. Instead, they should be brought urgently to the operating room for a formal airway examination, rigid bronchoscopy, and to make arrangements for an emergency tracheostomy. In the emergency room, refrain from using an endoscope or mouth exam to instrument the airway. Even in the unlikely event that a foreign body is not discovered, the patient in question needs to be further assessed in an operating room, where they can be safely assessed for respiratory distress and an unknown, unstable airway.

Aspiration of a foreign body can be the cause of persistent dyspnea, particularly in children and people with developmental delays who are not able to accurately describe what happened. This is more likely to occur in the smaller, farther-reaching airways, and the symptoms may be related to either a partial obstruction resulting in stridor, coughing, wheezing, and progressive symptoms as the surrounding respiratory epithelium becomes more reactive and edematous, or a complete occlusion of a terminal bronchus and development of pneumonia. The patient may experience dyspnea, coughing, or even complain of pain in the chest for a few weeks. Patients and their families may not be aware of or may have forgotten about the initial aspiration event in cases like these, which may present weeks or months later. Children's airway anatomy is different from adult anatomy. The glottis is the narrowest part of the adult airway, whereas the cricoid is the narrowest part in children. Particles of sufficient size could therefore be able to pass through children's vocal cords (glottis) and lodge in the subglottis near the cricoid, which could have fatal consequences.

When it comes to aspiration of foreign objects, children are slightly more likely to aspirate into the right mainstem bronchus. However, as adults age, this propensity increases because the right mainstem becomes the most dependent and direct portion of the adult airway due to its more vertical orientation, which parallels the orientation of the trachea. As mentioned above, the physical examination may reveal tripod posturing, drooling, stridor, or wheezing in cases of significant airway obstruction. Smaller airway aspiration may have a history suggestive of aspiration, even dating back several weeks, and symptoms may be more nebulous and subtle, such as focal wheezing or asthma-like symptoms. If a patient exhibits these symptoms and does not improve after receiving the recommended course of treatment for reactive airway disease and infectious causes, they should be evaluated formally using a bronchoscopy.

5.10.5. Evaluation

As previously mentioned, do not image or in any way agitate a patient who is in extremis or uncooperative as in a small child. Go straight to the operating room to have a rigid bronchoscopy performed under anesthesia, along with emergency tracheostomy supplies. Examining the patient with chest X-rays, PA, and lateral inspiratory-expiratory films can start if they are stable and cooperative. An obstruction on that side will be indicated by unilateral expansion, diaphragm flattening of the affected side, and mediastinal pushing away. On inspiratory-expiratory films, air trapping can also be seen as a sign of a foreign body obstruction-induced ball-valve effect. Additionally, these can identify and localize the foreign body if it is radiopaque. Get IV access and perform blood work, including electrolytes and a complete blood count, in case a general anesthetic is necessary. Regular venous blood gas testing is not very useful and ought to be avoided. A head and neck examination, either with or without flexible laryngoscopy, can reveal other mimicking conditions like tonsillitis or peritonsillar abscess, which can then be treated if the patient is stable and cooperative. Combining auscultation in the main lung fields with percussion and tactile fremitus assessment can reveal focal consolidations or wheezing. Only the most stable and comfortable patients, in whom the possibility of a foreign body is very low on the differential diagnosis, should undergo computed tomography. The mortality rate for an airway emergency in a radiology suite is high.

5.10.6. Treatment / Management

Airway control is critical for an active upper airway obstruction. Unless the patient is an adult, conscious, awake, giving consent, and not in the slightest uncomfortable, do not perform blind sweeping of the airway, direct visualization of the airway with any type of oral instrument or tongue blade, or attempt extraction with Magill forceps. For the vast majority of patients, these kinds of operations are best carried out in the operating room, where the conditions are more controlled. It may be necessary to intubate past the obstruction or force the blockage into one of the mainstem bronchi. If this is the case, it is best to determine that these maneuvers are required and to perform them in a fully-equipped operating room instead of an emergency department, as they are far more successful. If the patient presents with respiratory arrest and no other means of ventilation is available, an emergency cricothyroidotomy may be necessary. A thorough history and physical examination are crucial in determining the possibility of a lower airway obstruction. This is especially true in cases where a child has been unsupervised near small objects, has been observed aspirating or choking, or has developed a new cough or other respiratory symptoms that do not go away. An official interventional airway examination is necessary if the patient has received treatment but their symptoms have not improved. Rigid bronchoscopy is the gold standard for treatment; however, in certain centers, this procedure is done solely on the basis of history or suspicion because up to 15% of aspirations show normal physical examination and imaging results.

Under general anesthesia, rigid bronchoscopy is the definitive management for known radiopaque or suspected radiolucent foreign bodies. Retrieval and standard post-operative instructions, which may include oral or inhaled corticosteroids, are sufficient if the object has been acutely aspirated. Antibiotic therapy for post-obstructive infection can start at that point if there have been clinical indications of infection.

5.10.7. Differential Diagnosis

Asthma, pneumonia, tuberculosis, epiglottitis, retropharyngeal abscess, peritonsillar abscess, postviral pericarditis or pleuritis, and bronchiolitis are among the illnesses that can seem clinically similar to foreign body aspiration. Comparable symptoms of foreign body aspiration may be present in trauma injuries involving localized pulmonary, airway, or even diaphragmatic injury. This list demonstrates how wide the differential is because of the variety of complaints that are presented and how severe they are. This is one of the difficulties in diagnosing airway foreign bodies, especially in children or non-communicative individuals.

5.10.8. Prognosis

The prognosis for children who have aspirated foreign bodies is favorable provided it is removed promptly and without any issues. After aspirating a foreign body, the majority of patients who respond well to treatment in the emergency room have positive outcomes. Serious consequences may arise from acute aspiration of a larger object that obstructs the proximal airway or trachea.

5.10.9. Complications

Early intervention for aspirated foreign bodies has a roughly 25% complication rate during management, the great majority of which are mild. More serious side effects include bronchial injury, airway stenosis, abscess formation, pneumothorax, and hypoxic or anoxic brain injury (especially in cases of tracheal or mainstem bronchus obstruction). These complications are brought on by delayed intervention. These are also uncommon but important. With treatment for these delayed complications, children will probably recover, with the sad (very small) minority of cases resulting in death from respiratory compromise.

A Closer Look

Spasmodic Dysphonia

The voice muscles in the larynx, also known as the voice box, are affected by spasmodic dysphonia, also known as laryngeal dystonia. Your voice is produced when air from your lungs is forced between two elastic structures called vocal folds, which vibrate when you speak. Vocal fold vibrations are disrupted by the sudden, involuntary movements of the vocal fold muscles in spasmodic dysphonia. Other types of dystonia that result in recurrent spasms in the eyes, face, jaw, lips, tongue, neck, arms, or legs can also coexist with spasmodic dysphonia.

Speaking with spasmodic dysphonia results in voice breaks that can produce a breathy, tense, or tight sound. Some people only take pauses every few sentences. In more extreme situations, a person's speech may become extremely difficult to understand due to spasms that occur on every word. Vocal tremor, which is a trembling of the voice caused by a shaking of the larynx and vocal folds, can also occur in some people with spasmodic dysphonia. A person with spasmodic dysphonia will experience the condition for the rest of their life. When spasmodic dysphonia first appears, it may cause severe voice problems from the beginning of the disorder, or it may begin with mild symptoms that only happen sometimes before getting worse and happening more frequently over time. One uncommon condition is spasmodic dysphonia. Although anyone can get it, those between the ages of 30 and 50 are most likely to experience the initial symptoms. Women are more affected than men are.

Types of Spasmodic Dysphonia

- The most prevalent type of spasmodic dysphonia is adductor spasmodic dysphonia. The vocal folds slam and stiffen as a result of spasms in this disorder. The vocal folds' ability to vibrate and produce sounds is hampered by these spasms. An adductor spasmodic dysphonic person may have a strained, strangled voice. Because of muscle spasms, the person's speech may be jerky, with words being cut off or difficult to start. Whispering, crying, or laughing usually causes the voice to sound normal and eliminates the spasms. Stress frequently exacerbates the severity of muscle spasms.
- Less frequently occurs abductor spasmodic dysphonia. Spasms in this disorder result in the vocal folds staying open. When the vocal folds are too open, they are unable to vibrate. When speaking, the open position also permits air to exit the lungs. The voice consequently frequently sounds breathy and weak. Similar to adductor spasmodic dysphonia, laughing, crying, and whispering frequently cause the spasms to stop.
- It is extremely uncommon to have mixed spasmodic dysphonia, which combines the first two forms. The opening and closing muscles of vocal folds malfunction, resulting in characteristics of both adductor and abductor spasmodic dysphonia.
- **Causes:** It is believed that spasmodic dysphonia is caused by abnormal functioning

in the basal ganglia region of the brain, which is responsible for coordinating muscle movements throughout the body. Other areas of the brain linked to spasmodic dysphonia include the cerebral cortex, where commands to muscles are controlled and coordinated with sensory information. While the condition can sometimes be hereditary, a specific gene directly connected to spasmodic dysphonia has not been pinpointed yet. However, a mutation in a gene known to cause other types of dystonia has been linked to spasmodic dysphonia as well.

Diagnosis

- Due to the symptoms' commonality with other voice disorders, diagnosing spasmodic dysphonia can be challenging. The diagnosis typically comes after a team's examination, which includes:
- The otolaryngologist, a specialist in ear, nose, throat, head, and neck diseases, will perform a fiberoptic nasolaryngoscopy by passing a small lighted tube through the nose into the back of the throat. This procedure evaluates vocal fold anatomy and movements during speech and other larynx activities.
- A speech-language pathologist is a medical practitioner with training in diagnosing and treating disorders of the voice, speech, and language. The speech-language pathologist will evaluate any issues with voice.
- a physician with expertise in nervous system disorders, known as a neurologist. The neurologist will examine the brain for indications of movement disorders such as dystonia.

Treatment

At this time, there is no known cure for spasmodic dysphonia. However, treatment options are available to help alleviate symptoms. The most common form of treatment involves injecting small amounts of botulinum toxin directly into the affected muscles in the larynx. This toxin, produced by Clostridium botulinum, weakens the muscles by blocking the nerve impulse. Typically, these injections can improve the voice for a period of three to four months, after which symptoms gradually return. Follow-up injections are necessary to maintain improved speaking voice. Some initial side effects may include temporary weakness in the voice and swallowing difficulties, but these tend to improve within a few days to a few weeks. It is worth noting that botulinum toxin injections are more effective for adductor spasmodic dysphonia than for abductor spasmodic dysphonia, and may not be effective for all cases.

Voice therapy, in conjunction with botulinum toxin injections, may help alleviate symptoms in mild cases of spasmodic dysphonia. Psychological counseling can also be beneficial for individuals struggling to accept and cope with their voice issues. Augmentative and assistive devices can aid in communication for some individuals, while software and apps can translate text into synthetic speech. In cases where conventional methods have been ineffective, surgical interventions on the larynx may be considered. While some surgical treatments have shown positive results, outcomes vary among individuals and there is no consensus on the most effective approach. It is important for patients to consult with a physician to understand the potential risks and benefits of surgical treatment and to manage expectations.

Summary

- The cartilaginous larynx of the respiratory tract is situated in the anterior aspect of the neck. In humans and other vertebrates, the larynx's main job is to keep the lower respiratory tract safe from food particles that might enter the trachea during breathing.
- The larynx is made up of a mucous membrane, a cartilaginous skeleton, and a few muscles and ligaments that move and stabilize it.
- The laryngotracheal groove, a longitudinal notch, marks the location of the earliest human larynx, which originated in the first four weeks of intrauterine life on the primitive pharyngeal floor. Around the fifth week of embryonic life, this groove will eventually form the esophagotracheal septum, with the respiratory system located anteriorly and the esophagus on the dorsal side.
- Trauma to the larynx is rare but may prove to be fatal. There are two types of laryngeal trauma: penetrating and blunt.
- Inflammation of the larynx, or voice box, is known as laryngitis. In addition to a hoarse voice, other symptoms might include fever, coughing, frontal neck pain, and difficulty swallowing.
- Epiglottitis is an inflammatory disease of the epiglottis and surrounding structures, such as the vallecula, arytenoids, and aryepiglottic folds. It is typically caused by an infection.
- Acute laryngotracheobronchitis, also known as croup, is a contagious respiratory illness that affects infants and children. It can be brought on by an infection of either the trachea or the larynx.
- Diphtheria is a dangerous bacterial infection that primarily affects the throat and nose mucous membranes.
- Reinke's edema, also called polypoid corditis, is a condition in which swelling or polyps impair the superficial lamina propria, a structure necessary for regular voice function.
- Laryngitis sicca is characterized by extreme dryness of the larynx, nearly invariably accompanied by mucus crusting. It frequently causes voice hoarseness.
- The most prevalent granulomatous disease of the larynx, laryngeal tuberculosis (LT), has historically been linked to pulmonary tuberculosis (PT), though it can also occur locally as a primary lesion in the larynx without pulmonary involvement.
- Congenital anomalies can result from intrauterine events that impact fetal and embryonic growth, or they can be the outcome of errors in embryogenesis, known as malformations.
- A condition known as vocal cord paralysis causes you to lose control over the movement of the muscles that produce your voice. It occurs when your voice box's (larynx) nerve impulses are interfered with. The muscles of the vocal cord become paralyzed as a result.
- Male and female individuals can develop benign laryngeal tumors at any age. The most typical sign is a person's voice changing. The prognosis for this kind of tumor is typically favorable because it is not malignant.

- There are numerous causes for voice disorders in humans. A shift in voice quality is known as a voice disorder. Speech-language pathologists and medical professionals with training in ear, nose, and throat disorders diagnose and treat voice problems. The cause of the voice change determines the course of treatment. Interventions may involve medication, injections, surgery, or voice therapy.
- A tracheostomy, also known as a tracheotomy, is a surgically made opening in the neck that allows air to enter the trachea, or windpipe, and fill the lungs.
- A foreign body in the air can pose a serious risk to one's life. Both the diagnosis and treatment of patients with suspected airway foreign bodies—which are most frequently observed in patients with foreign body aspiration (FBA)—now revolve around flexible and rigid bronchoscopy.

References

1. Allen, E., et al. (2020). *Anatomy, Head and Neck, Larynx Recurrent Laryngeal Nerve*. StatPearls Publishing. Retrieved from: https://www.ncbi.nlm.nih.gov/books/NBK470179/ (accessed on 4 September 2024).
2. Boone, D. R. (2005). *The Voice and Voice Therapy* (7th ed.). Pearson/Allyn & Bacon.
3. Bruch, J. M., et al. (2020). *Hoarseness in Adults*. UpToDate. Retrieved from: https://www.uptodate.com/contents/search (accessed on 4 September 2024).
4. Colton, R. H. (2011). *Understanding Voice Problems: A Physiological Perspective for Diagnosis and Treatment*. Wolters Kluwer Health/Lippincott Williams & Wilkins.
5. Ferri, F. F. (2020). *Laryngitis*. In *Ferri's Clinical Advisor 2020*. Elsevier. Retrieved from: https://www.clinicalkey.com (accessed on 4 September 2024).
6. Gupta, G., et al. (2020). *Acute Laryngitis*. StatPearls Publishing. Retrieved from: https://www.ncbi.nlm.nih.gov/books/NBK534871/ (accessed on 4 September 2024).
7. Kahrilas, P. J. (2020). *Complications of Gastroesophageal Reflux in Adults*. UpToDate. Retrieved from: https://www.uptodate.com/contents/search (accessed on 4 September 2024).
8. Merck Manual Professional Version. (2020). *Croup*. Retrieved from: https://www.merckmanuals.com/professional/pediatrics/respiratory-disorders-in-young-children/croup?query=croup (accessed on 4 September 2024).
9. Rubin, J. S., Sataloff, R. T., & Korovin, G. S. (2014). *Diagnosis and Treatment of Voice Disorders*. Plural Publishing, Inc.
10. Stemple, J. C. (2009). *Clinical Voice Pathology: Theory and Management* (4th ed.). Plural Publishing.
11. Suárez-Quintanilla, J., et al. (2020). *Anatomy, Head and Neck, Larynx*. StatPearls Publishing. Retrieved from: https://www.ncbi.nlm.nih.gov/books/NBK538202/ (accessed on 4 September 2024).

Chapter

THYROID GLAND AND ITS DISORDERS

6

Contents

Introduction

The gland in the front of the neck that resembles a butterfly is called the thyroid. The hormones it produces are essential for controlling blood pressure, body temperature, heart rate, metabolism, and the body's response to other hormones. Triiodothyronine, or T3, and thyroxine (T4) are the two primary hormones that the thyroid produces. In addition, the gland generates calcitonin, which regulates the intracellular reabsorption of calcium by bone cells. Numerous conditions can cause the thyroid to produce too little (hypothyroidism) or too much (hyperthyroidism) thyroid hormone. Numerous other functions, including heart rate, mood, energy level, metabolism, bone health, and pregnancy, can be impacted by thyroid disorders (Figure 6.1).

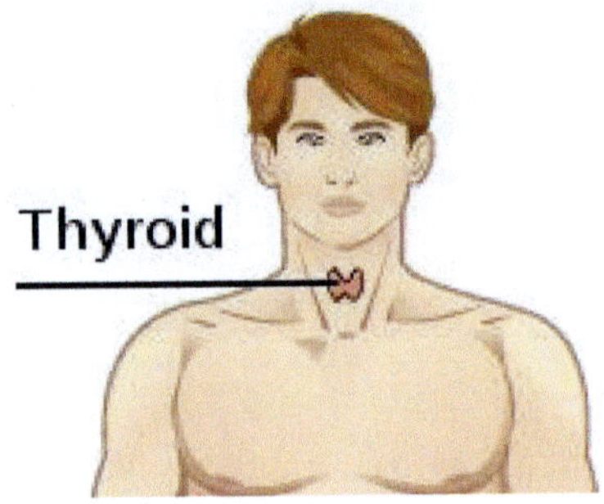

Figure 6.1. *The thyroid gland is a butterfly-shaped gland located in the neck below the Adam's apple.*

Source: By CFCF – Own work, CC BY-SA 4.0, https://commons.wikimedia.org/w/index.php?curid=41006760.

Orientation and Directional Terms

Term	Definition	Illustration
Hyperthyroidism	Hyperthyroidism can lead to Graves' disease, which has many symptoms, including sweating, arrhythmia (irregular heartbeat), weight loss, protruding eyes and nervousness.	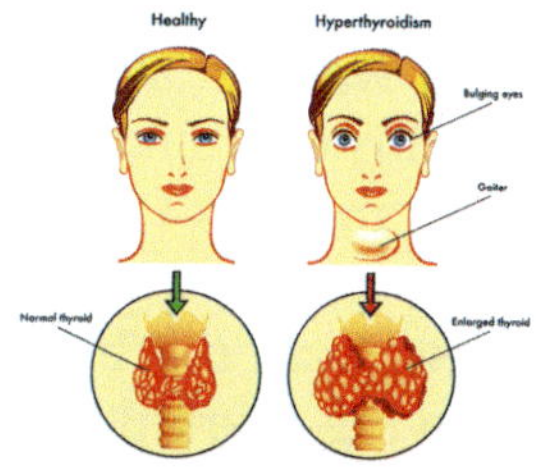
Hypothyroidism	Symptoms of hypothyroidism can include tiredness, weight gain, depression, abnormal bone development and stunted growth. The most common cause is autoimmune: the production of antibodies that attack the thyroid gland.	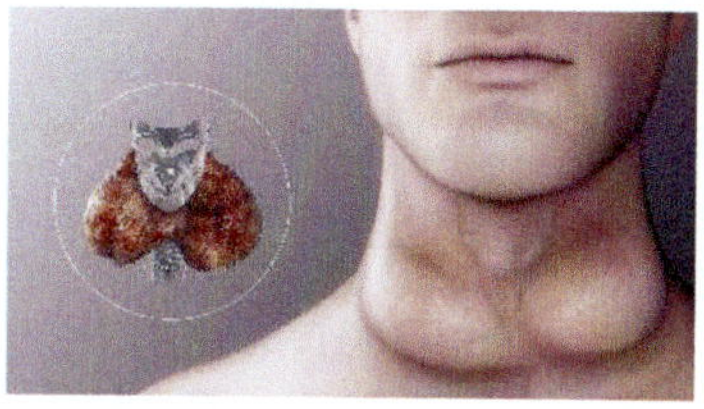
Hashimoto's Thyroiditis	Hashimoto's thyroiditis, an autoimmune disorder, is an inflammation of the thyroid gland. It can cause a goiter (swelling in the neck due to an enlarged thyroid gland) and other symptoms.	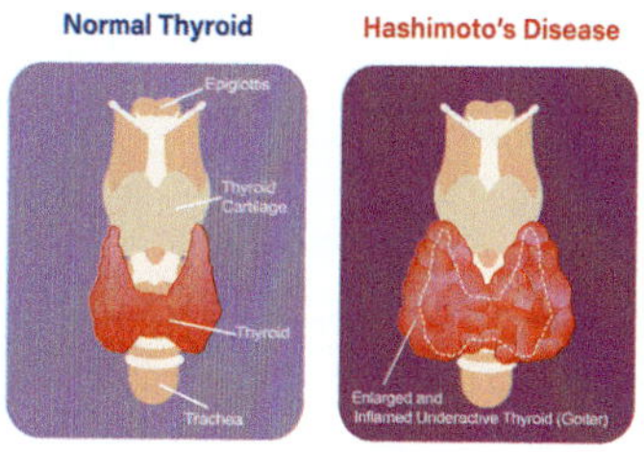
Thyroid Tumors	Thyroid nodules and adenomas, small, noncancerous growths, start in the cell layer that lines the inner surface of the thyroid gland. The adenoma itself may secrete thyroid hormone and may cause hyperthyroidism. Thyroid adenoma treatment may include surgery to remove the overactive nodule.	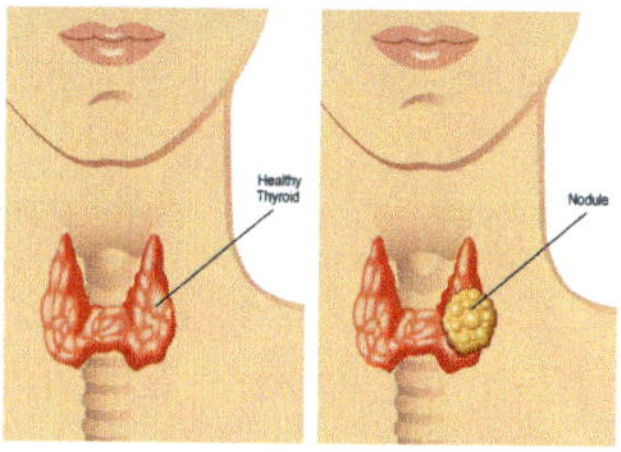
Thyroid Cancer	Thyroid cancer occurs more often in people who have undergone radiation to the head, neck or chest. However, it may also occur in those without any known risk factors. There are four main types of thyroid cancer: papillary thyroid cancer, follicular thyroid cancer, anaplastic thyroid cancer and medullary thyroid cancer. Most thyroid cancer can be treated successfully.	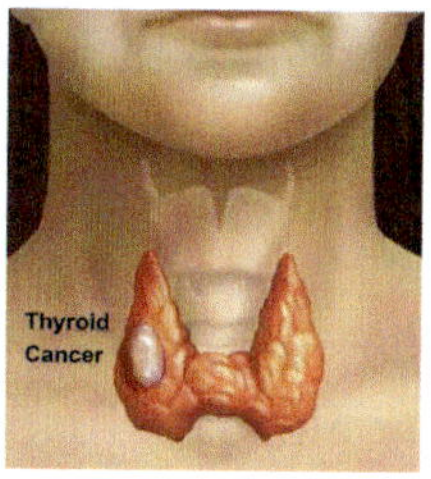

6.1. Surgical Anatomy of Thyroid Gland

The largest endocrine gland is the thyroid, and thyroid disorders are common health issues, particularly in women. The main way to treat thyroid conditions such as goiter, adenoma, and carcinoma is through surgery. To minimize surgical complications, safe thyroid surgery requires a deep understanding of thyroid anatomy. The anatomy of the thyroid, including its macroscopic and microscopic structure, thyroid embryology, vascular composition, and innervation, will all be covered in this section. Thyroid biopsy, ultrasound, and nuclear medicine imaging play a critical role in identifying thyroid nodules and distinguishing benign from malignant disease. The region of the body that typically divides the head from the torso is the neck. The laryngeal prominence is a thyroid cartilage prominence located in the midline in front of the neck. The hyoid bone is felt between the laryngeal prominence and the chin; the cricoid cartilage is felt in the midline below the thyroid cartilage. The thyroid gland's trachea and isthmus are palpable between the cricoid cartilage and the suprasternal notch. Located on the side of the neck, the quadrangular area is bordered anteriorly by a midline in front of the neck, posteriorly by the trapezius muscle, inferiorly by the clavicle, and superiorly by the lower border of the mandible and the mastoid process.

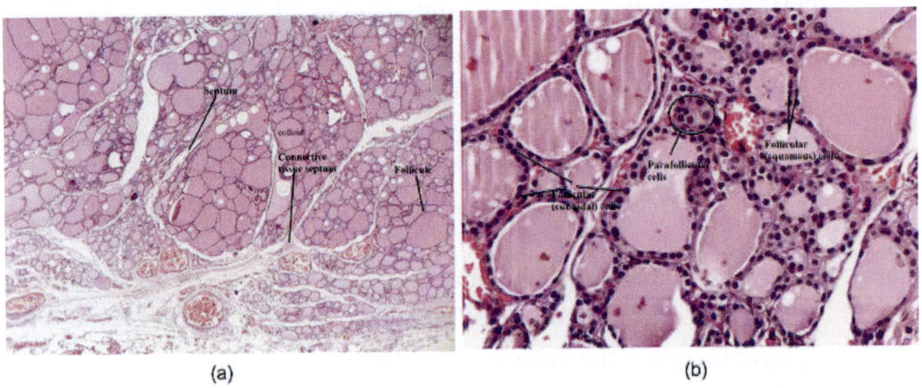

Figure 6.2. *a) General thyroid gland histology including fibrous capsule, septum, follicules and reticular fiber meshwork b) Thyroid gland cell types; parafollicular and follicular cells.*

Source: *Sinan Binboga, Eyup Gemici, and Elif Binboga, "Thyroid Anatomy," IntechOpen; 2019. Available from: http://dx.doi.org/10.5772/intechopen.85194.*

The external and internal jugular veins are the primary neck veins that return blood from the head and face. The primary arteries in the neck are the common carotids. The thyroid is situated in front of the neck, bridging the trachea, between the levels of the C5 and T1. These two levels are connected by an isthmus. Figure 6.2 provides the best understanding of the basic anatomy. In healthy individuals, the thyroid lobes differ significantly in size and form. Tall subjects have longitudinally elongated lateral lobes, while shorter subjects have a more oval-shaped gland. The thyroid gland in a newborn has an approximate diameter of 19 mm and an 8–9 mm anteroposterior (AP) diameter. At one year of age, the average length is 25 mm with a mean of 12–15 mm AP; in contrast, the average length in adults is roughly 40–60 mm with a mean of 13–18 mm AP. In women, the thyroid gland is a little bit heavier and larger. It displays slightly more growth during the menstrual cycle and pregnancy. The synthesis, storage, and secretion of thyroid hormones by the thyroid gland, an organ of the endocrine system, sustains bodily growth, development, and metabolism. These hormones consist of calcitonin, thyroxine (T4), and triiodothyronine (T3). T3 and T4 stimulate the metabolism of food into energy in cells. The regulation of calcium levels involves calcitonin to a minor extent. Thyroid gland dysfunction, which is controlled by the pituitary and hypothalamic glands, can lead to thyroid disorders.

6.1.1. Embryology of the Thyroid Gland

Prehistoric thyroid glands are among the earliest known endocrine organs. It is noticeable in the embryo on day 24 of development. It gradually moves to the final site between weeks four and seven of pregnancy. Up until week 10, it is connected to the tongue base via the thyroglossal duct and is formed from pharyngeal endoderm cells that originate from the foramen caecum in the tongue base. There is an isthmus connecting the two lobes, which are the lobus dexter and the lobus sinister. The hyoid bone is connected to a small lobe called "the pyramidal lobe," which is primarily descended from the left lobe of the thyroid. The cells that migrate from the neural crest and a fifth pharyngeal pouch structure combine to form the parafollicular thyroid ("C") cells that secrete calcitonin. This embryogenesis has a number of clinically significant pathologic effects, such as fistulas, medullary carcinoma, thyroglossal duct cysts, and hypothyroidism.

6.1.2. Histology of the Thyroid Gland

The thyroid gland is a special kind of endocrine gland that stores a lot of hormone in an inactive form in its follicles and extracellular components. The thyroid gland is surrounded by a fibrous capsule, and it is separated into lobules by a fine collagenous septum. Each lobule is made up of many thyroid follicles, which are densely packed, ring-shaped structures with an average diameter of 200 μm. The reticular fiber meshwork contains the embedded follicles (Figure 6.2a). The primary structural and functional elements of the gland are the thyroid follicles, which are the sites of T3 and T4 synthesis and release. Colloid, a gelatinous material containing T3 and T4 in their stored forms, fills each follicle. The colloid is primarily acidophilic in inactive glands and basophilic in active glands. This colloid exhibits vacuoles and is both less abundant in highly activated glands.

Thyroid cells come in different types, i.e., both parafollicular and follicular cells. The production of T3 and T4 is carried out by the follicular or principal cells. Typically, these cells are simple cuboidal cells, but depending on their secretion states, they can transform into simple squamous (inactive) or columnar (active) cells (Figure 6.2b). The follicular cells exhibit basophilic cytoplasm and a spherical nucleus with one or more unique nucleoli, according to HandE staining. The supranuclear position is where the Golgi apparatus is situated. From an ultrastructural perspective, the cells have short microvilli on the apical surface and organelles that exhibit both secretory and absorptive properties. Cells have a significant amount of rough endoplasmic reticulum in their basal locations. The apical region of cells is home to numerous endocytotic vesicles known as lysosomes, which are defined as colloidal resorption droplets, and small vesicles that morphologically resemble the Golgi apparatus.

The second type of thyroid cells are called parafollicular or clear cells (C cells), and they can be found inside the follicular epithelium or as tiny clusters next to the follicles. These cells are located on the basal follicular membrane and are comparatively large, oval or ellipsoid, with round nuclei and pale cytoplasm. These cells are known as "C" cells because of their large amounts of unstained cytoplasm, which makes them frequently difficult to identify in H and E sections. These cells create the hormone calcitonin, which is released in response to elevated blood calcium levels and which stops osteoclast activity.

6.1.3. Macroscopic Anatomy of the Thyroid Gland

The fascia surrounding the thyroid gland is made up of the anterior and posterior segments of the deep cervical fascia. The gland has an average size of 5 cm in length, 2.5 cm in width, and 1.5 cm in depth. It weighs roughly 10–20 g. During menstruation and pregnancy, the gland enlarges and becomes slightly heavier. The Ansa cervicalis, also known as the Ansa hypoglossi, innervates the thyroid lobes, which are situated lateral to the trachea and esophagus, anteromedial to the carotid sheath, and posteromedial to the strap muscles (sternohyoid, sternothyroid, and superior belly of the omohyoid) (Figure 6.3a). The gland is made up of two elongated lateral lobes with superior and inferior poles that are connected at the midline by an isthmus. Its shape can vary from an H to a U. The isthmus, which joins the two lobes, is between 12 and 15 high. The gland can occasionally exist as two distinct lobes without an isthmus (Figure 6.3b).

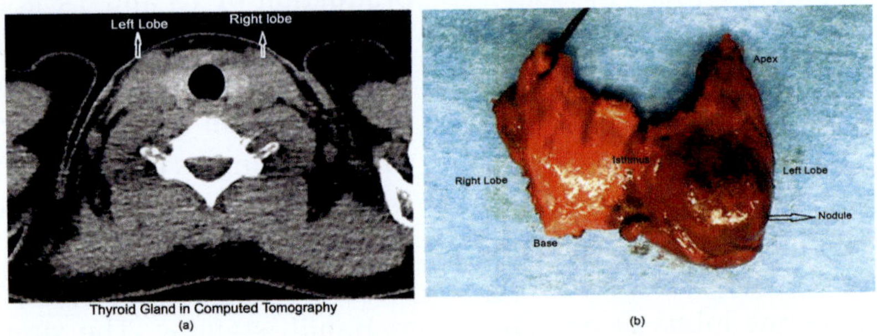

Figure 6.3. *a) Thyroid gland in computed tomography b) Macroscopic anatomy of the thyroid gland.*

Source: Sinan Binboga, Eyup Gemici, and Elif Binboga, "Thyroid Anatomy," IntechOpen; 2019. Available from: http://dx.doi.org/10.5772/intechopen.85194.

Roughly 50% of patients have a pyramidal lobe that extends toward the hyoid bone, to which it may be connected by a fibromuscular or fibrous band. ZTs, or Zuckerkandl tubercles, are the most lateral extension of the thyroid lobes. Recurrent laryngeal nerve (RLN) is located in close proximity to these tubercles, which are condensed thyroid parenchymas situated in the cricothyroid junction, where the medial thyroid connects to the ultimobranchial bodies. The lateral thyroid anlage and the median anlage of the fourth pharyngeal pouch fuse embryologically to form the ultimobranchial body, which gives rise to ZTs. This tissue's dissection is crucial because the RLN is situated beneath the ZTs in the thyroid gland's posterolateral region.

From the foramen cecum at the base of the tongue to the lower neck, the thyroglossal duct follows the thyroid's path. In humans, the most common congenital cervical anomalies are cysts of this duct. Although they rarely show symptoms, oral bacteria can sometimes infect them. Although duct carcinomas are exceedingly uncommon, 1–2%of them are discovered to be cancerous; these are typically papillary carcinomas, which account for 85% of cases. The thyroid lobes are encased in a thin layer of the deep cervical fascia, both in front and behind. The anterior and posterior suspensory ligaments, which connect this fascia to the capsule, are suspensory ligaments. From the superior medial aspect of each thyroid lobe to the thyroid cartilage and cricoid, the anterior suspensory ligament stretches. The cricoid cartilage and upper rings of the trachea are connected to the thyroid by the posterior ligament, also referred to as the Berry ligament. The Berry ligament has significant surgical implications because of its close attachment to the cricoid cartilage and the RLN. Typically, the RLN penetrates the posterior suspensory ligament deeply. There should be no force applied when the thyroid gland retracts on the medial side, as this could injure and stretch the RLN. Furthermore, bleeding may result from vena thyroidea media rupture. When performing the dissection and hemostasis to control bleeding, caution should be taken to avoid injuring any nerves. There are two parathyroid glands—two superior and two inferior. Little structures that are either embedded in the thyroid gland or located next to it are called parathyroid glands. Normally, the thyroid gland and two pairs of parathyroid glands are close by. The inferior glands have a higher likelihood of migrating to ectopic locations.

6.1.4. Microscopic Anatomy of the Thyroid Gland

Like other endocrine organs, the thyroid gland has a rich blood supply and a high degree of anastomosis, making it a highly vascular organ. Both the superior thyroid artery, the subclavian system, and the lower thyroid branch of the thyrocervical trunk supply the body's arteries bilaterally. There might just be one thyroid Ima artery that emerges from the brachiocephalic artery.

The ipsilateral external carotid arteries are the source of the superior thyroid arteries, which split into anterior and posterior branches at the peak of the thyroid lobes. Shortly after the origin of the subclavian arteries, the inferior thyroid arteries emerge from the thyrocervical. The inferior thyroid arteries pass through the midpoints of the thyroid lobes after emerging from the neck and the carotid sheath. In 1–4% of cases, a missing lower thyroid artery is replaced by or the arteries that originate directly from the aorta or innominate and enter the isthmus. Before the arterial branches are ligated, the recurrent laryngeal nerve (RLN) must be identified because the inferior thyroid artery passes through it. The aorta, intercostal arteries, and tracheobronchial arteries all directly branch into the inferior thyroid artery, which supplies the cervical esophagus with arterial blood via the subclavian artery.

The thyroid's three principal veins are the superior, middle, and inferior thyroid veins. The middle thyroid vein is not present with the superior thyroid vein, which drains to the internal jugular vein in conjunction with the superior thyroid artery. Several inferior thyroid vessels often empty into the brachycephalic or internal jugular veins.

6.1.4.1. Innervation of the Thyroid

The RLN branch of the vagus nerve is in charge of laryngeal motor function and sensation. The right RLN wraps around the right subclavian artery, while the left RLN loops from the vagus nerve to the back of the aorta. These nerves rise along the trachea close to the thyroid gland, so the surgeon must take care to protect them during a thyroidectomy. The RLN at the thyroid gland's entrance is closely associated with the inferior thyroid artery and its terminal branches. The nerve and an artery branch can occasionally be mistaken for one another. It is less rounded, elastic, and regular than the artery. The vasa nervorum is a tiny, red, curved vein that is typically visible in the nerve wall. The right RLN is more lateral and inclined than the left, rising straight up the tracheoesophageal groove. There are, however, a number of defined variations, so caution must be exercised in each instance. The RLN is embedded in the Berry ligament, the suspensory ligament, which is located behind the two upper tracheal rings. Tightly joining the thyroid to the trachea and esophagus, this ligament extends behind the recurrent nerve. A posterior artery is located here, close to the recurrent nerve. It is difficult to connect to this artery and provides a tiny branch to the thyroid gland (Figure 6.4).

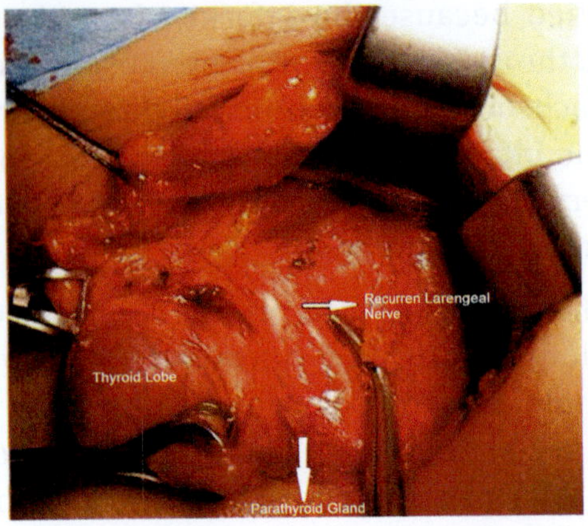

Figure 6.4. *Thyroid gland location with nerve and parathyroid gland.*

Source: Sinan Binboga, Eyup Gemici, and Elif Binboga, "Thyroid Anatomy," IntechOpen; 2019. Available from: http://dx.doi.org/10.5772/intechopen.85194.

Another branch of the vagus nerve is the superior laryngeal nerve. The external laryngeal nerve functions as the motor nerve, and the internal laryngeal nerve functions as the sensory nerve. The internal carotid artery divides into two arms on the pharynx side. The paralysis of the superior laryngeal nerve can result in a significant contraction of the pitch range, asymmetry in the vibratory phase of the vocal fold, and acoustic aperiodicity, all of which can contribute to an overall poor quality of voice. The external branch of the superior laryngeal nerve and the superior thyroid artery are closely related. High-pitched sounds could be caused by this nerve injury. It is advised to ligate the superior thyroid arteries as low as feasible during thyroidectomy to avoid harming the external branch of the superior laryngeal nerve. The cricothyroid artery, a branch of the superior thyroid artery, travels along the cricothyroid ligament toward the midline from its location in the cephalic region of the upper pole. During a cricothyroidotomy, this vessel could be harmed, which could result in bleeding. To control bleeding, great care should be used in large area hemostasis. Nerve damage can be avoided by ligating each vein individually. Below is a classification of the superior laryngeal nerve's external branch based on possible damage risk.

Type 1: The nerve traverses the superior thyroid vessels over 1 centimeter above the upper pole border of the thyroid.

Type 2a: Less than 1 cm above the thyroid upper pole border, the nerve crosses the vessels.

Type 2b: The nerve passes through the vessel just below the thyroid's upper pole border.

The lateral carotid artery, the medial trachea, the neck root, and the triangle the superior thyroid lobe forms can all be home to the recurrent laryngeal nerve (on the right, after it leaves the superior thoracic cavity). The tracheoesophageal groove is where the right recurrent laryngeal nerve normally enters the larynx at an angle of 0–30°. This angle ranges from 15 to 45° in the left recurrent laryngeal nerve. In 61% of cases, the recurrent laryngeal nerve travels through the posterior of the inferior thyroid artery, in 32% of cases, the anterior, and in 7% of cases, the artery's branches. The inferior laryngeal nerve is situated proximally by the lower parathyroid glands and distally by the upper parathyroid glands. 60%–70% of cases have the recurrent laryngeal nerve located in the tracheoesophageal groove, 25% in the lateral trachea, and 5% in the posterior trachea.

RLS splits into branches prior to entering the larynx in 35–80% of cases. Extralaryngeal branching typically occurs in two forms: motor and sensory branches. There have been descriptions of two to eight extralaryngeal branches in the literature, nevertheless. It is recognized macroscopically due to its linear extension and pale yellow color.

The inferior laryngeal nerves measure approximately 32 cm for the right and 43 cm for the left. The majority of nerve injuries occur on the left inferior laryngeal nerve because it has a longer course in the tracheoesophageal groove. In 0.3–0.8% of cases, nonrecurrent laryngeal nerve was reported. The nonrecurrent laryngeal nerve enters the larynx directly at the level of the cricothyroid joint without forming a loop after leaving the cervical portion of the vagus at the level of the thyroid gland or the larynx.

Thyroid surgery may make use of the intraoperative methylene blue spraying technique. The perilober region and thyroid lobe will be sprayed with methylene blue. It is possible to assess tissues, particularly parathyroides, the inferior thyroid artery, and the recurrent laryngeal nerve. The incidence of recurrent nerve damage following thyroid surgery ranges from 0% to 11%. While complications are negatively correlated with surgeon experience, they are more common following subtotal thyroidectomies and secondary surgeries than following total thyroidectomies and primary surgeries. Palpating the posterior cricoarytenoid muscle without the use of electromyography allowed for the monitoring of the vocal folds during surgery and the subsequent application of glottic pressure. Nonetheless, a significant drawback of this approach is that it is both challenging and produces less than ideal outcomes. Perioperative recurrent nerve monitoring resulted in a significant reduction in both surgical duration and postoperative complications. Surface electrodes built into endotracheal intubation tubes are used for measurements. The instrument sounds an alert to the surgeon. Furthermore, the surgeon will have legal support due to the ability to record the current modifications made to the device screen.

The choice of anesthesia is crucial for patients undergoing perioperative recurrent nerve monitoring. The outcomes will be entirely impacted by the muscle relaxant agent's ongoing effects. You can perform intubation without the need for a muscle relaxant. Additionally, agents that take effect quickly and degrade quickly can be used for it. Succinylcholine is frequently chosen for this reason since it functions as a short-acting depolarizing neuromuscular blocking agent.

Several techniques for recurrent nerve repair, including grafting and microsuturing glueing, have been proposed in the event of a nerve injury. When the defect is less than 5 mm and the primary repair can be finished without tension, direct microsuture is the preferred method. Following RLN transection, immediate reconstruction could be accomplished with three to four perineural stitches of 7-0 nylon thread, utilizing microsurgical instruments, and a direct, "end-to-end" anastomosis of neural stamps. The use of cyanoacrylate glue for nerve repair has also been suggested, but it has drawn criticism due to its toxicity, abnormally slow resorption, and potential for an inflammatory response in the perineural tissues. When the RLN's proximal stump is not suitable for grafting, the transverse cervical nerve, supraclavicular nerve, or Ansa cervicalis should be used. Commence by recognizing the Ansa cervicalis on the external jugular vein's surface. Its branches to the sternothyroid muscles may then be dissected. The distal RLN stump could be anastomosed to the proximal end of the major branch.

6.1.4.2. Lymphatics of the Thyroid

The thyroid gland's lymphatic drainage is

extensive and has a flexible flow pattern. The four distinct drainage patterns that make up the Hollinshead pattern are the median inferior drainage, right/left lateral drainage, posterior drainage, and median superior drainage. Originating from the upper middle edge of the lateral lobes and the upper edge of the isthmus, three to six lymphatic vessels are traversed by the median superior drainage. These lymphatic veins originate in the digastric nodes and travel upward toward the larynx. A portion of the lymphatics may enter one or both of the throat's (Delphian) nodes directly above the isthmus. Secondarily, from the Delphian nodes to the frontal side of the thyroid gland, or from the upper jugular nodes on either side of the neck, the anterior tracheal nodes under the thyroid travel downward via lymphatic channels.

Numerous lymphatic vessels that drain to the lower medial portions of the lateral lobes and the inferior portion of the isthmus make up the median inferior drainage. These lymphatic channels come to an end prior to the tracheal and brachycephalic nodes by following the inferior thyroid veins. The lymphatic bodies located at each lobe's lateral border are the source of the left and right lateral drainage patterns. The lower thyroid artery is at the bottom, and the superior thyroid artery and vein are ascending. The lymphatic ducts travel lateral, anterior, or posterior to the carotid sheath between these two groups in order to reach the internal jugular vein lymph nodes. Rarely, instead of flowing to the lymph node, these lymphatic vessels drain straight into the jugular vein, thoracic duct, or subclavian vein.

The lymphatic vessels that drain to the inferomedial regions of the lateral lobes and then into the lymph nodes along the RLN track are the starting point of the posterior drainage pattern. Seldom does a lymphatic body that ascends from the upper region of the lobe posteriorly reach the retropharyngeal nodes. There have been several hypothesized models of the thyroid gland's lymphatic drainage, and each one is accurate and understandable from the same perspective. An alternative drainage model that is more simplified states that the emergency lymphatic drainage first reaches the periglandular nodes, then the RLN-containing preterminal and paratracheal nodes, and finally the mediastinal lymph nodes. The impact of lymph node metastasis on prognosis and survival is still under debate, despite the fact that it is known to increase recurrence. Adjuvant treatment options for all patients with lateral LN recurrence include therapeutic neck dissection and RAI ablation therapy.

6.2. Physiology of the Thyroid

The production of thyroxine (T4), calcitonin, and triiodothyronine (T3) is the thyroid's main job. The thyroid gland produces the enzymes thyroxine (T4) and triiodothyronine (T3). T4 is considered a pro-hormone for T3, which has a higher metabolic activity. T4 is changed into T3 in tissues when deiodinase enzymes are active. Along with parathyroid hormone, which is released from the parathyroid, calcitonin, another hormone secreted by the thyroid gland, is in charge of regulating blood calcium levels.

6.2.1. Effect of Thyroid Hormones on Metabolism

The primary function of thyroid hormones T3 and T4 is to increase the basal metabolic rates of vitamins, proteins, and fats (Figure 6.5).

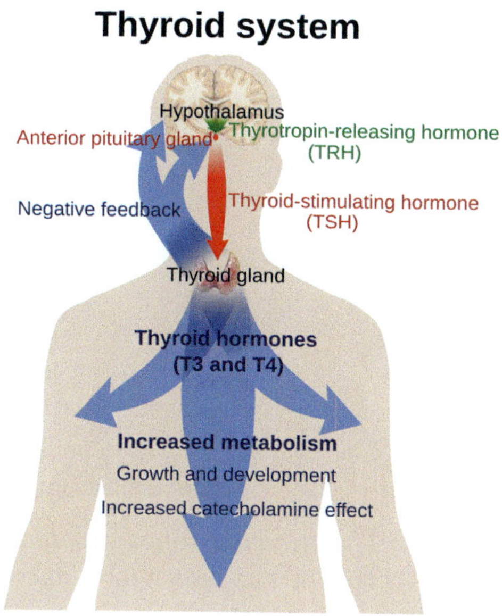

Figure 6.5. *Thyroid system: An overview of the thyroid system.*

Source: By Mikael Häggström – All used images are in public domain., Public Domain, https://commons.wikimedia.org/w/index.php?curid=8567011.

6.2.2. Effect of Thyroid Hormones on Body Temperature

The rate at which heat can leave the body is influenced by the dilatation of blood vessels, which is influenced by thyroid hormones. Heat can escape more quickly in blood vessels with greater dilating. When a person has hypothyroidism (a less active thyroid), their body temperature will drop; when they have hyperthyroidism (an overactive thyroid), their body temperature will rise.

6.2.3. Action of Thyroid Hormones on the Developing Fetus

For T3 and T4, the developing brain cells are a primary target. Given that they control actin polymerization during neuronal development, thyroid hormones are especially important for brain maturation during fetal development.

6.2.4. Action of Thyroid Hormones in Blood

T4 and T3 are partly bound to albumin, transthyretin, and thyroxine-binding globulin (TBG) in the blood. Just a very tiny portion of the hormone in circulation—T4 0.03% and T3 0.3%—is free. Hormonal activity is present only in the free fraction. Thyroid hormones are lipophillic, just like steroid hormones, and they can penetrate cell membranes to attach to intracellular receptors. These receptors can function as transcription factors on their own or in concert with other factors to modify DNA transcription.

6.2.5. Calcitonin Activity

There are three ways that calcitonin lowers blood calcium levels.

1. preventing the deterioration of bones caused by osteoclasts.
2. promoting osteoblastic activity in order to generate new bone.
3. inhibiting the kidneys' ability to reabsorb calcium.

6.2.6. Control of Thyroid Hormone Release

Thyroid-stimulating hormone (TSH), which is released from the anterior pituitary, controls the synthesis of thyroxine and triiodothyronine. Thyroid-stimulating hormone (TSH), which is secreted by the anterior pituitary gland, is the main hormone that controls the synthesis of thyroxine (T4) and triiodothyronine (T3). Thyrotropin-releasing hormone (TRH) is secreted by the hypothalamus in response to TSH release. Increased growth, development, metabolism, and the activation of multiple other thyroid hormone-regulated systems follow from this. Additionally, thyroid hormones give the anterior pituitary gland and hypothalamus negative feedback. TSH and TRH production are decreased in response to elevated blood thyroid levels. Additionally, too much TRH can prevent the body from producing more TRH.

6.3. Benign Disorders of the Thyroid

The thyroid needs iodine, a chemical element that occurs naturally in a variety of foods, in order to produce the T3 and T4 hormones. After absorbing iodine, the thyroid creates the hormones T3 and T4 via a series of chemical reactions. Another kind of endocrine gland, the parathyroid glands, are located next to the thyroid gland. The parathyroid hormone is a hormone that is produced by the four parathyroid glands. Three minerals—calcium, phosphorus, and magnesium—have different blood levels depending on this hormone. To keep bones healthy, these minerals are necessary components.

6.3.1. Hashimoto Thyroiditis

Hashimoto thyroiditis is an autoimmune disease caused by immune processes mediated by cells and antibodies that destroy thyroid cells. In developed nations, it is the most frequent cause of hypothyroidism. On the other hand, a diet low in iodine is the leading cause of hypothyroidism globally. Other names for this condition include chronic lymphocytic thyroiditis and chronic autoimmune thyroiditis. Antithyroid antibodies are formed as part of the disease's pathology, attacking thyroid tissue and leading to progressive fibrosis. The diagnosis is frequently difficult and may not come about until much later in the course of the illness. The most typical laboratory results show low levels of free thyroxine (fT4) and elevated thyroid-stimulating hormone (TSH), along with elevated antithyroid peroxidase (TPO) antibodies. However, patients may show hyperthyroidism-like signs, symptoms, and laboratory results early in the disease course, or normal values. This is due to the possibility of sporadic thyroid gland cell destruction (Figure 6.6).

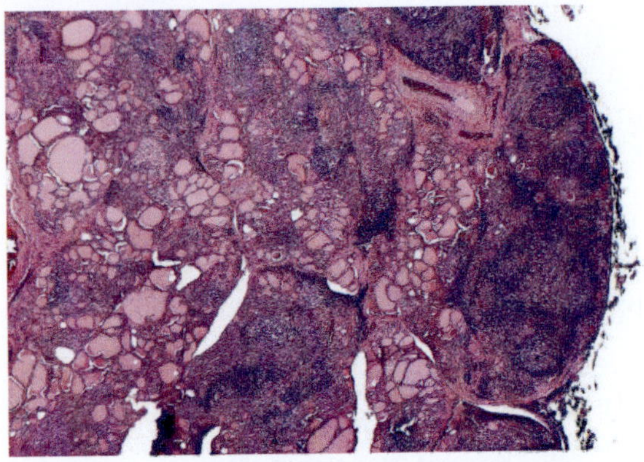

Figure 6.6. *The thyroid of a patient with Hashimoto's thyroiditis as seen with a microscope at low magnification.*

Source: By Librepath - Own work, CC BY-SA 3.0, https://commons.wikimedia.org/w/index.php?curid=45578566.

Affected women are more frequently than men. At least 10:1 is the female to male ratio. While some reports indicate that diagnoses occur more frequently in the fifth decade of life, the majority of women receive their diagnoses between the ages of 30 and 50. Levothyroxine at the suggested dosage of 1.6 to 1.8 mcg/kg/day is the mainstay of conventional treatment. The human body uses T3—the active form of thyroid hormone—to convert T4. Overdosing on supplements can have harmful and dangerous consequences, including osteoporosis and arrhythmias (of which atrial fibrillation is the most common).

6.3.1.1. Etiology

There is very little knowledge about the etiology of Hashimoto disease. Anti-thyroid peroxidase (anti-TPO) is the most frequently developed antibody to various thyroid antigens, which most patients develop antibodies to. Many also produce TSH receptor-blocking antibodies (TBII) and antithyroglobulin (anti-Tg). Thyroid tissue is attacked by these antibodies, which ultimately results in insufficient thyroid hormone production. Only a small portion of the population—between 10 and 15%—has a clinically noticeable illness and does not have serum antibodies. TPO antibody positivity foreshadows the clinical syndrome.

It may be associated with type 1 diabetes mellitus and autoimmune adrenal deficiency in Polyglandular Autoimmune Syndrome type 2. A number of other autoimmune conditions, including pernicious anemia, adrenal insufficiency, and celiac disease, are also linked to Hashimoto thyroiditis.

6.3.1.2. Pathophysiology

It is believed that Hashimoto disease develops due to an autoimmune process; characteristic features include lymphocyte infiltration and fibrosis. The current diagnosis is based on clinical symptoms that match elevated TSH with normal to low thyroxine levels in the laboratory. The lack of evidence supporting the involvement of antithyroid peroxidase (anti-TPO) antibodies in the etiology of autoimmune thyroid disease (AITD) is noteworthy, though. Anti-TPO antibodies have been demonstrated to bind and kill thyrocytes in vitro in addition to fixing complement. However, no relationship between the degree of disease severity and the concentration of anti-TPO antibodies in serum has been observed in human studies to date. However, we are aware that the active stage of the illness is associated with a positive serum anti-TPO antibody concentration. According to other theories, thyroid destruction is caused by immune complexes that contain antibodies directed against the thyroid.

6.3.1.3. Histopathology

The thyroid has a diffuse, symmetric enlargement on pathologic examination. The pyramidal lobe protrudes from the capsule, which is frequently intact. When sliced, the surface has a pale brown to yellow color that resembles lymph nodes. There could be interlobular fibrosis or not. In certain patients, the gland may develop atrophy and turn nodular or asymmetric. Nevertheless, the absence of necrosis or calcification would point to a different diagnosis.

6.3.1.4. History and Physical Examination

Hashimoto thyroiditis presents with a variety of organ system manifestations because of the nature of the illness. Patients may experience episodes of hyperthyroidism at first because the initial loss of thyroid cells may cause an increase in the amount of thyroid hormone released into the blood. After the antibody response has done enough damage, patients eventually show signs of hypothyroidism. These subtle, fluctuating symptoms have the potential to impact nearly every organ system in the body. Myxedema, or the edema-like skin condition brought on by increased glycosaminoglycan deposition, is the classic skin characteristic associated with hypothyroidism. That being said, this is rare and only happens in extreme situations. Dry and scaly skin can occur, particularly on the soles, palms, and extensor surfaces. Histologic analysis shows thinning of the epidermis. Water retention and pale skin are the results of increased dermal mucopolysaccharides. Hair can become dry, coarse, dull, and brittle as its growth rate slows. It is not unusual to have diffuse or partial alopecia.

In addition to lowering cardiac output by up to 50%, decreased thyroid function can raise peripheral vascular resistance by as much as 50% to 60%. A decrease in the thyroid hormone's direct chronotropic action on the sinoatrial cells may cause bradycardia. However, most patients have a few symptoms directly attributable to the cardiovascular system. Reduced muscle strength or increased muscle fatigue, along with limited pulmonary and cardiac reserve, are likely contributing factors to fatigue, exertional dyspnea, and exercise intolerance. Reduced endurance in hypothyroid rats has been demonstrated. This population has undergone biochemical changes that include decreased muscle pyruvate and palmitate oxidation, increased glycogen store utilization, and decreased fatty acid mobilization. Muscle weakness and myopathy are important features.

Subclinical presentation is another possibility. Weight gain, exhaustion, dry skin, and constipation are examples of early symptoms. Advanced symptoms can include menorrhagia, cold intolerance, decreased sweating, peripheral neuropathy, nerve deafness, decreased energy, depression, dementia, memory loss, muscle cramps, joint pain, hair loss, apnea, and pressure symptoms (like hoarseness) in the neck caused by goiter enlargement.

Physical findings may include:

- Cold and dry skin
- Edema of the face, especially periorbital, and nonpitting edema of the hands and feet.
- Brittle nails
- Bradycardia
- The delayed relaxation phase of tendon reflexes
- Elevated blood pressure
- Slow speech
- Ataxia
- Macroglossia

Additionally, it is rare for patients to have a buildup of fluid in the pericardial and pleural cavities. In terms of patient care, myxoedema coma requires management as an endocrine emergency due to its extreme clinical presentation.

6.3.1.5. Evaluation

An autoimmune disease characterized by insufficient thyroid hormone production is called Hashimoto thyroiditis. The biochemical picture shows that low free T4 causes an increase in thyroid-stimulating hormone (TSH). Primary hypothyroidism is confirmed by a low total T4 or free T4 level in the presence of an elevated TSH level. Practitioners of integrative and functional medicine may also measure reverse T3 and free T3 levels; Western medicine does not employ this method. Anti-thyroglobulin and anti-thyroid peroxidase antibodies point to Hashimoto thyroiditis. Nonetheless, 10% of patients might not have any antibodies. 30–40% of people have anemia. Hyponatremia may arise from reduced renal plasma flow, renal glomerular filtration rate (GFR), and renal free water clearance. There is usually an increase in creatine kinase. There could be an increase in prolactin. There may be elevated LDL, triglyceride, and total cholesterol levels. Thyroid ultrasound measures thyroid size, thyroid nodule presence, and echotexture; most of the time, it is not required to diagnose the condition.

6.3.1.6. Treatment / Management

Thyroid hormone replacement therapy is the cornerstone of treatment for hypothyroidism. Titrated levothyroxine sodium taken orally is the preferred medication. It can be taken once a day and has a half-life of seven days. To prevent less-than-ideal absorption, it shouldn't be administered with calcium or iron supplements, aluminum hydroxide, or proton pump inhibitors. For maximum absorption, it is best taken first thing in the morning on an empty stomach.

While 1.6–1.8 mcg/kg is the standard dose, individual patient dosages may differ. Patients under 50 years of age should start on the standard full dose; elderly and patients with cardiovascular diseases should use lower doses. It is advised to start patients over 50 at a dose of

25 mcg per day and to reevaluate them after six to eight weeks. On the other hand, higher doses of levothyroxine are required in patients with short-bowel syndrome in order to maintain a euthyroid state, and a 30% increase in thyroxine is required during pregnancy. A diet that is anti-inflammatory or autoimmune-supportive has less evidence. The underlying theory for the inflammation is related to leaky gut syndrome, which is characterized by an insult to the gut mucosa that permits the penetration of proteins through mucosal transporters that ordinarily prevent them from entering the bloodstream. Antibodies are thought to be produced against the antigens in a reaction akin to molecular mimicry. Unfortunately, thyroid peroxidase antibody formation may result from the antigen's strong structural similarity to the enzyme. The goal of an autoimmune diet is to reduce the intensity of the autoimmune response while also healing the gut.

6.3.1.7. Differential Diagnosis

- Euthyroid sick syndrome
- Goiter
- Graves' disease (diffuse toxic goiter)
- Hypopituitarism (panhypopituitarism)
- Lithium-induced goiter
- Nontoxic goiter
- Polyglandular autoimmune syndrome type 1
- Polyglandular autoimmune syndrome type 2
- Thyroid cancer (lymphoma)
- Toxic nodular goiter

6.3.1.8. Pearls and Other Issues

According to reports, 10–40% of patients with Hashimoto thyroiditis (HT), one of the most common autoimmune diseases, also have stomach issues. In about 40% of cases, Hashimoto thyroiditis coexists with autoimmune gastritis. The production of hydrochloric acid and intrinsic factor is impaired in chronic autoimmune gastritis (CAG), which is typified by the partial or total loss of parietal cells. The individuals proceed to experience iron-deficient anemia that is dependent on hypochlorhydria, which results in pernicious anemia and severe gastric atrophy.

When thyroid autoantibodies were discovered in a subgroup of patients with pernicious anemia and atrophic gastritis in the 1960s, the condition known as thyrogastric syndrome was first identified. According to the most recent guidelines, the two autoimmune disorders mentioned above have been combined into a syndrome that is now referred to as polyglandular autoimmune syndrome (PAS). Two or more endocrine and nonendocrine disorders define this. Since the primitive gut is where the thyroid gland develops, parietal cells that originate from the same endoderm share characteristics with thyroid follicular cells. For instance, both can concentrate and transfer iodine across the cell membrane via the sodium/iodide symporter. They also have polarized apical microvilli with enzymatic activity. In addition to being necessary for the synthesis of thyroid hormone, iodine also regulates the growth of gastric mucosal cells, provides an electron donor when gastric peroxidase is present, and aids in the elimination of free oxygen radicals.

It is significant to remember that patients with disorders of the gastric mucosa may experience difficulties with absorption because thyroxine is now available worldwide in pharmaceutical form. The majority of levothyroxine is produced by salinizing sodium hydroxide, which yields sodium levothyroxine. T4 is absorbed in all sections of the small intestine, with 62–84% of the dose being absorbed. With the exception of liquid-based or soft gel formulations, decreased gastric acid secretion can upset this proportion and result in problems with decreased absorption of the majority of pharmaceutical-grade forms of levothyroxine. Clinically speaking, it is critical to recognize the connection between autoimmune diseases of the thyroid and the stomach. In addition to thyroxine absorption problems, iron-deficiency anemia should prompt additional diagnostic testing.

6.3.1.9. Enhancing Healthcare Team Outcomes

Since there is no known treatment for Hashimoto thyroiditis, an interdisciplinary team comprising an internist, primary care physician, and endocrinologist is best suited to manage the condition. Monitoring thyroid hormone levels is essential. In certain individuals, the empirical prescription of a single standard dose of levothyroxine may result in hormone toxicity. Furthermore, lymphomas can develop in some patients, so it is important to have regular neck exams.

6.3.2. Hypothyroidism

Low thyroid hormone levels, with a variety of causes and symptoms, lead to hypothyroidism. Morbidity and mortality are increased by untreated hypothyroidism. Hashimoto thyroiditis, an autoimmune thyroid disease, is the most common cause of hypothyroidism in the United States, but iodine deficiency is the most common cause worldwide. The patient may present with myxedema coma or with an asymptomatic illness. These days, exogenous thyroid hormone can be used to treat hypothyroidism, which can be diagnosed with ease using straightforward blood tests.

6.3.2.1. Etiology

Primary and secondary (central) hypothyroidism are the two main categories into which hypothyroidism falls. When the thyroid gland is unable to produce enough thyroid hormone, the condition is referred to as primary hypothyroidism. When thyroid function is normal and the pathology is associated with the pituitary or hypothalamus, a condition known as secondary or central hypothyroidism is diagnosed. This type of hypothyroidism is less common.

Iodine deficiency is the most common cause of primary hypothyroidism in iodine-deficient regions of the world. In the iodine-sufficient regions and the United States, autoimmune thyroid diseases are the primary cause of hypothyroidism. The most prevalent cause of thyroiditis in Americans is Hashimoto's disease, which is closely linked to lymphoma. Both the creation of new iodine-deficient areas and iodine fortification can have a local impact on etiology.

Other common causes of hypothyroidism include:

- Medications like lithium, amiodarone, thalidomide, bexarotene, sunitinib, stavudine, interferon, perchlorate, rifampin, ethionamide, phenobarbital, phenytoin, carbamazepine, and interleukin-2.
- Thyroid radioactive iodine therapy
- Thyroid surgery
- Radiotherapy to the head or neck area
- disorders of the pituitary or hypothalamus that are iatrogenic, neoplastic, infiltrative, inflammatory, or genetic can cause central hypothyroidism.
- Anti-CTLA-4 and anti-PD-L1/

PD-1 therapy are two new classes of cancer drugs that have been linked to primary or secondary hypothyroidism.

About 10% of women experience postpartum thyroiditis, which typically manifests 8–20 weeks after the baby is delivered. Fewer women need thyroid hormone treatment than men. On the other hand, some women are more likely to experience recurrent postpartum thyroiditis or permanent hypothyroidism in subsequent pregnancies. About 80–90% of patients who receive radioactive iodine therapy for Grave disease typically develop permanent hypothyroidism 8–20 weeks after starting treatment. Hypothyroidism can also arise from head and neck radiation therapy. The de Quervain disease, subacute granulomatous thyroiditis is a relatively uncommon cause of primary hypothyroidism. It typically affects middle-aged women and is a self-limiting illness. AIRE gene mutation causes autoimmune polyendocrinopathy type-1, a combination of mucocutaneous candidiasis, Addison's disease, and hypoparathyroidism. A malfunction in the hypothalamic-pituitary axis results in secondary and tertiary hypothyroidism, which is also referred to as central hypothyroidism.

Among its reasons are the following:

- Pituitary tumors
- Tumors compressing hypothalamus
- Sheehan syndrome
- Thyroid releasing hormone (TRH) resistance
- TRH deficiency
- Lymphocytic hypophysitis
- Radiation therapy to the brain
- Drugs such as dopamine, prednisone, or opioids

6.3.2.2. Epidemiology

According to the NHANESIII (National Health and Nutrition Examination Survey) study, 0.3% of adults in the United States (12 years of age and older) have overt hypothyroidism, and 4.3% have subclinical hypothyroidism. Higher levels of thyroid-stimulating hormone (TSH) and the prevalence of antithyroid antibodies were linked to female gender and advancing age. Women who are small statured at birth and have a low body mass index as children are more likely to have hypothyroidism.

6.3.2.3. Pathophysiology

The most frequent cause of hypothyroidism is the inability of the thyroid gland to generate enough thyroid hormone, but thyroid dysfunction can also occasionally be brought on by pituitary and hypothalamic dysfunction. Thyrotropin-releasing hormone (TRH), which is secreted by the hypothalamus, causes the pituitary gland to release thyroid-stimulating hormone (TSH). The thyroid gland is stimulated by thyroid-stimulating hormone to produce and secrete primarily T4 (roughly 100–125 nmol per day) and comparatively smaller amounts of T3. T4 has a half-life of 7 to 10 days. Eventually, 5'-deiodination converts T4 to T3 peripherally. T3 and T4 levels primarily have a negative feedback loop that affects the synthesis of TRH and TSH. Hypothyroidism may arise from modifications to the anatomy or physiology of any of these organs or pathways. When T4 production declines, the pituitary gland secretes more TSH, which causes the thyroid parenchyma to enlarge and become more parenchymatic, increasing the production of T3.

6.3.2.4. Histopathology

Iodine turnover rises and organification is hampered by autoimmune thyroiditis. T-cell lymphocytic infiltration is the main result of parenchymal chronic inflammation. If this continues, dense fibrosis and atrophic thyroid follicles take the place of the initial lymphocytic hyperplasia and vacuoles. It is also possible to observe concurrent or related cancer, such as papillary thyroid cancer.

6.3.2.5. History and Physical

Since the signs and symptoms of hypothyroidism can be vague and mild, and because different patients may experience different symptoms, it is critical to keep a high index of suspicion. It is possible that typical symptoms like puffiness, reduced sweating, cold intolerance, and skin changes won't always be evident. Ask about changes in voice, hair loss, constipation, tiredness, cramping in the muscles, cold intolerance, sleep disturbances, irregular menstrual cycles, weight gain, and galactorrhea. Get a thorough medical, surgical, pharmaceutical, and family history as well. It is advisable to look for a history of unfavorable pregnancy and neonatal outcomes.

There may be signs of cognitive impairments like memory loss, psychosis, depression, or anxiety. Patients with pericardial effusion, rhabdomyolysis, and ascites are uncommon presentations. Additionally, patients may exhibit symptoms of sleep apnea, hyponatremia, hypercholesterolemia, congestive heart failure, prolonged QT interval, and carpal tunnel syndrome.

Hashimoto disease is difficult to differentiate clinically; however, some features are specific to this condition such as:

- Fullness of throat
- Fatigue
- Painless thyroid enlargement
- Episodic neck pains and/or sore throat

Since the symptoms of hypothyroidism are so subtle, a thorough physical examination may provide some clues. A physical examination might be important in the following situations:

- Enlarged thyroid gland
- Weight gain
- The slowness of speech and movements
- Dry skin
- Coarse and brittle hair
- Pallor and jaundice
- Dull facial expressions
- Macroglossia
- Bradycardia
- Pericardial effusion
- Prolonged ankle reflex relaxation time

On the other hand, the majority of patients' thyroid exams are normal.

6.3.2.6. Evaluation

Most patients have their serum TSH level checked for primary hypothyroidism. TSH levels are high and free T4 levels are low in overt hypothyroidism. TSH levels are high and free T4 levels are normal in subclinical hypothyroidism. Pituitary or hypothalamic origins can be the cause of central hypothyroidism. Since the amount of TSH produced can be physiologically inactive and influence the levels of bioactive TSH, free T4 should be used instead of TSH to diagnose central hypothyroidism (Figure 6.7).

Testing for autoimmune thyroid disorders should involve measuring anti-thyroid antibodies, such as thyroid peroxidase antibodies, and evaluating the results. Individuals who have thyroid peroxidase antibody positivity and subclinical hypothyroidism are more likely to develop overt hypothyroidism. Research indicates that within a 20-year period, half of the patients will experience primary hypothyroidism. There are no strict guidelines regarding the frequency of follow-up lab tests and clinical evaluations; instead, the decision to do so is based on clinical judgment. TSH testing ought to be reserved for hospitalized patients in cases where thyroid dysfunction is suspected. When sick patients experience slight TSH abnormalities while in the hospital, this should be interpreted as a sign of euthyroid illness. On the other hand, hypothyroidism is indicated by extremely high TSH values. Although "reverse T3" is not routinely measured in clinical practice, it will be elevated when a patient has euthyroid sickness. Anemia, elevated hepatic enzymes, elevated serum CK, and hyperlipidemia may all be found during a laboratory workup. Elevations may also be seen in BUN, creatinine, and uric acid levels. For hypothyroidism, imaging tests (ultrasounds) of the neck are not usually advised.

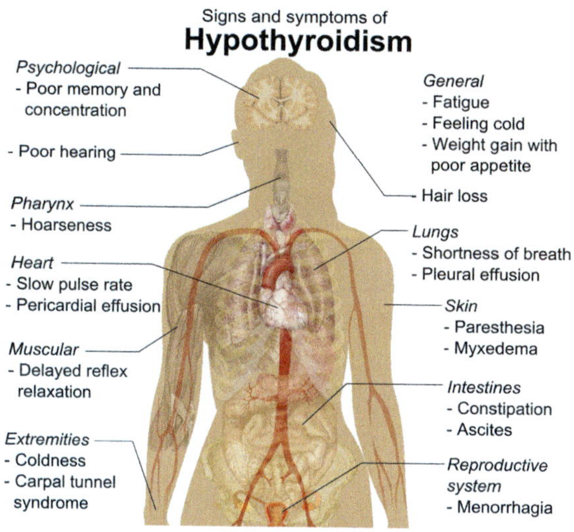

Figure 6.7. *Symptoms and signs of hypothyroidism.*

Source: By Mikael Häggström – Own work, CC0, https://commons.wikimedia.org/w/index.php?curid=30556160.

6.3.2.6.1. Screening for Hypothyroidism

The American Thyroid Association suggests that screening for thyroid disease should begin at age 35 and should continue every five years, despite the fact that there are no universal guidelines for this process.

Some people are more susceptible to hypothyroidism than others such as:

- Women over the age of 60
- Pregnancy
- Patients with a history of radiation therapy to the head and neck.
- Patients with type 1 diabetes and/or autoimmune disorders.
- Thyroid peroxidase antibody positivity.
- Family history

6.3.2.7. Treatment / Management

Levothyroxine monotherapy is the primary treatment for hypothyroidism. Treatment for thyroid replacement may make coexisting adrenal insufficiency worse. While waiting for results, patients with confirmed or suspected adrenal insufficiency should undergo testing and treatment. Subclinical hypothyroidism, which is treatable with treatment for adrenal insufficiency, is also linked to adrenal insufficiency. After receiving appropriate treatment for their adrenal insufficiency, patients with confirmed adrenal insufficiency should have their thyroid tests reevaluated. When a patient has severe hypothyroidism, as in myxedema coma, it is crucial to rule out or treat adrenal insufficiency.

The recommended daily replacement levothyroxine dose is 11.6 mcg/kg; however, it is crucial to lower this amount in older adults and people with atrial fibrillation. Levothyroxine should be taken 30 to 45 minutes before breakfast and at least 3 hours after dinner at bedtime, as these are the times that work best for the majority of patients, to aid in absorption. Furthermore, levothyroxine absorption is impacted by certain elemental supplements, including magnesium and calcium, to mention a couple. Proton pump inhibitors and other commonly used medications adversely affect the absorption of levothyroxine. It is imperative to uphold a uniform formulation or brand of levothyroxine. The generic formulations may differ slightly in dosage, which may have a clinical effect in a small number of extremely sensitive hypothyroid patients.

In hospitals, switching to intravenous (IV) thyroid replacement is recommended for patients who cannot take medication orally or who may have myxedema coma. The IV dose of levothyroxine is usually reduced to 50% of the oral dose, although the exact conversion percentage is debated among experts. Gel formulations like Triocent are used in cases of malabsorption syndromes. Some medications, such as sucralfate, calcium preparations, and bile acid sequestrants, can interfere with levothyroxine absorption. A levothyroxine absorption test may be performed to confirm if a patient is unable to absorb the medication.

According to the 2012 Clinical Practice Guidelines for Hypothyroidism in Adults from the American Association of Clinical Endocrinologists and the American Thyroid Association, treatment for hypothyroidism should be adjusted based on TSH levels. Free T4 levels can also be considered. Blood work should be done every 4 to 8 weeks until target levels are reached, especially after starting treatment, changing dosage, switching brands of medication, or starting/stopping medications that may impact thyroid levels. Once levels stabilize, monitoring can be extended to every 6 months, then every 12 months if levels remain stable, or more frequently as needed based on individual cases and clinical assessment. Central hypothyroiddism should be monitored based on free T4 levels rather than TSH.

Patients who have heart disease should be kept under observation in case atrial fibrillation or angina symptoms appear. A patient should have an osteoporosis screening if they are receiving excessive thyroid replacement therapy for a prolonged period of time. A normal TSH (or free T4 levels, if applicable), an improved sense of the patient's wellbeing, and a clinical improvement of the signs and symptoms are all outcomes of effective treatment. Since the symptoms of hypothyroidism are non-specific, however, it indicates that the patient's symptoms are not hypothyroidism-related if their lab results return to normal while receiving thyroid replacement therapy. Providers must handle this challenging scenario, and having excellent counseling skills will be very beneficial.

When biochemical euthyroidism is present and there are unresolved symptoms, a thorough workup for other differentials is advised. The routine use of levothyroxine and triiodothyronine (T3) preparations in the treatment of hypothyroidism is not well-supported by evidence. The FDA has approved treatments like Armor and Nature Thyroid, but it is crucial to realize that using these formulations raises the risk of cardiac arrhythmias. Furthermore, because of the T3 component, these formulations are not approved for use in patients with thyroid cancer, where stringent TSH goals are necessary, or in pregnant patients. When TSH and free T4 levels return to normal, non-endocrine causes should be taken into consideration if symptoms continue.

6.3.2.8. Differential Diagnosis

The differential diagnosis list is long because hypothyroidism presents with subtle signs and symptoms. Differential diagnosis is based on signs and symptoms. For example, iron deficiency anemia, depression, sleep apnea, and rheumatological diseases can all be indicated by fatigue.

The differentials may need to take into account the following disorders:

- Euthyroid sick syndrome
- Goiter

- Myxedema coma
- Anemia
- Riedel thyroiditis
- Subacute thyroiditis
- Thyroid lymphoma
- Iodine deficiency
- Addison disease
- Chronic fatigue syndrome
- Depression
- Dysmenorrhea
- Erectile dysfunction
- Familial hypercholesterolemia
- Infertility

6.3.2.9. Prognosis

Hypothyroidism may have a high morbidity and mortality rate if treatment is not received. Eventually, it may result in a coma or even death. If hypothyroidism is not treated in children, it can cause severe mental retardation. Heart failure is one of the main causes of death in adults. Most patients have an excellent prognosis with treatment, and the symptoms usually go away in a few weeks or months.

6.3.2.10. Complications

In an endocrine emergency, severe hypothyroidism may manifest as myxedema coma. Even in the intensive care unit (ICU), where timely diagnosis and treatment are crucial, mortality rates can still range from 25% to 60%. When there is encephalopathy, hypothermia, seizures, hyponatremia, hypoglycemia, arrhythmias, cardiogenic shock, respiratory failure, and fluid retention, myxedema crisis should be suspected.

Acute illnesses like sepsis, which may be brought on by higher metabolic demands, can also raise the risk of myxedema crisis. Other risk factors include undiagnosed hypothyroidism, treatment interruptions, and inadequate thyroid hormone dosages. In the intensive care unit, supportive care should be given for hypothermia, coexisting acute illnesses, ventilator support, fluid and electrolyte management, and vasopressors. Intravenous hydrocortisone at stress doses is the first step in thyroid replacement therapy. After clinical improvement, intravenous levothyroxine is administered and finally oral levothyroxine. Steroids are prescribed because these patients may be adrenal insufficient, and if the thyroid deficiency is corrected without treating the adrenal insufficiency, this could result in an Addisonian crisis. It is advised to screen for adrenal insufficiency but to wait for the results before beginning steroid treatment.

Improvements in cognitive function and cardiopulmonary health should follow if the treatment is successful. A concomitant improvement in laboratory abnormalities ought to be observed, encompassing an upward trend in free T4, which ought to be assessed every one to two days throughout the first treatment phase. Until there is some initial improvement, low-dose intravenous liothyronine (T3) may be considered. Since TSH can take up to 4 weeks to normalize, it might not be useful in these situations and may not reflect changes. One should think about consulting an endocrinologist.

6.3.2.11. Enhancing Healthcare Team Outcomes

Hypothyroidism impairs the functioning and general well-being of patients in all age groups by affecting various organ systems and daily activities. The primary care physician or endocrinologist is the best person to manage this disorder. Levothyroxine monotherapy is the course of treatment. A team-based, patient-centered approach is necessary for effective treatment. It is crucial to rule out nonendocrine pathologies as a possible explanation for the nonspecific symptoms when a patient's symptoms are not well controlled even after their thyroid labs have returned to normal. It is also advised to consult an endocrinologist in complex situations like preconception, pregnancy, congenital and pediatric hypothyroidism, treatment failure, problems with thyroid replacement absorption, co-occurring cardiac or other endocrine disorders, trouble interpreting thyroid test results, and drug-induced hypothyroidism. Psychiatrists, cardiologists, obstetricians, gynecologists, and intensivists are among the other professionals who might be required.

Collaborating closely with a pharmacist can be beneficial in identifying potential drug and food interactions, assessing the impact of levothyroxine formulation modifications, and exploring the reasons behind unusually high levothyroxine dosage requirements or erratic TSH levels. Particularly in the inpatient setting, such as in myxedema coma, prompt notification of abnormally high TSH levels by laboratory staff and careful observation of vital signs and mental state by nurses can promote early treatment and better outcomes. When myxedema coma results in severe, long-term hypothyroidism that causes hemodynamic instability, rapid response teams can be used effectively. Improving patient outcomes requires close interprofessional communication with all the teams involved.

6.3.3. Graves' Disease

An immune system ailment called Graves' disease causes hyperthyroidism or an excess of thyroid hormones. Hyperthyroidism can be caused by several conditions, but Graves' disease is a common one. Graves' disease can have a wide range of signs and symptoms because thyroid hormones have an impact on numerous bodily systems. Graves' disease can strike anyone, but it disproportionately affects women and those under 40. The main objectives of treatment are to lessen the severity of symptoms and decrease the quantity of thyroid hormones that the body produces.

6.3.3.1. Etiology

It is more common in patients with a positive family history, similar to all autoimmune diseases. Compared to dizygotic twins, it occurs more frequently in monozygotic twins. Environmental factors such as stress, smoking, infection, iodine exposure, postpartum, and immune reconstitution following highly active antiretroviral therapy (HAART) can trigger it.

6.3.3.2. Epidemiology

Between 60–80% of cases of hyperthyroidism are caused by Graves' disease, which is also the most common cause of hyperthyroidism. In the United States, hyperthyroidism affects 1.2%of the population overall, with an incidence ranging from 20 to 50 per 100,000. Most people with it are between the ages of 20 and 50. Females are more likely than males to have Graves' disease. According to certain data, the lifetime risk for men and women is 0.5%and 3%, respectively. The Nurses' Health Study II (NHSII) data showed that among women aged 25 to 42, the 12-year incidence reached 4.6/1,000.

6.3.3.3. Pathophysiology

Graves' disease is a condition that is triggered by thyroid stimulating immunoglobulin (TSI), also known as thyroid stimulating antibody (TSAb). B lymphocytes are the main producers of TSI within the thyroid cells, although it can also be produced in lymph nodes and bone marrow. T lymphocytes stimulate the B lymphocytes after being sensitized by an antigen in the thyroid gland. Thyroid stimulating immunoglobulin binds to the thyroid-stimulating hormone (TSH) receptor on the thyroid cell membrane, leading to the stimulation of thyroid-stimulating hormone activity. This stimulation results in increased synthesis of thyroid hormones and growth of the thyroid gland, causing hyperthyroidism and enlarged thyroid (thyromegaly). Various environmental factors, such as pregnancy (especially after giving birth), excess iodine intake, infections, stress, smoking, and interferon alfa, can trigger immune responses in susceptible genes, ultimately leading to the development of Graves' disease.

Thyroid stimulating antibodies and cytokines secreted by cytotoxic T lymphocytes (killer cells) cause inflammation, cellular proliferation, and increased growth of extraocular muscles, retro-orbital connective, and adipose tissues, which in turn causes Graves' orbitopathy (ophthalmopathy). These cytokines and thyroid-stimulating antibodies cause the synthesis of excess hydrophilic glycosaminoglycans (GAG) and retro-orbital fat growth by activating preadipocytes and periorbital fibroblasts. Glycosaminoglycans trap water, which results in muscle swelling. Proptosis, diplopia, congestion, and periorbital edema result from these modifications. It ultimately results in irreversible muscle fibrosis if untreated.

Although the pathophysiology of other uncommon Graves' disease manifestations, such as pretibial myxedema and thyroid acropachy, is unclear, it is thought to be caused by fibroblasts being stimulated by cytokines. Increased sensitivity to catecholamines is thought to be linked to several hyperthyroidism symptoms, including tachycardia, sweating, tremors, lid lag, and stare.

6.3.3.4. History and Physical

The majority of Graves' disease patients exhibit the typical hyperthyroidism signs and symptoms at first. It is uncommon for Graves' disease to initially manifest as just Graves orbitopathy or pretibial myxedema. The severity, duration, and age of hyperthyroidism all affect presentation. Elderly people may exhibit non-specific signs and symptoms such as fatigue, weight loss, and new-onset atrial fibrillation, or their symptoms may be mild or masked. Another name for the atypical presentation of elderly hyperthyroidism is apathetic thyrotoxicosis.

Heat intolerance, sweating, exhaustion, weight loss, palpitations, hyperdefecation, and tremors are typical presentations in younger patients. Additional symptoms include loss of libido, hyperkinesia, anxiety, insomnia, dyspnea, muscle weakness, pruritus, polyuria, oligomenorrhea or amenorrhea in females, and fullness in the neck. Ocular pain, conjunctival redness, swelling of the lids, and double vision are examples of eye symptoms. Those under 60 years old have a higher prevalence of palpable goiter. 10% or more of patients may gain weight. Tachycardia, systolic hypertension with elevated pulse pressure, atrial fibrillation, fine tremors, hyperkinesia, hyperreflexia, warm and moist skin, palmar erythema and onycholysis, hair loss, diffuse palpable goiter with thyroid bruit, and altered mental status are among the physical signs of hyperthyroidism (Figure 6.8).

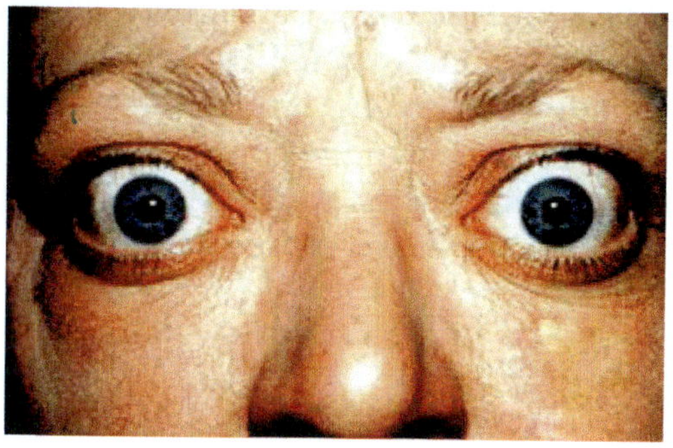

Figure 6.8. *The classic finding of exophthalmos and lid retraction in Graves' disease.*

Source: By Jonathan Trobe, M.D. – University of Michigan Kellogg Eye Center – The Eyes Have It, CC BY 3.0, https://commons.wikimedia.org/w/index.php?curid=16115992.

Ophthalmopathies such as chemosis, scleral injection, exposure keratitis, proptosis, periorbital edema, and eyelid retraction are indicators of Graves' disease extrathyroidal manifestations. Although rare—occurring in only 2–3% of cases—thyroid dermopathy results in noticeable skin thickening, mostly over the tibia.

The thicker, harder-to-pinch skin has an orange complexion. Subperiosteal bone formation and metacarpal bone swelling, also referred to as osteopathy or thyroid acropachy, are examples of bone involvement. Rare are clubbing and onycholysis (Plummer nails).

6.3.3.5. Evaluation

The first step in diagnosing Graves' disease is a complete medical history and physical examination. A family history of Graves' illness should be mentioned in the history.

6.3.3.5.1. Thyroid Function Tests to Diagnose Hyperthyroidism

Thyroid-stimulating hormone (TSH) testing is the first step in diagnosing hyperthyroidism. One must order Free T4 (FT4) and Free T3 (FT3) if TSH is suppressed. It is possible to order total T4 (thyroxine) and total T3 (triiodothyronine) if free hormone assays are not available. A lowered TSH combined with either a high FT4 or FT3 or both will validate the hyperthyroidism diagnosis. Only TSH is suppressed in subclinical hyperthyroidism; FT4 and FT3 are normal.

6.3.3.5.2. Tests to Differentiate Graves from Other Causes of Hyperthyroidism

A thorough history and physical examination can clearly identify Grave's disease. A positive family history of Graves' disease, orbitopathy, a diffusely enlarged thyroid with or without bruit, and pretibial myxedema are among the characteristics that are suggestive of the disease. Nonetheless, the tests listed below can be requested if the diagnosis is in doubt because one or more of these characteristics are absent.

1. **Measurement of TSH receptor antibody (TRAb):** Thyroid stimulating immunoglobulin (TSI) and thyrotropin-binding inhibiting (TBI) immunoglobulin or thyrotropin-binding inhibitory immunoglobulin (TBII) are the two available assay procedures. To diagnose Graves' disease, third-generation assay measurement of TRAb has a 97%sensitivity and 99%specificity.

   The following circumstances call for TRAb measurement:

   - pregnancy-related hyperthyroidism when a thyroid uptake scan is not advised.
   - Given that these antibodies cross the placenta, pregnant women with h/o Graves' disease should be monitored for potential fetal and neonatal hyperthyroidism.
   - Patients without biochemical hyperthyroidism who may have Graves' orbitopathy.
   - Individuals with recent high iodine load for whom a thyroid uptake scan is unreliable, e.g., recent imaging studies using iodinated contrast, and recent use of amiodarone.
   - to ascertain the treatment-related prognosis for hyperthyroidism.

2. Radioactive iodine uptake scan using I-123 or I-131: In a toxic nodule, the uptake is focal and referred to as a "hot nodule," but in Graves' disease, the uptake is high and diffuse. Heterogeneous absorption characterizes toxic multinodular goiter. In factitious hyperthyroidism, subacute or silent thyroiditis, and recent iodine overload, there will be minimal radioactive iodine uptake.
3. Thyroid Doppler Ultrasonography: In most cases, the thyroid gland in people with Graves' disease is hypervascular.

4. The T3/T4 ratio (ng/mcg) or FT3/FT4 ratio (SI unit) greater than 0.3 indicates Graves' disease and can be used to distinguish Graves' disease from thyrotoxicosis caused by thyroiditis.

6.3.3.5.3. Other Tests

If a patient has orbitopathy but not hyperthyroidism, an orbit CT or MRI can be used to diagnose Graves orbitopathy. Microcytic anemia, thrombocytopenia, bilirubinemia, elevated transaminases, hypercalcemia, elevated alkaline phosphatase, and low levels of HDL and LDL cholesterol are all possible symptoms of hyperthyroidism in patients.

6.3.3.6. Treatment / Management

Graves' disease treatment is based on how the condition manifests. The goal of treatment is to reduce thyroid hormone secretion and quickly control symptoms. For symptomatic patients, especially those with a heart rate greater than 90 beats per minute, those with a history of cardiovascular disease, and elderly patients, a beta-adrenergic blocker should be initiated. Because it is convenient to take once daily and is cardioselective (beta-1 selective), atenolol 25 mg to 50 mg may be regarded as the best beta blocker. Propranolol 10 mg to 40 mg taken orally every six to eight hours is advised by some prescribers because of its potential to prevent the peripheral conversion of T4 to T3. Following that, calcium channel blockers such as verapamil and diltiazem can be used to regulate heart rate if a beta blocker is used.

There are three options to reduce thyroid hormone synthesis. These options are:

1. Antithyroid medications that prevent the production and release of thyroid hormone.
2. Treatment of the thyroid gland with radioactive iodine (RAI).
3. Total or subtotal thyroidectomy.

There are advantages and disadvantages to each of the three options, and it is unclear which is the best. Making a customized decision after thoroughly going over all three options with the patients is crucial.

6.3.3.6.1. Anti-Thyroid Drugs (Thionamides)

The anti-thyroid medications methimazole (MMI) and propylthiouracil (PTU) are marketed in the United States. Carbamazole, a methimazole derivative that is quickly converted to methimazole, is also obtainable outside of the United States. These thioamides prevent the thyroid gland's thyroglobulin from being iodinated by Thyroid Peroxidase (TPO), which prevents the thyroid gland from producing T4 and T3. Propylthiouracil also partially inhibits the peripheral conversion of T4 to T3.

Methimazole is the recommended medication for non-pregnant patients because of its once-daily dosage, decreased frequency of adverse effects (particularly hepatotoxicity), and quicker return of normal thyroid function. Propylthiouracil is required during the first trimester of pregnancy because its side effects are less likely to be teratogenic. Methimazole can be started during the second trimester of pregnancy. Propylthiouracil is advised by the American Thyroid Association (ATA) for individuals with thyroid storm and for those who refuse surgery or radioactive iodine (RAIA) but have mild reactions to methimazole therapy.

Patients should be made aware of the potential side effects of thionamide therapy, such as hepatotoxicity, allergic reactions, and neutropenia, prior to beginning treatment. It is recommended to obtain a liver function test and a complete blood count with differentials. If the absolute neutrophil count (ANC) is less than 1000/ml or the baseline transaminase level is greater than five times the upper limit of normal, thionamide should not be started.

- **Methimazole Dosage:** If FT4 is one to one and a half times the upper limit of normal (ULN), start with 5 mg to 10 mg oral daily; if FT4 is one and a half to two times ULN, start with 10 mg to 20 mg oral daily; if FT4 is more than two to three times ULN, start with 30 mg to 40 mg oral daily. PTU should be started at 50 mg to 150 mg orally three times per day, depending on the severity of hyperthyroidism. The dose of thioamide can be reduced and maintained at maintenance levels once TFTs reach euthyroid status, provided that thyroid function improves. Usually, propylthiouracil is maintained at 50 mg twice or three times per day, and methimazole is kept at 5 to 10 mg daily. Adverse effects: Prickly and rash (3–6%), hepatocellular injury (2–7% propylthiouracil, 0% methimazole), agranulocytosis (0–7%, ANC < 500/ml), and vasculitis (occasionally lupus and pANCA-positive small vessel vasculitis; more with propylthiouracil than methimazole) are among the severe side effects. With methimazole therapy, hypoglycemia has sporadically been reported.
- **Follow-Up and Monitoring:** For the purpose of adjusting the thionamide dosage, check thyroid function tests (TFTs) every four to six weeks. We can lower the thionamide dosage by 30 to 50%after TFTs get better, up until a maintenance dose is reached. TFTs can be checked every three months for up to 18 months after starting a maintenance dose; after that, every six months is acceptable. Keep an eye out for side effects and run blood tests when necessary, depending on clinical data. If transaminase is more than three times the upper limit of normal, stop taking the thionamide. It is not required to regularly check the results of complete blood counts and liver function tests. For minor cutaneous reactions, thionamides can be continued with or without concurrent antihistamine use; however, if the issue continues, other options for treatment, such as surgery or RAI therapy, should be taken into consideration.
- **Treatment Duration:** If TSH and TRAb levels return to normal during follow-up, we may be able to discontinue long-term thionamide therapy for patients receiving maintenance doses after 12 to 8 months. We can repeat TFTs every two to three months for the first six months following treatment cessation, then every four to six months for an additional 6 months, and finally every 6 to 12 months if patients continue to be clinically and biochemically euthyroid. It is sufficient to monitor TSH annually if it stays normal for a year without treatment.

6.3.3.6.2. RAI Therapy

Patients who are over the age of 21, are not expecting to become pregnant within the next 6 to 12 months after treatment, have dangerous comorbid conditions that make surgery risky, or are not prescribed thioamides should all use this treatment option. It should not be administered to patients with moderate to severe Graves orbitopathy, those who cannot follow radiation safety guidelines, those who are pregnant, nursing, or who have coexisting thyroid cancer.

Preparation: Patients with a high risk of complications from hyperthyroidism and those with very high thyroid hormone levels should be considered for beta-adrenergic blockade and pretreatment with methimazole (propylthiouracil pretreatment has a high failure rate for RAI treatment). Three to five days prior to receiving RAI treatment, methimazole should be stopped if it has been started. For high-risk patients, it can be resumed three to seven days following therapy. RAI treatment must be preceded by a pregnancy test.

Dosage: I-131 is taken by mouth as a liquid or capsule. One can use a fixed dose or calculate the I-131 dose. The calculated dosage takes into account local factors, RAI uptake, and thyroid volume. I-131 at a fixed dose of 10–25 mCi is possible. Following radiation therapy, the patient should receive written radiation safety instructions to prevent radiation exposure to family members, neighbors, and pregnant women in particular.

Follow-up and monitoring: For six months, or until the patient develops hypothyroidism, TFTs should be checked every four to six weeks. The patient can have TFTs every 6 to 12 months once they are on a stable levothyroxine dose. After six months of RAI therapy, hyperthyroidism may still exist, indicating a potential need for additional RAI treatment. This can be regarded as treatment failure.

6.3.3.6.3. Thyroidectomy

Patients with a very large goiter (greater than 80 grams), compressive symptoms in the anterior neck, large thyroid nodules (greater than 4 cm), cold nodules, co-existing parathyroid adenoma, very high TRAb, and moderate to severe Graves orbitopathy are recommended to have a thyroidectomy.

Preparation:

- To reach a near- or fully euthyroid state prior to surgery, use thionamides.
- Use Beta-blockers as needed.
- To reduce vascularity, use potassium iodide, one to two drops of SSKI, or five to seven drops of Lugol's solution mixed in water or juice three times a day, beginning 7 to 10 days prior to surgery.
- Check your levels of calcium and vitamin D and replenish as necessary.
- Post-Op Follow-Up:

After surgery, beta-blockers should be weaned off and thionamides should be discontinued. Starting at 1.6 micrograms per kilogram of body weight, levothyroxine is dosed every six to eight weeks depending on TSH levels.

6.3.3.6.4. Other Adjunct Treatment for Graves Hyperthyroidism

Sodium ipodate, iopanoic acid, and iodinated contrast agents prevent peripheral T4 conversion to T3. Since they can result in resistant hyperthyroidism, they are used in conjunction with methimazole rather than alone. The United States does not have access to them. For mild hyperthyroidism, iodide (SSKI drops) can be used, particularly following RAI treatment. Other agents that have been tried include carnitine, cholestyramine, lithium, and glucocorticoids. Rituximab is expensive, but it can cause remission in Graves' disease patients.

6.3.3.6.5. Treatment of Graves Orbitopathy (GO)

Patients with Graves orbitopathy should aim for rapid attainment of euthyroid level. If a patient smokes, they ought to be counseled to stop. The degree of orbitopathy determines the course of treatment. For patients with mild orbitopathy who undergo RAI treatment, prednisone 0.4 mg/kg/day to 0.5 mg/kg/day should be started one to three days after treatment and continued for one month. Over a two-month period, it should be gradually reduced. Artificial tears should be used to treat mildly active Graves orbitopathy, and glucocorticoid therapy may also be an option. When you sleep, elevate your head to relieve orbital congestion. Treatment with selenium may not be beneficial. All cases of Graves orbitopathy should be referred to ophthalmology as soon as possible.

Treatment for moderate to severe active Graves orbitopathy involves intravenous (IV) methylprednisolone 500 mg/wk for six weeks, followed by 250 mg/wk for six weeks, or up to 100 mg of oral prednisone daily for one to two weeks, then tapered over 6 to 12 weeks. The FDA has approved the use of tepretumumab for the treatment of moderate to severe active graves orbitopathy if glucocorticoids are ineffective. Orbital irradiation, rituximab, and emergency orbital decompression are further options. Depending on the severity, treatment for inactive Graves orbitopathy includes eyelid repair, elective orbital decompression, strabismus correction, and interval close clinical monitoring.

6.3.3.6.6. Treatment of Dermopathy and Acropachy

Treatment for gravis dermopathy is typically not necessary. Topical high potency glucocorticoids combined with occlusive dressings may be considered as a form of treatment. Treating B-cells with rituximab may be helpful, but it is still in the experimental stage. Acropachy does not currently have a treatment option.

6.3.3.7. Differential Diagnosis

- Exogenous thyroid hormone
- Hashimoto thyroiditis
- Hyperemesis gravidarum
- Papillary Thyroid carcinoma
- Pheochromocytoma
- Pituitary resistance to thyroid hormone
- Postpartum thyroiditis
- Radiation-induced thyroiditis
- Silent thyroiditis
- Struma ovarii
- Subacute thyroiditis
- Thyrotropin producing pituitary adenomas
- Toxic multinodular goiter

Complications

- Thionamide-related agranulocytosis.
- Exacerbation of hyperthyroidism

Enhancing Healthcare Team Outcomes

Since Graves' disease affects many organs and presents in a variety of ways, an interprofessional team is best suited to manage this complex disorder. Graves' disease has a well-documented natural history, and all patients eventually develop hypothyroidism and need hormone replacement treatment. In a similar vein, the disorder's ocular symptoms eventually go dormant. Following ablation, some patients may experience a recurrence of hyperthyroidism, necessitating additional radioactive iodine therapy. Relapses are common because antithyroid medications only manage the disease's symptoms rather than curing it. Radioactive iodine is the most effective treatment for the condition. Every patient should receive education regarding the warning signs and symptoms of both hyper- and hypothyroidism, as well as the adverse effects of any medications. More importantly, during treatment, the patient needs to be strongly advised not to take any over-the-counter drugs that contain ephedrine or pseudoephedrine.

6.4. Malignant Disorders of Thyroid

Thyroid cancer accounts for two to three new cases per 100,000 annually. In females compared to males, it is two to four times more common. There is also a genetic component to their development.

6.4.1. Papillary Thyroid Carcinoma

Roughly 80% of thyroid cancer cases are of the most common type, called papillary thyroid cancer. With over 20,000 new cases annually, it is one of the cancer types with the fastest rate of growth. It is actually the most common cancer in women under 25 and the eighth most common cancer among women overall. Papillary thyroid cancer can strike anyone at any age, but most cases occur before the patient turns 40. Radiation exposure and a family history of thyroid cancer are risk factors for papillary thyroid cancer, but it is crucial to remember that most patients have no risk factors at all. Thankfully, papillary thyroid cancer has the best prognosis of any thyroid cancer type, and most patients can be cured with proper and timely treatment. At the time of diagnosis, up to 20% of patients will have lymph nodes that are involved. However, in thyroid cancer, involved lymph nodes typically have almost no effect on survival, unlike other cancers where involved lymph nodes mean a very poor prognosis. The likelihood of recurrence may rise in lymph nodes that are involved (i.e., cancer returning), but they have no effect on the prognosis. The majority of people who have papillary thyroid cancer will not pass away from it.

6.4.1.1. Signs and Symptoms

The majority of papillary thyroid cancers are asymptomatic i.e., they exhibit no symptoms. Many patients won't even be aware of their presence. Large nodule patients may feel a palpable mass (i.e., a tangible mass) or an apparent mass (i.e., a mass visible to them). Excessive nodules may result in compressive symptoms, such as pressure or shortness of breath when lying flat, difficulty swallowing, and food or pills getting stuck in the throat. When an advanced cancer is spreading (i.e., patients may experience difficulty swallowing or hoarseness as a result of the invaders' invasion of nearby structures. Large neck lymph nodes that are firm, non-tender, growing, and/or do not shrink with time are all indicative of cancer. Individuals should get medical attention as soon as possible if they have compressive symptoms, enlarged lymph nodes, hoarseness, or a nodule that is growing quickly.

6.4.1.2. Diagnosis

A thorough medical history and physical examination should be carried out upon the discovery of a thyroid nodule. The doctor is specifically searching for the following cancer risk factors: age under 20, age over 70, male gender, radiation exposure to the head, neck, and/or chest in the past, extremely hard nodules, enlarged lymph nodes, and/or hoarseness. A TSH level should be taken following the history and physical examination to determine whether the patient is euthyroid (i.e., thyroid function that is normal), hyperthyroid (i.e., The thyroid may be hyperactive (overactive) or hypothyroid (i.e., hypoactive thyroid). Patients with hyperthyroidism rarely develop cancer, whereas hypothyroid patients may experience a marginally elevated cancer risk. The majority of thyroid cancer patients are euthyroid.

An ultrasound (USG) of the neck is the next test in the work-up for thyroid cancer. A USG is not associated with any radiation. The greatest test for examining the thyroid is a USG, which gives the physician detailed information about the nodule(s), including its size, number, presence of calcifications (calcium deposits), and echotexture (i.e., the USG image's brightness and darkness), borders, form, and whether the object is solid or cystic (i.e., liquid-filled. The general USG findings that raise the possibility of thyroid cancer are microcalcifications (i.e., microcalcifications), nodules that are hypoechoic, hypervascularity (i.e., increased suspicious lymph nodes, erratic borders, and more blood vessels than usual.

A fine-needle aspiration biopsy (FNAB) is the most effective method of determining whether a thyroid nodule is cancerous or benign. In this test, the nodule is felt with the fingers or by USG, and a tiny needle (similar to the ones used for blood draws) is inserted into it. The nodule's cells are extracted and placed into the needle (i.e., aspirated) and examined under a microscope by a medical professional with specialized training known as a cytologist. Nodules larger than 1 cm should generally be biopsied, though there are several guidelines regarding which nodules should be biopsied. Nodules larger than 0.5 cm on a USG should be biopsied if the patient has thyroid cancer risk factors (such as radiation therapy exposure or a family history of thyroid cancer).

The FNAB may produce one of four outcomes:

- **Non-Diagnostic:** This indicates that insufficient cells were extracted to enable a diagnosis. This occurs in 5–10% of FNAB cases, even in the best of hands. The FNAB will usually be conducted again. A second biopsy will often be taken if the nodule grows. In some circumstances, a patient may receive a diagnosis immediately after surgery, particularly if there is a high risk of cancer or if the patient has previously experienced two or more non-diagnostic FNAB.
- **Benign:** This indicates that the nodule has a 97% chance of not being cancerous. Patients who have had a benign biopsy are typically monitored with a USG and physical examination six months later, as well as at other regularly scheduled times. Even if a benign nodule is not causing symptoms, it may still require surgery if it is large or unsightly.
- **Malignant:** This indicates a 97% probability that the nodule is cancer, most commonly papillary thyroid cancer. The FNAB may, in a far less frequent instance, reveal medullary or anaplastic thyroid cancer. The nodule may occasionally be reported by the cytologist as suspicious for thyroid cancer, indicating an 80–90% probability of cancer, most often papillary thyroid cancer. Most cancer patients who have a FNAB will undergo a total thyroidectomy (i.e., Thyroidectomy (complete or partial), with or without lymph node excision.
- **Indeterminate:** This category comprises a variety of readings, such as atypical cells or atypical lesions, Hurthle cell lesion, Hurthle cell neoplasm, and follicular lesion. It is therefore unclear to the cytologist whether the nodule is cancerous, even though the cells

do not appear normal. With an indeterminate biopsy, there is a 15–20% chance of thyroid cancer. In other words, 1 in 5 patients who have an indeterminate biopsy will have cancer. The only way to make a clear diagnosis of cancer or no cancer is to remove half or all of the thyroid and see if the cells in the nodule are invading (i.e., growing) outside of the nodule into the surrounding thyroid or outside of the thyroid.

6.4.1.3. Treatment

The three primary components of papillary thyroid cancer treatment are as follows.

6.4.1.3.1. Surgery

Almost always, a total thyroidectomy is the best course of treatment for papillary thyroid cancer (i.e., thyroid extraction in its entirety). In certain extremely rare circumstances, some physicians will only remove the cancerous half of the thyroid (i.e., thyroid lobectomy), although the majority of medical professionals advise a full thyroidectomy due to:

- Mostly, multifocal papillary thyroid cancers (i.e.in multiple thyroid locations).
- If there is no normal thyroid tissue left to absorb the radiation, post-operative RAI ablation therapy is more effective.
- Monitoring for relapse (i.e., cancer recurrence) using the thyroglobulin blood test is more precise. Proteins produced by thyroid cells—both healthy and malignant—include thyroglobulin. Thyroglobulin should be almost zero in the absence of any normal thyroid tissue; if it increases, it is most likely a sign of recurrent cancer. In cases where only half of the normal thyroid gland remains, interpreting the levels becomes more challenging. An increase in the level could indicate the return of the cancer or the growth of the normal thyroid lobe.
- The rate of recurrence (i.e., compared to lobectomies, patients who have undergone a total thyroidectomy have a decreased risk of cancer recurrence.

At the Thyroid Center, generally remove the thyroid gland entirely to stop cancer from coming back or spreading to the other side, but the patient ultimately decides how much surgery is necessary. Prior to the operation, a lymph node mapping (i.e., a USG exam of the central and lateral compartments of the neck) should be done to see if there are suspicious lymph nodes that may need to be removed along with the thyroid. The most common location to have involved lymph nodes is in the central neck compartment (i.e., the lymph nodes surrounding the thyroid). If there are suspicious looking nodes on lymph node mapping or on inspection in the operating room, a therapeutic central neck dissection (i.e., removal of the central neck lymph nodes) should be performed. In an operation known as a prophylactic central neck dissection, some surgeons recommend removing all of the central neck lymph nodes, regardless of whether they appear suspicious or not, in an effort to reduce the recurrence rate.

Nonetheless, the majority of surgeons think that a central neck dissection ought to be reserved for the following reasons:

1. There is virtually no change in the recurrence rate.
2. Prophylactic central neck dissections

have a much higher rate of complications than therapeutic central neck dissections.

6.4.2. Follicular Carcinoma

About 10 to 15% of thyroid cancers are follicular thyroid cancers, which are the second most common type of thyroid cancer. Similar to papillary thyroid cancer, follicular carcinoma (also known as follicular thyroid cancer) is referred to as a "well differentiated" thyroid cancer; however, it is usually a little more aggressive and malignant than papillary cancer. Compared to papillary thyroid cancer, follicular thyroid cancer is more common in older adults and less common in younger ones. Follicle thyroid cancer is less common than papillary thyroid cancer and is primarily caused by radiation exposure. The degree of vascular invasion is a common factor in determining death from follicular thyroid cancer (discussed below). Age plays a significant role in the prognosis. When it comes to follicular cancer, patients over 55 typically have a more aggressive disease course and their tumors usually do not concentrate iodine as well as those of younger patients. Follicle thyroid cancer frequently exhibits vascular invasion, which makes distant metastasis more frequent than in papillary thyroid cancer. Even in cases where the thyroid cancer is small, distant spread is possible. The bladder, skin, liver, brain, lung, and bone are possible distant spread sites. Compared to papillary thyroid cancer, lymph node involvement is much less common (approximately 8–10%) in cases of follicular thyroid cancer.

6.4.2.1. Characteristics of Follicular Thyroid Cancer

- Peak onset ages 40 through 60
- There are three times as many females as males.
- The prognosis is directly correlated with the size of the tumor (less than 1.0 cm, or 3/8 inch, is good).
- Rarely associated with radiation exposure
- Spread to lymph nodes is uncommon (~12%)
- There is often invasion of the thyroid gland's vascular structures (arteries and veins).
- In contrast to papillary cancer, distant spread (to the lungs or bones) is more frequent but less common.
- The overall cure rate is high (almost 95% for small lesions in younger patients), but it declines with age.

6.4.2.2. Management of Follicular Thyroid Cancer

When it comes to treating well-differentiated thyroid carcinomas (follicular and papillary), there is a great deal of disagreement. Certain experts argue that if the tumors are small and do not invade other tissues, as is typically the case, then the tumor-containing half of the thyroid, or the thyroid lobe, can be removed with the same degree of success as the thyroid as a whole. Advocates of conservative surgical therapy point out that although small amounts of tumor cells are present in up to 88%of the thyroid tissues in the opposite lobe, the clinical tumor recurrence rate is only 5–20%. Additionally, they cite studies that demonstrate patients undergoing total thyroidectomy—a procedure that involves surgery on both sides of the neck—have a higher risk of hypoparathyroidism and recurrent laryngeal nerve injury. Proponents of total thyroidectomy, or more aggressive surgery, point to a number of large studies that demonstrate that the incidence of permanent hypoparathyroidism and recurrent nerve injury is relatively low (approximately 1%) in skilled hands. More importantly, these studies demonstrate that when tumors are larger than 1.0 cm, patients who undergo total thyroidectomy followed by radioiodine therapy and thyroid suppression have a significantly lower recurrence rate and lower mortality. It is important to keep in mind that minimizing the quantity of normal gland tissue that is radioiodine-absorbing is also an advantageous goal.

It is important to remember that the frozen section method, which involves quickly examining the tumor under a microscope to check for signs of cancer, might not be accurate in providing a firm diagnosis of follicular cancer at the time of surgery. Put differently, without specific biopsy sample preparation, it is challenging for the pathologist to promptly and accurately diagnose follicular thyroid cancer. Other forms of thyroid cancer do not present with this issue. The following is a typical treatment plan based on these studies, as well as the natural history and epidemiology of follicular carcinoma mentioned above: hemi-thyroidectomy (removal of one half of the thyroid) may be used to treat follicular carcinomas that are well-circumscribed, isolated, minimally invasive, and less than 1 cm in young patients (< 40). Complete thyroidectomy and excision of any enlarged lymph nodes in the lateral or central neck regions should likely be the course of treatment for everyone else.

6.4.2.3. The Use of Radioactive Iodine Post-Operatively

The cellular mechanism that allows thyroid cells to absorb iodine makes them special. Thyroid cells use the iodine to produce thyroid hormone. Iodine is rarely absorbed or concentrated by other body cells. This fact allows doctors to treat patients with thyroid cancer with radioactive iodine. Radioactive iodine comes in a variety of forms, one of which is harmful to cells. Since follicular cancer cells absorb iodine, it is possible to target them with a toxic isotope (I-131) to kill them. Again, not every patient with papillary thyroid cancer requires this treatment, but older patients, those with larger tumors, those that have spread to lymph nodes or other regions, and tumors that appear aggressive under the microscope may all benefit from it. This is highly customized, and neither this page nor any other on this website is meant to offer advice. There are far too many variables at play. However, there are very few to no possible side effects from this kind of targeted therapy, including no weight loss, nausea, or hair loss.

High TSH levels increase the uptake of radioactive iodine; therefore, patients should refrain from thyroid hormone replacement and follow a low-iodine diet for at least two weeks before starting therapy. It is typically administered six weeks after surgery, though this can vary. If necessary, it can be repeated every 12 months (within certain dose limits). Every patient with follicular thyroid cancer has ongoing disease and hormone monitoring. A yearly blood thyroglobulin level test and high-resolution neck ultrasound surveillance should be provided to patients. Serum thyroglobulin is quite helpful in the follow-up of well-differentiated carcinoma (if a total thyroidectomy has been performed), but it is generally not useful as a screen for the initial diagnosis of thyroid cancer. A high level of serum thyroglobulin, which was previously low after a total thyroidectomy, is almost definitely a sign of recurrence, especially if it increases gradually with stimulation of TSH. Even if an iodine scan is negative, a value higher than 10 ng/ml is frequently linked to a structural (identifiable) recurrence. Diagnostic imaging should be conducted in response to elevated thyroglobulin levels in order to identify any potential local, regional (lymph node), or distant site structural abnormalities. Low levels of unstimulated thyroglobulin in the range of 1–3 pg/ml might not be linked to any discernible structural disease.

6.4.3. Hurthle Cell Carcinoma

Thyroid gland cancer is an uncommon type of cancer known as hurthle cell cancer. The thyroid is a gland at the base of the neck that resembles a butterfly. Hormones secreted by it are vital for controlling the body's metabolism. Hurthle cell carcinoma is also referred to as oxyphilic cell carcinoma. Thyroid cancers come in a variety of forms, this one included. Compared to other thyroid cancer forms, this one may be more aggressive in its nature. The most typical course of treatment involves thyroid gland removal via surgery.

6.4.3.1. Symptoms

Hurthle cell cancer is not always symptomatic; occasionally, it is discovered during a physical examination or imaging test that is being performed for another purpose.

When they manifest, these are possible signs and symptoms to look out for:

- A lump in the neck, just below the Adam's apple
- Pain in the neck or throat
- Hoarseness or other changes in your voice
- Shortness of breath
- Swallowing difficulty

It is not a given that these symptoms and indicators indicate Hurthle cell cancer. These might be signs of other illnesses, like goiter, or an enlargement of the thyroid gland as well as thyroid inflammation.

6.4.3.2. Causes

The cause of Hurthle cell cancer is unknown. The genesis of this cancer is due to mutations in the DNA of thyroid cells. The instructions that tell a cell what to do are encoded in its DNA. The mutations in the DNA instruct the thyroid cells to proliferate and grow rapidly. The cells acquire the capacity to survive when other cells would eventually perish. The growing cells combine to form a mass known as a tumor, which has the ability to invade, kill, and spread to other areas of the body.

6.4.3.3. Risk Factors

Some of the factors that can elevate the risk of developing thyroid cancer include:

- Being female
- Being older
- Having a background of radiation therapy to the head and neck region
- having thyroid cancer in one's family.

6.4.3.4. Complications

Possible complications of Hurthle cell cancer include:

- **Difficulties Breathing and Swallowing:** These may happen if the cancer spreads and puts pressure on the windpipe (trachea) and food tube (esophagus).
- **Cancerous Growth:** Treatment and recovery from Hurthle cell cancer can be more challenging when the disease spreads (metastasizes) to other tissues and organs.

6.4.3.5. Diagnosis

Following are some of the tests and procedures used to diagnose Hurthle cell cancer.

- **Physical Exam:** Your doctor will examine your neck, measuring the thyroid's size and determining whether or not the lymph nodes are enlarged.
- **Blood Tests:** Blood tests may identify variations in your thyroid

function, providing additional details about your health to your provider.

- **Imaging Tests:** Your doctor may use imaging tests, such as CT and ultrasound, to find out if your thyroid has a growth.
- **Examining the vocal cords (laryngoscopy):** During a laryngoscopy procedure, your doctor will use a light and a tiny mirror to look into the back of your throat in order to visually inspect your vocal cords. Alternately, your doctor might employ fiber-optic laryngoscopy. A tiny camera and light are inserted into a thin, flexible tube that is inserted through your mouth or nose and into the back of your throat. Then, while you speak, your healthcare provider can observe how your vocal cords move.

If there is a chance that the cancer cells have spread to the vocal cords, such as if you have worrying changes in your voice, this procedure may be advised.

- Removing a sample of thyroid tissue for testing (biopsy). In a thyroid biopsy, ultrasound images are used to guide the insertion of a thin needle through the neck skin. A sample of thyroid tissue is taken using a syringe that has a needle attached to it. Experts in the analysis of blood and bodily tissue, known as pathologists, examine the sample in a lab for indications of cancer.

6.4.3.6. Treatment

The standard course of treatment for Hurthle cell cancer is thyroid surgery. It might be advised to try other treatments, based on your circumstances.

6.4.3.6.1. Surgery

The most popular treatment for Hurthle cell cancer is thyroidectomy, which involves removing the thyroid completely or almost completely. In order to reduce the risk of harming the small adjacent glands (parathyroid glands), the surgeon removes all or almost all of the thyroid gland during a thyroidectomy, leaving tiny edges of thyroid tissue close by. The body's calcium levels are controlled by the parathyroid glands. If surrounding lymph nodes appear to have been affected by the cancer, they may be removed. Thyroidectomy-related risks include the following.

- Damage to the recurrent laryngeal nerve, which regulates the voice box, may result in hoarseness that is either temporary or permanent or in vocal loss.
- Parathyroid gland damage may necessitate medication to control blood calcium levels.
- Excessive bleeding

Following surgery, your doctor will prescribe levothyroxine (Synthroid, Unithroid, and other brands) to replace the hormone that the thyroid produces. This hormone is something you will always need to take.

6.4.3.6.2. Radioactive Iodine Therapy

In radioactive iodine therapy, a radioactive liquid-containing capsule is swallowed. Following surgery, radioactive iodine therapy may be suggested in order to help destroy any thyroid tissue that remains, as this tissue may contain remnants of cancer. If Hurthle cell cancer has spread to other bodily regions, radioactive iodine therapy may also be employed. Radiation therapy may have the following short-term side effects:

- Dry mouth

- Decrease in taste sensations
- Neck tenderness
- Nausea
- Fatigue

6.4.3.6.3. Radiation Therapy

High-powered energy beams, like protons or X-rays, are used in radiation therapy to destroy cancer cells. While receiving radiation therapy, you lie down on a table and a machine revolves around you, applying radiation to particular areas of your body. If Hurthle cell cancer spreads or if cancer cells are still present after surgery and radioactive iodine treatment, radiation therapy might be a possibility.

Side effects may include:

- Sore throat
- Sunburn-like skin rash
- Fatigue

6.4.3.6.4. Targeted Drug Therapy

Medication used in targeted drug treatments targets particular vulnerabilities in cancer cells. If your Hurthle cell cancer spreads to other parts of your body or comes back after receiving other treatments, targeted therapy might be an option for you.

Depending on the medication, side effects could include:

- Diarrhea
- Fatigue
- High blood pressure
- Liver problems

Research on targeted drug therapy is a current focus in cancer treatment. Physicians are researching a plethora of novel targeted therapy medications for use in thyroid cancer patients.

6.4.4. Anaplastic Carcinoma

A malignant neoplasm that arises from the unchecked proliferation of transformed cells of epithelial origin, or that exhibits some epithelial characteristics, but does not exhibit any cytological or architectural features characteristic of more differentiated tumors, such as the glandular formation or unique cellular junctions characteristic of squamous cell carcinoma and adenocarcinoma, respectively, is referred to as anaplastic carcinoma. A tumor's anaplasia can be focal or diffuse.

6.4.4.1. Signs and Symptoms

Anaplastic cancers often grow very quickly (sometimes over a few weeks), unlike most thyroid cancers which do not cause symptoms. These tumors cause compressive symptoms, such as difficulty swallowing, food or pills getting stuck in the throat, and pressure or shortness of breath when lying flat. Most often, patients report feeling a solid mass or seeing a visible mass (i.e., a mass visible to them). When an advanced cancer is spreading (i.e., patients may experience difficulty swallowing or hoarseness as a result of the invaders' invasion of nearby structures. Individuals should seek immediate medical attention if they have compressive symptoms, enlarged lymph nodes, hoarseness, and/or a rapidly expanding mass in the neck, especially if they are known to have a thyroid goiter.

6.4.4.2. Diagnosis

Anaplastic thyroid cancer screening should begin right away in patients with a history of a fast expanding neck mass, whether or not they are experiencing compressive symptoms. Anaplastic cancer-like symptoms can be present in other types of thyroid cancer, particularly medullary thyroid cancer and thyroid lymphoma. Anaplastic cancer and other causes can frequently be distinguished by a FNAB, however occasionally a core needle biopsy i.e., the required method is either a surgical biopsy or a biopsy using a big needle. It is critical to determine the disease's extent following the diagnosis of anaplastic thyroid cancer. If the tumor has spread to other parts of the body, a CT scan of the neck and chest can reveal its size as well as whether or not it is affecting the surrounding structures, such as the muscles, trachea, or esophagus. You can find out if the cancer has affected the vocal cords by having a flexible laryngoscopy, which is a procedure where a scope is put down the throat.

6.4.4.3. Treatment

Complete surgical excision is the best treatment for anaplastic thyroid cancer. Complete resection is rarely achievable, and even patients with potentially curable disease will typically have invasion into surrounding structures like the esophagus, windpipe, and large blood vessels. To further treat their disease, patients with resected anaplastic thyroid cancer will probably need to enroll in a clinical trial for radiation therapy or chemotherapy. A tiny proportion of patients diagnosed with early-stage cancer that is curable may continue to live for many years after receiving their diagnosis. Nonetheless, the majority of patients will have incurable illness (i.e., not be fully surgically removed) at the time of diagnosis. Choosing the best course of action to enhance the patient's quality of life and make their remaining days as comfortable and meaningful as possible is crucial for patients with incurable diseases.

For certain patients, palliative surgery may be appropriate (i.e., therapy aimed at enhancing quality of life but not targeting cure). For example, a tracheostomy tube (i.e., an oxygen-supplying tube inserted under the skin into the trachea) and/or a feeding tube i.e., a feeding tube inserted under the skin and into the stomach. Opting for hospice care, on the other hand, allows patients to receive all treatments with the goal of maximizing their level of comfort during their remaining days.

6.4.5. Medullary Carcinoma

Less than 2% of thyroid cancers in the US are attributed to a rare type of cancer called medullobular thyroid cancer (MTC). The parafollicular C cells of the thyroid gland, which release the hormone calcitonin, are the source of MTC. The parathyroid hormone, a protein hormone secreted by parathyroid cells, and the calcitonin hormone cooperate to control the body's calcium levels. Compared to thyroid follicular cells, which are linked to differentiated thyroid cancer, parafollicular C cells are not the same. The primary distinction is that parafollicular C cells are unable to absorb iodine, which may result in fewer treatment options for kids with medullary thyroid cancer that recurs or is persistent.

6.4.5.1. Causes of Medullary Thyroid Cancer

A mutation in a particular gene known as a RET proto-oncogene, which enables impacted cells to grow and multiply quickly and operate uncontrollably, is the cause of medullary thyroid cancer. The aberrant RET genes can be inherited from one generation to the next or they can arise spontaneously (referred to as a de novo mutation). Because the RET proto-oncogenes are inherited in an autosomal dominant pattern, there is a 50% chance that a child of a parent with a particular RET gene will also inherit that gene and develop medullary thyroid cancer.

Medullary thyroid cancer in children is frequently linked to multiple endocrine neoplasia, type 2 (MEN2), an uncommon hereditary cancer syndrome. Thyroid gland and other endocrine tissue tumors occur in people with multiple endocrine neoplasia (MEN). This can be classified as type 1 or type

2 MEN depending on the precise mutations that cause the disorder and the tissues that are impacted. Thyroid cancer in any form is not linked to MEN1. Patients who carry a MEN2 gene mutation have an almost 100% chance of developing medullary thyroid cancer. The RET protein is constantly active, which sends signals to cells encouraging them to proliferate and aid in the development of cancer. Based on the specific RET mutation and family history, an estimate can be made regarding the timing of the development of medullary thyroid cancer. Guidelines that describe the known risk as moderate, high, or highest for people with each gene mutation known to cause MTC were recently released by the American Thyroid Association.

6.4.5.2. Signs and Symptoms of MTC

Similar to differentiated thyroid cancer, medullary thyroid cancer shares symptoms with other types of thyroid cancer.

Symptoms may include:

- A visible lump (nodule)
- A lump that is felt when you swallow.
- Persistently enlarged lymph nodes or hoarseness.

Patients with MEN2 type B and medullary thyroid cancer may also have other physical characteristics. The most typical symptoms in infants are constipation and alacrima, or the inability to cry.

Symptoms in school-age children consist of:

- An elongated face (marfanoid facies)
- Mucosal neuromas are nodules that can be found on the lips, tongue, or inside the mouth's cheeks.
- Droopy or swollen-appearing eyelids or lips
- Scoliosis
- Constipation

Children of school age who experience constipation and abdominal distension should also be assessed for Hirschsprung's disease, a rare intestinal disorder that is frequently linked to MEN2 type A.

6.4.5.3. Testing and Diagnosis of MTC

Clinical experts may use a variety of diagnostic tests including:

- To find out how effectively your child's thyroid is functioning, have a blood test to measure the levels of thyroid-stimulating hormone (TSH) and calcitonin.
- To find out the size, number, shape, and location of any thyroid nodules and abnormal lymph nodes, undergo a thyroid ultrasound, also known as a thyroid scan.
- Fine-needle aspiration (FNA), which involves removing thyroid and potentially lymph node cells for microscopic examination.

6.4.5.4. Treatment for Medullary Thyroid Cancer

Radioactive iodine (RAI) therapy is an ineffective treatment for medullary thyroid cancer because it targets tumor cells that have spread outside of the thyroid gland because the cancer is thought to have originated from the parafollicular cells of the thyroid gland, which do not absorb iodine. Currently under the scanner are a number of additional chemotherapy drugs, but so far these only appear to slow tumor growth. None seem to result in a healing.

6.4.5.4.1. Surgery

A total thyroidectomy, which involves surgically removing the entire thyroid gland, is the only treatment that is effective for medullary thyroid cancer. The aim of treatment for individuals with a confirmed RET mutation is thyroid gland excision prior to the onset and metastasis of medullary thyroid cancer. Your child will spend two to three days in the hospital following surgery. This gives your child time to heal, makes sure their pain is managed, and keeps an eye out for any possible surgical side effects, like low calcium levels or damage to the RLN. The majority of patients experience a reduction in pain during the first few days following surgery, return to school in four to five days, and resume full activity in two weeks. Usually measuring 3 to 4 centimeters in length, the surgical scar is hidden in a skin fold to minimize visibility. The use of steri-strips and absorbable sutures (stitches) eliminates the need for suture removal (Figure 6.9).

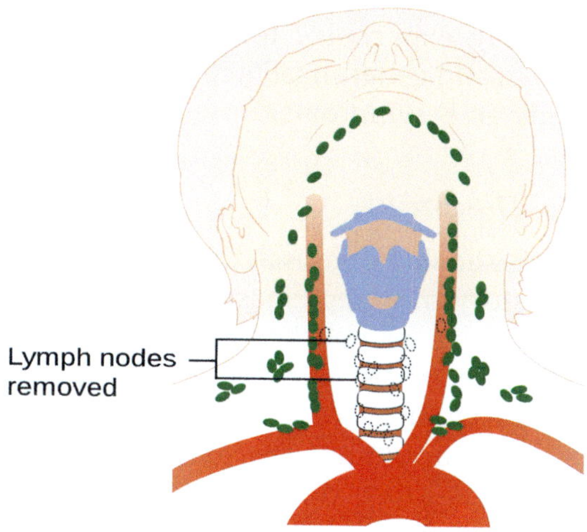

Figure 6.9. *A surgery for MTC showing the central lymph nodes and thyroid gland removed.*

Source: By Cancer Research UK – Original email from CRUK, CC BY-SA 4.0, https://commons.wikimedia.org/w/index.php?curid=34333127.

6.4.5.4.2. Hormone Replacement Therapy

Your child will no longer be able to produce thyroid hormone on their own following a thyroidectomy. To get their thyroid-stimulating hormone (TSH) and thyroxine hormone (T4) in normal ranges, your child will need to take thyroid hormone.

6.4.5.4.3. Thyroid Hormone Suppression

Higher dosages of thyroid hormone replacement therapy are prescribed for patients with thyroid cancer in an effort to bring the TSH below the normal limit and the T4 high-normal or slightly above it. This is known as suppressive therapy, and it is employed because TSH has the ability to promote the growth of both healthy and thyroid cancerous cells. Suppressive therapy reduces the likelihood that any cancer cells that remain will proliferate. Children who receive higher dosages of thyroid hormone replacements may exhibit mild hyperthyroidism symptoms, such as the following.

- Anxiousness, irritability and/or nervousness
- Poor, restless sleep
- Increased activity (fidgetiness, hyperactivity, restlessness)
- Fatigue
- A greater desire to eat whether or not one loses weight.
- Increased daily frequency of bowel movements.
- Intolerance to heat (constantly feeling warm).
- Reduced or subpar academic performance; possibly late-onset attention deficit disorder-related difficulties focusing.

6.4.5.5. Follow-up Care for MTC

The majority of kids with medullary thyroid cancer will require ongoing care well into adulthood. Your child will need physical examinations and laboratory testing every three to six months for the first few years following surgery. After some time has passed and there is no sign of a recurrence, annual follow-up exams may be necessary. A follow-up plan will be tailored by your child's medical team based on their condition and results. Many children will experience remission following surgery and hormone replacement therapy, meaning they won't have any clinical, imaging, or laboratory test evidence of medullary thyroid cancer. On the other hand, some people may experience recurrent or persistent thyroid cancer, which has the potential to spread to other organs. 6 to 12 months following the start of treatment, persistent thyroid cancer is defined as disease-related findings from imaging, laboratory testing, and/or physical examination. A patient is said to have recurrent thyroid disease if their clinical condition reappears after they have been thought to be disease-free for at least six months.

6.4.5.6. Outlook for Medullary Thyroid Cancer

There is no chance of recurrence for patients who had their thyroid gland removed prior to the development of medullary thyroid cancer. The likelihood of remission for patients treated after the development of medullary thyroid cancer varies and is primarily based on the extent of the cancer's spread. It could take years or even decades for the tumor to spread further, even in patients with widespread cancer.

6.4.6. Lymphoma

Lymphoma is a rare disease where lymphocytes, which are blood cells that defend against infection, transform into cancer cells. When this occurs in the thyroid, it is known as thyroid lymphoma. This form of cancer is uncommon, making up only 1–2% of all thyroid cancers and lymphomas outside of the lymph nodes. Typically affecting older individuals, with an average age in their late 60s, thyroid lymphoma has a favorable prognosis when diagnosed and treated correctly.

6.4.6.1. Signs and Symptoms

Thyroid lymphomas often grow very quickly (sometimes over a few weeks), in contrast to the majority of thyroid cancers that do not cause symptoms. These compressive symptoms include trouble swallowing, food or pills getting stuck in the throat, and pressure or shortness of breath when lying flat. Most often, patients report feeling a firm mass or seeing a visible mass (i.e., a mass visible to them). Patients may experience difficulty swallowing or hoarseness in certain instances. Individuals should get medical attention as soon as possible if they have compressive symptoms, enlarged lymph nodes, hoarseness, or a neck mass that is growing quickly. Similar to other types of lymphoma, patients may experience fever, night sweats, weight loss, and generalized itching throughout their body as B-symptoms.

6.4.6.2. Diagnosis

Individuals should be assessed right away if they have a history of a neck mass that is growing quickly, whether or not they have compressive symptoms. Anaplastic and advanced medullary thyroid cancers are two more types of thyroid cancer that can mimic a thyroid lymphoma in appearance. Because the two conditions have very different prognoses and treatments, it is imperative to distinguish between anaplastic thyroid cancer and thyroid lymphoma. Occasionally, a FNAB can differentiate thyroid lymphoma from other causes, but on occasion, a core needle biopsy (i.e., large-needle biopsy), and frequently a surgical biopsy is required. In order to stage a patient with thyroid lymphoma, a full body PET scan may be performed to check for lymphomas elsewhere in the body.

6.4.6.3. Treatment

The majority of thyroid lymphomas are treated with chemotherapy. Usually, after receiving a few chemotherapy doses, the thyroid lymphoma becomes smaller. Surgery is rarely required when treating thyroid lymphoma because chemotherapy works so well. While receiving chemotherapy, the lymphoma may shrink with the use of external beam radiation.

6.4.7. Metastases to Thyroid

Thyroid cancer that has spread from the thyroid gland to distant parts of the body is referred to as metastatic thyroid cancer, or stage 4 thyroid cancer. Thyroid cancer is at its most advanced stage at this point. There will probably be a lot of symptoms at this point in the disease. Actually, symptoms usually show up earlier and are often detectable prior to the thyroid cancer spreading.

6.4.7.1. Symptoms

Thyroid cancer usually manifests as a lump or nodule at the base of the neck. This lump may be visible and palpable to you, or it may be discovered by your doctor during a standard examination. Before the cancer has spread, additional signs of thyroid cancer could exist, such as:

- Changes in your voice or constant hoarseness
- Pain or soreness in the front of the neck
- A persistent cough
- Trouble swallowing
- Difficulty breathing

Other symptoms may appear when thyroid cancer spreads and metastasizes to other parts of the body. Symptoms of metastatic thyroid cancer comprise:

- Fatigue
- Nausea and vomiting
- Loss of appetite
- Unexpected weight loss

Early detection of thyroid cancer increases treatment options, improves prognosis, and enhances quality of life, similar to other forms of cancer. To get an accurate diagnosis and treatment plan, it is critical to see a doctor as soon as you notice any symptoms that could indicate thyroid cancer.

6.5. Thyroid Nodule and Its Management

Thyroid nodules are lumps, either solid or fluid-filled, that develop inside your thyroid, a small gland situated just above your breastbone at the base of your neck. The majority of thyroid nodules are asymptomatic and not dangerous. The proportion of thyroid nodules that are cancerous is quite low. Usually, a thyroid nodule is not noticeable to you until it is found by your doctor during a standard physical examination. Alternatively, your physician might find it when doing a scan for a different medical condition. On the other hand, some thyroid nodules might grow to the point of being noticeable or interfere with breathing or swallowing. The type of thyroid nodule you have will determine your treatment options.

6.5.1. Symptoms

The majority of thyroid nodules show no symptoms at all. However, on rare occasions, some nodules grow to such a size that they can:

- Be felt
- Be seen, often as a swelling at the base of your neck

- Press on your windpipe or esophagus, causing shortness of breath or difficulty swallowing

Thyroid nodules can occasionally produce more thyroxine, a hormone secreted by the thyroid gland.

The excess thyroxine may result in hyperthyroidism, which is characterized by symptoms like:

- Unexplained weight loss
- Increased sweating
- Tremor
- Nervousness
- Rapid or irregular heartbeat

Thyroid nodules rarely develop into cancer. But assessing your symptoms by themselves won't help you identify which nodules are cancerous. When your doctor finds a thyroid cancerous nodule, it may be small because most of these nodules grow slowly. Rarely, aggressive thyroid cancers can have large, firm, fixed nodules that grow quickly.

- ***When to See a Doctor:*** Even though the majority of thyroid nodules are benign and cause no issues, you should still get your neck swollen abnormally and consult your doctor if you experience any difficulty breathing or swallowing. It is critical to assess the risk of cancer. Seek medical attention if you experience any of the following hyperthyroidism signs and symptoms.
  - Unexpected loss of weight even though your appetite is unchanged or has grown.
  - A pounding heart
  - Trouble sleeping
  - Muscle weakness
  - Nervousness or irritability

See your doctor if you experience any of the following symptoms or indicators that hypothyroidism, or insufficient production of thyroid hormone by the thyroid gland, is present.

- Feeling cold
- Feeling tired more easily
- Dry skin
- Memory problems
- Depression
- Constipation

6.5.2. Causes

Thyroid gland nodules can arise from many conditions, such as:

- **Hypertrophy of Healthy Thyroid Tissue:** Thyroid adenoma is the term used to describe an overgrowth of normal thyroid tissue. Although the cause of this is unknown, it is not cancerous and is not taken seriously unless its size results in bothersome symptoms.

Hyperthyroidism is a result of certain thyroid adenomas.

- **Thyroid Cyst:** Thyroid adenomas that are degenerating are the most common cause of fluid-filled cavities in the thyroid called cysts. In thyroid cysts, solid materials are frequently combined with fluid. Cysts are typically not cancerous, but sometimes, they may contain solid cancerous elements.
- Chronic inflammation of the thyroid brought on by Hashimoto's disease can lead to enlarged nodules. This is frequently linked to hypothyroidism.
- **Multinodular Goiter:** Any

enlargement of the thyroid gland, which may result from a thyroid condition or an iodine shortage, is referred to as a goiter. A multinodular goiter has several different nodules inside of it; however, its etiology is unclear.

- **Thyroid Cancer:** There is little likelihood that a nodule is malignant. On the other hand, a large, hard nodule that hurts or causes discomfort is cause for concern. Your doctor should probably check it out for you.

A family history of thyroid or other endocrine cancers, as well as radiation exposure from medical therapy or nuclear fallout, are among the factors that raise your risk of thyroid cancer.

- **Iodine Deficiency:** Thyroid nodules can occasionally develop on your thyroid gland as a result of a diet low in iodine. In the United States, however, where iodine is frequently added to table salt and other foods, iodine deficiency is rare.

6.5.3. Complications

Some thyroid nodules can cause the following complications:

- **Problems Swallowing or Breathing:** Either a multinodular goiter or large nodules can obstruct breathing or swallowing.
- **Hyperthyroidism:** An overabundance of thyroid hormone in the body can result from a nodule or goiter producing thyroid hormone. Weight loss, muscular weakness, heat intolerance, and nervousness or irritability are all possible side effects of hyperthyroidism.

  An irregular heartbeat, weak bones, and thyrotoxic crisis—a rare but potentially fatal worsening of signs and symptoms—are possible side effects of hyperthyroidism that call for prompt medical attention.
- Problems related to thyroid nodule surgery. You might require lifetime thyroid hormone replacement therapy if your doctor advises surgery to remove a nodule.

6.5.4. Diagnosis

One of your doctor's primary objectives when evaluating a lump or nodule in your neck is to rule out cancer. However, the proper functioning of your thyroid will also be of interest to your doctor.

Tests consist of:

- **Physical Exam:** Since swallowing causes a thyroid gland nodule to move up and down, your doctor will probably ask you to swallow while doing an examination of your thyroid.

  Additionally, your doctor will be checking for hyperthyroidism symptoms and signs like tremors, hyperactive reflexes, and an irregular or fast heartbeat. Additionally, he or she will look for hypothyroidism symptoms like dry skin, swollen faces, and a slow heartbeat.
- **Thyroid Function Tests:** You can find out if you have hyperthyroidism or hypothyroidism by having tests that measure your blood levels of thyroid-stimulating hormone (TSH) and hormones produced by your thyroid gland.

- **Ultrasound**: With this imaging method, images of your thyroid gland are created using high-frequency sound waves. The most accurate way to determine the form and composition of nodules is through a thyroid ultrasound. It can be used by medical professionals to identify solid nodules from cysts or to ascertain whether there are multiple nodules. It can also serve as a guide for medical professionals when doing a fine-needle aspiration biopsy.
- **Fine-Needle Aspiration Biopsy:** To ensure there is no cancer present, nodules are frequently biopsied. Your doctor will remove a sample of cells from the nodule by inserting a very thin needle into it during the procedure.

  The procedure takes about 20 minutes, is typically performed in your doctor's office, and carries minimal risks. Your doctor will frequently use ultrasonography to help guide the needle's placement. After that, your doctor sends the samples to a lab for microscopic analysis.
- **Thyroid Scan:** To assess thyroid nodules, your doctor might advise a thyroid scan. An isotope of radioactive iodine is injected into a vein in your arm during this test. After that, you lie on a table and a computer screen displays an image of your thyroid taken by a special camera.

The reason why hot nodules, or overproducing thyroid nodules, appear on the scan is that they absorb more isotope than normal thyroid tissue does. Nearly invariably, hot nodules are not malignant. Less isotope-absorbing nodules, or "cold nodules," can occasionally be malignant. Nevertheless, it is impossible to differentiate between cancerous and non-cancerous cold nodules using a thyroid scan.

6.5.5. Treatment

The type of thyroid nodule you have will determine how it is treated.

6.5.5.1. Treating Benign Nodules

Treatment choices for a thyroid nodule that is not cancerous include:

- **Watchful Waiting:** Your doctor might advise you to monitor your thyroid nodule if a biopsy reveals that it is not cancerous.

This typically entails routine physical examinations and thyroid function testing. An ultrasound might also be a part of it. A second biopsy is probably in order if the nodule gets bigger. A benign thyroid nodule may never require treatment if it stays untreated.

- **Thyroid Hormone Therapy:** Your doctor might suggest thyroid hormone therapy if the results of your thyroid function test show that your gland is not producing enough thyroid hormone.
- **Surgery:** Surgery might occasionally be necessary for a noncancerous nodule if it is so big that it interferes with swallowing or breathing. Large multinodular goiters may also be surgically removed by doctors, especially if they are obstructing the esophagus, blood vessels, or airways. Surgery is required to remove nodules that a biopsy deems suspicious or indeterminate so that they can be inspected for indications of cancer.

6.5.5.2. Treating Nodules that Cause Hyperthyroidism

Your doctor may advise treating hyperthyroidism if a thyroid nodule is producing an excessive amount of thyroid hormones, surpassing the normal levels produced by your thyroid gland. This could consist of:

- **Radioactive Iodine:** Radioactive iodine is used by doctors to treat hyperthyroidism. Your thyroid gland absorbs radioactive iodine when it is taken as a liquid or in the form of capsules. As a result, the nodules shrink and the hyperthyroidism symptoms go away, usually in two to three months.
- **Anti-Thyroid Medications:** In certain situations, your physician might advise taking an anti-thyroid drug, like methimazole (Tapazole), to lessen hyperthyroidism symptoms. It is crucial to go over the advantages and disadvantages of the treatment with your doctor because it is typically long-term and may have major negative effects on your liver.
- **Surgery:** In case radioactive iodine treatment or antithyroid medication is not working for you, you might be a good candidate for thyroid nodule removal surgery. Your doctor will probably go over the risks of surgery with you.

6.5.5.3. Treating Cancerous Nodules

Surgery is often required to treat a cancerous nodule.

- **Observation:** Your doctor may decide to closely monitor any cancerous nodules before treating them because very small cancers have a low chance of spreading. A thyroid specialist's assistance is frequently sought when making this choice. Performing blood tests and keeping an eye on ultrasounds are examples of observation.
- **Surgery:** Surgical removal is a common treatment for cancerous nodules. Previously, a procedure known as a near-total thyroidectomy was the norm for removing the majority of thyroid tissue. However, some cancerous nodules may now benefit from a more restricted surgical procedure that involves only removing half of the thyroid. Depending on the severity of the illness, a near-total thyroidectomy may be necessary.

  The nerve that regulates your voice cords and the parathyroid glands, which are four tiny glands on the back of the thyroid that help regulate your body's calcium levels, are two of the risks associated with thyroid surgery. You will require levothyroxine therapy for the rest of your life following thyroid surgery in order to provide your body with thyroid hormone. Your thyroid specialist will assist you in figuring out how much is right to take, as managing your cancer risk may involve more than just hormone replacement.
- **Alcohol Ablation:** Alcohol ablation is an additional treatment option for some small cancerous nodules. To destroy the cancerous thyroid nodule, a tiny amount of alcohol is injected into it using this technique. Frequently, several therapy sessions are needed.

A Closer Look

Thyroidectomy

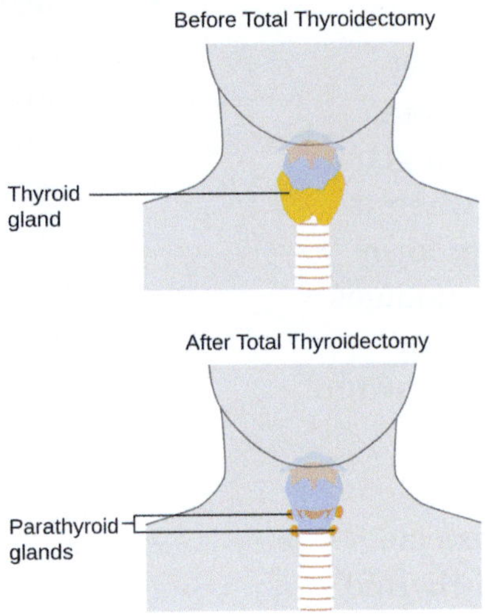

Source: By Cancer Research UK – Original email from CRUK, CC BY-SA 4.0, https://commons.wikimedia.org/w/index.php?curid=34333179.

Thyroidectomy is the surgical excision of the thyroid gland, which is situated in the front of the neck, all or in part. Thyroid hormone is released by the thyroid gland and regulates a number of vital bodily processes. Those with hyperthyroidism, a condition in which the thyroid gland produces excessive amounts of thyroid hormone, thyroid tumors, or thyroid nodules may benefit from a thyroidectomy. An autoimmune condition, an excess of iodine in the diet, a benign pituitary tumor, an overabundance of thyroid medication, a swelling (goiter) in the thyroid gland, or an inflammatory process can all lead to hyperthyroidism.

Risks of thyroidectomy:

- Voice changes, such as hoarseness
- Sore throat
- Bleeding and blood clots
- Scar tissue or adhesions that call for additional surgery.
- Injuries to the windpipe or esophagus.
- Hypoparathyroidism: An excessive amount of parathyroid hormone can cause abnormally low calcium levels in the blood.

Before the Procedure: The physician will request laboratory and imaging examinations, such as:

- Ultrasound, magnetic resonance imaging, or computed tomography (CT) for thyroid imaging (MRI).
- Blood test(s) for other factors, including thyroid hormone levels.
- The laryngoscope is a tool used for voice cord examination.

If you are susceptible to infections due to a medical condition that compromises your immune system, the surgical team may prescribe you an antibiotic before your procedure. Antiemetics, or medications to lessen nausea and vomiting, may be prescribed to you. To maintain thyroid hormone balance both during and after surgery, the doctor will prescribe medication to patients who have hyperthyroidism.

Types of Thyroidectomy

- **Traditional Thyroidectomy:** Assume a semi-seated position in the operating room, with your shoulders and neck supported, and your chin tilted back if desired. You are unconscious and pain-free during the majority of thyroidectomies because they are done under general anesthesia. To minimize the visibility of the scar, the surgeon creates a tiny incision in the neck skin as near to a natural crease as possible. The thyroid gland's lobes, as well as any surrounding lymph nodes that might be impacted by illness, are removed by the surgeon after he or she parts a thin layer of muscle to release the thyroid gland. After that, the surgeon fixes the anterior neck muscles back into place. Sutures or glue are used to close the skin.
- **Scarless (Transoral) Thyroidectomy:** A more recent method involves using the mouth to gain access to the thyroid gland. Since the outside of the neck is not incised, this surgery leaves no visible scar.
- **Thyroidectomy: Recovery and Next Steps:** While some patients stay overnight in the hospital, others go home the same day of surgery. The body will need thyroid hormone replacement in the form of pills (whether of synthetic or natural origin) to maintain the proper balance of essential functions after the thyroid gland is surgically removed.

Summary

- The largest endocrine gland is the thyroid, and thyroid disorders are common health issues, particularly in women. The main way to treat thyroid conditions such as goiter, adenoma, and carcinoma is through surgery.
- The thyroid gland is a special kind of endocrine gland that stores a lot of hormones in an inactive form in its follicles and extracellular components. The thyroid gland is surrounded by a fibrous capsule, and it is separated into lobules by a fine collagenous septum.
- The production of thyroxine (T4), calcitonin, and triiodothyronine (T3) is the thyroid's main job. The thyroid gland produces the enzymes thyroxine (T4) and triiodothyronine (T3).
- Thyroid-stimulating hormone (TSH), which is released from the anterior pituitary, controls the synthesis of thyroxine and triiodothyronine. Thyroid-stimulating hormone (TSH), which is secreted by the anterior pituitary gland, is the main hormone that controls the synthesis of thyroxine (T4) and triiodothyronine (T3).
- The thyroid needs iodine, a chemical element that occurs naturally in a variety of foods, to produce the T3 and T4 hormones. After absorbing iodine, the thyroid creates the hormones T3 and T4 via a series of chemical reactions.
- Thyroid cancer accounts for two to three new cases per 100,000 annually. In females compared to males, it is two to four times more common. There is also a genetic component to their development.
- Thyroid nodules are lumps, either solid or fluid-filled, that develop inside your thyroid, a small gland situated just above your breastbone at the base of your neck.

References

1. Agrawal, P. (2015). Congenital hypothyroidism. *Indian Journal of Endocrinology and Metabolism, 19*(2), 221–227.
2. Ajmani, S. N., Aggarwal, D., Bhatia, P., Sharma, M., Sarabhai, V., & Paul, M. (2014). Prevalence of overt and subclinical thyroid dysfunction among pregnant women and its effect on maternal and fetal outcome. *Journal of Obstetrics and Gynaecology of India, 64*(2), 105–110. https://doi.org/10.1007/s13224-013-0487-y.
3. Braverman, L. E., & Utiger, R. D. (2000). *Werner & Ingbar's the Thyroid: A Fundamental and Clinical Text* (8th ed., pp. 837-838). Lippincott Williams & Wilkins.
4. Duntas, L. H., et al. (2011). The interface between thyroid and diabetes mellitus. *Clinical Endocrinology, 75*(1), 1–9.
5. Haddow, J. E., et al. (2011). Maternal thyroid deficiency during pregnancy and subsequent neuropsychological development of the child. *New England Journal of Medicine.*
6. Hage, M., et al. (2011). Thyroid disorders and diabetes mellitus. *Journal of Thyroid Research, 2011*, Article ID 43946.
7. Jameson, J. L., & Weetman, A. P. (2008). Disorders of the thyroid gland. In A. Fauci, E. Braunwald, D. L. Kasper, S. L. Hauser, D. L. Longo, J. L. Jameson, et al. (Eds.), *Harrison's Principles of Internal Medicine* (17th ed., pp. 2224–2247). The McGraw-Hill Companies Inc.

8. Jayakumar, R. V. (2012). Guidelines for management of thyroid disorder in pregnancy. *Indian Thyroid Society*.
9. Jayakumar, R. V., et al. (2012). Thyroid disorders and dyslipidemia. *Indian Thyroid Society*.
10. Kadiyala, R., et al. (2010). Thyroid dysfunction and diabetes. *International Journal of Clinical Practice, 64*(8), 1130–1139.
11. Kochupillai, N., et al. (2000). Clinical endocrinology in India. *Current Science, 79*(8), 25.
12. Laloo, D. (2012). Thyroid dysfunction in type 2 diabetes mellitus patients: A retrospective study. *Indian Journal of Endocrinology and Metabolism, 16*(Suppl 2), S334, S335.
13. Marieb, E., & Hoehn, K. (2007). Regulation and integration of the body: The endocrine system. In *Human Anatomy and Physiology* (7th ed., pp. 620–625). Pearson Education Inc.
14. Poongothai, S., Pradeepa, R., Ganesan, A., & Mohan, V. (2009). Prevalence of depression in a large urban South Indian population—The Chennai Urban Rural Epidemiology Study (CURES–70). *PLoS ONE, 4*(9), e7185.
15. Shah, S. N., & Joshi, S. R. (2011). Indian thyroid guidelines 2011. *Supplement to Journal of the Association of Physicians of India*, *59*, 68.
16. Stagnaro-Green, A. (2011). Overt hyperthyroidism and hypothyroidism during pregnancy. *Clinical Obstetrics and Gynecology, 54*(3), 478–487.
17. Stagnaro-Green, A., et al. (2012). Approach to the patient with postpartum thyroiditis. *Journal of Clinical Endocrinology & Metabolism, 97*(2), 334–342.
18. Unnikrishnan, A. G. (2013). Prevalence of hypothyroidism in adults: An epidemiology study in 8 cities of India. *Indian Journal of Endocrinology and Metabolism, 17*(4), 647–652.

Chapter

DISEASES OF THE ESOPHAGUS

7

Contents

Introduction

A group of illnesses known as esophageal disorders impact the function of the esophagus. The portion of the digestive system that facilitates food movement from your mouth to your stomach is called the esophagus, sometimes known as the food pipe. Various illnesses that impact the esophagus can result in dysphagia, or trouble swallowing. Gastroesophageal reflux disease is the most prevalent esophageal disorder. Acid reflux, or too much stomach acid flowing back into the esophagus, can lead to inflammation and GERD (Figure 7.1).

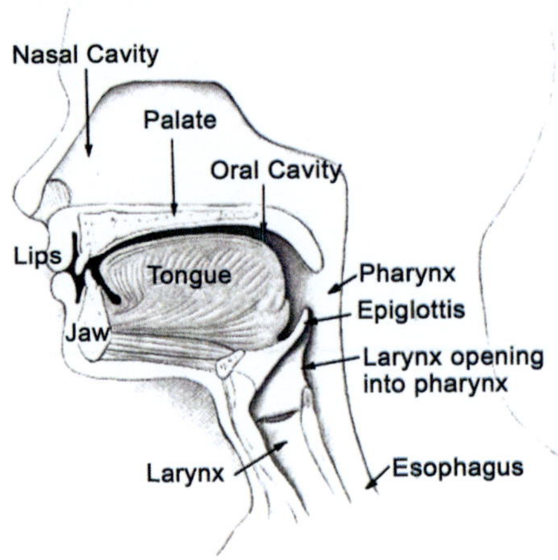

Figure 7.1. *Head and neck. The esophagus is at the bottom.*

Source: By Arcadian – http://training.seer.cancer.gov/head-neck/anatomy/overview.html, Public Domain, https://commons.wikimedia.org/w/index.php?curid=1678037.

Orientation and Directional Terms

Term	Definition	Illustration
GERD	The most common esophageal disorder occurs when the lower esophageal sphincter doesn't close properly. As a result, stomach acid and contents flow backward into your esophagus.	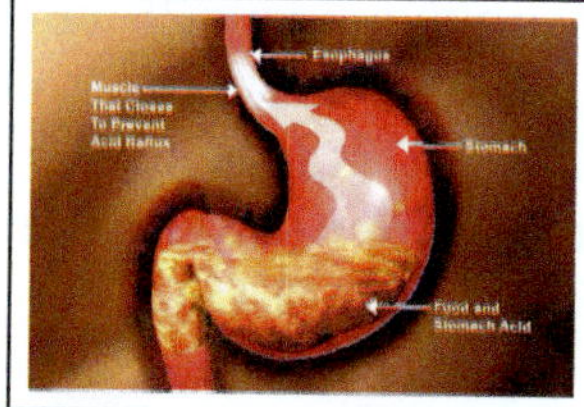
Achalasia	The lower esophageal sphincter doesn't open or relax, preventing food from going into the stomach. Experts believe achalasia may be an autoimmune disease, but the exact cause is unknown. Something damages the nerves that control the muscles in the esophagus.	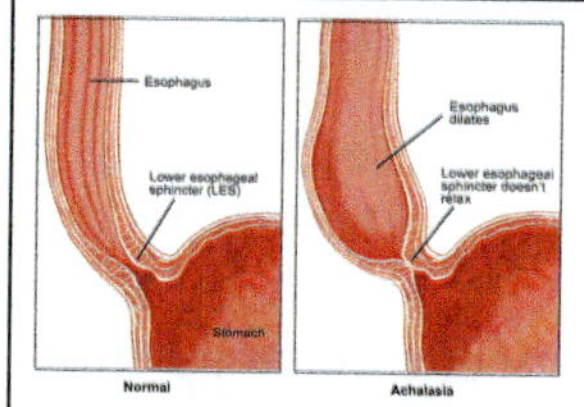
Barrett's esophagus	For people with chronic, untreated acid reflux, the lining of the bottom part of their esophagus starts looking like the stomach lining, and the cells start to resemble intestinal cells. These changes take place where the esophagus and stomach meet. This condition is associated with a higher risk of esophageal cancer.	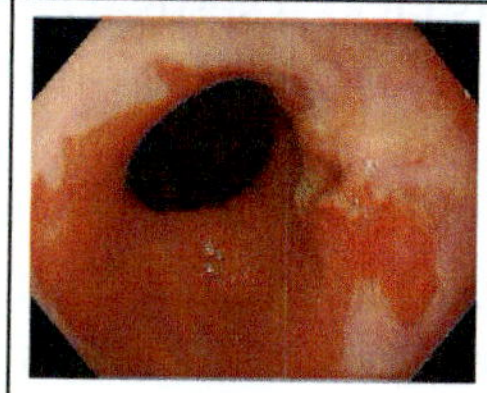
Eosinophilic esophagitis	White blood cells called eosinophils become overabundant in the esophagus. The result is inflammation or swelling of the esophageal lining (esophagitis). This condition is more common in patients with multiple allergies.	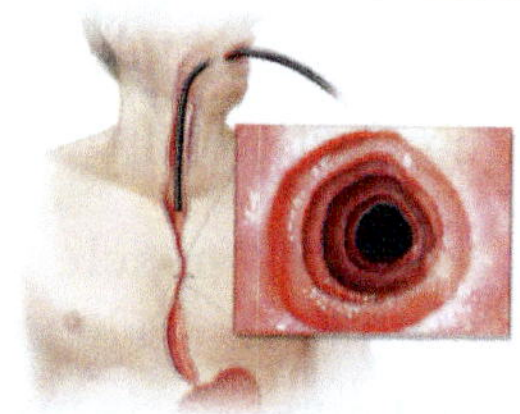
Esophageal diverticulum	An outpouching occurs in a weak spot in the esophagus. People with achalasia are more prone to developing diverticula.	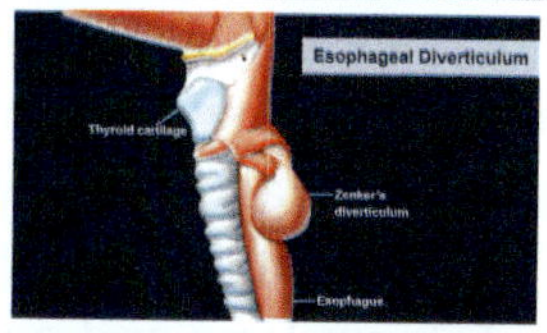
Esophageal spasms	Abnormal muscle spasms (contractions) occur in the esophagus. This rare, painful condition keeps food from reaching the stomach.	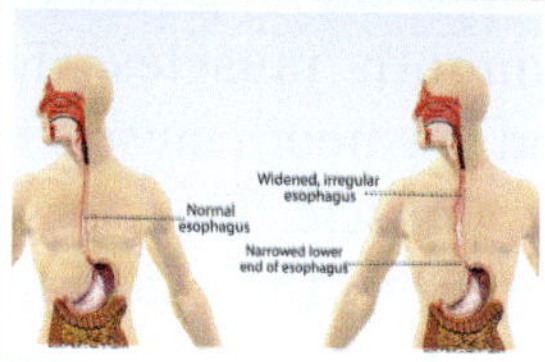
Esophageal strictures	The esophagus becomes too narrow. Foods and liquids pass through slowly to the stomach.	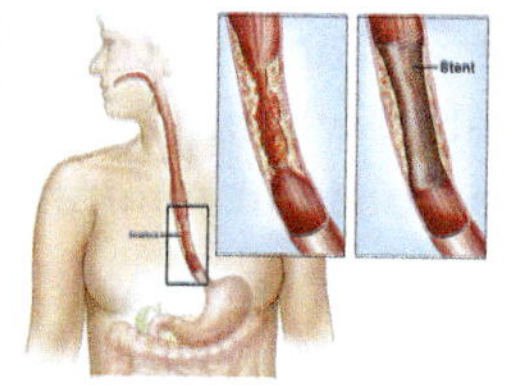

7.1. Anatomy and Physiology of the Esophagus

The esophagus is a 25 cm long fibromuscular tube that carries food from the throat to the stomach. It starts at the cricoid cartilage's inferior border (C6) and ends at the stomach's cardiac orifice (T11).

7.1.1. Anatomy

The adult esophagus is a tubular organ that measures between 18 and 26 centimeters in length. The muscularis propria, submucosa, and mucosa make up the esophageal wall. The esophagus lacks a serosal covering, in contrast to other parts of the gastrointestinal tract, and its outer wall is only slightly bound by connective tissue. The mucous membrane, lamina propria, and muscularis mucosae are the three sublayers that make up the stratified squamous epithelium that makes up the esophageal mucosa. There are glands in the esophageal submucosa, but they are not as numerous as those found in the remaining portion of the stomach.

A circular muscle layer encircled by a longitudinal muscle layer makes up the esophageal muscularis propria. The distal two-thirds of the esophagus, the thoracic esophagus, is made up of smooth muscles, while the proximal esophagus, or cervical esophagus, is made up of striated muscle. There is a segment that is 4–6 cm long and contains both striated and smooth muscles. The transition from striated to smooth muscle is gradual. This mixed zone of muscle fibers made up about 35% of the length of the esophagus. This segment is typically found at the aortic arch level. This anatomical zone is confirmed by esophageal manometry, which shows that the contraction wave's amplitude minimums in this area.

At the T4 vertebral level, the esophagus runs posterior to the right of the aortic arch. The diaphragmatic hiatus and the level of T8 are where the esophagus lies anterior to the aorta. Subsequently, the esophagus passes through a diaphragmatic aperture anterior to the descending aortic aperture. The esophagus is attached to the diaphragm by normal anatomy, but because it must expand to accommodate luminal contents, it does not tightly fill the hiatus. The phrenoesophageal membrane's elastic tissue gradually diminishes with age or other factors, making it more lax and raising the possibility of a hiatal hernia.

Both sympathetic and parasympathetic nerves innervate the esophagus. The parasympathetic nerve supply supplies motor innervation to the esophageal muscles and secretomotor innervation to the glands. It is derived from the nucleus ambiguus and the dorsal motor nucleus of the vagus (DMN). The intermediolateral cell columns of the T1–T10 spine provide the sympathetic nerve supply, which controls esophageal sphincter tone, blood vessel contractions, muscle wall relaxation, and an increase in glandular function.

The vagus nerves are primarily responsible for the motor innervation of the esophagus. Lower motor neurons in the brainstem's nucleus regulate the striated muscle portion of the esophagus, i.e., center for swallowing. The somatic type nerve fibers end on motor endplates found in striated muscle fibers. The DMN is where the nerve fibers in the smooth muscle segment begin.

Preganglionic neurons of the DMN are divided into two categories. In the myenteric (Auerbach's) plexus, short latency fibers in the caudal part of the DMN form synapses with postganglionic nitrergic inhibitory neurons, while long latency fibers in the rostral part of the DMN form synapses with postganglionic cholinergic excitatory neurons. The submucosal (Meissner's) plexus's ganglia control the muscularis musosae's secretion and contraction.

The proximal esophageal striated muscle has a scattered myenteric plexus, but its significance is still unknown.

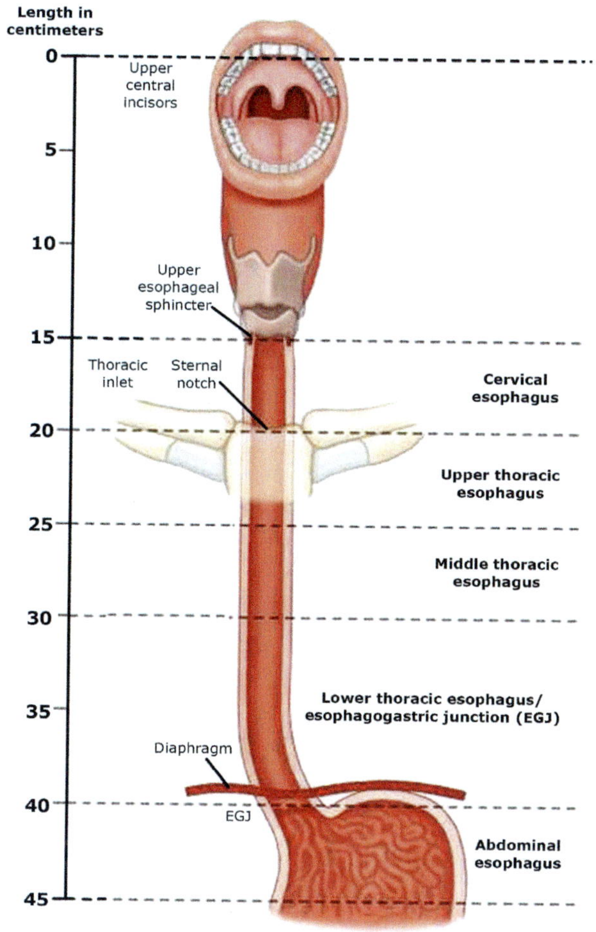

Figure 7.2. *Length of esophageal parts.*

Source: Murat Ferhat Ferhatoglu and Taner Kıvılcım, "Anatomy of Esophagus," InTech; 2017. DOI: 10.5772/intechopen.69583.

Three sources supply the esophagus with arterial blood supply: the paired aortic esophageal arteries or terminal branches of bronchial arteries supply the thoracic esophagus with arterial blood supply; the left gastric artery and a branch of the left phrenic artery supply the most distal segment of the esophagus with arterial blood supply; and the upper esophageal sphincter (UES) and the cervical esophagus with arterial blood supply. All of the extramural vessels are connected by a continuous, dense network of arteries in the submucosa, which provides the esophagus with an abundant blood supply. The azygous system drains blood from the proximal and distal esophagus, and the superior vena cava receives the blood directly. The mid-esophagus sends venous blood to the left gastric vein, a branch of the portal vein. Esophageal varices associated with portal hypertension can arise from the submucosal vein connections in the distal esophagus between the portal and systemic venous systems (Figure 7.2).

7.1.2. Physiology

The most common perception of esophageal physiological issues is dysphagia, or difficulty swallowing. The physiology of the esophagus is hampered by obstructive esophageal lesions and disorders of esophageal motility, which cause a sensation of dysphagia. Disorders pertaining to motility stem from issues with the esophageal muscles or the nerves that supply them. On the other hand, obstructive lesions cause the esophageal lumen to mechanically narrow. Both cause dysphagia as a result of changed food passage through the esophagus. Oropharyngeal dysphagia is a condition that causes difficulty starting a swallow due to issues in the oropharynx. Food gets lodged in the chest during swallowing due to esophageal dysphagia, which is an issue of the esophagus.

7.1.2.1. Cellular Level

There are four layers that make up the esophageal wall: adventitia, muscularis propria, submucosa, and mucosa. The innermost layer that lines the esophageal lumen is called the mucosa. It begins with a mucous membrane made of skin-like stratified squamous epithelium. The mucous membrane is followed by a thin layer of connective tissue known as the lamina propria. Lastly, the deepest portion of the mucosa is formed by a muscularis mucosa, which is mainly composed of smooth muscles arranged erratically. The submucosa is the layer that lies below the mucosa and is primarily made up of connective tissue, tiny mucous glands, and blood vessels. Additionally, it has a nerve plexus known as Meissner's or submucosal plexus. The muscularis propria, which is more intricate than the preceding layers, is located beneath the submucosa. The muscularis propria, also known as the muscularis externa, consists of an outer longitudinal layer and an inner circumferential layer that may or may not be made of smooth or striated muscle. In the proximal esophagus, smooth muscles are more common than striated muscles, and vice versa in the distal esophagus. There is a transition zone between the proximal and distal ends that is made up of both muscle types. The myenteric or Auerbach's plexus is a different nerve plexus found in the muscular layer. The adventitia, an external fibrous layer that joins the esophagus to other external structures, is the last outermost layer.

7.1.2.2. Development

During the fourth week of pregnancy, the developing foregut initiates the formation of the esophagus. In the coming weeks, it will rapidly divide and differentiate from what is currently just a tiny tube dividing the stomach from the pharynx. In the sixth week, blood vessels, ganglion cells in the myenteric plexus, and circular muscle fibers start to develop. The epithelium is simple columnar around the eighth week of pregnancy. Until roughly the 17th week of pregnancy, when the number of ciliated cells begins to decline, things usually remain this way. Full formation of the non-keratinized stratified squamous epithelium occurs at birth.

7.1.2.3. Organ Systems Involved

The esophagus facilitates the passage of a bolus from the throat into the stomach. The esophagus is thus impacted by events that take place both upstream, in the mouth, and downstream, in the stomach. The diaphragm and the trachea are also very close to the esophagus; the latter surrounds the LES through its crural portion, and the former is located anterior to it. In order to facilitate the passage of the food bolus to the stomach, the LES high-pressure region must relax, and this is mediated by the crural diaphragm.

7.1.2.4. Function

7.1.2.4.1. Upper Esophageal Sphincter (UES)

Between the pharynx and the upper portion of the esophagus is a high-pressure region known as the upper esophageal sphincter. The sphincter has strong elastic and tonic qualities because of its composition, which is a blend of muscles and cartilages. The sphincter's ability to remain wide-open in response to a stimulus is another benefit of its distinct composition. The purpose of the UES is to prevent food from refluxing back into the airways. Significant amounts of air are also kept from entering the gastrointestinal tract by it. The arytenoid and interarytenoid muscles, along with the cricoid cartilage, comprise the anterior portion of the sphincter. The majority of the posterior and lateral walls of the sphincter are made up of the thyropharyngeus and cricopharyngeus muscles; the former makes up the upper two-thirds of the sphincter, while the latter occupies the lower one-third. The sphincter opens widely when the hyoid muscle, which pulls the larynx forward, contracts and the cricopharyngeus and thyropharyngeus relax.

The food bolus stimulates sensory receptors in the oropharynx once it gets there. Afferent nerve fibers from the receptors subsequently carry the signal to the brainstem's swallowing center. After the brainstem has processed the information, smooth muscle cells in the UES receive efferent fibers. The food bolus passes the UES when the cricopharyngeus and thyropharyngeus muscles relax in response. The stimulus causes the UES to open as well as swallowing, stopping breathing, and peristaltic motions down the esophagus. It is important to note that, as opposed to being stimulatory, the signals that travel to the thyropharyngeus and cricopharyngeus muscles are inhibitory. Stated differently, they prevent tonic contractions of these muscles, which cause the LES to open.

The hyoid muscle contracts in response to efferent signals, which raises the hyoid. The contraction of the hyoid muscles occurs nearly concurrently with UES relaxation. These three forces work in concert with the propulsion force to enable the food bolus to cross the pressure barrier of the UES region and enter the esophagus. In addition, the bolus volume is crucial in modulating the UES physiology. It sets the time interval between opening of the UES and movement of the pharynx. Pharyngeal movements begin more quickly at higher volumes. Furthermore, the time interval between the UES opening and pharyngeal movements lengthens when the bolus thickness increases.

7.1.2.4.2. Peristalsis

The bolus enters the esophagus after passing through the UES. The striated muscles that make up the upper part of the esophagus are primarily controlled by central control mechanisms. Both intrinsic and central control mechanisms regulate the smooth muscle that makes up the lower portion of the esophagus. Peristalstic movements, like the swallowing reflex, that come from the brainstem are referred to as central control mechanisms. Peripheral control mechanisms, on the other hand, are intrinsic to smooth muscles because of their abundant nerve plexuses and relate to peristaltic movements that originate from the esophagus itself. The esophagus is made up of four layers: mucosa, submucosa, muscularis propria, and serosa. The muscularis propria layer consists of an outer longitudinal and an inner circular muscular layer. While the exact function of longitudinal muscles in esophageal physiology is not completely understood, recent studies suggest that they help reduce tension during circular muscle contractions, enhancing peristaltic movements. Circular muscle fibers, on the other hand, play a defined role in esophageal physiology by contracting radially to propel the food bolus distally through peristalsis. Primary peristalsis is initiated by the entry of the bolus into the esophagus, triggering esophageal contractions. Secondary peristalsis, on the other hand, is induced by distension. During peristalsis, the area in front of the bolus relaxes while the area behind it contracts, allowing the bolus to move forward smoothly. Nervous inputs help coordinate these contractions and relaxations, ensuring the seamless movement of food along the esophagus.

The intricate process of primary peristalsis in the esophagus is regulated by brainstem-derived central control mechanisms. The way smooth muscles in the lower esophagus react to food is slightly different from that of the striated muscles in the upper esophagus. A peristaltic wave is produced by the sequential activation of lower motor neurons in the nucleus ambiguous of the brainstem in striated muscles. However, in smooth muscles, the activation of inhibitory neurons located in the caudal dorsal motor nucleus (cDMN) results in the simultaneous inhibition of the entire esophagus. The process of simultaneously producing a peristaltic wave in the smooth muscle of the esophagus is known as deglutitive inhibition. The lower than the upper portions of the esophagus experiences a longer-lasting inhibition. Peristalstic contraction is induced as the inhibition ends by successive activation of excitatory neurons in the rostral dorsal motor nucleus (rDMN).

The rostral part of the DMN (rDMN) contains vagal preganglionic neurons, which are the source of the excitatory pathway in smooth muscles. The medulla's ventral floor of the fourth ventricle contains the DMN, a vagal nerve nucleus. Acetylcholine (ACh) and substance P are released by excitatory postganglionic neurons, which are attached to the rDMN preganglionic neurons. In contrast, the cDMN's preganglionic vagal fibers are a part of the inhibitory pathway. These fibers project to postganglionic inhibitory neurons containing substance P (SP), adenosine triphosphate (ATP), vasoactive intestinal peptide (VIP), and nitric oxide (NO).

Remarkably, when there is food remnants in the esophagus, the intrinsic nervous system and vaso-vagal reactions can coordinate the process of secondary peristalsis in the esophagus. In most cases, secondary peristalsis happens when a swallow is not made. It may be just as strong and quick as the main peristalsis. Secondary peristalsis in skeletal muscles is centrally mediated and proceeds similarly to primary peristalsis, with unclear nerve innervations originating from the nucleus. Secondary peristalsis in smooth muscles is regulated by a peripheral mechanism. When food boluses or distention occur in the esophagus, sensory neurons are activated, initiating the peripheral mechanism. An interneuron receives the signal from an excited sensory neuron and forwards it to a motor neuron. The motor neuron then produces a secondary peristaltic wave by releasing nitric oxide (NO) distally and acetylcholine (ACh) proximally. The peripheral mechanism both generates and locally confines this peristaltic wave in smooth muscle.

7.1.2.4.3. LES

The bolus needs to go through the LES in order to enter the stomach after it reaches the end of the esophagus. The esophagus and stomach are separated by a high-pressure zone that is formed by the LES and the crural diaphragm. They serve as an anti-reflux barrier, shielding the esophagus from the digestive juice's acidic qualities. They also make it possible for the bolus to enter the stomach. Smooth muscles in the LES aid in maintaining the sphincter's tight closure. The LES's smooth muscles relax in response to direct inhibitory signals, which opens the sphincter and lets the food bolus pass. However, the LES lacks dilator muscles, so opening is dependent only on smooth muscle relaxation.

The myogenic tone of the smooth muscles, the inhibitory nitrergic nerves, and the excitatory cholinergic nerves work together to determine the pressure in the LES. The sphincter's tonic contraction is brought about by the myogenic tone, an innate characteristic of the smooth muscle cells in the LES. It occurs as a result of the LES smooth muscle cells' more depolarized resting membrane potentials, which cause basal tone production and action potentials that resemble spikes to occur spontaneously. Acetylcholine is released by excitatory cholinergic nerves (ACh) to initiate smooth muscle contraction. As such, they promote contraction and strengthen the LES's tonic, myogenic characteristic. The inhibitory nitrergic (NO) pathway, on the other hand, promotes inhibition and releases NO. As a result, it conflicts with the LES's contractile qualities. Contraction is preferred over relaxation when these forces are combined. Because of its myogenic nature, the LES therefore stays contracted even in cases where it is completely denervated.

A bolus in the pharynx stimulates pharyngeal receptors, which send signals to the brainstem, causing esophageal peristalsis and LES relaxation. The DMN is connected to the nucleus tractus solitarius, which receives the sensory stimulus. The smooth muscles are not directly innervated by the DMN's vagal efferent nerves. Rather, they send a signal to the myenteric plexus, which uses nitric oxide (NO) to mediate LES relaxation. Motor neurons, both excitatory and inhibitory, make up the myenteric plexus. The stimulus's location determines whether an inhibitory or excitatory response occurs. Whereas the neurons of the excitatory pathway originate in the rostral DMN, those of the inhibitory pathway originate in the caudal DMN. The most important inhibitory postganglionic neurotransmitter is nitric oxide (NO). On the other hand, tachykinin and ACh are important excitatory ones.

The LES temporarily relaxes in addition to its stimulus-triggered relaxation to permit gas to escape from the stomach. One vital physiological function of the LES is transient lower esophageal sphincter relaxation (TLESR). The brain receives information from afferent nerves in the pharynx, larynx, and stomach to mediate the TLESR reflex. The swallow reflex and the efferent nerves use the same pathway to initiate LES relaxation.

As was previously mentioned, the smooth muscles of the LES and the crural diaphragm combine to form the high-pressure zone between the esophagus and the stomach. Just as smooth muscle relaxation facilitates the passage of a food bolus into the stomach, the crural diaphragm also plays a crucial role in this process. It also aids in controlling the esophageal reflux disease's rate of occurrence. The phrenoesophageal ligament connects it to the LES, allowing the two structures to move in unison during breathing but separating during peristalsis and temporary LES relaxation. The crural diaphragm, a crucial component of the LES, needs to loosen up in order for a food bolus to travel from the esophagus to the stomach and back again. Uncertainty surrounds the exact process by which the crural diaphragm relaxes. It is widely recognized, nevertheless, that nicotinic acetylcholine receptors on the phrenic nerve are what allow diaphragmatic contractions to occur.

7.1.2.5. Pathophysiology

Dysphagia, or difficulty swallowing, is the term used to describe the subjective perception of abnormal difficulty swallowing. It may happen at the beginning of the swallow or soon after. The former, as the name suggests, is called oropharyngeal dysphagia and happens when there is an issue at the oropharynx level. Esophageal dysphagia is the term for the latter condition, which is brought on by issues in the esophagus. The causes of esophageal dysphagia are multifactorial. The two most common causes of dysphagia are physical obstruction and motor issues. The UES, the esophagus, or the LES may be the site of them. Some common causes of dysphagia due to motor impairments are scleroderma, diabetes mellitus, achalasia, and diffuse esophageal spasm. Conversely, disorders causing dysphagia as a result of an obstructive process include Schatski's rings, reflux esophagitis, esophageal carcinoma, and peptic strictures. Esophageal blockages first result in trouble swallowing liquids, which later develops into dysphagia for both liquids and solids. On the other hand, dysphagia with solids and liquids is initially brought on by motor disease.

7.2. Disorders of the Esophagus

The esophagus, which is the tube that transports food from your mouth to your stomach, is impacted by esophageal disorders. The most typical kind is GERD. Heartburn and difficulty swallowing are symptoms of disorders such as GERD, achalasia, and Barrett's esophagus, which also raise the risk of esophageal cancer. Medication can be helpful, as can dietary and lifestyle modifications.

7.2.1. GERD

Acid reflux from the stomach constantly running back into the esophagus, the tube that connects your mouth and stomach, is known as gastroesophageal reflux disease (GERD). The lining of your esophagus may become irritated by this backwash, or acid reflux. Periodically, a lot of people experience acid reflux. GERD can develop, though, if acid reflux occurs frequently over an extended period of time. With medication and lifestyle modifications, the majority of people are able to control their GERD discomfort. Even though it is rare, some people may require surgery to relieve their symptoms.

7.2.1.1. Symptoms

The following are typical GERD signs and symptoms.

- A burning feeling in your chest (heartburn), usually after eating, and possibly more severe at night or while you're sleeping.
- Food or sour liquid regurgitated, or backwashed.
- Upper abdominal or chest pain
- Trouble swallowing (dysphagia)
- Sensation of a lump in your throat

In addition to these symptoms, you may have acid reflux during the night.

- An ongoing cough
- Inflammation of the laryngitis, or vocal cords.
- New or worsening asthma

When to See a Doctor: If you experience arm, jaw, or chest pain, or shortness of breath, get medical attention right away. These could be heart attack warning signs and symptoms.

Schedule a visit with your physician if you:

- Suffer from frequent or severe GERD symptoms.
- Utilize over-the-counter heartburn remedies more than twice a week.

7.2.1.2. Causes

Frequent stomach acid reflux or reflux of nonacidic content is the cause of GERD. The lower esophageal sphincter, a circular band of muscle that surrounds the bottom of your esophagus, relaxes during swallowing to let food and liquids pass into your stomach. The sphincter then shuts once more. Stomach acid can return to your esophagus if the sphincter weakens or fails to relax as it should. The lining of your esophagus becomes irritated by this continuous backwash of acid, which frequently results in inflammation (Figure 7.3).

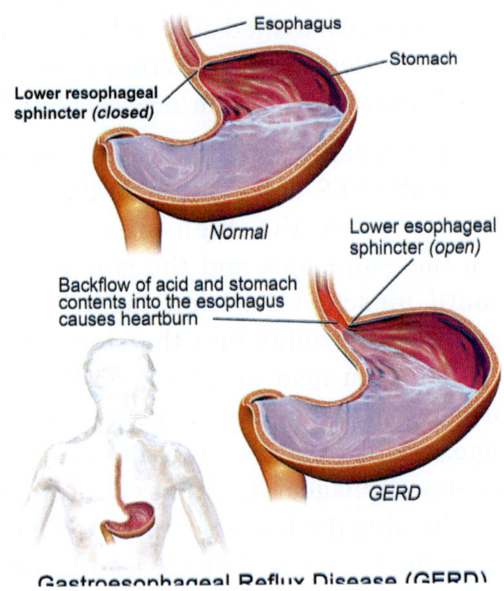

Figure 7.3. *A comparison of the healthy condition vs. GERD.*

Source: *By BruceBlaus – Own work, CC BY-SA 4.0, https://commons.wikimedia.org/w/index.php?curid=44923646.*

7.2.1.3. Risk Factors for GERD

Over 60 million American adults—many of whom are pregnant—have heartburn at least once a month, and over 15 million adults experience it daily. Unbelievably, more babies and kids than previously believed have GERD, according to recent studies. It may result in recurrent episodes of vomiting. Coughing and other respiratory issues may also result from it. According to certain medical professionals, a hiatal hernia may weaken the LES and increase the likelihood of reflux disease. A hiatal hernia occurs when the upper portion of the stomach passes through a tiny diaphragmatic hiatus opening and up into the chest. The muscle that divides the abdomen from the chest is called the diaphragm. The lower end of the esophagus is supported in part by the diaphragm's opening, according to recent research.

Heartburn or reflux is rare in many patients with hiatal hernias. However, a hiatal hernia may make it easier for stomach contents to reflux into the esophagus. A hiatal hernia can result from sudden physical exertion, vomiting, coughing, or straining that increases pressure in the abdomen. Many 50 and older adults in otherwise good health have a small one. Hiatal hernias can affect people of any age, but they typically affect those in their middle years. Most of the time, hiatal hernias heal on their own. However, it might be required if there is a risk that the hernia could become strangulated or twisted in a way that would cut off the blood supply. If you have one and severe GERD or esophagitis (esophageal inflammation), you might also need to treat it. Your physician might operate to reduce the size of the hernia or avoid strangulation.

There are several other factors that can increase your risk of developing GERD:

- Being overweight or obese
- Pregnancy
- Delayed stomach emptying (gastroparesis).
- Disorders of the connective tissue, like lupus, scleroderma, and rheumatoid arthritis.

If you already have acid reflux, certain dietary and lifestyle choices may exacerbate it:

- Smoking
- Some foods and beverages, such as chocolate, fried or fatty foods, coffee, and alcohol.
- Large meals
- Eating too soon before bed
- Specific drugs, such as aspirin.

7.2.1.4. GERD Symptoms

Acid reflux disease, also known as heartburn, is the most typical GERD symptom. Usually, it feels like a searing pain in your chest that travels up to your neck and throat from behind your breastbone. A lot of people report feeling as though food is returning to their mouths, leaving behind an acidic or bitter taste. Heartburn can cause pressure, burning, or pain that lasts for up to two hours. Usually, it gets worse after eating. Additionally, bending over or lying down can cause heartburn. Many people find that standing up straight or taking an antacid that removes acid from the esophagus helps them feel better.

There are distinctions between the pain of heartburn and that of heart disease or a heart attack, which is sometimes the case. While resting may lessen heart disease pain, exercise may exacerbate it. Physical activity has a lower correlation with heartburn pain. You can't tell the difference, though, so if you experience any chest pain, get medical attention straight away. Other than pain, you might experience:

- Nausea
- Bad breath

- Trouble breathing
- A hard time swallowing
- Vomiting
- Wearing away of tooth enamel
- A lump in your throat

You might also have the following if you experience acid reflux at night:

- A lingering cough
- Laryngitis
- Asthma that comes on suddenly or gets worse
- Sleep problems

7.2.1.5. GERD Treatment and Home Remedies

The goal of GERD treatment is to reduce reflux or the harm that refluxed materials cause to the lining of the esophagus. To treat your symptoms, your doctor might suggest over-the-counter or prescription drugs.

- **Antacids:** These medications can help prevent heartburn by neutralizing stomach and esophageal acid. A lot of people discover that over-the-counter antacids offer fleeting or incomplete relief. For certain people, combining an antacid with a foaming agent is helpful. Scientists believe that these substances create a foam layer over the stomach to prevent acid reflux.
- However, prolonged antacid use can cause a buildup of magnesium in the body, altered calcium metabolism (a change in how the body breaks down and uses calcium), and diarrhea. For those with kidney disease, an excess of magnesium can be dangerous. See your doctor if you require antacids for a period longer than two weeks.
- **H2 blockers:** In cases of persistent reflux and heartburn, the physician might suggest drugs that lower stomach acid. Among these medications are H2 blockers, which assist in preventing the stomach's production of acid. Cimetidine (Tagamet), famotidine (Pepcid), and nizatidine are examples of H2 blockers.
- **Proton Pump Inhibitors (PPIs):** These medications, also called acid pumps, inhibit a protein required for the production of stomach acid. PPIs consist of pantoprazole (Protonix), rabeprazole (Aciphex), omeprazole (Prilosec), lansoprazole (Prevacid), esomeprazole (Nexium), and dexlansoprazole (Dexilant).
- **Prokinetics:** Rarely, these medications can speed up stomach emptying, reducing the amount of acid that remains in your stomach. They might also be beneficial for symptoms like nausea, vomiting, and bloating. They may, however, also have detrimental side effects. Many are unable to handle them, and those who are able to ought to use them sparingly. Domperidone and metoclopramide (Clopra, Maxolon, Metozolv, Reglan) are two examples of prokinetics.

7.2.1.6. Diet and Lifestyle Changes

Doctors advise you to modify your lifestyle in a few ways to help reduce your GERD symptoms.

- **Avoid Foods and Beverages Triggers:** Foods like chocolate, peppermint, fatty foods, caffeine, and alcoholic beverages should be avoided as they can relax the LES. Citrus fruits and juices, tomato products, and pepper are among the foods and drinks that should be avoided if they cause symptoms due to their potential to irritate a damaged esophageal lining.

- **Eat Smaller Servings:** Reducing the size of meals may also aid in symptom management. Additionally, eating meals two to three hours before going to bed allows your stomach to partially empty and reduce acid production.
- **Eat slowly:** Take your time at every meal.
- **Chew Your Food Thoroughly:** If you put down your fork after a bite, it might help you remember to do this. Only pick it back up after you've fully chewed and swallowed that bite.
- **Stop Smoking:** Smoking cigarettes weakens the LES. It is critical to give up smoking in order to lessen GERD symptoms.
- **Elevate Your Head:** Reflux of stomach contents into the esophagus can be lessened by elevating the head of your bed on 6-inch blocks or by sleeping on a specially made wedge. Never elevate yourself with pillows. That just causes the stomach to become more compressed.
- **Stay at a Healthy Weight:** Symptoms are frequently made worse by obesity. When they lose weight, many overweight people experience relief.
- **Wear Loose Clothes:** Wearing clothing that clings to your waist puts strain on your lower esophagus and belly.
- **Acupuncture:** Acupuncture treatment prevented reflux in the test group more effectively than proton pump inhibitors, with longer-lasting effects.

7.2.1.7. Severe GERD Diagnosis

Tests may be necessary for a more accurate diagnosis if you have severe, chronic reflux disease or if your symptoms do not improve after treatment. To accomplish this, your physician might perform one or more of the following procedures:

- **Endoscopy:** Your doctor will insert an endoscope, a tiny illuminated tube with a tiny video camera on the end, into your esophagus to check for tissue irritation or inflammation (esophagitis). A small tissue sample may be removed for additional testing (biopsy) if the results are unusual or dubious.
- **Upper GI Series:** One of your doctor's initial tests might be this one. This type of X-ray displays your stomach, duodenum, and upper portion of your small intestine. It can help rule out other conditions, like peptic ulcers, but it provides limited information about potential reflux.
- **Esophageal Manometry and Impedance Study:** This test looks for signs of low esophageal pressure. It may also reveal abnormalities in the contraction of your esophageal muscles.
- **pH Testing:** Your doctor may use

this test to measure the acid levels in your esophagus if a definitive diagnosis is difficult to make. It monitors your esophageal acid production during meals, physical activity, and sleep. This is a more useful tool now that longer-term pH tracking has been done using newer methods.

7.2.1.8. Surgery for Severe GERD

Surgery for GERD may be necessary if you have a hiatal hernia, damage to your esophagus that does not go away with medicine, and a need for frequent, high doses of PPIs to manage your symptoms. But you ought to exhaust all other treatment options first.

- **Fundoplication:** The lower esophageal pressure is increased during this procedure. The top of your stomach will be wound around the LES by the doctor. This stops reflux by tightening the muscle and increasing pressure in your lower esophagus. Either open surgery or a laparoscope—small incisions made in the abdomen—will be used to accomplish this.
- **Transoral Incisionless Fundoplication (TIF):** In a more recent version of the procedure, the stomach is wrapped around the LES with plastic fasteners using an endoscope, a tiny tube with a camera. Compared to a standard fundoplication, it is less invasive.
- **Stretta Procedure:** In a more recent version of the procedure, the stomach is wrapped around the LES with plastic fasteners using an endoscope, a tiny tube with a camera. Compared to a standard fundoplication, it is less invasive.
- **LINX Surgery:** Your esophageal-gastric junction is bandaged by your physician with magnetic titanium beads. The beads' magnetic pull keeps it just tight enough to prevent reflux but loose enough to allow food to pass through into the stomach.

7.2.1.9. GERD Complications

Serious complications can sometimes result from GERD.

- **Esophageal Ulcer:** Your esophagus is eroded by stomach acid until an open sore appears. These sores may bleed and are frequently painful. They could make swallowing difficult.
- **Esophageal Stricture:** Scar tissue forms and the lower portion of your esophagus is damaged by stomach acid. The accumulation of scar tissue causes the esophagus to narrow, making it difficult to swallow food.
- **Barrett's Esophagus:** Acid reflux modifies the esophageal lining's cellular composition. The lining thickens and becomes crimson. This illness is associated with an increased risk of esophageal cancer.
- **Lung Problems:** Reflux can irritate and hurt your throat if it reaches the back. It can then enter the lungs through perspiration from there. You might get hoarse if this occurs. It is also possible that you have a persistent cough and chest congestion. You run the risk of developing pneumonia, bronchitis, and asthma if your lungs become inflamed.

7.2.1.10. GERD Outlook

GERD is rarely fatal, but it can make daily activities more difficult. You ought to feel better if you comprehend the underlying causes and receive the right care.

7.2.2. Achalasia

Achalasia is a rare condition that impacts the esophagus, the tube connecting the throat and stomach. This disorder causes abnormal muscle contractions in the esophagus, preventing the proper movement of food towards the stomach. Additionally, the lower esophageal sphincter, located at the bottom of the esophagus, fails to relax and allow food to pass into the stomach. Achalasia usually affects adults between the ages of 30 and 60, with a peak in the 40s, and it is more common in men than women.

7.2.2.1. Achalasia Causes

Although achalasia's causes are unknown, researchers are investigating a number of theories. One has to do with the deterioration of the nerve cells that lie in the space between the esophageal muscles' layers. Food can be forced into and into the stomach by the esophagus thanks to these nerve cells. A possible correlation between parasitic or viral infections and achalasia has been suggested by certain studies.

Individuals diagnosed with achalasia may exhibit a higher likelihood of presenting symptoms of prior infections, including antibodies to the measles virus, human papillomavirus, and herpes simplex virus. Additionally, there is evidence that suggests achalasia could be an inflammatory autoimmune disorder, meaning the body could attack itself to cause the condition. Scientists have observed immune system activity in the nerve cells that supply strength to the esophageal muscles. Additionally, autoimmune diseases like uveitis, type I diabetes, rheumatoid arthritis, systemic lupus erythematosus, and Sjögren's syndrome are three to six times more common in patients with achalasia.

7.2.2.2. Achalasia Symptoms

Food buildup in the esophagus that prevents it from passing into the stomach can contribute to certain symptoms of achalasia. The esophagus widens and may twist as it fills up. The abnormal contractions of the esophageal muscles are linked to additional symptoms of achalasia.

Achalasia symptoms usually appear during or right after meals. Among them are:

- The most common symptom of achalasia is the sensation that food or liquids are difficult to swallow and are "sticking" or getting caught in the esophagus on the way down to the stomach.
- Regurgitation, or the backflow of food and liquids into the mouth following swallowing.
- Chest pain, which can be very intense and cause a person to wake up.
- Heartburn
- Coughing, especially at night
- Choking or aspirating food particles or liquids into one's airways.

One or more of the initial symptoms of achalasia, such as regurgitation and chest pain, are also linked to gastroesophageal reflux disease (GERD). The two situations are not the same, though. Too much slack in the lower esophageal sphincter allows stomach acid to pass through and cause GERD. The sphincter is overly constricted in achalasia. The symptoms of achalasia can worsen. Severe achalasia can cause severe exhaustion, weight loss, malnourishment, and chest pain. Food particles can cause pneumonia, an inflammation of the airways that can be fatal, if they get into the airways as a result of coughing or choking during eating.

7.2.2.3. Types of Achalasia

There are differences in the way esophageal muscles contract in individuals with achalasia. The lower esophageal sphincter, which regulates the passage between the esophagus and the stomach, malfunctions to relax at the appropriate moment in all cases of achalasia. Three types of achalasia have been identified by medical professionals based on concurrent problems.

- Chalasia type 1 is also referred to as classic achalasia at times. When food falls because of gravity alone, it is because the esophageal muscles contract very little.
- The esophagus becomes compressed in Type 2 achalasia as a result of increased pressure inside it. Compared to type I, this is the most prevalent type of achalasia and frequently results in more severe symptoms.
- Due to abnormal contractions at the base of the esophagus where it joins the stomach, type III achalasia is also known as spastic achalasia. The most severe kind of achalasia is this one. The pain in the chest that the contractions can produce can wake someone up from sleep and mimic the signs of a heart attack.

7.2.2.4. Achalasia Diagnosis

Apart from a comprehensive physical assessment and a review of your medical background and symptoms, your physician might suggest the following tests to aid in the diagnosis of achalasia.

- Using pharyngeal and esophageal manometry, you can monitor and document variations in the pressure in your throat and esophagus while you swallow. Because manometry can identify the location and degree of muscle contractions that impair swallowing ability—or lack thereof—some believe it to be the most accurate test for achalasia.
- **Upper endoscopy:** This procedure uses an endoscope, a thin tube with a camera inserted through the mouth, to examine the stomach and esophagus. This test aids in identifying esophageal abnormalities such as tumors and strictures, or narrowing. Your doctor may take a biopsy or remove any abnormal tissue for additional examination during an endoscopy.
- To assess the level of acidity in the esophagus over an extended period of time and rule out other conditions like GERD, use wireless pH testing or 24-hour pH impedance testing.
- Barium swallow is an imaging test that produces images of the upper gastrointestinal (GI) tract using X-rays and the contrast medium barium. A significant narrowing of the esophagus, sometimes referred to as an achalasia bird beak, may be detected by this test.

7.2.2.5. Achalasia Treatment

Although there are currently no cures for achalasia, there are a number of ways to manage the condition's symptoms, including dilation, surgery, injections of botulinum toxin, and medication. The aim of treatment is to help the sphincter relax and permit food to pass into the stomach while also returning the esophageal contractions to normal (Figure 7.4).

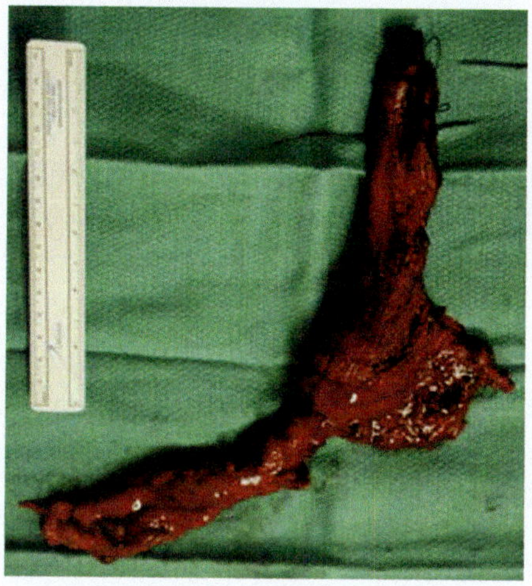

Figure 7.4. *Transhiatal oesophagectomy specimen from a patient with late-stage achalasia. Diverticulum at the left lower end of the esophagus.*

Source: By Science Direct - https://www.sciencedirect.com/science/article/pii/S1743919110004875#bib8, CC BY-SA 4.0, https://commons.wikimedia.org/w/index.php?curid=113067898.

7.2.2.5.1. Dilation of the Esophageal Sphincter

Dilation refers to the act of widening a passageway. In a dilation procedure for achalasia, a gastroenterologist gently inflates a balloon close to the lower esophageal sphincter while the patient is sedated and an endoscope is inserted into the mouth and esophagus. By doing this, you can stretch the sphincter muscles and lower the pressure inside the esophagus, allowing food and liquids to pass through more easily. Probably the most popular method of treating achalasia is balloon dilation. Following the procedure, the majority of patients (65–80%) report a significant improvement in their ability to swallow. The relief, though, might only last temporarily, as achalasia symptoms can recur and necessitate additional care.

7.2.2.5.2. Achalasia Surgery — Esophageal Myotomy

A gastroenterologist performs a myotomy to prevent the lower stomach, esophageal sphincter, and esophageal muscles from tightening. A procedure known as a laparoscopic Heller myotomy, or peroral endoscopic myotomy, can be used to perform an achalasia myotomy through the mouth using an endoscope, or through multiple small abdominal incisions. Not enough muscle is disrupted by a lower esophageal sphincter myotomy to cause acid reflux, but enough is to relieve the symptoms of achalasia. Although this is the most long-term treatment for achalasia, not all patients should go for it.

7.2.2.5.3. Botulinum Toxin Injections

It has been demonstrated that some achalasia patients respond well to botulinum toxin injections into the lower esophageal sphincter. Patients who are older or not suitable candidates for dilation or myotomy benefit most from these treatments. Injections of botulinum toxin for achalasia relieve the sphincter's surrounding nerves and cause it to become numb, allowing it to relax. Using an endoscope, a special needle is inserted to administer the injections. Their short-lived impact lasts roughly a year. It might be required to administer shots again. There have been reports of skin rashes following this treatment, and some patients may have mild chest pain.

7.2.2.5.4. Medications for Achalasia

In general, achalasia cannot be effectively treated with medication. Lower esophageal sphincter temporary relaxation is possible with certain medications that contain calcium channel blockers or nitrates. But they have to be taken before every meal, and generally speaking, the negative effects outweigh the positive ones.

7.2.2.6. Living with Achalasia

Following achalasia treatment, you should work with your doctor to look into other options if your symptoms persist. Changing your eating habits, diet, or other aspects of your lifestyle may improve your quality of life.

7.2.3. Barrett's Esophagus

Barrett's esophagus is a disorder where acid reflux damages the lining of the esophagus, the flat, pink tube that connects the mouth to the stomach. As a result, the lining thickens and turns red. The lower esophageal sphincter (LES) is a vital valve that sits between the esophagus and the stomach. Gastroesophageal reflux disease (GERD) is a condition caused by acid and chemical damage to the esophagus caused by the LES failing over time. Heartburn and regurgitation are common symptoms of GERD. Barrett's esophagus is a condition where the lining of the lower esophagus changes as a result of GERD in certain individuals.

An increased risk of esophageal cancer is linked to Barrett's esophagus. Despite the low risk of esophageal cancer, it is crucial to have frequent examinations with meticulous imaging and thorough esophageal biopsies to screen for precancerous cells (dysplasia). To stop esophageal cancer, precancerous cells can be treated if they are found.

7.2.3.1. Symptoms

The most common cause of Barrett's esophagus is chronic GERD, which can manifest as any of the following symptoms:

- Frequent reflux of stomach contents and heartburn.
- Having trouble swallowing food.
- Less commonly, chest pain

It is interesting to note that barely any symptoms of acid reflux are reported by about half of patients with Barrett's esophagus. As a result, you should talk to your doctor about any concerns you may have with your digestive system, including Barrett's esophagus.

When to See a Doctor: Consult your physician regarding your risk of Barrett's esophagus if you have experienced heartburn, regurgitation, or acid reflux for longer than five years.

Seek immediate help if you:

- Experience chest pain, which could indicate a heart attack.
- Have difficulty swallowing
- Are throwing up blood in the form of coffee grounds or red blood.
- Are voiding tarry, bloody, or black stools.
- Are gaining weight inadvertently.

7.2.3.2. Causes

It is unknown what specifically causes Barrett's esophagus. Although GERD is common in people with Barrett's esophagus, many also have silent reflux, or no reflux symptoms at all. Barrett's esophagus is caused by stomach acid and chemicals that wash back into the esophagus, damaging tissue and altering the swallowing tube's lining whether or not GERD symptoms are present.

7.2.3.3. Risk Factors

The following variables raise your risk of Barrett's esophagus:

- **Family History:** If esophageal cancer or Barrett's esophagus is there in your family, your chances of developing these conditions rise.

- **Being Male:** Men are far more likely to develop Barrett's esophagus.
- **Being White:** Compared to people of other races, white people are more likely to contract the illness.
- **Age:** Although it can happen at any age, adults over 50 are more likely to have Barrett's esophagus.
- **Chronic Heartburn and Acid Reflux:** Barrett's esophagus is more common in people with GERD that is unresponsive to proton pump inhibitor treatment or in people with GERD that needs ongoing medication.
- Current or past smoking.
- **Being Overweight:** Your risk is further increased by abdominal body fat.

7.2.3.4. Complications

Barrett's esophagus is not a serious medical emergency. However, in a small percentage of cases, Barrett's esophagus can result in precancerous changes. Less than 1% of individuals with Barrett's esophagus go on to develop esophageal adenocarcinoma, a dangerous and potentially fatal esophageal cancer. This is a very tiny increase in risk if you have Barrett's esophagus. Regular checkups will help your doctor detect precancerous and cancerous cells early on, when the disease is easier to treat and before they can spread.

7.2.3.5. Diagnosis

The most common method for identifying Barrett's esophagus is endoscopy. Your throat is examined with an endoscope, a lit tube with a camera at the end, to look for indications of shifting esophageal tissue. Normal esophageal tissue has a glossy, pale appearance. The tissue in Barrett's esophagus has a velvety, red appearance. Your esophagus will be biopsied, or tissue removed, by your doctor. To ascertain the extent of change, the biopsied tissue can be examined.

7.2.3.5.1. Determining the Degree of Tissue Change

The level of dysplasia in your esophageal cells is assessed by a pathologist, a medical professional who specializes in analyzing tissue in a lab. It is best to have two pathologists agree on your diagnosis because dysplasia in the esophagus can be challenging to diagnose, with at least one of them specializing in gastroenterology pathology.

You could categorize your tissue as:

- If Barrett's esophagus is present but there are no precancerous alterations in the cells, there is no dysplasia.
- Low-grade dysplasia, in which cells exhibit minute indications of cancerous alterations.
- Elevated dysplasia, if numerous alterations are seen in the cells. It is believed that high-grade dysplasia is the last stage before cells transform into esophageal cancer.

7.2.3.5.2. Screening for Barrett's Esophagus

According to the American College of Gastroenterology, screening may be advised for men who have experienced GERD symptoms at least once a week that do not improve after taking a proton pump inhibitor medication and have at least two of the following risk factors:

- Barrett's esophagus or esophageal cancer in the family.
- Caucasian
- Above 50 years old
- A current or past smoker
- Increased abdominal girth

Despite the fact that women are much less likely than men to have Barrett's esophagus, if they have uncontrolled reflux or other risk factors, they should get screened.

7.2.3.6. Treatment

The degree of aberrant cell growth in your esophagus and your general state of health will determine how you are treated for Barrett's esophagus.

7.2.3.6.1. No Dysplasia

Your doctor will likely recommend:

- Routine endoscopy to keep an eye on the esophageal cells. You will likely have a follow-up endoscopy in a year if your biopsies reveal no dysplasia, and then every three to five years if no changes take place.
- **GERD Treatment:** Your signs and symptoms may be lessened by medication and lifestyle modifications. To treat a hiatal hernia or tighten the lower esophageal sphincter, which regulates the flow of stomach acid, surgery or endoscopic procedures may be necessary.

7.2.3.6.2. Low-Grade Dysplasia

Low-grade dysplasia is thought to represent the initial stage of precancerous alterations. If low-grade dysplasia is discovered, a qualified pathologist should confirm it. Your doctor might suggest an additional endoscopy in six months for low-grade dysplasia, along with additional follow-up every 6 to 12 months. However, if the diagnosis is confirmed, treatment might be advised due to the risk of esophageal cancer.

Among the recommended therapies are:

- **Endoscopic Resection:** This procedure helps identify dysplasia and cancer by removing damaged cells with the help of an endoscope.
- Heat is applied during radiofrequency ablation to eliminate abnormal esophageal tissue. It might be advised to undergo radiofrequency ablation following endoscopic resection.
- Cryotherapy involves applying a cold liquid or gas to abnormal cells in the esophagus using an endoscope. The cells are first allowed to thaw before being frozen once more. The aberrant cells are harmed by the freezing and thawing cycle.

After you've had three or four months of treatment to lower stomach acid, another endoscopy is done if there is noticeable esophageal inflammation at the first one.

7.2.3.6.3. High-Grade Dysplasia

Most people believe that high-grade dysplasia is a sign of esophageal cancer. Your doctor might therefore suggest radiofrequency ablation, cryotherapy, or endoscopic resection. Surgery is an additional option that entails cutting out the damaged section of your esophagus and joining the remaining section to your stomach. Following treatment, Barrett's esophagus recurrence is possible. Find out from your doctor how frequently you must return for additional testing. Your doctor may prescribe lifelong medication to lower acid and promote esophageal healing if your course of treatment involves anything other than surgery to remove abnormal esophageal tissue.

7.2.3.7. Lifestyle and Home Remedies

Controlling acid reflux is another treatment objective that can be attained by modifying one's lifestyle.

You may attempt to:

- Make dietary adjustments. Reflux can be made worse by chocolate, caffeine, fatty meals, spicy foods, and peppermint.
- Steer clear of tobacco, alcohol, and caffeinated drinks.
- Lose weight. The risk of reflux is increased by being overweight because excess weight around the abdomen can compress the stomach and push acid up into the esophagus.
- Elevate the head of your bed while you sleep. Elevating your head during sleep could potentially mitigate the risk of stomach acid refluxing up into the esophagus.
- Adjust the time you eat. Eat frequently in small portions rather than in large ones, and avoid lying down for at least three hours after eating.
- Drink a lot of water when taking any medications.

7.2.4. Eosinophilic Esophagitis

One known chronic allergic/immune esophageal condition is eosinophilic esophagitis (EoE). The tube that transports food from the mouth to the stomach is called the esophagus. Eosinophils, a type of white blood cell, are abundant in the lining of the esophagus in patients with eosinophilia (EoE). Eosinophils can release inflammatory substances into the tissues around them. Eosinophils are typically absent from the esophagus. An individual suffering from eosinophil accumulation and inflammation in the esophagus is known as an EoE patient. Symptoms arise from the ongoing inflammation caused by EoE. Its symptoms change as people age. Young children may refuse to eat or may not develop normally. Children of school age frequently experience a decrease in appetite, recurrent stomach pain, difficulty swallowing, or vomiting. Adults and teenagers may experience similar symptoms, although they frequently have trouble swallowing solid, dry, or dense foods. The esophagus becomes inflamed, and in severe cases, the esophagus narrows to the point where food becomes lodged, causing difficulty swallowing. A "food impaction" is defined as food that has become firmly lodged in the esophagus. If the food does not pass into the stomach or is not quickly vomited up, it may be a medical emergency.

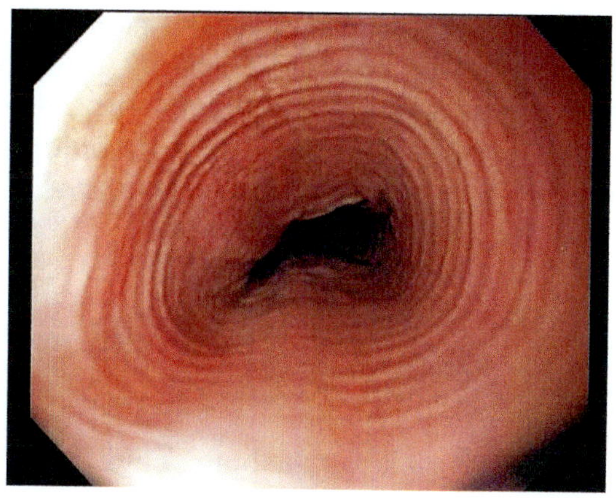

Figure 7.5. *Endoscopic image of esophagus in a case of eosinophilic esophagitis. Concentric rings are termed trachealization of the esophagus.*

Source: By Samir at the English-language Wikipedia, CC BY-SA 3.0, https://commons.wikimedia.org/w/index.php?curid=5161861.

A growing number of patients with EoE are being seen by gastroenterologists and allergists.

This is because EoE is occurring more frequently and doctors are more aware of it. EoE is thought to be a chronic illness that does not go away with treatment. In conditions other than EoE, eosinophils can be discovered in the esophageal tissue. Acid reflux disease is a typical example. To properly diagnose EoE, other conditions involving eosinophils in the esophagus must be ruled out (Figure 7.5).

7.2.4.1. Diagnosing Eosinophilic Esophagitis

To diagnose esophageal biopsies and upper endoscopy, respectively, is currently required. A flexible tube with a light source and a camera lens is inserted down the esophagus during an endoscopy procedure to allow your doctor to check for inflammation in the esophagus. Biopsies are tiny samples of esophageal tissue, about the size of a pen tip, that are taken and examined under a microscope to check for other indications of inflammation and the presence of eosinophils. To diagnose EoE, gastroenterologists, allergists, and pathologists adhere to specific criteria. These include EoE-conforming symptoms combined with results from the upper endoscopy and a pathologist's review of the esophageal tissue biopsies that corroborate EoE.

7.2.4.1.1. Eosinophilic Esophagitis and Allergies

Atopic patients make up the bulk of EoE patients. Atopic individuals are those who exhibit signs of one or more allergy disorders. These consist of food allergies, atopic dermatitis (eczema), asthma, and allergic rhinitis. Others in the family may also experience EoE. Since many EoE patients are atopic, an allergist may initially see them, suspecting EoE, and then refer them to a gastroenterologist for confirmation of the diagnosis. Alternatively, you might be referred to an allergist for assessment and management of EoE and any associated allergic diseases if a gastroenterologist diagnoses you with EoE. Visiting an allergist will give you, your family, and the gastroenterologist information that will enable appropriate treatment of any allergic aspects of EoE. Planning diet therapy and the eventual reintroduction of foods into your diet can be aided by an allergist as well.

7.2.4.1.2. Eosinophilic Esophagitis: Environmental Allergies

Environmental allergies to dust mites, molds, animals, pollens, and other substances may contribute to EoE. Some patients may experience a worsening of their EoE during the pollen season. The EoE evaluation frequently includes allergy testing for these common environmental allergies.

7.2.4.1.3. Eosinophilic Esophagitis: Food Allergies

For the majority of patients, food allergies are the primary cause of EoE. Experts in diagnosing and treating EoE associated with food allergies are allergists. However, there is a complicated connection between food allergies and EoE. When a person with a traditional immunoglobulin E (IgE)-mediated food allergy has experienced a severe allergic reaction, such as hives or vomiting, minutes after consuming the offending food, it is simple to identify the triggers. It is more challenging to determine the role of foods in EoE because the reactions are delayed and sometimes take days to manifest, making it more challenging to identify a single food as the trigger. Foods including dairy, wheat, eggs, and soy are known to be the most frequent causes of Epstein-Barr syndrome. Sadly, blood allergy testing, skin testing, and patch testing cannot consistently detect food triggers for Epstein-Barr syndrome. This is due to the fact that, in addition to traditional IgE-mediated food allergies, the majority of food allergy reactions in EoE are delayed and primarily caused by immune mechanisms. One or more foods may set off an allergic reaction in a person with EoE. After a person's diet is altered to exclude the offending food or foods, the symptoms of esophageal inflammation usually go away in a few weeks. Additional biopsies are required to determine which food(s) is(are) causing EoE and to determine whether a diet is effective in treating the condition, as symptoms may not always indicate whether inflammation is present in the esophagus.

7.2.4.2. Eosinophilic Esophagitis: Treatment

A treatment plan that suits you can be found with the assistance of your doctor. Depending on what is causing your EoE and how severe your symptoms are, a different treatment plan will be recommended. Therapies could consist of:

7.2.4.2.1. Empiric Elimination Diets

Removing the main dietary allergens is regarded as a reasonable approach to treating EoE. Typically, foods like dairy, wheat, eggs, and soy are off -limits. Although these diets can be very challenging to follow, particularly without the assistance of a dietitian with experience treating EoE, they are very helpful in treating EoE. Foods are usually reintroduced one at a time, with follow-up endoscopies to help identify the precise foods causing endoerosis. As an alternative, if the inflammation does not go down, diets can begin with cutting out dairy products only and then add other foods.

7.2.4.2.2. Elemental Diets

All dietary sources of allergens are eliminated during this stringent elimination diet. The patient is fed only an amino acid formula, or occasionally they are allowed to eat one or two simple foods selected for their low potential to cause EoE. The diet is altered to exclude all other foods. Very young children on this diet may require a feeding tube because they frequently cannot drink enough formula to receive enough nutrition. Children with multiple EoE food triggers who have not responded to other forms of treatment are typically the target audience for this approach.

7.2.4.2.3. Medical Therapy

The only medication for treating eosinophilic esophagitis that the Food and Drug Administration (FDA) has approved to date is dupixent (dupilumab). It has recently been approved for use in patients who weigh at least 40 kilograms, or roughly 88 pounds, and who are 12 years of age or older. Weekly injections of the monoclonal antibody (also known as a biologic) drug dupixent are given. It makes it easier for patients to swallow food and lessens the inflammation brought on by the condition. It has been demonstrated that other drugs lessen eosinophil counts in the esophagus and alleviate symptoms. In certain EoE patients, proton pump inhibitors (PPIs), which decrease stomach acid production, have also been shown to lessen esophageal inflammation. PPIs are therefore frequently used as an initial treatment for EoE. Other forms of therapy, such as swallowed topical corticosteroids or food elimination diets, are taken into consideration because not all patients respond to PPIs. Careful observation by a medical professional experienced in treating EoE is crucial.

Corticosteroids are useful drugs for treating EoE because they reduce inflammation. The most common treatment is to swallow small doses of corticosteroids so they come into contact with the esophageal inner lining. There are various types of corticosteroids that can be swallowed. To lower the risk of steroid side effects, the dose of swallowed corticosteroid is lowered to the lowest dose required to maintain control of EoE once esophageal inflammation has been sufficiently controlled.

7.2.4.2.4. Working with Your Doctors

EoE is a complicated illness. Patients should pay close attention to their gastroenterologist's advice when it comes to managing endometriosis (EoE) and determining when endoscopies are necessary to monitor the condition's improvement or worsening. To determine whether allergies are a factor, patients must also collaborate closely with their allergist or immunologist. Additionally, an allergist/immunologist can help you manage related conditions like asthma, eczema, and allergic rhinitis and determine which foods you should avoid. Your allergist and gastroenterologist must collaborate and reach a consensus regarding the management of your EoE. Working with a dietitian who is knowledgeable about elimination diets used to treat EoE is highly recommended if you are on a diet to treat your EoE.

7.2.4.3. Risk Factors

EoE it is far more common in people with atopic dermatitis, asthma, and food or environmental allergies. There are additional conditions that can lead to an increase in eosinophils within the esophagus. Your medical professional must assess you for these potential ailments. Another risk factor for the illness is a family history of EoE.

7.2.4.4. Complications

Eosinophilic esophagitis in certain individuals can result in the following:

- Esophageal scarring and narrowing. This makes swallowing challenging and increases the possibility of food becoming lodged in your throat.
- Damage to the esophagus. Endoscopy can result in perforations or tears in the tissue lining the esophagus due to esophageal inflammation. Tearing may also be related to retching, which some people get when food gets lodged in their esophagus.

7.2.5. Esophageal Cancer

The development of cancer cells in the esophagus, a tube-like structure that connects your throat to your stomach, results in esophageal cancer. Food travels down the esophagus from the mouth to the stomach. The cancer begins in the inner layer of the esophagus and has the potential to metastasize—travel throughout the esophageal layers and other parts of the body. The two primary forms of esophageal cancer exist. Squamous cell carcinoma is one kind. The inner esophagus is lined with squamous cells, and cancer that develops from these cells can spread throughout the esophagus. Adenocarcinoma is the term for the other kind. This type of cancer arises from gland cells. The squamous cells that typically line the esophagus are replaced by gland cells in esophageal adenocarcinomas. This usually happens in the lower esophagus close to the stomach, and it is thought to be mostly caused by the lower esophagus being exposed to acid.

7.2.5.1. Symptoms

Esophageal cancer symptoms and signs include:

- Dysphagia, or difficulty swallowing.
- Weight loss that happens naturally.
- Burning or pressure in the chest.
- Intensifying heartburn or dyspepsia.
- Coughing or hoarseness

Most of the time, early esophageal cancer shows no symptoms at all.

- **When to See a Doctor:** If you are concerned about any persistent signs or symptoms, schedule an appointment with your doctor. Your risk of developing esophageal cancer is increased if you have been diagnosed with Barrett's esophagus, a precancerous condition brought on by persistent acid reflux. Consult your doctor about the symptoms and indicators that could indicate that your illness is getting worse. People with Barrett's esophagus may be candidates for esophageal cancer screening. Talk to your doctor about the benefits and drawbacks of screening if you have Barrett's esophagus.

7.2.5.2. Causes

The exact cause of esophageal cancer is unknown. DNA alterations, or mutations, in esophageal cells lead to esophageal cancer. The alterations cause uncontrollably growing and dividing cells. The abnormal cells build up to form a tumor in the esophagus, which can spread to other parts of the body and invade neighboring structures.

7.2.5.3. Types of Esophageal Cancer

The type of cells involved in esophageal cancer determines the classification of the disease. The kind of esophageal cancer you have affects the available treatments. Esophageal cancer comes in various forms.

- **Adenocarcinoma:** The cells of the mucus-secreting glands in the esophagus are where adenocarcinoma starts. The lower part of the esophagus is where adenocarcinomas most frequently occur. The most prevalent type of esophageal cancer in the US is called adenocarcinoma, and it mainly affects white men.
- **Squamous Cell Carcinoma:** The thin, flat cells that border the esophageal surface are called squamous cells. Most cases of squamous cell carcinoma are found in the middle and upper regions of the esophagus. Globally, squamous cell carcinoma is the most common type of esophageal cancer.
- **Other Rare Types:** Sarcoma, lymphoma, melanoma, small cell carcinoma, and choriocarcinoma are a few uncommon types of esophageal cancer.

7.2.5.4. Risk Factors

Chronic esophageal irritation is thought to be a factor in the alterations that lead to esophageal cancer.

The following are some of the factors that irritate the esophageal cells and raise your risk of esophageal cancer:

- Suffering from GERD, or gastroesophageal reflux disease.
- Smoking
- Possessing Barrett's esophageal cells, which are precancerous in nature.
- Being obese
- Drinking alcohol
- Having bile reflux
- Experiencing dysphagia due to a non-relaxing esophageal sphincter (achalasia).
- Drinking hot beverages on a regular basis.
- Eating insufficient amounts of veggies and fruits.
- Receiving radiation therapy to the upper abdomen or chest.

7.2.5.5. Complications

As esophageal cancer spreads, it may result in complications like these.

- **Obstruction of the Esophagus:** Food and liquids may become more difficult to pass through your esophagus if you have cancer.
- **Pain:** Pain can arise from advanced esophageal cancer.
- **Bleeding in the Esophagus:** Hemorrhage may result from esophageal cancer. Bleeding typically occurs gradually, but occasionally it can happen suddenly and severely.

7.2.5.6. Prevention

- **Quit smoking:** If you smoke, discuss quitting methods with your physician. There are options for counseling and medication to assist with quitting. Don't start using tobacco if you don't already.
- If you use alcohol at all, do so in moderation. If you decide to use alcohol, use it sparingly. This translates to up to one drink for women and up to two for men per day for healthy adults.
- Eat more fruits and vegetables.
- Maintain a healthy weight. Speak with your doctor about weight loss techniques if you are obese or overweight. Aim for a slow and steady weight loss of 1 or 2 pounds a week.

7.2.5.7. Diagnosis

Esophageal cancer is diagnosed using the following tests and procedures:

- **Barium Swallow Study:** You will swallow a barium-containing liquid during this study, and you will then get X-rays. Your esophagus's interior is coated with barium, which causes any changes to the tissue to show up on an X-ray.
- **Examining Your Esophagus with a Scope (Endoscopy):** A flexible tube with a video lens, called a videoendoscope, is passed down your throat and into your esophagus by your doctor during an endoscopy. Your doctor looks for cancer or irritated areas in your esophagus with the endoscope.
- **Obtaining a Tissue Sample for Examination (Biopsy):** To take a sample of suspicious tissue for a biopsy, your doctor may use an endoscope, a special scope that is inserted down your throat and into your esophagus. A lab receives the tissue sample to search for cancerous cells.

7.2.5.7.1. Determining the Extent of the Cancer

In order to ascertain whether your cancer has spread to your lymph nodes or other parts of your body, your doctor might advise further testing if esophageal cancer is diagnosed.

Tests may include:

- Bronchoscopy
- Endoscopic ultrasound (EUS)
- Computerized tomography (CT)
- Positron emission tomography (PET)

Your doctor stages your cancer based on the data gathered from these procedures. Roman numerals 0 through IV represent the stages of esophageal cancer; the lowest stage signifies a small cancer that only affects the outermost layers of the esophagus. When a cancer reaches stage IV, it is thought to be advanced and to have spread to other bodily parts. As medical professionals advance in the diagnosis and treatment of cancer, the system for staging the disease keeps changing and growing more intricate. Your doctor determines the best course of treatment for you based on the stage of your cancer (Figure 7.6).

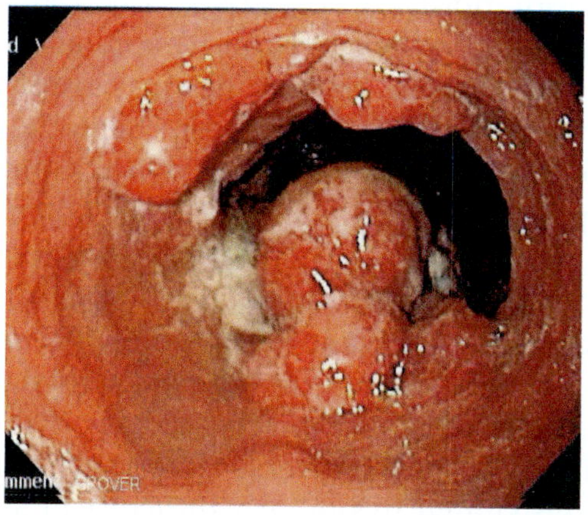

Figure 7.6. *Endoscopic image of an esophageal adenocarcinoma.*

Source: By Samir – http://en.wikipedia.org/wiki/Image:Esophageal_adenoca.jpg, CC BY-SA 3.0, https://commons.wikimedia.org/w/index.php?curid=2587715.

7.2.5.8. Treatment

The kind of cells causing your esophageal cancer, its stage, your general health, and your treatment preferences will all influence the treatments you receive.

7.2.5.8.1. Surgery

Cancer removal surgery can be used either as a stand-alone treatment or in conjunction with other therapies.

The following procedures are used to treat esophageal cancer:

- **Surgery to Cut Out Tiny Tumors:** In case your esophageal cancer is localized to the outermost layers and hasn't spread, your surgeon might suggest excising the cancer along with the surrounding healthy tissue margin. An endoscope that is inserted down your throat and into your esophagus can be used for surgery.
- An esophagectomy involves surgery to remove a portion of the esophagus. An esophagectomy involves the removal of the cancerous section of your esophagus, a portion of your stomach, and any surrounding lymph nodes by the surgeon. Your stomach is reconnected to the remaining esophagus. To accomplish this, the stomach is typically pulled up to meet the remaining esophagus.
- Surgery known as an esophagogastrectomy involves removing a portion of your stomach and esophagus. A larger portion of your stomach, adjacent lymph nodes, and a portion of your esophagus are removed by the surgeon during an esophagogastrectomy. After that, the remaining portion of your stomach is raised and joined to your esophagus again. You may use a portion of your colon to help connect the two if needed.

Serious side effects from esophageal cancer surgery include bleeding, infection, and leakage from the site where the stomach and remaining esophagus are reattached. Your esophagus can be removed surgically through an open procedure involving large incisions or laparoscopically, using a series of small skin incisions to insert special surgical instruments. Your surgeon's unique management strategy and the specifics of your case will determine how your surgery is carried out.

7.2.5.8.2. Treatments for Complications

Treatments for dysphagia, or difficulty swallowing, may involve the following.

- **Relieving Esophageal Obstruction:** If your esophagus has become narrowed due to esophageal cancer, a surgeon may insert a metal tube (stent) to keep the esophagus open using an endoscope and specialized instruments. Surgery, radiation therapy, chemotherapy, laser therapy, and photodynamic therapy are further options.
- **Providing Nutrition:** If you are experiencing difficulty swallowing or are undergoing esophageal surgery, your physician might suggest a feeding tube. After cancer treatment, a feeding tube allows nutrition to be given directly to your stomach or small intestine, allowing your esophagus to heal.

7.2.5.8.3. Chemotherapy

Chemotherapy is a medication used to destroy cancer cells with chemicals. In patients with esophageal cancer, chemotherapy medications are usually administered either before (neoadjuvant) or after (adjuvant) surgery. Radiation therapy and chemotherapy can also be used in tandem. Chemotherapy may be used alone in patients with advanced cancer that has spread outside of the esophagus to help relieve the disease's symptoms. The specific chemotherapy drugs you are prescribed will determine the side effects you experience.

7.2.5.8.4. Radiation Therapy

High-energy beams, like protons and X-rays, are used in radiation therapy to destroy cancer cells. Usually, radiation is directed toward your cancer by a machine outside of your body (external beam radiation). Or, less frequently, radiation therapy (brachytherapy) can be applied inside your body in the vicinity of the cancer. For patients with esophageal cancer, chemotherapy is most frequently combined with radiation therapy. It is usually used either before or occasionally following surgery. Additionally, radiation therapy is used to treat complications resulting from advanced esophageal cancer, such as tumor growth that prevents food from reaching the stomach. Radiation to the esophagus can cause adverse effects such as skin reactions similar to sunburn, difficulty or agony when swallowing, and harm to neighboring organs like the heart and lungs.

7.2.5.8.5. Combined Chemotherapy and Radiation

The efficacy of radiation therapy and chemotherapy combined may be increased. You might only receive combined chemotherapy and radiation therapy, or you might receive combined therapy and surgery at the same time. However, the chance and intensity of side effects are increased when radiation and chemotherapy are administered together.

7.2.5.8.6. Targeted Drug Therapy

Treatments with targeted drugs concentrate on particular flaws in cancer cells. Targeted drug therapies have the ability to kill cancer cells by obstructing these vulnerabilities. Targeted medications are typically used in conjunction with chemotherapy to treat esophageal cancers that are advanced or resistant to other forms of treatment.

7.2.5.8.7. Immunotherapy

A medication called immunotherapy strengthens your body's defenses against cancer. Because cancer cells produce proteins that make it difficult for immune system cells to identify cancer cells as dangerous, your body's disease-fighting immune system may not attack cancer. Immunotherapy functions by obstructing that procedure. Immunotherapy may be used to treat esophageal cancer in cases where it has progressed, returned, or spread to other body parts.

7.2.6. Esophageal Diverticulum

A pouch that extends outward in a vulnerable area of the esophageal lining is called an esophageal diverticulum. Anywhere in the esophageal lining between the throat and stomach can have this pocket-like structure. All ages can be affected by esophageal diverticula, but middle-aged and older people are the most common victims. In general, esophageal diverticula are uncommon; they are seen in less than 1% of upper gastrointestinal X-rays and less than 5% of patients who report having trouble swallowing.

Aspiration pneumonia, which is brought on by breathing in regurgitated diverticula content, dysphagia, regurgitation, and other gradually worsening symptoms are the most common complaints associated with esophageal diverticula. These diverticula typically grow slowly over many years. An obstruction near the diverticulum may make it difficult for a person to swallow when their esophageal diverticula symptoms worsen; in rare cases, the esophagus may burst. An esophageal diverticulum can rupture or cause an obstruction, both of which are dangerous complications that need to be treated right away.

Diverticulum-induced regurgitation frequently happens while you're lying down at night. This can result in lung abscesses, choking, and aspiration pneumonia, a lung infection brought on by secretions or foreign objects getting into your trachea and lungs. Squamous cell carcinoma is rare, but it can occur in 0–5% of people with diverticula. Long-term food retention is assumed to be the cause of this chronic diverticula irritation. It is crucial to remember that surgically treating diverticula is not justified by a fear of cancer.

7.2.6.1. Symptoms

The esophagus's internal pressure to push food into the stomach is thought to have the ability to herniate the lining of the esophagus through a weak spot in the wall, resulting in the formation of a pouch or diverticulum. Usually, there is obstruction at the distal end. Esophageal diverticula are more common in patients with esophageal motility disorders, such as achalasia, which can result in regurgitation of food, difficulty swallowing, and, in certain cases, pain that feels like a spasm.

Esophageal diverticula symptoms include:

- Dysphagia is a condition marked by difficulty swallowing and a sensation of food getting stuck in the throat.
- Aspiration of secretions or foreign objects into the lungs and trachea is known as pulmonary aspiration.
- Aspiration pneumonia is an infection of the lungs brought on by pulmonary aspiration.
- Spitting up saliva and food that has been swallowed.
- Pain when swallowing
- Cough

- Neck pain
- Weight loss
- Bad breath (halitosis)

A gurgling sound as air moves through the diverticulum may be heard by some people. Boyce's sign is what this is called.

7.2.6.2. Tests

The following are the most often utilized tests for esophageal diverticulum diagnosis and evaluation.

- **Barium Swallow:** After the patient swallows a liquid or other form of barium preparation, X-ray technology is used to assess the preparation's passage through the esophagus.
- **Gastrointestinal Endoscopy:** An endoscope is a thin, flexible tube that is inserted into the digestive system to project images of the inside onto a screen.
- **Esophageal Manometry:** This test assesses the timing and force of contractions in the esophagus and the relaxation of muscular valves.
- **24-h pHmetry:** A test to determine whether reflux disease (GERD) is present in the body.

7.2.6.3. Treatment

Modest cases of esophageal diverticulum can be managed with dietary modifications, thorough chewing, drinking lots of water after meals, and eating a bland diet. In the event that a patient's symptoms worsen, a number of surgical options are available to remove the diverticula, fix the defects, and enhance the patient's quality of life.

Treatment of diverticula require:

- An examination of the diverticula;
- Repair of the weakened wall; and
- Relief of obstruction

The size and location of diverticula determine the recommended surgical treatment, which may involve one or more of the following.

- **Cricopharyngeal Myotomy:** This surgical procedure, known as transoral robotic surgery, can be performed in an open or minimally invasive manner to remove small diverticula. The precise wrist-like movement of the robot during transoral robotic surgery enables the surgical removal of the tumor by moving in multiple directions through confined spaces and around corners. Utilizing instruments attached to the robotic arms and 3-D imaging, the surgeon guides the procedure from the command console, increasing precision.
- **Diverticulopexy with Cricopharyngeal Myotomy:** This procedure, which is used to remove larger diverticula, entails suturing the diverticular sac to the esophageal wall in order to suspend it.
- **Diverticulectomy and Cricopharyngeal Myotomy:** Since nearly a century ago, diverticulectomy has been used to treat Zenker's diverticula, which are the most common type of esophageal diverticula. Zenker's diverticula are typically located in the back of the throat, directly above the esophagus. This procedure is advised for diverticula larger than 4 centimeters, as it involves the complete excision of the diverticular sac.

- **Endoscopic Diverticulotomy (Dohlman Procedure):** The diverticular pouch and the cervical esophagus are separated by this procedure's division of the septum. Food can freely flow from the pouch into the esophagus due to the septum's division.

Patients can benefit greatly from minimally invasive (Laparoscopic) procedures like endoscopic diverticulotomy.

- Several small scars rather than a single, large abdominal scar.
- Shorter hospital stay
- Reduced postoperative pain
- Shorter recovery time
- Faster return to routine, including eating a regular diet.

Your medical team will go over the potential dangers and advantages of each procedure with you.

7.2.7. Esophageal Spasms

Painful contractions in the muscular tube that connects your stomach and mouth are known as esophageal spasms. The esophagus is the name of this tube. Esophageal spasms can cause abrupt, excruciating chest pain that subsides over a few minutes to several hours. It could be confused by some with angina, or heart pain. Esophageal spasms usually happen infrequently and may resolve on their own. However, there are instances when the spasms are frequent, which can obstruct the esophagus from receiving food or liquids. There are treatments available if your inability to eat or drink is caused by esophageal spasms.

7.2.7.1. Symptoms

Symptoms of esophageal spasms include:

- A tightness in your chest. Since the pain is frequently severe, you might confuse it for angina, another name for heart pain.
- Difficulty swallowing liquids and solids; occasionally associated with difficulty swallowing particular substances. The more frequent offenders are red wine and extremely hot or cold liquids.
- The sensation that something is lodged in your throat.
- Regurgitation is the term for the process of sending food and liquids back up your esophagus.

When to See a Doctor

A heart attack can also be the cause of the tightness in the chest that is linked to esophageal spasms. If you feel like your chest is tightening, get help right away.

7.2.7.2. Causes

The exact cause of esophageal spasms is unknown. Nonetheless, it seems that they are connected to abnormal nerve activity in the muscles that govern your swallowing motion. Food is often moved into your stomach by a series of well-coordinated muscle contractions in a healthy esophagus. The muscles that line the walls of your lower esophagus work in unison to move food down to your stomach when you have esophageal spasms. Distal esophageal spasm and hypercontractile esophageal spasm, also known as jackhammer esophagus, are the two types of esophageal spasms.

7.2.7.3. Risk Factors

There are no known risk factors for esophageal spasms.

7.2.7.4. Diagnosis

Your health care provider might recommend:

- **Esophageal Manometry:** This test assesses the force and coordination of the esophageal muscles, the rhythmic contractions of the esophageal muscles during swallowing, and the degree to which the lower esophageal sphincter relaxes or opens during swallowing.
- Upper digestive system X-rays, also known as esophagrams. After consuming a chalky liquid that coats and fills the inside lining of your digestive tract, X-rays are taken. Your doctor can see the outline of your stomach, upper intestine, and esophagus thanks to the coating.
- **Upper Endoscopy:** To examine the inside of your stomach and esophagus, your healthcare provider puts a thin, flexible tube down your throat that is fitted with a light and camera. We refer to this device as an endoscope. A tissue sample can be taken during an endoscopy in order to test for additional esophageal disorders. We refer to this tissue sample as a biopsy.

7.2.7.5. Treatment

The frequency and intensity of your esophageal spasms will determine how you are treated. Your doctor may initially advise avoiding extremely hot or cold foods if your spasms are sporadic in order to see if that helps.

Your doctor may suggest the following if your spasms make it difficult for you to eat or drink.

- **Managing Any Underlying Conditions:** There are situations when heartburn or gastroesophageal reflux disease (GERD) are linked to esophageal spasms. Proton pump inhibitors may be suggested by your physician as a GERD treatment. An antidepressant like imipramine (Tofranil) may occasionally be recommended. This medication might lessen esophageal pain perception.
- **Medications that Ease the Muscles Used in Swallowing:** Spasms can be lessened in severity by using peppermint oil, onabotulinumtoxin A (Botox) injections, or calcium channel blockers like diltiazem (Cardizem, Tiazac, and other brands).
- **Surgery (Myotomy):** In the event that medication is ineffective, your physician may suggest a lower esophageal slitting procedure. The myotomy procedure can help lessen the force of esophageal contractions. Since there are no long-term studies on this strategy, myotomy is typically not advised for esophageal spasms. If alternative therapies prove ineffective, it may be taken into consideration.
- **Peroral Endoscopic Myotomy (POEM):** It is a minimally invasive procedure. An endoscope is inserted through your mouth and down your throat using this new technique. This makes it possible for a surgeon to cut into the lining of your esophagus. The lower end of the esophagus's muscle is then cut by the surgeon, just like in a typical myotomy. POEM is typically only considered in cases where other

treatments have failed, much like standard myotomy.

7.2.8. Esophageal Strictures

A peptic stricture, also known as a benign esophageal stricture, is a narrowing or tightening of the esophagus that results in difficulty swallowing.

- **Signs and Symptoms:** Heartburn, an acidic or bitter taste in the mouth, choking, coughing, shortness of breath, frequent burping or hiccups, difficulty swallowing, vomiting blood, or weight loss are all signs of esophageal strictures.
- **Causes:** It may be brought on by or linked to lye ingestion, esophagitis, a malfunctioning lower esophageal sphincter, disordered motility, or a hiatal hernia. Following esophageal surgery and other treatments like laser therapy or photodynamic therapy, strictures may develop. A scar forms as the area heals, pulling and tightening the tissue and making swallowing difficult.
- **Diagnosis:** It can be identified by an endoscopy, a computerized tomography scan, a biopsy, or an X-ray taken while the patient is swallowing barium (referred to as a barium study of the esophagus).
- **Treatment:** In cases where esophagitis is the result of an underlying infection, treating the infection is the usual course of action (usually with antibiotics). A bougie, a weighted tube designed to dilate the constricted areas in the esophagus, can be inserted by a surgeon to open the stricture. In some cases, additional medications can be used to treat it. For example, a H2 antagonist (e.g., ranitidine) or a proton-pump inhibitor (e.g., omeprazole) can treat underlying acid reflux disease.

7.2.9. Hiatal Hernias

A hiatal hernia happens when the upper portion of the stomach pushes up into the chest through a tiny opening in the diaphragm, the muscle that divides the abdomen from the chest. This is in contrast to ventral hernias, which protrude through the abdominal wall. Acid and other contents are retained when there is a hiatal hernia because the stomach is compressed by this diaphragmatic opening. These acids and other chemicals have an easy time refluxing or regurgitating back up into the esophagus. Hiatal hernias come in four different varieties. Type I, or sliding hiatal hernias, account for the great majority of cases of hiatal hernias. This kind has a tiny diaphragmatic hole through which the stomach periodically slides up into the chest. Paraesophageal hernias are the term for hiatal hernias of types II, III, and IV. They arise from the protrusion of the stomach into the chest next to the esophagus.

7.2.9.1. Hiatal Hernia Causes

Hiatal hernia's precise etiology is unknown. Weakness of the supporting tissue could be the cause of the condition. You are more susceptible to the issue as you get older, become obese, and smoke. Hiatal hernias occur frequently. People over 50 years old are more likely to experience this issue. Acid reflux, or the backflow of stomach acid into the esophagus, may be connected to this illness. Most often, this condition is congenital, meaning it affects the child from birth. It frequently happens with gastroesophageal reflux in babies.

7.2.9.2. Hiatal Hernia Diagnosis

A medical professional may employ several diagnostic methods to find a hiatal hernia, but they will start with a physical examination and medical history. The supplier will ask about and/or search for:

- Acid reflux
- Sour or acidic taste in the back of the throat or mouth.
- Anemia
- Belching
- Difficulty swallowing
- Fatigue
- Heartburn

Additional diagnostics may include:

- To determine the position and location of the stomach organs, obtain a barium X-ray or CT scan of the upper digestive tract.
- **Endoscopy Examination:** To check for inflammation, your doctor will insert a thin, flexible tube called an endoscope—which is fitted with a light and video camera—down your throat, into your esophagus, and into your stomach.

7.2.9.3. Hiatal Hernia Treatments

Acid reflux and other hiatal hernia symptoms can be managed with medication and lifestyle modifications. In order to repair the hiatal hernia, surgery might be required. Your doctor will choose the best course of action for your hiatal hernia based on a number of criteria, such as your overall health, the location and size of the hernia, and the severity of any associated symptoms like acid reflux. Emergency surgery is always the first line of treatment for any rotation or twisting of the stomach or other abdominal organs that results in excruciating pain, blockage, or even possible strangulation with loss of blood supply.

7.2.9.3.1. Hiatal Hernia Lifestyle and Medication Treatments

Many people with hiatal hernias either have mild symptoms, such as heartburn, or no symptoms at all. Generally speaking, lifestyle modifications and medications like these can be used to manage the symptoms of hiatal hernias.

- Consuming food at least three to four hours prior to dozing off.
- Consuming modest to tiny amounts of food.
- Avoiding fatty foods, acidic foods like citrus fruits or juices, foods with caffeine, and alcoholic beverages.
- Achieving or keeping a healthy weight.
- If over-the-counter antacids or antihistamines do not relieve your symptoms, your doctor may recommend a stronger medication to help manage them.
- Sleeping with one's head slightly raised.
- Smoking cessation

7.2.9.3.2. Hiatal Hernia Surgical Treatments

When a hiatal hernia is repaired surgically, the stomach and any surrounding tissue are typically pulled down from the chest cavity and back into the abdomen through tiny incisions. In order to treat reflux, the surgeon may also reconstruct an esophageal valve and reduce the size of the diaphragm opening. An alternative is to repair a hiatal hernia through the chest.

7.3. Dysphagia

The medical term for difficulty swallowing is dysphagia. Dysphagia is sometimes a painful disorder. Swallowing may not always be feasible. Occasionally having trouble swallowing—for example, when you eat too quickly or don't chew your food thoroughly enough—usually doesn't mean anything serious. However, persistent dysphagia may be a dangerous illness that requires medical attention. Although dysphagia can occur at any age, older adults are more likely to experience it. Treatment for swallowing issues is based on the underlying cause, which varies.

7.3.1. Symptoms

The following are possible signs of dysphagia:

- Discomfort when swallowing.
- Not being able to swallow.
- Having the sensation that food is lodged in one's chest, throat, or behind the breastbone.
- Drooling.
- Hoarseness.
- Food regurgitating, also known as refluxing.
- Frequent heartburn.
- Backflow of food or stomach acid into the throat.
- Weight loss.
- Gagging or coughing during ingestion.

When to See a Doctor: Consult a medical professional if you experience weight loss, regurgitation, vomiting, or frequent difficulties swallowing due to dysphagia. Make an emergency help call right away if breathing becomes difficult due to a blockage. Visit the closest emergency room if you can't swallow because you feel like food is lodged in your chest or throat.

7.3.2. Causes

Swallowing is a multi-muscled, multi-nerve process. Dysphagia can be brought on by any illness that weakens or damages these muscles and nerves or narrows the esophagus or back of the throat. Generally speaking, dysphagia fits into one of the following groups.

7.3.2.1. Esophageal Dysphagia

The feeling that food sticks or gets trapped in the base of the throat or in the chest after swallowing is known as esophageal dysphagia.

Esophageal dysphagia has many causes, including:

- **Achalasia:** Swallowing difficulties are caused by the condition achalasia. The esophagus has difficulty forcing food and liquids into the stomach when there is damage to its muscles or nerves. Time usually makes achalasia worse.
- **Esophageal Spasm:** This disorder results in irregularly timed, high-pressure esophageal contractions, usually following swallowing. The lower esophageal wall's involuntary muscles are impacted by esophageal spasm.
- **A Narrowed Esophagus:** Large food fragments can become trapped in a narrowed esophagus known as a stricture. Narrowing can be caused by tumors or scar tissue, which are frequently brought on by GERD.
- **Esophageal Tumors:** Swallowing difficulties usually worsen over time when esophageal tumors are present. The esophagus gradually narrows due to growing tumors.
- **Foreign Bodies:** Food or other objects can occasionally cause a

partial blockage in the esophagus or throat. The risk of food particles getting lodged in the throat or esophagus may be higher in older adults wearing dentures and in those who have trouble chewing their food.

- **Esophageal Ring:** Occasionally, a small area of narrowing in the lower esophagus can make it difficult to swallow solid food.
- **GERD:** The tissues lining the esophagus may sustain damage from stomach acid backing up into it. This may result in lower esophageal spasm, scarring, or constriction.
- **Eosinophilic Esophagitis:** Immune system illness is known as eosinophilic esophagitis. It is brought on by an accumulation of white blood cells in the esophagus known as eosinophils.
- **Scleroderma:** Tissues become stiffer and harder due to the development of scar-like tissue brought on by scleroderma. The lower esophageal sphincter may become weaker as a result. Acid backs up into the esophagus as a result, frequently causing heartburn.
- **Radiation Therapy:** This cancer treatment may cause esophageal scarring and inflammation.

7.3.2.2. Oropharyngeal Dysphagia

When swallowing, food may be difficult to pass from the mouth into the throat and esophagus due to conditions that weaken the throat muscles. When trying to swallow, a person may choke, gag, cough, or feel as though food or liquids are going up their nose or down their trachea, or windpipe. Pneumonia may result from this. Oropharyngeal dysphagia can be caused by the following factors:

- **Neurological Disorders:** Dysphagia can be brought on by a number of illnesses, including Parkinson's disease, muscular dystrophy, and multiple sclerosis.
- **Neurological Damage:** Swallowing can be impacted by sudden neurological damage, such as that caused by a stroke or injury to the brain or spinal cord.
- Zenker diverticulum is another name for pharyngoesophageal diverticulum. Food particles get trapped in a little pouch called a diverticulum that forms in the throat, usually right above the esophagus. This can cause gurgling sounds, bad breath, and frequent coughing or clearing of the throat.
- **Cancer:** Swallowing problems may result from specific cancers and some cancer treatments, such as radiation.

7.3.3. Risk Factors

The risk factors for dysphagia are as follows:

- **Aging:** Swallowing problems are more common in older adults. This is caused by esophageal wear and tear, natural aging, and an increased risk of certain illnesses like Parkinson's disease and stroke. Disphagia, however, is not regarded as a typical aging symptom.
- **Certain Health Conditions:** Dysphagia is more common in people with specific neurological or nervous system disorders.

7.3.4. Complications

Difficulty swallowing can lead to:

- Dehydration, malnourishment, and weight loss. It may be challenging to consume enough food and liquids if you have dysphagia.
- **Aspiration Pneumonia:** Aspiration pneumonia can occur when food or liquid gets into the airway during attempts to swallow, causing bacteria to enter the lungs.
- **Choking:** Choking can occur from food getting lodged in the throat. Death may result if food completely obstructs the airway and no one performs a successful Heimlich maneuver to clear the airway.

7.3.5. Diagnosis

You will be questioned by your doctor regarding your symptoms. They'll probably ask you to name any foods or liquids that you find difficult to swallow. If you experience frequent heartburn or pain when swallowing, they will want to know. In addition, your doctor might inquire as to whether you have coughed up any blood. Your doctor may prescribe tests to determine the cause of your dysphagia if they believe you may have it. A barium swallow test is one that you might undergo. You will be required to consume a liquid that has a trace amount of barium throughout this test. Then, using an X-ray machine, the doctor can see it move through your body. This test can determine whether your dysphagia is being caused by an esophageal blockage or by another issue.

An endoscopy might also be necessary. The physician uses a flexible tube with a light at the end for this examination. They'll examine the stomach, esophagus, and the first segment of the small intestine. A biopsy is a tiny sample of tissue that the doctor may take in order to rule out cancer or other potential causes of your dysphagia. It is likely that you'll receive a sedative medication. You ought to feel more at ease and relaxed throughout the test as a result. You won't feel any pain when the tube is inserted because your throat will also be numbed. After the test and biopsy, your throat might become a little irritated.

7.3.6. Treatment

Treatments vary depending on the kind of dysphagia. A range of tests enable medical professionals and speech-language pathologists to examine different phases of the swallowing process when diagnosing and treating swallowing disorders. The Flexible Endoscopic Evaluation of Swallowing with Sensory Testing (FEESST) is one test that looks at how the swallowing mechanism reacts to stimuli like food, liquids, or a puff of air. It does this by using a lighted fiberoptic tube, or endoscope, to view the mouth and throat.

During a video fluoroscopic swallow study (VFSS), a physician will have you swallow multiple foods or liquids and the mineral barium to enhance visibility of the digestive tract. The test results will be a videotaped X-ray of the entire swallowing process. These pictures assist in determining the stage of the swallowing process at which you are having difficulty. Using this technique, speech-language pathologists investigate potential modifications that could provide a safe swallowing strategy. The modifications could involve the size, texture, or posture of the food, as well as behavioral techniques like the "chin tuck," which is the tactic of tucking your chin to prevent food particles and other materials from entering your trachea during swallowing. Despite rehabilitation techniques, if you are still unable to swallow safely, you may require short-term medical or surgical intervention while you heal. In chronic illnesses like Lou Gehrig's disease or amyotrophic lateral sclerosis (ALS), a feeding tube may be required in the stomach.

Treatment for some individuals may include muscle exercises to strengthen weak facial muscles or improve coordination, while others may need to learn specialized eating techniques. For example, some may need to eat with their head turned to one side or facing forward. Modifying food preparation or avoiding certain foods can also be beneficial in some cases, such as adding thickeners to drinks for those who have difficulty swallowing thin liquids. Others may need to avoid hot or cold foods. In some cases, individuals may no longer be able to consume enough food and liquids orally, requiring alternative methods for nourishment, such as a feeding tube system.

7.3.7. Prevention

While it is not possible to completely prevent swallowing difficulties, you can lower your chance of experiencing them on occasion by eating slowly and thoroughly chewing your food. See a medical practitioner, nevertheless, if you exhibit dysphagia symptoms.

7.4. Foreign Bodies

When a patient is evaluated for a foreign body in the esophagus, it is usually because they have accidentally swallowed a known object. In these cases, the patient is stable and exhibiting only mild symptoms. The difficulties arise from patients who are unable or unwilling to provide a history of the object consumed or the time it occurred, such as newborns, children, mentally impaired patients, psychiatric patients, and prisoners. Additionally, this can be a challenging condition to assess and treat due to the broad range of potential complications, as well as the wide range of possible symptoms and clinical presentations.

7.4.1. Etiology

The esophagus, which runs from the hypopharynx to the stomach in adults, is about 20 to 25 cm long. The esophagus is composed of two layers: an inner layer of mucosa and a muscular layer that consists of outer longitudinal and inner circular muscles. The lower third's muscles are involuntary smooth muscles, whereas the upper third's voluntary striated muscles enable the start of swallowing. The esophagus is the most common location in the gastrointestinal tract for an acute foreign body or food impaction, and 80–90% of swallowed objects that make it to the stomach will eventually pass without any medical attention.

There are many different objects that can accidentally be swallowed, but common items that get stuck in the esophagus include pieces of food (especially meat), fish or chicken bones, dentures, and coins. The types of objects that are ingested vary depending on the region and culture. For instance, in southern China, fish bones were the most commonly found foreign objects in the esophagus.

7.4.2. Epidemiology

Approximately 80% of patients who present to emergency rooms with an esophageal foreign body are children. These are usually inadvertent ingestions of small objects like coins, jewelry, toys, crayons, sharp objects like pins and needles, batteries, large food boluses, fish and chicken bones, and so on. The most frequent foreign object that kids swallow is coins. The majority of such cases have typical anatomy. However, abnormalities like eosinophilic esophagitis, prior esophageal atresia repair, and prior Nissen fundoplication increase the risk of impactions.

Similar unintentional foreign body ingestions also happen to adults; however, food boluses, primarily consisting of meat, are the most frequent cause of impaction in adults. It is estimated that there are 13.0 points of food impaction per 100,000 people annually. 80–90% happen in the distal esophagus and are linked to abnormalities in anatomy or motor function. Diverticula, webs, rings, strictures, tumors, eosinophilic esophagitis, achalasia, scleroderma, or esophageal spasms are examples of these anomalies. Because of this, it is advised that adults who have experienced food impaction in the past, even if it goes away on its own, have a follow-up esophageal evaluation.

7.4.3. Pathophysiology

The middle esophagus, where the esophagus crosses over the aortic arch, the lower esophageal sphincter (LES), and the upper esophageal sphincter (UES), which includes the cricopharyngeus muscle, are the three main areas of physiologic narrowing in the normal esophagus. Roughly 74% of foreign bodies in children are entrapped at the UES level. About 68% of adult obstructions are related to pathologic abnormalities and occur at the distal esophagus.

Local mucosal injury, such as abrasions, lacerations, necrosis, and stricture formation, is one possible consequence. Aside from esophageal injury, other serious complications include tracheoesophageal fistula, esophageal perforation, airway obstruction, and vascular injury (e.g., aortoesophageal fistula), mediastinitis, pericarditis, vocal cord injury, or retropharyngeal abscess. Three unique categories of foreign body ingestions that carry a higher risk of complications are sharp-pointed objects, multiple magnets, and button batteries (sometimes referred to as "disc" or "coin" batteries). The positive and negative poles of a button battery create an electrical current if it gets lodged in the esophagus. In addition to producing hydroxide ions that quickly raise the local pH and cause thermal injury, this current can also cause caustic alkaline injury. Within 15 minutes, an injury starts, and within hours, a perforation may result. Chronic stricture formation and localized esophageal mucosal necrosis are examples of complications. Esophageal perforation and erosion into nearby structures like the mediastinum, trachea, or vascular structures are more severe complications.

Multiple magnets cause issues, but a single small, smooth magnet will typically pass through without any issues. It is possible for tissue to become stuck between the magnets, which could result in volvulus, pressure ischemia, perforation, fistula formation, or obstruction. Sharp-pointed objects that become lodged in the esophagus also pose a greater risk of puncturing and must be removed right away.

7.4.4. History and Physical

The kind and quantity of objects consumed, the location, the amount of time since ingestion, and the patient's current signs and symptoms are all important considerations when evaluating patients who have ingested foreign bodies. These variables will assist in ascertaining whether the patient can be safely managed with observation and follow-up, or if the object needs to be retrieved emergently or urgently.

The majority of adults and older kids can recall the specifics of when they first consumed a foreign body. The most typical symptoms are dysphagia, or difficulty swallowing, or a sensation of a foreign body. Usually, symptoms appear within minutes to hours. The patient can locate foreign bodies in the upper esophagus more precisely. On the other hand, an ache, discomfort, or chest pain may be indicative of an impaction in the mid or lower esophagus. Hypersalivation, retrosternal fullness, regurgitation, choking, gagging, hiccups, and retching are additional symptoms. Patients who experience dysphagia may have more serious issues, such as an esophageal laceration or perforation. During examination, the patient might show signs of anxiety and difficulty swallowing. In the event that the patient is unable to swallow saliva, a complete obstruction is present and requires immediate medical attention.

It is possible that prisoners, mentally ill people, infants, and younger kids won't or won't be able to provide history. One must exercise a high degree of suspicion in these circumstances. Symptoms in infants and early children can include drooling, gagging, poor feeding, or irritability. Additionally, a foreign body lodged in the esophagus may press against the trachea, resulting in respiratory symptoms like stridor, coughing, dyspnea, or wheezing. Airway foreign bodies, however, would also have to be taken into account. Airway patency, vital signs, the patient's capacity to manage secretions, and the search for signs of complications like hematemesis, abnormal breath sounds, tenderness in the neck, chest, or abdomen, or subcutaneous air should be the primary focus of the physical examination.

7.4.5. Evaluation

Should a radio-opaque object be suspected, routine X-rays are typically the first course of action. This will assist in identifying the item, its location, and any potential issues. An XX-ray of the chest (posterior-anterior (PA) and lateral views) is usually sufficient, but depending on the clinical presentation, an X-ray of the neck and abdomen may be required. If flat objects, such as coins, bottle caps, or disc batteries, become lodged in the esophagus and appear round on the frontal (PA) view, they are typically oriented in the coronal plane. On the other hand, they orient in the sagittal plane and appear round on the lateral view if they are lodged in the trachea. If an X-ray shows a circular, "coin-like" object, it needs to be carefully examined to look for a "halo" or "double-ring" appearance, which would indicate that it is a button battery that needs to be removed right away. About 80% of coins and button batteries can be distinguished from one another using a chest X-ray's sensitivity, specificity, and accuracy. Food, wood, plastic, and aluminum cannot be seen on standard X-rays because they are not radio-opaque. X-rays may or may not show glass and bones. If routine X-rays reveal nothing and there is still a high level of suspicion regarding a foreign body, a diagnostic endoscopy or CT scan may be necessary. CT scans are helpful in identifying complications like perforation and have a high sensitivity for identifying foreign bodies.

7.4.6. Treatment / Management

Treatment and management are determined by the type of foreign body, its location, its degree of obstruction, and its duration, assuming that the airway is stable and that no complications are developing. The preferred method is endoscopic removal, which has a success rate of over 90% and a minimal rate of complications of less than 5%. There are three categories for endoscopic management: emergency, urgent, and nonurgent.

- Emergent:
  - Esophageal obstruction: incapacity to manage oral discharge.
  - The esophagus contains disk batteries.
  - Sharp objects lodged in the esophagus.
- Urgent (within 12 to 24 hours):
  - Objects in the esophagus that are not sharp.
  - Food impacts that are not totally blocked.
  - Sharp-pointed objects in the stomach or duodenum
  - Objects longer than 6 cm that are situated above the duodenum.

- A number of magnets (or one magnet plus an additional ferromagnetic object that is reachable with an endoscope).
- Coins in esophagus

- Nonurgent:
  - Anything bigger than 2.5 cm in diameter that is inside the stomach.
  - If asymptomatic, disk battery in the stomach for up to 48 hours.
  - Blunt items that don't pass through the stomach after three to four weeks.

Numerous medical management modalities have been investigated. Theoretically, drugs that relax the LES's smooth muscles might permit smooth, blunt objects to enter the stomach on their own. The most often talked about medication is glucagon; a sitting patient should receive a dose of 0–25 mg–2 mg intravenously (IV) over a period of 1–2 minutes. After a minute, this is followed by drinking carbonated beverages or water orally to encourage LES relaxation and esophageal distention. Glucagon may result in vertigo and nausea. Vomiting has the potential to loosen the object but also raises the possibility of an esophageal rupture. Unfortunately, the majority of glucagon studies have a number of flaws, such as small sample sizes, non-generalizable exclusion criteria, or inadequate power to assess side effects. As a result, most findings indicate little to no benefit over placebo. It is not advised to use papain, an ingredient found in meat tenderizers, for meat bolus impactions due to potential complications and a theoretical risk of esophageal damage.

It is truly an emergency and must be removed right away if a disc battery becomes lodged in the esophagus. The main cause for concern is the potentially fatal consequence of an aortoesophageal fistula, which is most likely to occur in children under five years old, as well as in cases of prolonged impact, impaction at the level of the aortic arch, and any degree of hematemesis. An interdisciplinary approach involving pediatric gastroenterology, pediatric surgery, cardiothoracic surgery, radiology, anesthesia, and operating room or cardiac catheterization lab management may be necessary in these particular cases. Children who are asymptomatic and have a coin lodged in their esophagus can be treated urgently and monitored for up to 24 hours without experiencing any more problems. Coin location is significant because within 16 hours of ingestion, 10% of coins in the proximal esophagus, 26% of coins in the middle esophagus, and 43% of coins in the distal esophagus pass spontaneously.

7.4.7. Differential Diagnosis

A foreign body sensation that persists after the passage of an object can be brought on by esophageal abrasions. Within 12 to 24 hours, the patient can be reassessed if they are stable and tolerant of oral intake; if not, further testing, such as an endoscopy or CT scan, may be required.

Other medical conditions that could result in a foreign body sensation even in the absence of a foreign body include:

- Infection caused by viruses like Cytomegalovirus (CMV), Herpes simplex virus (HSV), or Candida.
- Esophagite (acid reflux, pill esophagitis, eosinophilic esophagitis).
- Esophageal spasm
- Globus pharyngeus, also known as globus hystericus, is an unexplained sensation of a lump or foreign body in the throat.

Once more, if the patient is stable and able to take oral medication, start treating the underlying condition appropriately and/or set up a follow-up.

7.4.8. Prognosis

Within three to seven days, 80–90% of ingested foreign bodies will pass on their own. Short- and long-term follow-up is necessary for children whose disc battery-induced esophageal injury is to look for complications related to erosion or perforation and esophageal stricture. Adults with food impactions will require evaluation and treatment of the underlying abnormalities because they will exhibit abnormalities 85–90% of the time.

7.4.9. Enhancing Healthcare Team Outcomes

It takes an interprofessional team and interprofessional approach to manage foreign bodies in the esophagus. The majority of patients will show up at the emergency room, so the triage nurse needs to be knowledgeable about the warning signs and symptoms of an esophageal foreign body. These patients require admission right away. While the workup is ongoing, emergency department nurses must support the clinical team by keeping the parents informed about their child's condition and keeping an eye out for respiratory distress in the patient. It is strongly advised to consult with the relevant specialist as soon as the diagnosis is made. The majority of foreign bodies in the esophagus pass through on their own, but 3–10% might need medical attention. For some, an endoscopy may be necessary to remove the foreign object, while surgery may be necessary for others.

It is the responsibility of all clinicians and nurses working together as an interprofessional team to teach patients and caregivers to keep small objects out of children's reach prior to discharge. It is important to inform the parent about the symptoms of an esophageal foreign body and when to get medical attention. The only way to reduce this condition's morbidity is by using an interprofessional approach. When foreign bodies are found in the esophagus, the majority of patients have excellent outcomes.

A Closer Look

Plummer–Vinson (Patterson– Brown–Kelly) Syndrome

Dysphagia, iron-deficiency anemia, glossitis, angular stomatitis, koilonychia (nail-spooning), and achlorhydria are among the classic symptoms of this syndrome. The alimentary tract's mucous membrane undergoes atrophy. It mostly affects women over 40 years old. A web can be observed in the postcricoid region during barium swallowing and oesophagoscopy. This area has subepithelial fibrosis, which is the cause. In roughly 10% of cases, postcricoid carcinoma will develop in those with this syndrome. Moreover, it increases the risk of developing carcinoma in the stomach, pharynx, esophagus, buccal mucosa, and tongue.

Treatment

1. To treat anemia with parenteral or oral iron. Iron levels in the serum have greater significance than hemoglobin levels. Correction of related B12 and B6 deficiencies is also necessary.
2. Dilatation caused by oesophageal bougies in the webbed area.

Summary

- The esophagus is a 25 cm-long fibromuscular tube that carries food from the throat to the stomach. It starts at the cricoid cartilage's inferior border (C6) and ends at the stomach's cardiac orifice (T11).
- The most common perception of esophageal physiological issues is dysphagia, or difficulty swallowing. The physiology of the esophagus is hampered by obstructive esophageal lesions and disorders of esophageal motility, which cause a sensation of dysphagia.
- The esophagus, which is the tube that transports food from your mouth to your stomach, is impacted by esophageal disorders.
- Acid reflux from the stomach constantly runs back into the esophagus, the tube that connects your mouth and stomach, which is known as gastroesophageal reflux disease (GERD).
- Achalasia is a rare condition that impacts the esophagus, the tube connecting the throat and stomach. This disorder causes abnormal muscle contractions in the esophagus, preventing the proper movement of food towards the stomach.
- Barrett's esophagus is a disorder where acid reflux damages the lining of the esophagus, the flat, pink tube that connects the mouth to the stomach.
- Eosinophils, a type of white blood cell, are abundant in the lining of the esophagus in patients with eosinophilia (EoE). Eosinophils have the ability to release inflammatory substances into the tissues around them.
- The development of cancer cells in the esophagus, a tube-like structure that connects your throat to your stomach, results in esophageal cancer.
- A pouch that extends outward in a vulnerable area of the esophageal lining is called an esophageal diverticulum. Anywhere in the esophageal lining between the throat and stomach can have this pocket-like structure.
- Painful contractions in the muscular tube that connects your stomach and mouth are known as esophageal spasms.
- A peptic stricture, also known as a benign esophageal stricture, is a narrowing or tightening of the esophagus that results in difficulty swallowing.
- A hiatal hernia happens when the upper portion of the stomach pushes up into the chest through a tiny opening in the diaphragm, the muscle that divides the abdomen from the chest. This is in contrast to ventral hernias, which protrude through the abdominal wall.
- The medical term for difficulty swallowing is dysphagia. Dysphagia is sometimes a painful disorder. Swallowing may not always be feasible.
- When a patient is evaluated for a foreign body in the esophagus, it is usually because they have accidentally swallowed a known object. In these cases, the patient is stable and exhibiting only mild symptoms.

References

1. Castell, D. O., & Richter, J. E. (2004). *The Esophagus* (4th ed.). Lippincott Williams & Wilkins.
2. Galloro, G. (2019). *Revisiting Barrett's Esophagus*. Springer International Publishing. https://doi.org/10.1007/978-3-319-92093-1.
3. Katzka, D. A., & Metz, D. C. (2003). *Esophagus and Stomach*. Mosby.
4. Richter, J. E., & Castell, D. O. (2012). *The Esophagus*. Wiley-Blackwell. https://doi.org/10.1002/9781444346220.
5. Tilanus, H. W., & Attwood, S. E. A. (2001). *Barrett's Esophagus*. Springer Netherlands. https://doi.org/10.1007/978-94-017-0829-6.
6. Tilanus, H. W., & Attwood, S. E. A. (2001). *Barrett's Esophagus*. Kluwer Academic Publishers.

Chapter

RECENT ADVANCES

8

Contents

Introduction

Issues related to the ears, nose, and throat come up from time to time in life. Small illnesses like colds and pharyngitis incapacitate us momentarily but serve as a wonderful reminder of how wonderful health is. We take for granted the senses—hearing, sight, smell, unrestricted breathing, speaking, singing, and the effortless, effortless ability to swallow our own saliva. When these fundamental processes are compromised by disease, life becomes very challenging. While thousands of patients face these issues each year, some have been partially alleviated by recent advancements in otolaryngology. These issues have the potential to ruin the lives of patients for decades.

Orientation and Directional Terms

Term	Definition	Illustration
Buccal Mucosa	The buccal mucosa is the lining of the cheeks and the back of the lips, inside the mouth where they touch the teeth.	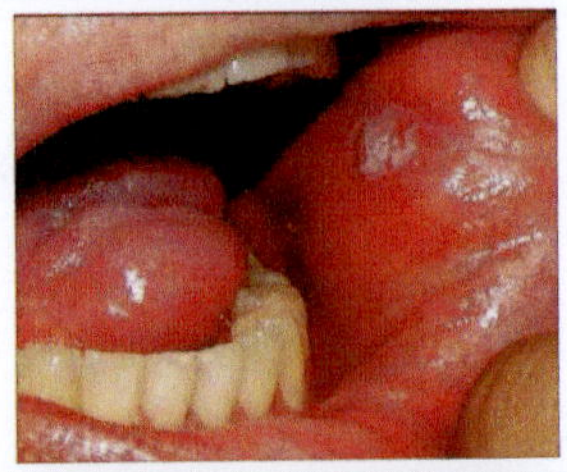
Gingiva	The gingiva, also known as the gums, is the pink-colored keratinized mucosa that surrounds and protects the teeth.	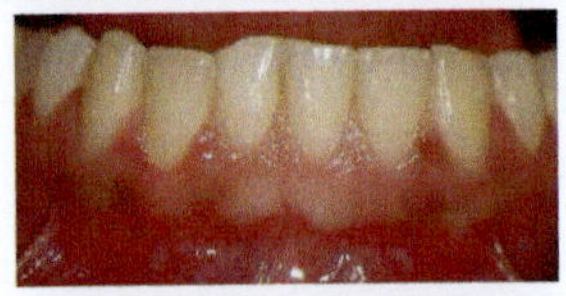
Floor Of the Mouth	The floor of the mouth is a horizontally aligned U-shaped space situated in the part of the oral cavity that lies beneath the tongue.	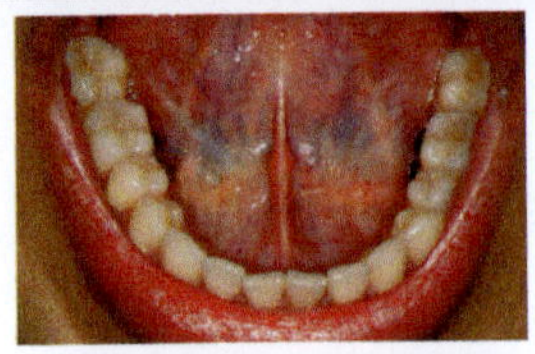
Retromolar Trigone	The retromolar trigone (RMT) is a small triangular subsite of the oral cavity. It is the portion of mucosa that lies behind the third molar tooth covering the anterior ramus of the mandible.	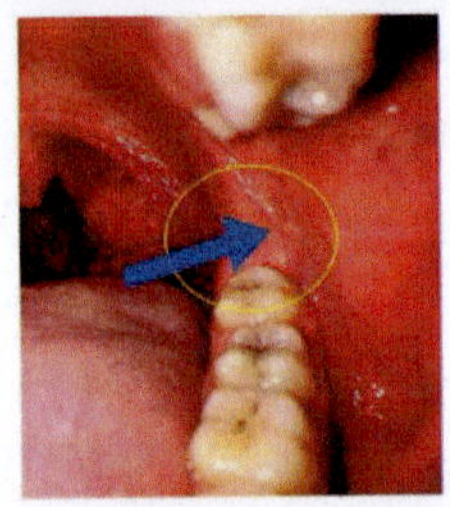
Hard Palate	The hard palate formally separates the oral cavity from the nasal cavities, forming the floor of the nasal cavity and the roof of the oral cavity.	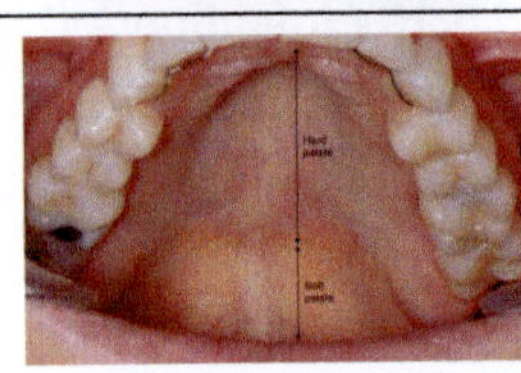

8.1. Laser Surgery, Radiofrequency Surgery, Hyperbaric Oxygen Therapy, and Coblation

8.1.1. Laser Surgery

In laser surgery, surgical operations are performed using specific light beams rather than tools.

8.1.1.1. Laser Physics

A simple laser is made up of two parallel mirrors, one of which is partially transmitting and partially reflecting, enclosing a laser medium, which sets the system's wavelength. An electrical source is used to excite the medium until the population inversion occurs, or when there are more atoms in the excited state than in the ground state. Upon activation, excited photons are spontaneously released in all directions by the laser medium. A tiny portion of these photons, nevertheless, move unison along the laser system's centerline between the mirrors. These photons are then reflected by the mirrors, amplifying the stimulated emission process. Then, a strong, coherent photon beam that manifests as laser light is released by the partially transmitting mirror (Figure 8.1).

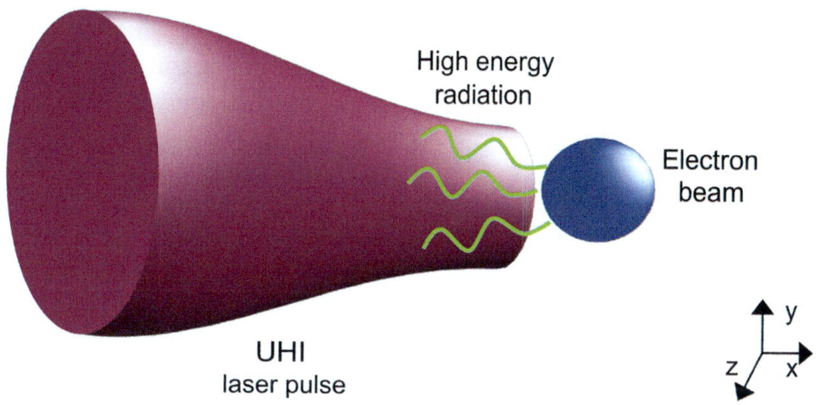

Figure 8.1. *An ultra-high intensity laser pulse colliding with an energetic electron beam.*

Source: *Vladisavlevici I-M, Vizman D, d'Humières E. (2022). Laser driven electron acceleration from near-critical density targets towards the generation of high energy γ-photons. Photonics, 9(12), 953. https://doi.org/10.3390/photonics9120953.*

8.1.1.2. Laser-Tissue Interaction

The characteristics of the tissue and the laser both affect how a laser affects a sample of tissue. The structure, water content, density, heat capacity, thermal conductivity, and the tissue's capacity to absorb, scatter, or reflect energy are among its characteristics. The laser's power, density, energy content, and wavelength are its properties that are involved. The primary biological targets that are targeted have very different light-absorbing spectra, and the wavelength of the incident photon energy determines their optimal absorption spectra. Melanin and hemoglobin are the primary target chromophores (any material that absorbs light) for visible light and some near-infrared lasers, whereas water is the only chromophore for CO_2 lasers. The target tissue must contain chromophores that absorb a particular laser wavelength, and these chromophores should not be present in the surrounding tissue, in order to achieve selective photo thermolysis (using energy at high peak powers and short pulse widths to destroy the intended target alone) without harming the surrounding tissue.

The most widely used lasers in medicine are the CO_2, Nd:YAG, and Argon lasers. The CO_2 laser emits light at a wavelength of 10,600 nm using carbon dioxide gas as its medium. Despite being tissue-selective, CO_2 lasers cannot be used for selective photothermolysis because their chromophore, water, is ubiquitous. Deeper tissue damage is avoided because all of the incident energy is absorbed in the tissue water up to a certain depth. Since CO_2 lasers operate in the invisible infrared wavelength range, precise treatment necessitates the use of an aiming beam. When the laser is focused on the tissue, it produces a very high power density that causes the tissue to instantly evaporate and be ablationed. The surgeon can quickly switch the laser from incision mode to bulk vaporization or coagulation by defocusing the beam because the irradiance of the laser beam is proportional to the inverse of the square of the beam diameter. There are several beam modes available for the CO_2 laser, and each one interacts with tissue in a unique way. The most basic mode is continuous wave (CW), which involves emitting the laser beam, running it for a predetermined amount of time, and then shutting it off. However, more modern lasers are quasi-CW (ultrapulsing), which means they generate brief pulses with high peaks and long intervals between them. The benefit of this is that because each pulse is delivered faster than the target tissue cools, it allows for more precise incisions with less heat build-up.

Neodymium ions are coated on a single YAG crystal bar, which serves as the active medium of the Nd:YAG laser. The neodymium ions in this system determine the wavelength of light it produces, which is 1,060 nm (5). The interaction between the Nd:YAG laser and tissue primarily results in a scattering effect because there are no important tissue chromophores at this wavelength. Reflection from scattering makes it impossible to create the usual narrow, cohesive beam. As a result, the tissue heats up more slowly and the laser's penetration ability is reduced. This characteristic of the Nd: YAG laser makes it perfect for many endoscopic procedures across different specialties, as well as hemostasis and tumor necrosis. Ion lasers function similarly to gas lasers, with the exception that they ionize the active medium. Examples of these lasers are argon and krypton. This requires a big power source and excites ions rather than atoms. The two most potent beams are in the blue (488 nm) and green (514 nm) regions of the spectrum. They can produce wavelengths anywhere between 250 and 530 nm and operate in both pulsed and continuous wave (CW) modes.

8.1.1.3. Clinical Applications of Lasers

The use of lasers has grown in popularity in modern medicine as less invasive methods for treating various pathologic processes are constantly being explored. Apart from their operational utility in the operating room, lasers are extensively employed in ophthalmology, lithotripsy, cancer diagnosis and treatment, as well as dermatology and cosmetic activities.

8.1.1.3.1. Lithotripsy

For the past few decades, laser lithotripsy has been a commonly used method for the fragmentation of biliary and urinary stones. Lasers can either have a primarily photothermal effect or a photoacoustical/photomechanical effect (also known as laser-induced shockwave lithotripsy). The most widely used shockwave laser for lithotripsy is the 1-μsec pulsed-dye laser, which has been the subject of extensive research. This apparatus produces the monochromatic light that breaks up the calculi by excite rating coumarin dye. Its safe use is made possible by the green light it emits at 504 nm, which is mostly absorbed by the yellow-colored urinary calculi and does not significantly harm nearby tissues. The excited ions that are released when the stone absorbs the laser's energy rapidly expand and pulse, encircling the stone and producing a shock wave that shatters the calculus into pieces. As nonabsorbent colorless calculi like those made of cystine are unabsorbent to this laser, photosensitizers, or dye, have been used as irrigation fluids and absorbents to effectively start the fragmentation process. This method is also used by the Q-switched Nd:YAG laser to achieve lithotripsy, although the shockwaves it produces are stronger.

In contrast, the long-pulsed Holium:YAG laser fragments calculi primarily through photothermal mechanisms (Figure 8.2A). Water can absorb a great deal of the 2,100 nm wavelength of light that the laser produces. As a result, in the right conditions, the fluid absorbs the energy and becomes heated. The result is a cloud of vapor that separates the water and lets the laser light that is still in direct contact with the calculus surface pierce it, causing it to shatter.

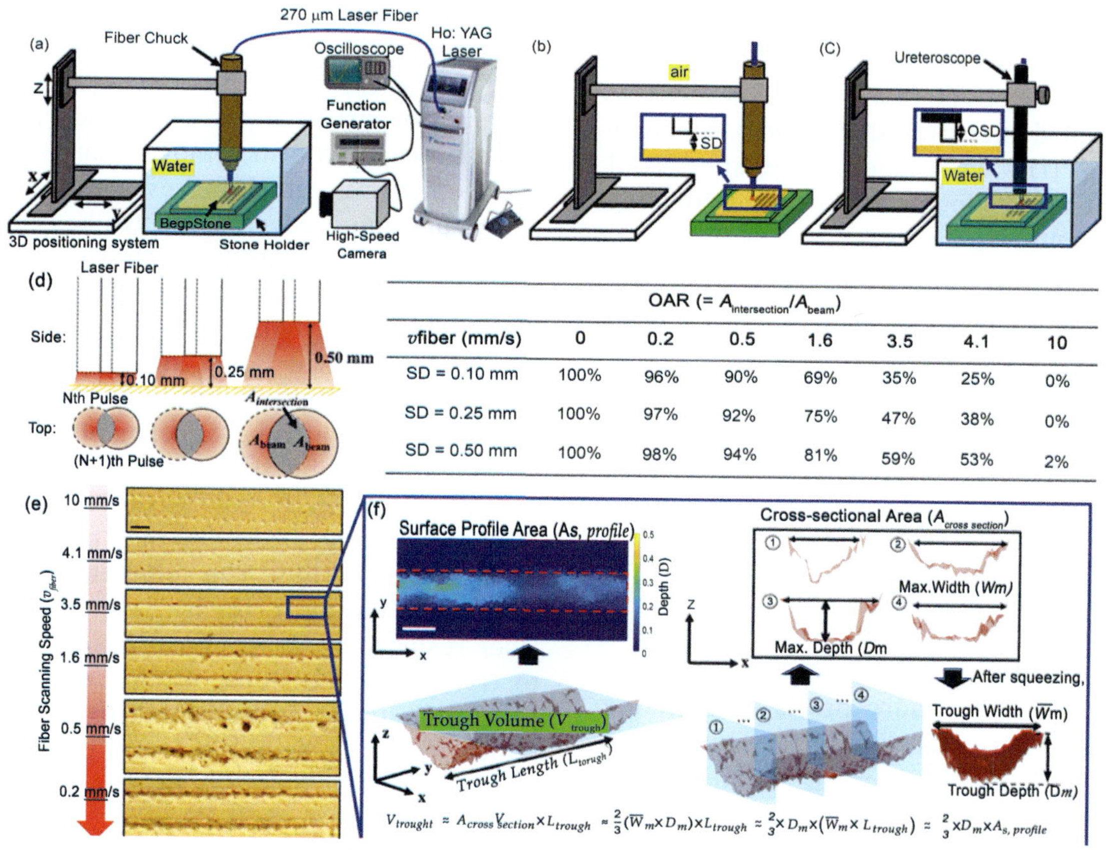

Figure 8.2. *Demonstrates a Ho: YAG lithotripsy laser.*

Source: *Chen J, Li D, Yu W, Ma Z, Li C, Xiang G, Wu Y, Yao J, Zhong P. (2022). The effects of scanning speed and standoff distance of the fiber on dusting efficiency during short pulse holmium: YAG laser lithotripsy. Journal of Clinical Medicine, 11(17), 5048. https://doi.org/10.3390/jcm11175048.*

8.1.1.3.2. Oncology

Cancers that develop in different organ systems can now be treated with lasers in a safe manner. For patients who are not the best candidates for surgery, laser interstitial thermal therapy (LITT) is the recommended course of treatment in neurosurgery. Lasers have proven to be a safe and effective tool in neurosurgery since their inception. They have been used to treat hard and hemorrhagic tumors like meniniomas, tumors of the deep skull base, and tumors deep within the ventricles, as well as unresectable gliomas. Currently, a variety of superficial gastrointestinal cancers, such as early gastric cancer, superficial esophageal cancer, colorectal adenoma, and high-grade Barrett's esophagus, are being successfully treated with mucosal ablation techniques that use lasers. Additionally, it has been demonstrated that photodynamic therapy (PDT) with lasers is a successful treatment option for particular kinds of lung cancer lesions.

Since direct laser ablation produces photochemical, photomechanical, and photothermal effects, it has been used to directly destroy cancer cells. The photochemical reactions that take place eventually result in the formation of toxic radicals, which cause tissues to die; the photomechanical reactions stress the tissue and cause it to fragment; and the photothermal reactions cause heating and coagulation, which kill cells. PDT was created almost a century ago with the goal of improving this procedure and more precisely targeting the intended tumor cells. Since then, it has become extremely popular. In this treatment method, a photosensitizing medication is first administered, and then the target area is exposed to visible light with an absorbance wavelength matching the photosensitizing medication. Following activation, the photosensitizer forms an excited singlet state before changing into a triplet state. In the presence of oxygen, these states give rise to reactive oxygen species, which are lethal to cancerous cells. On the other hand, localized light-absorbing dye is used in selective photothermal therapy to increase the tumor cell destruction by laser.

8.1.1.3.3. Aesthetic and Reconstructive Surgery

Lasers are an extremely useful tool in reconstructive and cosmetic surgery because of their exceptional capacity to target particular tissue layers and structures. Since it is known to reduce the effects of photoaging by inducing new collagen formation, laser resurfacing has become a major tool in anti-aging medicine. Ablative CO_2 and Er:YAG laser systems were used in the early skin resurfacing procedures to target a particular area of the dermis. But these procedures also remove a large portion of the epidermis, which causes a longer healing period and more adverse effects like erythema and infections. To address these problems, nonablative lasers were later developed, mainly releasing infrared light. Examples of these lasers are intense pulsed light, Nd:YAG, diode, and Er:glass lasers. These systems aim to target the dermal water, which heats collagen and causes remodeling during the process. No external wound is created and tissue evaporation is prevented by a system that concurrently cools the epidermis. The foundation for skin resurfacing has most recently been fractionated laser resurfacing. Fractionated lasers are used to treat small portions of skin at a time by producing tiny thermal damage zones (also known as "microscopic thermal zones") with fine beams of high-energy light.

In cosmetic surgery, laser-assisted lipolysis—which employs an optical fiber placed inside a 1-mm cannula—has also grown in popularity. Because the cannula is so small, a smaller incision is required, which minimizes bleeding and scarring. Because they have the lowest absorption coefficient in fat tissue among all the lasers available for medical use, 920 nm lasers are able to reach deeper tissue layers. The highest absorption coefficient in fat is found in those whose wavelengths fall between 1,320 and 1,444 nm. This results in a lower penetration depth and permits superficial treatment of fat tissues. Because fat tissue absorbs light at a wavelength that allows for good penetration depth and medium absorption, the Nd:YAG laser (1,064 nm) is the most commonly used system for laser lipolysis. This results in only a moderate temperature elevation and less tissue damage. Furthermore, there is substantially less blood lost during the procedure because the laser light at this wavelength causes the coagulation of tiny blood vessels.

Lastly, lasers are a perfect tool for treating vascular defects like port-wine stains because of their capacity to target pathologic vasculature specifically. Patients had few options for treating these kinds of abnormalities before lasers were used. For this purpose, however, hemoglobin-absorbing lasers are currently preferred over melanin-absorbing lasers, causing minimal damage to the epidermis. Longer wavelength lasers, which can penetrate deeper into tissue, have also been introduced more recently.

8.1.1.3.4. Ablation of Conductive Pathways

Catheter ablation devices were developed for circumferential PV isolation (PVI) after it was found that the pulmonary veins (PV) are a major source of ectopic beats that cause the paroxysms of atrial fibrillation (AF). One of the endoscopic ablation systems (EAS) that is frequently used to treat atrial fibrillation (AF) these days is the laser balloon catheter. The apparatus is made up of a catheter that is continuously flushed with deuterium oxide and has a compliant balloon at the tip. After the catheter is inserted into the left atrium, the ablation target inside the heart can be directly seen thanks to the endoscope that is inserted into the catheter shaft. A 980 nm diode laser, housed in the central lumen, is used for ablation. It emits laser energy perpendicular to the catheter shaft, covering a 30° angle arc and enabling circular ablation around each PV. Deuterium oxide is not absorbed by lasers at this wavelength.

Consequently, it passes through tissue beyond the endothelium and is absorbed by water molecules, which causes coagulation necrosis and heating. It is possible to titrate the energy delivered by varying the power (5.5–12 W) within a range of predetermined levels. Depending on which cardiac wall is being targeted, the energy levels change. Another popular laser system for this purpose is the Nd:YAG laser.

To effectively produce a full conduction block, the heart's transmural lesion needs to be made fully. MRI-guided laser-induced thermal therapy (MRgLITT) is a frequently used disconnection tool or method of ablating the epileptic foci in neurological surgery for treating refractory epilepsy. With the help of imaging technology and a diode laser operating at 980 nm, MRgLITT can deliver intraoperative data that is required for managing the energy dosage. Since their creation, lasers have been used in medicine far and wide, often being necessary. Laser therapy has improved many diseases, from potentially fatal illnesses to psychologically upsetting cosmetic flaws, eventually helping patients and doctors alike. Up until now, the development of laser technology has resulted in less invasive procedures, quicker recovery periods, and lower risks to the health of the patient. The use of lasers in medicine is expected to grow as their accuracy and safety continue to increase, offering safer procedures, better disease clearance, and higher levels of patient satisfaction.

8.1.2. Radiofrequency Surgery

Surgically, tissues have had their volume reduced by using radio waves. It has been applied to the base of the tongue to relieve sleep apnea, the inferior turbinates to relieve nasal obstruction, and the soft palate to relieve upper airway resistance, primary snoring, and sleep apnea. Additionally, it has been applied to the management of lingual thyroid. The radiofrequency (RF) device produces very high frequency electromagnetic waves that range from 350 kHz to 4 MHz. 460 kHz is often utilized. Depending on the ablation site, multiple probes are used to deliver radiofrequency. When the probe is inserted into the tissues, it heats them up, agitates the ions within, and causes tissue necrosis and protein coagulation without burning. In three weeks, there will be a decrease in tissue size and subsequent scar formation. The standard range for temperature control is 80–85°C. The power (measured in Watts), temperature (in degrees Celsius), resistance (measured in Ohms), treatment time (measured in seconds), and total energy delivered (measured in joules) are the key radiofrequency parameters (i.e., Watt × seconds); all of them are controllable within the apparatus.

Additionally, tonsillotomies, myringotomies, uvulopalatoplasty, correction of rhinophyma, and cosmetic removal of skin lesions have all been accomplished with radiofrequency using various types of electrodes. Tissues are cut and coagulated with radiofrequency, causing the least amount of charring and lateral tissue damage. It is a minimally invasive procedure that can be carried out outside. Problems are not very many. The processes are economical.

8.1.2.1. Radiofrequency Tonsillectomy

To prepare the tonsil for tonsillar dissection, the tonsils were exposed on both sides, and the plane was cut or opened using the Rf needle or to-bite radiofrequency forceps. Hemostasis was simultaneously achieved during dissection by using the same technique. Post-operative pain scores were low and bleeding was minimal if the procedure was performed correctly. After surgery, the fossa stiffens and deepens. Rf settings are as follows: 2–3 for cutting and 5–6 for coagulation.

8.1.2.2. Radiofrequency Adenoidectomy

It can be carried out following the coagulation of the adenoid using bipolar forceps and the retracting of the lower palate using tongue depressors or tourniquets. A ball point or Rf needle can also be used to dissect the adenoid's lower edge. Little bleeding occurs, and the wound heals quickly. There were no instances of post-operative hemorrhage. Perfect for recurring head pain with the Rf setting: 5–6 in the coagulation mode.

8.1.2.3. Radiofrequency Somnoplasty

The goal of temperature-controlled Rf volumetric palate tissue reduction is to scar or stiffen the soft palate. Energy delivery to the soft palate is accomplished at different points using the Sutter Rf bipolar probe. Blanching must not be done. The subsequent six-week period saw a stiffening. The operations can be performed in-office and under local anesthesia; there was very little pain and no bleeding during the process. Even after just one sitting, there was a subjective reduction in snoring.

8.1.2.4. Radio Frequency Tongue Base Reduction

By applying radiofrequency (Rf) energy to various posterior tongue base sites using Sutter RF bipolar probes, a temperature-controlled, volumetric reduction of the tongue base is accomplished. There is a noticeable decrease in tongue base tissue after three application sessions. No cases of infection or tongue base edema were observed. Both local and general anesthesia are options for the procedure. Radiofrequency UP3 (Rf -ssisted uvulopalatopharyngoplasty) is accomplished by tonsillectomy with pillar suturing and uvular and lateral incisions made while Rf is in cutting mode. The widening, contracture, and stiffening that occurs after surgery aid in the successful outcome. The uvular and lateral cuts made during RAUP (Rf-Assisted Uvulopalatoplasty) are used to redefine the posterior pillars and treat snoring, perhaps combined with a tonsillectomy. Fibrosis-induced healing and the subsequent removal of superfluous mucosa are the reasons it produces the desired effect. In most cases, a subjective reduction in snoring is attained. Rf is utilized in the cutting mode.

8.1.3. Hyperbaric Oxygen Therapy in ENT

Hyperbaric oxygen therapy has gained popularity as an adjuvant therapy for otolaryngology, head and neck surgery. It is recommended for the management of ischemic facial cutaneous flaps, necrotizing anaerobic wound infections, and osteoradionecrosis of the mandible. Patients can heal more quickly if you raise the tissue oxygen level.

Hyperbaric Oxygen Therapy (HBOT) is defined as an intervention in which an individual breathes nearly 100% oxygen intermittently while inside a hyperbaric chamber that is pressurized to greater than sea level pressure [1 atmosphere absolute (ATA), which converts to 101.325 kilopascals (kPa)]. For clinical purposes, the pressure must equal or exceed 1.4 ATA (141.86 kPa) while breathing near 100% oxygen. By breathing 100% oxygen at high pressure, the oxygen dissolved in the plasma increases and consequently increases the oxygen that reaches the tissues. Three centuries ago, compressed gas was first used in medicine. The history of this type of treatment has seen both advancements and setbacks because of a dearth of scientific proof. Only in the past 40 years has solid science been available to back up some of its current uses.

8.1.3.1. Mechanisms of Action of HBOT

One of the most intriguing mechanisms that HBOT induces is angiogenesis, which is mediated by the release of omnipotent stem cells that can differentiate into endothelial cells as well as the production of key angiogenesis mediators like VEGF and HIF-1 alpha. Furthermore, it seems that HBOT-induced hyperoxia enhances microcirculation by causing red blood cells to become more distorted and by lowering blood viscosity. HBOT is also known to play a role in wound healing, where it is thought to produce reactive nitrogen and oxygen species. When combined, these function as growth factors, sand signal transducers, attenuate cell apoptosis, and minimize inflammation. Importantly, HBOT also works in concert with antibiotics to reduce wound infection by directly affecting anaerobic bacteria and indirectly affecting aerobic bacteria by boosting polymorphonuclear leukocytes' capacity for microbicidal activity.

8.1.3.2. Clinical Applications of HBOT in Otorhinolaryngology

In 2016, the European Committee on Hyperbaric Medicine (ECHM) reviewed the current indications for HBOT. HBOT is highly recommended as the primary treatment approach in otolaryngology for the following conditions: treating mandibular osteoradionecrosis; treating idiopathic sudden sensorineural hearing loss (ISSNHL); treating any case of compromised skin grafts and flaps (as soon as possible after the diagnosis of compromised grafts/tissues); and treating both pre- and postoperatively in cases where there is an increased risk for compromised skin grafts and flaps (e.g., a patient with weakened immunity, an infected or radioactive wound bed). Although there is not enough evidence to support this last indication, experts also recommend HBOT for treating soft tissue radio necrosis of the head and neck region, treating radio induced lesions of the larynx, and treating osteoradionecrosis in other bones. Its potential benefit in minimizing post-radiation sequelae has been the subject of recent studies. To increase the range of applications for this type of treatment, more randomized, controlled studies are necessary.

8.1.3.3. Adverse Effects

The side effects of HBOT are rare and usually temporary, making it a reasonably safe treatment option. The two primary mechanisms by which these complications can arise are either the toxic effects of oxygen or the effect of pressure on enclosed gas spaces. Ophthalmologic (for instance. severe cataract development, reversible myopia), and otorhinolaryngologic complications (e.g., sinus squeeze and ear barotrauma) are rare but typically mild and temporary injuries. Chest pain exacerbation, pulmonary edema, and retinal abnormalities are among the more serious, though less common, side effects of HBOT.

8.1.3.4. Contraindications

Untreated tension pneumothorax is the only complete contraindication. If oxygen hyperbaric therapy is being considered for treatment, there are a few relative contraindications that need to be aware of. Congestive heart failure, hyperthyroidism, convulsive disorders, febrile illness, and pulmonary diseases, chronic obstructive pulmonary disease) claustrophobia, and pregnancy are not suitable. A well-known therapeutic approach, hyperbaric oxygen therapy has been refined and updated in light of recent scientific discoveries. Its low cost and absence of severe side effects make it a great choice for treating a variety of surgical and medical conditions. More controlled and randomized studies are required in accordance with the evidence-based medicine principle before its indications can be expanded to include different kinds of clinical conditions.

8.1.4. Coblation

Coblation is a cutting-edge technique that uses natural saline and mild radiofrequency energy to rapidly and efficiently remove and shrink bulky tongue base tissue as well as soft palate tissue. Given that coblation does not function by means of heat, the surrounding healthy tissue is preserved, facilitating a quick and simple recovery. Surgeons in the fields of ear, nose, and throat (ENT) and other medicine have performed over two million procedures successfully using the tried-and-true, patented Coblation process. With a quick and easy procedure, coblation-assisted soft palate treatment is a medical innovation that can help you stop snoring.

This revolutionary treatment:

- Results in a 1–4 week improvement in snoring that is noticeable.
- Short general anesthesia is used for palate surgery.
- A brief general anesthetic is necessary before tongue base surgery.
- In some offices, the procedure typically takes less than 10 to 15 minutes. (After the procedure, patients usually return home shortly after).

8.2. Cryosurgery

Tissues that are quickly frozen to -30°C or lower and then slowly thawed are destroyed. This information has been applied to the management of a variety of head and neck lesions, such as benign, premalignant, and malignant neoplasms. The agents that are used to freeze the tissue are either applied through a closed system, like a cryoprobe, or through an open method, like liquid nitrogen spray or carbon dioxide snow. Based on the Joule-Thomson effect, a cryoprobe i.e., cooling results from compressed gas expanding quickly through a tiny hole. Presently in use probes have a tip temperature of -70°C or lower and come in a variety of sizes and designs to accommodate various cryoapplications. Additionally, some probes include thermocouples that can be used to track temperature by inserting them into the tissue. The closed systems that are clinically available use carbon dioxide, nitrous oxide, or liquid nitrogen.

8.2.1. Mechanism of Tissue Destruction

There are multiple ways that freezing results in cell death.

- **Dehydration:** As a result of the pure water inside and outside the cell crystallizing, the concentration of electrolytes rises. With the crystallization of the buffering materials, the medium's pH also shifts. Cell death is also caused by toxic concentrations of dissolved gases and urea.
- **Denaturation:** Lipoproteins make up cell membranes. Their denaturation allows cations to pass through the cell membrane. Cell lysis results from the thawing of cells that are now swollen with cations.
- **Thermal Shock:** This stops the cell's ability to breathe.
- **Vascular Stasis:** A vascular or arterial blockage of blood supply results in an ischemic infarct. After cryoapplication, capillary microthrombosis appears a few hours later. This mechanism explains why vascular tumors can be effectively treated with cryosurgery, e.g., glomus tumors, angiofibromas, or hemangiomas.
- **Cryoimmunization:** In experiments, autoantibodies unique to the frozen tissues have been observed. This is intended to offer tissue-specific immunity against recurrent tumor challenges.

8.2.2. Technique

Both local and mild general anesthesia can be used during cryotherapy treatments. Sometimes numbness results from freezing alone, so no anesthetic is needed.

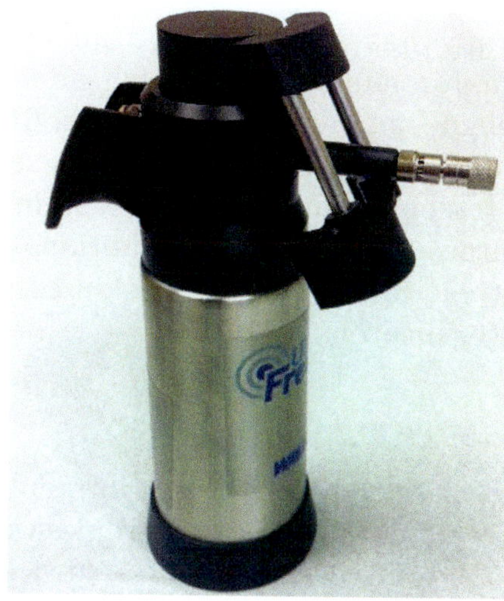

Figure 8.3. *Cryogun used to spray liquid nitrogen.*

Source: By Warfieldian – Own work, CC BY-SA 3.0, https://commons.wikimedia.org/w/index.php?curid=15833003.

Insulation is required in the area that will be frozen. The tissues are placed inside or on top of a suitable cryoprobe, rapidly frozen for three to eight minutes, and then allowed to slowly thaw. The process is carried out one or two more times. Normal tissue should be present around the frozen area. It is possible to implant a thermocouple to guarantee freezing at a suitable depth. Following cryotherapy, the secondary intention is used to allow the area to heal. In three to six weeks, the necrotic slough peels off. It might take more cryotherapy cycles to get the desired outcome (Figure 8.3).

8.2.3. Uses of Cryotherapy

8.2.3.1. Benign Vascular Tumors

It has been discovered that cryotherapy is effective in treating hemangiomas affecting the skin, mouth, or oropharynx. Additionally, it has been used as a supplement to treat vascular tumors like glomus tumors and angiofibromas.

8.2.3.2. Premalignant Lesions

Cryotherapy has proven to be an effective treatment for leukoplakia, which affects the cheek, tongue, and floor of the mouth. Because there is no lesion recurrence, better quality regenerated epithelium, and less scarring than electrosurgery, it is preferred. Additionally, it is used to treat solar keratosis, a skin condition that is precancerous.

8.2.3.3. Malignant Lesions

Skin cancers like Bowen disease (intraepithelial carcinoma) and basal cell carcinoma have been treated successfully with a cure rate of 94–97%. Because cartilage does not necrotize when frozen, cryotherapy is especially helpful in cases where a tumor is located over it. Multiple skin cancers can also benefit from it. This treatment approach should not be used for recurrent skin cancers or lesions with ill-defined margins. Cryotherapy has proven to be very effective in treating advanced cancers as well as recurrent or residual tumors. Debulking the tumor mass is the goal in these situations in order to aid respiration or deglutition, lessen the tumor's propensity to bleed, and alleviate pain. Curative cryotherapy has a limited role in treating primary malignant lesions of the oral cavity and oropharynx, however some success has been documented in treating early lesions ($T_1 N_0$) affecting the palate, tongue, and floor of the mouth. Because of this, cryotherapy should only be applied very sparingly to patients who fall into other high-risk categories and whose other conditions have limited their time to live.

8.2.3.4. Other Uses

Nasal turbinates have undergone cryotherapy to shrink and open up the airway. It has also been used to manage rhinorrhea and sneezing in cases of allergic rhinitis. In patients at low risk, tonsils have been cryodestroyed.

8.2.4. Advantages of Cryotherapy

1. Beneficial for patients with low risk and suitable for both local and no local anesthesia application.
2. Useful for individuals suffering from coagulopathies or bleeding disorders.
3. Can be used to treat multiple cancers and to palliate recurrent cancers when a second radiation treatment is not recommended.
4. Minimal pain or discomfort following treatment.
5. Leaves little scars behind.
6. Useful in locations known to form keloid formation, e.g., anterior region.
7. It is an outpatient procedure.

8.2.5. Disadvantages of Cryotherapy

1. If the lesion is small, there is no tissue available for a biopsy.
2. It is impossible to evaluate the tumor's margins to determine if they are free of cancerous cells.

3. No command over the freezing depth.
4. Cryotherapy for skin lesions results in hair follicle destruction, depigmentation, and hair loss.
5. The part must be anesthetized if the lesion is close to the nerve, e.g., either digital or ulnar.

Many of the indications for cryotherapy will decline with the introduction of laser therapy, but its lower cost will be a significant consideration in developing nations.

8.3. Radiotherapy in Head and Neck Cancer

As part of radiation therapy, high-energy particle beams are directed toward the tumor through the skin. The beams damage the DNA of the cancer cells as soon as they arrive at the tumor, destroying the cells. Radiation therapy is well-known for being especially successful in treating tumors of the head and neck. There are several ways to treat head and neck cancer with radiation therapy. Following head and neck surgery, it might be advised to stop the cancer from returning. It is also possible to treat someone just with radiation. Some patients may get radiation treatment in addition to chemotherapeutic measures or other medication therapies.

8.3.1. General Management of Specific Cancers by Region

8.3.1.1. Paranasal Sinuses

The standard treatment for these tumors is total surgical resection. For locally advanced primary tumors (T3 or T4 lesions), positive or close surgical margins, and unfavorable pathologic findings (high-grade perineural, lymphatic, and vascular invasion), postoperative radiation therapy is recommended. For diseases that cannot be cured, definitive radiation therapy or a chemotherapy and radiation regimen may be utilized. When patients with cancers of the paranasal sinus and nasal cavity receive combination therapy instead of radiotherapy alone, the 5-year local control rate is higher (79% vs. 48%).

8.3.1.2. Nasal Cavity

Because surgical excision of the nasal vestibule carcinoma results in an associated deformity, radiotherapy is generally preferred over surgery in this case. Excision via surgery is limited to minor, superficial lesions only. 97% of patients receiving definitive radiation therapy achieved local control. Both radiation and surgery are equally effective for patients with early-stage nasal cavity carcinoma. Surgery plus postoperative radiation therapy is the recommended course of treatment for advanced-stage nasal cavity cancers. Patients with early-stage lesions were able to achieve locoregional control rates of 60–80% with definitive radiation, while patients with advanced-stage lesions were able to achieve similar rates with combined surgery and postoperative radiotherapy.

8.3.1.3. Oral Cavity

The oral cavity includes the upper and lower lips, buccal mucosa, gums, ridge, trigone, floor, palate, and front of the tongue. Surgery and radiotherapy are typically used to treat oral cavity cancers, with the choice depending on expected outcomes. Treatment may vary based on complications, cosmetic changes, and functionality. The T and N classification of the patient also influences the treatment plan. For early-stage cancers, surgery or radiotherapy alone may be curative, while advanced tumors often require a combination approach. Some T3 lesions without lymph node involvement may only need one type of treatment. Chemotherapy can be beneficial for advanced cases. Surgery can quickly remove tumors with fewer dental and salivary issues. Advances in microvascular reconstruction techniques have improved outcomes for advanced diseases. Radiotherapy preserves anatomy and function, but can cause dry mouth, taste changes, and tissue damage.

8.3.1.3.1. Lip

Regarding local control, radiotherapy and surgery are comparable treatments for early-stage cancers. The degree of illness, the patient's preferences, the state of their health, and the expected functional and cosmetic outcomes all play a role in the selection of local treatment modalities. With surgical excision, some very small or superficial cancers can be treated more quickly and effectively without causing functional deformities or unsatisfactory cosmetic results. When a tumor occupies the commissure, definitive radiotherapy is recommended for moderately sized infiltrative cancers because surgical excision often fails to produce satisfactory functional and cosmetic outcomes. The final course of treatment could involve either interstitial implants, external beam radiation, or both, depending on the size of the tumors. For smaller lesions, interstitial irradiation is appropriate. Positive margins, perineural invasion, cervical lymph node metastases, and locally advanced disease all suggest postoperative radiotherapy. Patients with early-stage disease and a clinically negative neck can avoid elective neck irradiation, while those with advanced or recurrent diseases should have it. Local control rates with irradiation exceed 80%, and the 5-year survival rate is in excess of 95%.

8.3.1.3.2. Buccal Mucosa

Buccal mucosa tumors in their early stages are frequently treatable with radiation therapy or surgery. Definitive radiation therapy is recommended for intermediate tumors and those involving the oral commissure due to its high local control rate, good functional and cosmetic outcomes, and favorable side effects. Radical surgery and reconstruction are usually advised for locally advanced lesions involving the bones, gingiva, and buccogingival sulcus. Postoperative radiotherapy is then usually advised. After surgery, usually two to six weeks later, postoperative radiotherapy can begin as soon as wound healing is satisfactory. A prospective randomized trial evaluating the role of postoperative radiotherapy in patients with stage III and IV carcinoma of the buccal mucosa showed that the 3-year disease-free survival rate was 68% versus 38% for patients with and without postoperative radiotherapy. The 3-year overall survival rates were 94% versus 84%, respectively.

8.3.1.3.3. Oral Tongue

Surgery is often used to treat minor oral tongue lesions. Definitive radiotherapy is preferred for small lesions that are posteriorly located or poorly defined. Radiotherapy and surgery are usually the best treatments for locally advanced lesions. In addition, postoperative radiation therapy is advised in cases of perineural or lymphovascular invasion, as well as close or positive margins. Chemotherapy and radiation therapy may be used in cases that are not treatable. For patients receiving definitive radiotherapy, the reported local control rates were 79 to 83% for T1 lesions and 64 to 74% for T2 lesions.

8.3.1.3.4. Gingiva

The best course of treatment for gingival carcinoma is surgery due to the tumors' frequent involvement of the bone and the possibility of bone exposure following radiation. Radiation therapy alone can be used to treat small superficial gingival tumors that do not invade the bone. In patients with locally advanced diseases, postoperative radiation therapy is added. The whole mandible should be covered by the radiation portals when receiving radiotherapy. The neck lymphatics may be exposed to radiation therapy in patients with advanced primary lesions or positive neck lymph nodes. The reported local control rates are 71.5% for T1, 70% for T2, and 59% for T3 tumors.

8.3.1.3.5. Floor of the Mouth

Radiotherapy or surgery are easily used to treat lesions on the floor of the mouth that are in the early stages. For lesions that invade the tongue, definitive radiotherapy may be an option; however, it is not recommended for lesions that adhere to the mandible. For operable advanced-stage diseases, particularly for lesions involving the mandible, multiple cervical lymph nodes, and the tongue musculature, a combination of surgery and postoperative radiotherapy is advised. An alternate form of treatment for diseases that are locally advanced and incurable may involve the use of chemotherapy and radiation. For carcinomas of the floor of the mouth, interstitial implants, intraoral cone irradiation, and external beam radiotherapy are the available radiotherapy modalities. For small, superficial, or exophytic tumors, intraoral cone irradiation and interstitial implants are appropriate treatments. The reported 5-year local control rates were 93% for T1 lesions and 88% for T2 lesions.

8.3.1.3.6. Retromolar Trigone

Radiotherapy or surgery are used to treat diseases in their early stages. Generally speaking, surgical excision is the recommended method. Advanced localized illnesses necessitate both surgery and radiation therapy after surgery. The reported ultimate local control rates of patients treated with definitive radiotherapy and surgical salvage of irradiation failure is 100% for T1, 94% for T2, and 92% for T3 tumors.

8.3.1.3.7. Hard Palate

Hard palate cancers are typically treated with surgical excision. Postoperative radiation is added for high-grade mucoepidermoid and adenoid cystic carcinoma.

8.3.1.4. Nasopharynx

Nasopharyngeal carcinoma is generally very difficult to surgically treat because of its anatomic location and early propensity to involve retropharyngeal lymph nodes. Intensity-modulated radiation is gradually displacing conventional radiotherapy as the cornerstone of treatment. For primary nasopharyngeal tumors, surgery is not recommended; however, neck dissection following radiotherapy is recommended for persistent neck lymphadenopathy. A randomized Intergroup trial demonstrated that in terms of 5-year progression-free and overall survival rates, radiotherapy plus concurrent and adjuvant chemotherapy outperformed radiotherapy alone for patients with locoregionally advanced diseases.

Additionally, radiotherapy is the cornerstone of salvage treatment for locally recurrent disease. Brachytherapy with intracavitary insertion or interstitial implants has been used as a boost treatment modality after external beam irradiation in the treatment of primary or recurrent disease because of the quick fall-off of radiation dose with increasing distance from the radioactive source. Brachytherapy is generally not recommended for nasopharyngeal tumors that extend intracranially.

8.3.1.5. Oropharynx and Soft Palate

Excellent local control has been achieved for soft palate tumors in their early stages through definitive radiotherapy or surgery. Because the functional outcome is likely better and the treatment results are satisfactory, radiotherapy is typically preferred. Patients who have locally advanced lesions typically have postoperative radiotherapy after surgical excision. According to a recent randomized trial, concurrent chemoradiotherapy did not statistically increase severe late morbidity and instead improved overall survival and locoregional control rates when compared with radiotherapy alone. Thus, for locally advanced oropharyngeal cancers, concurrent chemoradiotherapy should be taken into consideration as an alternate course of treatment.

8.3.1.6. Tonsillar Region

Treatment options for tonsillar tumors in their early stages include surgery and definitive radiotherapy. Primary radiotherapy is the recommended and final treatment for the majority of tonsillar region T1, T2, and exophytic T3 tumors. Because radiotherapy produces a better functional outcome, it is preferred. Avoid irradiating the contralateral parotid gland in order to lower the incidence of xerostomia. Postoperative radiation therapy in conjunction with surgery is advised for lesions in the tonsillar region that are locally advanced. According to reports, the 5-year local control rates for T1 through T4 patients treated with definitive radiotherapy and surgical salvage of irradiation failure are 92%, 89%, 77%, and 65%, respectively. The 5-year disease-specific survival rates by 1997 American Joint Committee on Cancer stage were as follows: I, 100%; II, 86%; III, 82%; and IVa, 63%. For advanced disease treated with surgery followed by postoperative radiotherapy, local control was achieved in 94% of T3 lesions and 75% of T4 lesions.

8.3.1.7. Base of the Tongue

Early lesions of the tongue base may be treated with radiation therapy or surgery. Definitive radiation therapy is typically used to treat most patients due to its improved quality of life and functional outcomes. It is customary to recommend surgery and postoperative radiation therapy for patients with advanced disease. As an alternative course of treatment, a nonsurgical strategy like concurrent chemoradiotherapy for organ preservation may be taken into account. Definitive radiotherapy has achieved a local control rate of ~80 to 90% for T1 to T2 lesions and 70 to 85% for T3 lesions. For locally advanced cancers of the base of the tongue treated with surgery and postoperative radiotherapy, the 7-year local control rates have been reported to be 94% for T3 tumors and 75% for T4 tumors.

8.3.1.8. Oropharyngeal Wall

Early pharyngeal wall lesions may respond to radiotherapy or surgery. Because radiotherapy produces good results and causes less functional impairment, it is preferred. The best course of treatment for locally advanced lesions is surgery plus postoperative radiation. For pharyngeal wall cancers, the reported local control rates after radiotherapy were ~100% for T1, 67 to 92% for T2, 43 to 80% for T3, and 17 to 50% for T4 tumors.

8.3.1.9. Hypopharynx

Preserving swallowing function and optimizing control rates are the main objectives of treatment for hypopharyngeal cancer. Radiation therapy or surgery on its own is recommended for piriform sinus carcinomas classified as T1 or T2. For T1 and T2 lesions, the final local control rates that were reported for patients who received radiotherapy in addition to surgical salvage were 95% and 91%, respectively. Radiation therapy plus radical surgery is the usual treatment for diseases that have progressed locally. Certain establishments favor employing irradiation and saving radical surgery for situations where larynx preservation is not an option. The European Organization for Research in Cancer Therapy (EORTC) conducted a randomized trial of larynx-conserving treatment, which involved induction chemotherapy followed by definitive radiotherapy in patients who responded completely to chemotherapy, or surgery in patients who did not respond well. The results of the trial showed that the larynx-preserving procedures allowed two thirds of the survivors to keep their larynxes and had survival rates comparable to conventional treatment.

Tumors located on the back of the throat are often deemed inoperable, and doctors typically recommend definitive radiotherapy with or without chemotherapy. If surgery is chosen as the main treatment, patients usually receive postoperative radiotherapy as well. For patients treated with radiotherapy alone, 5-year local control rates of 70 to 100% for early lesions and 20 to 50% for advanced lesions have been reported.

8.3.1.10. Larynx

The maintenance of the airway and preservation of speech function are the primary considerations when selecting a treatment modality for laryngeal cancer. Radiation therapy or surgery are the most effective treatments for most cases of early-stage laryngeal cancer. For T1 and T2 glottic tumors, definitive radiation therapy is generally the preferred treatment. After radiotherapy fails, surgery is saved for salvage. It is not recommended to electively irradiate the neck lymphatics because early glottic cancers rarely spread to the local lymph nodes. Five-year local control rates for T1 glottic tumors were 78 to 93% after definitive radiotherapy. For T2 glottic tumors treated with radiotherapy alone, 5-year local control rates of 72 to 73% have been reported. Individuals with T3 lesions primarily affecting one side of the larynx are counseled to consider surgical salvage or definitive radiotherapy. It is nearly always necessary to perform a total laryngectomy followed by postoperative radiation therapy for advanced T3 and T4 glottic tumors. For patients whose tumors are medically inoperable or who refuse laryngectomy, definitive radiotherapy or concurrent chemoradiotherapy is recommended. Surgery is saved for cases of treatment failure and is now reserved for patients with locally advanced carcinoma of the larynx who have not responded well to chemotherapy or radiotherapy.

Radiation therapy or surgery can be used to treat supraglottic cancers in their early stages. The voice may be preserved through radiotherapy or surgery. The outcomes of definitive radiotherapy and patients undergoing supraglottic laryngectomies are similar. With a 5-year local control rate of 58% for T1 lesions, supraglottic cancers respond to radiation therapy less favorably than glottic cancers. Surgery and postoperative radiation therapy are frequently needed for locally advanced supraglottic cancers. Although they are not common, subglottic cancers are usually treated with surgery. In cases where there is cartilage invasion or positive surgical margins, postoperative radiotherapy is recommended.

8.3.1.11. Salivary Glands

Radiotherapy is a treatment option for malignant tumors of the salivary glands that are either inoperable or have recurred after being previously unirradiated. Postoperative radiotherapy is generally indicated for the following conditions: high-grade lesions, such as adenoid cystic carcinoma; perineural and vascular invasion; positive or close surgical margins; and regional lymph node metastasis. Postoperative radiotherapy significantly improved survival and local control in patients with advanced-stage malignant salivary gland tumors, according to a matched-pair analysis. For patients receiving postoperative radiotherapy, the 5-year local control and survival rates were higher than for those undergoing surgery alone (local control rates 51% vs. 17%; survival rates 51% vs. 10%).

8.3.1.12. Thyroid Gland

The cornerstones of thyroid cancer treatment are radioiodine therapy and surgery. For some patients, radiotherapy may be an option. The indications for radiotherapy for patients with differentiated thyroid cancers include inoperable lesions, recurrence following maximal radioiodine therapy, tumors exhibiting low radioiodine uptake, and bulky residual tumors following surgery that are unlikely to absorb enough radioiodine to achieve a therapeutic radiation dose. When a tumor is inoperable, radiotherapy is used to treat medullary carcinoma. The best treatment for anaplastic thyroid cancer involves a combination of surgery, radiation, and chemotherapy.

8.3.2. Intensity-Modulated Radiation Therapy

The planning and administration of radiotherapy treatments have been significantly enhanced by recent developments in radiation physics, computer technology, imaging technology, and radiotherapy facilities. With the help of technological advancements like inverse treatment planning and the linear accelerator equipped with a multileaf collimator, intensity-modulated radiation therapy (IMRT) has been successfully implemented. Using a computer-controlled multileaf collimator and computer-optimized inverse treatment planning, IMRT is a sophisticated type of three-dimensional conformal radiotherapy. By using these techniques, it is possible to modulate the radiation intensity to deliver a higher dose to targets with a sharply conformal target volume coverage, while also significantly reducing the dose to the surrounding normal tissues. As a result, there are methods for administering radiation therapy that maintain the greatest amount of vital organs and functions. In recent times, IMRT has been widely used to treat head and neck cancers, which have shown to be the best candidates for its application. Organ motion in the head and neck region is essentially nonexistent. The targets are close to a number of radiosensitive critical organs, including the brain stem, spinal cord, and parotid gland. High levels of accuracy in patient preparation and immobilization, the best imaging modalities, sufficient target volume delineation, and the right calculation of dose-volume constraints are all necessary for the successful application of IMRT. Despite intensive research, the ideal fractionation scheme for IMRT has not been determined with certainty. Further investigation is required to assess various fractionation schemes.

8.3.3. Brachytherapy

Treatment with radioactive sources nearby the target of radiation is referred to as brachytherapy. Interstitial implantation is the surgical implantation of radioactive sources or applicators intended to contain radioactive sources. The procedure for intravitreal brachytherapy involves putting applicators containing radioactive sources into a bodily cavity close to the targets. Radiology staff members' exposure to radiation may be significantly decreased with the development of computer-controlled remote after loading devices. The most often utilized isotope for long-term interstitial brachytherapy is iodine-125 seeds. The most often utilized radioactive isotope for intracavitary and temporary interstitial brachytherapy is iridium-192.

8.3.4. Radiation Dose

The size, location, and lymph nodes in the neck of the primary tumors determine the ideal radiation dosage. Primary tumors and gross lymphadenopathy typically require 70 Gy or more in total, divided into 2 Gy daily fractions. A minimum of 50 Gy is needed to reach low-risk neck nodal regions with radiation. Higher radiation doses (60–66 Gy) are typically needed for microscopic disease in postoperative radiotherapy to reduce the risk of locoregional failure due to disruption of the normal vasculature, scarring, and relative hypoxia in the postoperative tumor bed.

8.3.5. Fractionation

For all head and neck cancers, no single fractionation schedule has been shown to be the most effective. Conventional fractionation involves five treatments per week, with daily fractions of 1.8–2 Gy. Alternative schedules for the delivery of radiation therapy have been developed in an effort to enhance treatment outcomes for head and neck cancers. Hyperfractionation and accelerated fractionation are the two main modified fractionation schedules that have been studied over the last 20 years. The hyperfractionation schedule maintains or slightly shortens the total treatment time by administering two or more small-dose fractions on each treatment day. By using smaller-dose fractions, the tolerance of late-responding normal tissues is increased and a higher biologically effective dose can be administered to the tumors. According to certain randomized trials, the hyperfractionation schedule was linked to survival and locoregional control rates that were significantly higher than those of the standard fractionation schedule. Hyperfractionation is linked to more severe acute mucositis when taking into account the normal tissue effect, but the incidence of late complications was within the range seen with traditional fractionation schedules.

A schedule known as "accelerated fractionation" shortens the treatment period overall while maintaining or slightly reducing the number of dose fractions, total dose, and dose size per fraction. Accelerated fractionation is primarily justified by the idea that shorter treatment durations reduce the chance of tumor cell regeneration during the course of treatment. Clinical studies on accelerated fractionation revealed that locoregional control and survival rates significantly improved with shorter treatment durations. Severe acute mucositis was brought on by the accelerated schedules, but there was no discernible rise in late complications. Normal tissue repair of sublethal radiation injuries requires a minimum of 4 hours and 5 minutes between fractions for both hyperfractionation and accelerated fractionation schedules.

8.3.6. Dental Care

It is imperative to receive proper dental care prior to starting radiation therapy. Every patient needs to have a dental examination prior to starting radiation treatment. A thorough examination of the oral cavity's soft tissues and teeth is necessary. It is not advised to routinely extract every tooth in the irradiated volume. The only teeth that require extraction are those that are not viable in the long run. If teeth are extracted either before or after radiation, prophylactic antibiotics are usually prescribed. Regular dental follow-up exams are crucial both during and following radiation treatment. Every patient should receive instruction in proper oral hygiene practices. To reduce the risk of dental caries, fluoride-containing toothpaste, topical fluoride applications, and frequent mouth irrigation with a salt and baking soda solution should all be continued long after radiation therapy.

8.3.7. Complications

Acute and late complications can arise from the extensive treatment volume used for head and neck cancers. Patients who are receiving chemotherapy at the same time as other medical conditions, such as diabetes, have higher rates of complications. Radiation-related complication rates can be decreased with the use of contemporary three-dimensional conformal radiation techniques.

8.3.7.1. Acute Complications

Acute mucositis is caused by direct damage to the mucosa from radiation therapy and is the most common side effect that limits the dose. Symptoms include throat and mouth soreness. Patients should be taught an oral hygiene routine to prevent this. The goal of radiotherapy is to have patchy or confluent mucositis (grade 2 to 3) and avoid ulcerative mucositis (grade 4) which may require hospitalization or parenteral nutrition. Pain, often caused by mucositis, is a common complication that can be treated with conservative medical methods.

Radiation may have an impact on the taste buds that line the tongue. It is said that the sweet sense is more impacted than the salty sense. Following radiation therapy, taste changes may resolve in a few months, but for some patients, the change in taste is permanent. Foods that still have some taste sensation should be encouraged to be consumed by these patients, as should prolonged chewing of food to increase its contact with the taste buds. Oral candidiasis is a common side effect during radiation therapy for head and neck cancers because of radiation-induced xerostomia and the ensuing changes in the oral pH values and oral flora. Antifungal medications applied topically or taken systemically can effectively manage this complication.

Almost every patient will experience an acute skin reaction during radiation therapy to some extent. The course and intensity of skin reactions to radiation therapy can be influenced by the following parameters: total dose, daily fraction size, radiation type (photon or electron), beam energy, and beam modifiers. Steroid-containing creams or lotions can be used on skin lesions, but in order to reduce the risk of superimposed infection, they shouldn't be applied to moist desquamation areas. By the fourth week of treatment, irradiated hair-bearing areas typically epilate, losing their ability to sweat and secrete sebaceous glands. During radiation therapy, laryngeal edema and hoarseness are frequent acute morbidities. It is important to take precautions to prevent potentially fatal airway blockages.

As treatment goes on, patients typically experience nutritional issues. Patients receiving radiation therapy for head and neck cancers may have reduced saliva production, mucositis-related pain, acute oral cavity and pharyngeal mucositis, taste loss or impairment, and decreased saliva production. Dietitian counseling can be beneficial as it offers suggestions for a well-balanced diet. Patients may be advised to eat more frequently and in smaller quantities. Meals that are liquid or semiliquid, or foods that have been moistened with soups and sauces, are advised for patients who have trouble chewing and swallowing. If the patient's severe mucositis prevents them from eating enough, nutritional supplements administered through a nasogastric tube or percutaneous gastrostomy may be a viable option to help them meet their dietary needs.

8.3.7.2. Late Complications

Radiation-related complications most frequently associated with xerostomia by far. Xerostomia typically appears by the third week of radiation therapy and lasts until the end of the course of treatment. The radiation dosage and the size of the main salivary glands within the radiation fields have a major impact on the severity of xerostomia. After radiation treatments of 35 Gy, salivary gland function is typically permanently lost. Poor sleep quality, altered taste perception, poor oral hygiene, poor dental health, difficulty swallowing, and nutritional deficiencies are all caused by xerostomia. It may result in low social engagement and a low quality of life. A lot of work has gone into treating or preventing this issue. Salivary gland parenchymal damage has been shown to be considerably reduced by radioprotective agents like amifostine. Whether or not amifostine administration carries a risk of tumor protection is still unknown. There have been reports of xerostomia benefits from acupuncture and oral pilocarpine. It has been tried to stop radiation-induced xerostomia by surgically transferring submandibular glands. There has been evidence that salivary toxicity can be reduced when IMRT is used for head and neck cancers. Reducing the mean dose to the parotid gland to less than 26 Gy is the aim of planning.

Reduced salivary flow and changed salivary consistency lead to dental caries. The incidence of dental problems can be decreased with dental prophylaxis using topical fluoride and proper dental care. Prior to radiotherapy, the carious teeth should be extracted. Because aggressive extraction of carious teeth predisposes to osteoradionecrosis, it is imperative that the teeth be kept in good condition after radiotherapy.

After head and neck radiation, patients may develop osteoradionecrosis as a result of reduced vascular supply, fewer osteoblasts and osteoclasts, altered bone metabolism, and impaired healing ability in response to various injuries. Patients with osteoradionecrosis usually affect the mandible and maxilla. Bone complications can range from mild exposure to severe bone necrosis that results in osteomyelitis and excruciating pain. Osteoradionecrosis development is also linked to brachytherapy administered in close proximity to the mandible. The radiation dose to the irradiated bones is typically correlated with the risk and severity of osteoradionecrosis. With appropriate dental care, osteoradionecrosis incidence can be decreased. Conservative care, most likely including antibiotics and analgesics, is the standard for managing osteoradionecrosis. By promoting angiogenesis, neovascularization, and osteoblast and fibroblast activity, hyperbaric oxygen can be beneficial. Trismus may occur from radiation to the temporomandibular joint and masticator spaces. Both fibrosis of the temporomandibular joint and contraction of the pterygoid muscles can result in trismus. Exercises for the mandible may stop the trismus from getting worse. Occasionally, surgery is recommended to treat severe trismus. Using a large fraction size frequently led to subcutaneous fibrosis of the soft tissues. The incidence of soft tissue fibrosis may be decreased by using daily fractions less than 2 Gy.

Patients whose larynxes were part of the irradiated volume may experience laryngeal edema long after radiation treatment is finished. Persistent laryngeal edema affects approximately 15% to 25% of cases. A higher incidence of laryngeal edema was linked to larger radiation doses, large field sizes, large fraction sizes, and advanced tumor invasion. According to reports, the prevalence of severe laryngeal edema ranges from 1.5 to 4.6%. Conservative measures and careful follow-up examination can be used to manage persistent laryngeal edema following radiotherapy. If an infection is suspected, empirical antibiotics may be administered. When there is a significant compromise to the airway, steroids should be administered. Suspected persistent or recurrent disease is warranted if the primary tumors initially involved the larynx and the laryngeal edema is progressive and resistant to conservative treatment. In case of positive biopsies, salvage surgery is recommended. Rarely, there are cases of crayonrecrosis, skin necrosis, soft tissue necrosis, laryngeal stricture, and carotid stenosis. Radiation to the neck can result in hypothyroidism. Hypopituitarism may be caused by radiation fields that cover the cavernous sinus, base of the skull, and sphenoid sinus.

Patients who received radiation treatment to their middle and inner ears may develop chronic otitis media and hearing loss. Patients who received more than 50 Gy to the cochlea had a significantly higher incidence of hearing impairment, which was related to radiation dose. Patients treated with a combination of radiation and the ototoxic drug cisplatin are more likely to experience hearing loss. Cataract formation may occur following dosages lower than 10 Gy. Irradiation of the lacrimal glands may result in painful dry eyes.

Neurologic side effects from radiation treatment for head and neck cancer are the most serious. Entrapment in the lateral retroparotid and parapharyngeal spaces, as well as soft tissue fibrosis along the nerves' path, can cause injury to the cranial nerves, particularly to nerves IX to XII. Radiation retinopathy, or damage to the optic nerve, can happen if the orbit and optic chiasm are exposed to radiation and the radiation dose is not kept within tolerable limits. Blindness could then ensue. After 50 Gy, optic nerve injury is possible, and the incidence rises with high daily fractions. Radiation from concave pharyngeal tumors can cause damage to the brain stem and spinal cord. There have also been reports of some patients developing transverse radiation myelitis. These potentially fatal side effects may be avoided with the use of conformal radiotherapy, magnetic resonance imaging, and computed tomography scans.

The alimentary tract has been rebuilt using a range of abdominal viscera following head and neck surgery. Surgeons are very concerned about how postoperative radiation therapy will affect the displaced visceral grafts. The introduction of IMRT has made radiation delivery extremely precise. Technological developments in radiotherapy are ongoing. Real-time image-guided IMRT can be obtained through the innovative technique of image-guided radiation therapy. Proton therapy will become more widely used as manufacturing standardization drives down facility costs. Radiation therapy advancements over the last 10 years have improved head and neck cancer patients' prognosis. Regretfully, increased morbidity and a lower quality of life have resulted from these advancements. Future studies will focus on investigating cutting-edge tactics to increase head and neck cancer patients' chances of survival and quality of life.

8.4. Chemotherapy for Head and Neck Cancer

Head and neck squamous cell carcinoma (HNSCC) is the sixth most common cancer worldwide, with 700,000 cases diagnosed per year. Although there have been advances in multimodality therapy, the overall 5-year survival rate remains approximately 40% to 50%.

8.4.1. Chemotherapy and Chemoradiation

Chemoradiation refers to the combination of chemotherapy and radiation therapy administered concurrently. In this method, chemotherapy not only helps radiation therapy work better, but it also directly treats the tumor. Thyroid cancers that have metastasized to the liver, lungs, or bones can be eradicated with these medications.

On a treatment schedule known as a cycle, many chemotherapy medications are administered intravenously (IV) through a vein. Depending on the type of head and neck cancer a person has, the length of time and number of cycles vary. Doctors typically recommend a mix of medications. The optimal chemotherapy regimen for you is decided by your doctors working together as a team.

8.4.2. Targeted Drugs

In order to treat head and neck cancer, doctors may recommend a targeted medication like cetuximab. These medications, known as monoclonal antibodies, are derived from immune proteins that specifically target tumor antigens, which either trigger the body's defense mechanism against foreign objects or stop the development of blood vessels that sustain tumors. These medications, which are administered intravenously (IV) block a chemical that signals cancer cells to proliferate and divide. Tumors may consequently shrink. Radiation therapy and targeted medications are occasionally used in tandem. Doctors may recommend a combination of standard chemotherapy drugs and targeted drugs for more advanced cancers.

8.4.3. Immunotherapy

Your doctor may recommend immunotherapy to help in the fight against cancer by utilizing the body's own immune system. This treatment may involve the use of pembrolizumab, an anti-PD1 immunotherapy that targets cells with DNA repair defects. Nivolumab, another option, is often prescribed for patients with squamous cell carcinoma that has recurred or spread following chemotherapy. This medication works as a checkpoint inhibitor, boosting the immune system's response to cancer by activating T-cells, a crucial white blood cell that aids in combating diseases.

8.4.4. Managing Side Effects of Medications

Fatigue, appetite loss, neuropathy, and hearing loss are among the most frequent side effects of chemotherapy for head and neck cancer. Itching and a rash are linked to cetuximab. Your doctor might suggest other medications, change the dosage of the drugs, or suggest support services to minimize side effects.

8.5. HIV Infection/AIDS and ENT Manifestations

The acquired immunodeficiency syndrome (AIDS) and the human immunodeficiency virus (HIV) have become global threats to human survival over the past 20 years. Pneumocystis carinii pneumonia (PCP), a rare infection that is rarely seen in healthy young people, was the reason five young homosexual men in Los Angeles were hospitalized in 1981. This discovery marked the beginning of the unraveling of a medical mystery involving an apparently new disease. There are no documented cases of immune function recovery brought on by therapy or by chance, which has had a devastating effect on the AIDS-affected population. While the overall mortality rate is estimated to be between 50 and 60%, patients who have a full-blown illness are likely to die 100% of the time.

HIV infection has been linked to a number of head and neck issues. Studied found that 41% of HIV-positive patients who presented for the first time had issues with their heads and necks. Individuals infected with HIV are susceptible to both common and uncommon diseases. For a clinician treating an HIV-positive patient, it can be costly and overwhelming to take into account all of these illnesses when making a differential diagnosis. The majority of HIV-related otolaryngologic symptoms fall into one of three groups: infections, neoplasms, or primary neurological damage.

8.5.1. Epidemiology

According to estimates from the World Health Organization, between 38 and 100 million people worldwide were HIV positive as of 2,000. Three types of epidemiological patterns are identified for the AIDS pandemic, which is best understood as a sequence of discrete epidemics that overlap in space and time. The type that is most common in Western Europe, North Africa, and North America is one kind. In these areas, intravenous drug users and homosexual or bisexual men are the main carriers of HIV infection. Sub-Saharan Africa and the majority of South America exhibit the second epidemiological pattern. These areas have a heterosexual spread mode with no sex preference. Three patterns have been identified: young heterosexual men, female commercial sex workers, and intravenous drug abuse. This third pattern is found in Asia and the Middle East. There are four known ways to get HIV: through sexual or intimate contact with an HIV-positive person; intravenous drug abuse using a contaminated needle or syringe; maternal transmission to the fetus during pregnancy, to the newborn at birth, or through breast milk; and, finally, transfusion of infected blood and blood products. Free HIV-positive cells can be found in a number of bodily fluids, including blood, cerebrospinal fluid (CSF), genital secretions, amniotic fluids, bronchial lavage fluids, urine, milk, tears, and saliva. However, other bodily fluids—aside from blood, genital secretions, and CSF—contain very little free infectious virus.

8.5.2. Pathophysiology

HIV is the etiologic agent of AIDS. The virus prefers T-cells, specifically the CD4 and CDS receptors that are frequently present on helper inducer T-lymphocytes. Although they have comparatively few CD4 surface receptors, monocytes and macrophages can also become HIV-positive. The AIDS virus is a type of retrovirus, which means that it can enter the host genome by converting from single-stranded RNA to double-stranded DNA. The virus is known as a provirus and the host cell is irreversibly infected with HIV once the new viral DNA has been integrated into the DNA of the cell. There are two types of HIV: HIV1 and HIV2. Another retrovirus that causes a less severe form of AIDS is HIV2. With only a few cases documented in the United States, it is almost entirely found in Africa.

8.5.3. Diagnosis

Viral culture, antigen testing, and antibody testing are the three main categories of HIV infection testing. The enzyme-linked immunosorbent assay (ELISA), which uses antibody testing, is the test most frequently used to diagnose HIV infection. The most common method for confirming this is the Western blot technique. The specificities and sensitivities of the two tests are both higher than 99%. This kind of antibody testing performs reasonably well across nearly all age groups. Immunoglobulin G is the antibody that is tested for because it can pass through the placenta. Maternal HIV antibodies can be found in the infant up until the age of 15 to 18 months if the mother has the virus. Positive tests in children under the age of 18 months may or may not indicate HIV infection. These kids should undergo testing later on.

8.5.4. Clinical Manifestations According to Anatomic Sites

8.5.4.1. The Ear

Otitis externa—also known as seborrheic dermatitis—is characterized by recurrent super infections of the skin surrounding the external canal. It is treated with 0.5% steroid cream three times a day. Pneumocystis carinii or Mycobacterium tuberculosis infections are another type of otitis externa. Since patients with pulmonary pneumocystitis began receiving prophylactic treatment, there has been a marked increase in the number of extrapulmonary infections. Both *Mycobacterium tuberculosis* and *Pneumocystis carinii* typically resolve clinically quickly with appropriate therapy.

Acute recurrent otitis media and serous otitis media are rather common, particularly in children, and are typically caused by pathogens that are common in immunologically normal patients. After experiencing one episode, these kids are more likely to experience subsequent acute otitis media, which typically responds fairly well to the standard treatment plan. Vertigo and sensori neural hearing loss are the most prevalent inner ear conditions associated with HIV. The hearing loss can be unilateral or bilateral and it occurs in 21- 49% of HIV infected patients. Vertigo is frequently a symptom of subacute encephalitis or HIV-disease dementia complex.

8.5.4.2. Nose and Paranasal Sinuses

The most prevalent ways that HIV illness manifests itself are nasal obstruction, allergic rhinitis, and sinusitis. The Waldeyer ring is frequently involved in nasal obstruction. These children's recurrent adenoton-sillar hypertrophy may result in sleep apnea symptoms, which can be effectively treated with an adeno-tonsillectomy. Prospective studies of HIV-positive patients reported a 30–60%prevalence of sinusitis. Research also found that men with HIV had a two-fold increase in the incidence of allergic symptoms due to an increase in Ig-E production. Additional studies have confirmed these elevated Ig-E levels. Patients with later stages of HIV disease are more likely to be diagnosed with aspergillosis, an extremely aggressive infection with a generally poor prognosis. The treatment for this IgE-mediated allergic rhinitis is the same as for patients with oilier allergies. Although infections typically occur in the lungs, they have also been documented in the skin, kidney, heart, and paranasal sinuses. Treatment consists of early systemic antifungal medication administration along with adjunctive surgery.

8.5.4.3. Throat

For patients with HIV, oral candidiasis is the most prevalent fungal infection. About 20% of individuals with AIDS have esophageal candidiasis, which typically results in severe dysphagia, odynophagia, and dehydration. Treatment for oral candidiasis is comparable, but systemic therapy is frequently needed. These patients also frequently experience recurrent aphthous mouth ulcers. Oral hairy leukoplakia, which is clinically described as a white thickening of the mucosa, is thought to have been observed in about 25% of HIV-positive patients. Epstein-Barr virus (EBV) opportunistic infection is thought to be the causative factor. Biopsy or in-situ hybridization of scrapings from suspected lesions that have undergone cytospin analysis is used to make the diagnosis. The medication used is acyclovir.

8.5.4.4. The Face

According to one report, 7.2% of HIV patients experience facial nerve paralysis. The most common diagnosis for patients with seventh nerve palsy who are HIV-positive is idiopathic facial nerve palsy, also known as Bells palsy. This condition can be unilateral or bilateral. Typically, the nerve heals in three weeks to three months when corticosteroids and cyclovir are used as regular therapy. The Ramsay-Hunt syndrome, also known as the herpes zoster infection, is more common in HIV-positive individuals than in non-infected ones. Corticosteroid is also very effective and should be initiated as soon as possible.

8.5.4.5. Neoplasms

The most frequent cancer linked to HIV infection is Kaposi sarcoma. It is rare in hemophiliacs but occurs in 4% of intravenous drug abusers and 43% of homosexual or bisexual men. Clinical suspicion frequently enables biopsy-based confirmation of the diagnosis. Non-Hodgkins lymphoma is the second most frequent cancer linked to HIV infection. The majority of patients have fever, weight loss, and night sweats at first. Chemotherapy is the mode of treatment. Diffuse persistent lymphadenopathy, involving two or more extrainguinal sites for more than three months, is suggestive of lymphadenopathy caused by HIV. Before any other symptoms manifest, this syndrome affects up to 70% of HIV-positive patients. They can have a diameter of up to 5 centimeters and are typically symmetrically distributed and soft.

8.5.4.6. Salivary Glands

An increasing number of studies have reported the presence of parotid gland enlargement as a symptom of HIV infection. Cystic parotid enlargement accounts for 6% of those with HIV infection. Children are more likely to develop parotid cysts. They are deliberate and painless, expanding and are typically two-sided. Usually, the affected lobe is only the superficial one. CT scan, ultrasound, and biopsy are used for diagnosis. The histology report from the biopsy typically resembles benign lymph epithelial lesions. The presence of CD8 T-cells is confirmed by a CD4/CDS count. Rarely is a parotidectomy necessary. Radiation therapy at low doses causes symptoms to clear up quickly and the chance of recurrence to decrease.

The goal of current AIDS research is to extend the life expectancy and enhance the quality of life for those who suffer from this illness. Compared to 10 years ago, doctors are seeing more advanced disease today. An overview of the complexity of otolaryngologic manifestations in HIV infections is provided in research. AIDS can cause a variety of intricate symptoms that affect the head, neck, nose, and ears. The disease's infectious form may have detrimental effects on society. Since early and accurate diagnosis is crucial for providing the patients with concrete, effective treatment, doctors need to be well-versed in the possibility that H1V/A1DS may be the cause of otolaryngologic symptoms and signs. It is still clinically significant to identify each of these manifestations in the early stages of HIV disease diagnosis. In order to lower the risks of transmission to healthcare professionals, the Centers for Disease Control (CDC) formally introduced guidelines for standard (universal) precautions that must be followed to prevent the spread of HIV.

In order to prevent HIV/AIDS, society must be made aware of the behaviors that encourage the spread of the virus. Treatment for HIV infections and AIDS must target both the virus itself and any potential or current opportunistic bacterial superinfection.

A Closer Look

Anticancer Drugs

Any medication that effectively treats malignant, or cancerous, disease is an anticancer medication. Anticancer medications fall into various major categories, such as hormones, alkylating agents, antimetabolites, and natural products. Furthermore, a number of medications that do not belong to those classes but exhibit anticancer activity are nonetheless used to treat malignant illnesses. Although it more correctly refers to the use of chemical compounds to treat disease generally, the term "chemotherapy" is often associated with the use of anticancer drugs.

One of the first drugs that was used clinically in modern medicine for the treatment of cancer was the alkylating agent mechlorethamine, a nitrogen mustard that in the 1940s was found to be effective in treating lymphomas. The first medication to treat a solid tumor was the antimetabolite methotrexate, which was introduced in 1956. The following year, 5-fluorouracil was introduced as the first member of a new class of compounds called pyrimidine analogs, which were designed to fight tumors. Since then, numerous anticancer medications have been created and successfully used.

The type, location, and severity of the cancer, as well as whether or not radiation therapy or surgery is appropriate, all play a role in the decision to use a particular anticancer medication. The majority of anticancer medications are injected intravenously, though some can also be taken orally, injected intramuscularly, or administered intrathecally (within the spinal cord). Cancer treatment is made more difficult by the fact that the drugs used to treat it target human cells—albeit genetically altered cells that are proliferating quickly and uncontrollably. Nonetheless, some anticancer medications have the ability to distinguish between cancerous and normal tissue cells to some extent, and the apparent selectivity of agents may actually be influenced by the pace at which cancer cells proliferate. For example, alkylating agents appear to be particularly toxic to cells during the synthesis, or S, stage of the cell cycle, when DNA is replicating, and unpaired nucleotides, the nitrogen-containing units of DNA and RNA, are most susceptible to alkylation (the addition of an alkyl group). Alkylating agents act on cells at all stages of the cell cycle. Targeted cancer therapies, which have a relatively high degree of specificity for cancer cells, were developed in the late 20th and early 21st centuries as a result of the discovery of molecular characteristics specific to cancer cells.

Reducing the severity of side effects related to anticancer drug use is largely dependent on how specific the drug is. Anticancer agents can cause numerous side effects, some of which are life-threatening, and are generally toxic to normal cells due to the similarities between cancer cells and normal human cells. Hair loss, mouth and mucous membrane sores, cardiac abnormalities, bone marrow toxicity, and extreme nausea and vomiting are a few examples of these adverse effects. Both anemia and a weakened immune system are brought on by the bone marrow toxicities. Another possibility is permanent infertility. To make the medication more tolerable for the patient, these side effects might necessitate lowering the dosage or altering the dosage schedule.

Rarely, long-term anticancer medication use can result in the emergence of secondary malignancies. The degree of carcinogenicity (cause of cancer) of an anticancer drug depends on the kind of agent, the primary cancer it is used to treat, and the total cumulative dose given. Myelodysplastic syndrome and acute leukemias are common secondary cancers linked to anticancer drug therapy; the risk of these conditions is heightened by the use of alkylating agents and topoisomerase inhibitors (e.g., etoposide).

Combining different agents can help minimize the side effects of anticancer medications, often allowing for lower dosages of each medication to be administered. Combining different treatments may also lessen the likelihood of cellular resistance, a condition that permits tumors to evade therapy and grow even after a period of remission (absence of disease activity). Multidrug therapy operates under the assumption that distinct anticancer drug classes act at distinct stages of the cell cycle (e.g., cellular growth, division, and resting phases). As a result, one medication may be used to halt the growth of cancer cells at one stage, and another medication may act at a different stage. Cancer chemotherapy often involves not only intricate drug regimens but also surgery to decrease the number of cancer cells and radiation therapy to kill more cells.

Summary

- In laser surgery, surgical operations are performed using specific light beams rather than tools.
- Surgically, tissues have had their volume reduced by using radiowaves. It has been applied to the base of the tongue to relieve sleep apnea, the inferior turbinates to relieve nasal obstruction, and the soft palate to relieve upper airway resistance, primary snoring, and sleep apnea. Additionally, it has been applied to the management of lingual thyroid.
- As an adjuvant therapy for otolaryngology, head and neck surgery, hyperbaric oxygen therapy has gained popularity. It is recommended for the management of ischemic facial cutaneous flaps, necrotizing anaerobic wound infections, and osteoradionecrosis of the mandible. Patients can heal more quickly if you raise the tissue oxygen level.
- Coblation is a cutting-edge technique that uses natural saline and mild radiofrequency energy to rapidly and efficiently remove and shrink bulky tongue base tissue as well as soft palate tissue. Coblation does not function by means of heat.
- Tissues that are quickly frozen to -30°C or lower and then slowly thawed are destroyed. This information has been applied to the management of a variety of head and neck lesions, such as benign, premalignant, and malignant neoplasms.
- Both local and mild general anesthesia can be used during cryotherapy treatments. Sometimes numbness results from freezing alone, so no anesthetic is needed. Insulation is required in the area that will be frozen.
- As part of radiation therapy, high-energy particle beams are directed toward the tumor through the skin. The beams damage the DNA of the cancer cells as soon as they arrive at the tumor, destroying the cells. Radiation therapy is well-known for being especially successful in treating tumors of the head and neck.
- With the help of technological advancements like inverse treatment planning and the linear accelerator equipped with a multileaf collimator, intensity-modulated radiation therapy (IMRT) has been successfully implemented.
- Treatment with radioactive sources nearby the target of radiation is referred to as brachytherapy. Interstitial implantation is the surgical implantation of radioactive sources or applicators intended to contain radioactive sources. The procedure for intravitreal brachytherapy involves putting applicators containing radioactive sources into a bodily cavity close to the targets.
- For all head and neck cancers, no single fractionation schedule has been shown to be the most effective. Conventional fractionation involves five treatments per week, with daily fractions of 1.8–2 Gy.
- Chemoradiation refers to the combination of chemotherapy and radiation therapy administered concurrently. In this method, chemotherapy not only helps radiation therapy work better, but it also directly treats the tumor. Thyroid cancers that have metastasized to the liver, lungs, or bones can be eradicated with these medications.

- HIV is the etiologic agent of AIDS. The virus prefers T-cells, specifically the CD4 and CDS receptors that are frequently present on helper inducer T-lymphocytes.
- Viral culture, antigen testing, and antibody testing are the three main categories of HIV infection testing. The enzyme-linked immunosorbent assay (ELISA), which uses antibody testing, is the test most frequently used to diagnose HIV infection. The most common method for confirming this is the Western blot technique.

References

1. Fletcher, J. (2018). *Tonsillectomy: Procedure and Recovery*. MedicalNewsToday. Retrieved from: https://www.medicalnewstoday.com/articles/tonsillectomy (accessed on 4 September 2024).
2. Fosen, K. M., & Thom, S. R. (2014). Hyperbaric oxygen, vasculogenic stem cells, and wound healing. *Antioxidants & Redox Signaling, 21*(11), 1634–1647.
3. Godman, C. A., Chheda, K. P., Hightower, L. E., Perdrizet, G., Shin, D. G., et al. (2010). Hyperbaric oxygen induces a cytoprotective and angiogenic response in human microvascular endothelial cells. *Cell Stress & Chaperones, 15*(4), 431–442.
4. Hopf, H. W., Gibson, J. J., Angeles, A. P., Constant, J. S., Feng, J. J., et al. (2005). Hyperoxia and angiogenesis. *Wound Repair and Regeneration, 13*(5), 558–564.
5. Howell, R. S., Criscitelli, T., Woods, J. S., Gillette, B. M., & Gorenstein, S. (2018). Hyperbaric oxygen therapy: Indications, contraindications, and use at a tertiary care center. *AORN Journal, 107*(4), 442–453.
6. Lam, G., Fontaine, R., Ross, F. L., & Chiu, E. S. (2017). Hyperbaric oxygen therapy: Exploring the clinical evidence. *Advances in Skin & Wound Care, 30*(4), 181–190.
7. Machiels, J. P., Leemans, C. R., et al. (2020). Squamous cell carcinoma of the oral cavity, larynx, oropharynx, and hypopharynx. *Annals of Oncology, 31*(11), 1462–1475.
8. Mathieu, D., Marroni, A., & Kot, J. (2017). Tenth European Consensus Conference on Hyperbaric Medicine: Recommendations for accepted and non-accepted clinical indications and practice of hyperbaric oxygen treatment. *Diving and Hyperbaric Medicine, 47*(1), 24–32.
9. McMonnies, C. W. (2015). Hyperbaric oxygen therapy and the possibility of ocular complications or contraindications. *Clinical and Experimental Optometry, 98*(2), 122–125.
10. Raggio, B. S., & Winters, R. (2018). Modern management of osteoradionecrosis. *Current Opinion in Otolaryngology & Head and Neck Surgery, 26*(4), 254–259.
11. Ranganathan, K., & Hemalatha, R. (2006). Oral lesions in HIV infection in developing countries: An overview. *Advances in Dental Research, 19*, 63–68.
12. Ravi, P., Vaishnavi, D., Gnanam, A., & Krishnakumar, R. V. B. (2017). The role of hyperbaric oxygen therapy in the prevention and management of radiation-induced complications of the head and neck: A systematic review of literature. *Journal of Stomatology, Oral and Maxillofacial Surgery, 118*(6), 359–362.
13. Sen, C. K., Khanna, S., Gordillo, G., Bagchi, D., Bagchi, M., et al. (2002). Oxygen, oxidants, and antioxidants in wound healing: An emerging paradigm. *Annals of the New York Academy of Sciences, 957*, 239–249.
14. Sharkey, L. S. (2000). Current indications for hyperbaric oxygen therapy. *ADF Health, 1*, 64–72.

15. Singh, S., & Gambert, S. R. (2014). Hyperbaric oxygen therapy: A brief history and review of its benefits and indications for the older adult patient. *Annals of Long-Term Care, 22*(7–8), 37–42.

16. Sultan, A., Hanna, G. J., Margalit, D. N., Chau, N., Goguen, L. A., et al. (2017). The use of hyperbaric oxygen for the prevention and management of osteoradionecrosis of the jaw: A Dana-Farber/Brigham and Women's Cancer Center multidisciplinary guideline. *The Oncologist, 22*(3), 343–350.

17. Thom, S. R. (2011). Hyperbaric oxygen: Its mechanisms and efficacy. *Plastic and Reconstructive Surgery, 127*(1 Suppl), 131S–141S.

18. Weaver, K. L. (2014). *Hyperbaric Oxygen Therapy Indications* (13th ed., pp. 9–11). Best Publishing Company.

19. Whiteside, T. L. (2005). Immunobiology of head and neck cancer. *Cancer Metastasis Reviews, 24*(1), 95–105.

20. Whitlock, J. (2019). *Tonsillectomy Surgery*. Verywell. Retrieved from: https://www.verywellhealth.com/tonsillectomy-surgery-4171140 (accessed on 4 September 2024).

21. Ztürk, F., Ermertcan, A. T., & İnanır, I. (2013). Hyperbaric oxygen therapy for the management of chronic wounds. *Cutaneous and Ocular Toxicology, 32*(1), 72–77.

Chapter

9

CLINICAL METHODS IN ENT AND NECK MASSES

Contents

Introduction

The clinical method is how doctors learn details about their patients, whether they are ill or well, and incorporate those details into the diagnostic and treatment process in tandem with knowledge of pathophysiology, disease, and technology. The clinical method's shortcomings as it is currently taught and applied cause issues for medical professionals, patients, and the healthcare system as a whole, particularly in primary care. Three issues exist. First, as the basis of primary care, knowledge about people—which is typically lacking from the approach—is just as crucial as knowledge about diseases. Second, talking to and examining patients continues to yield a large portion of the data needed for primary care diagnostic and treatment decisions. The clinical judgment of individual physicians is a crucial component of the clinical method that is often overlooked, despite its direct impact on patients' health and well-being.

Orientation and Directional Terms

Term	Definition	Illustration
Laryngeal Mirror	Tool used to exam the larynx and other areas of the throat. The laryngeal mirror reflects the inside of the mouth and throat for the physical examination. It may be used to visualize the throat for the application of anesthesia or to remove tissue from the mouth.	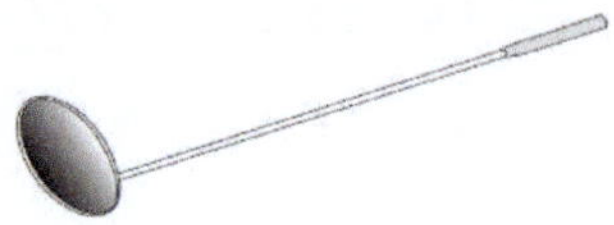
Nasal Speculum	Tool inserted into the nostril to assist the physician with the visual inspection of the lining of the nose, nasal membranes and septum.	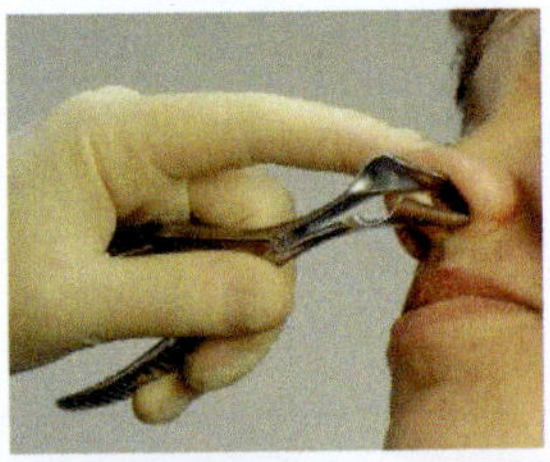
Otoscope	Allows the physician to view the ear canal and tympanic membrane. The otoscope has a magnifying lens, light and cone-shaped insert to examine the inner ear.	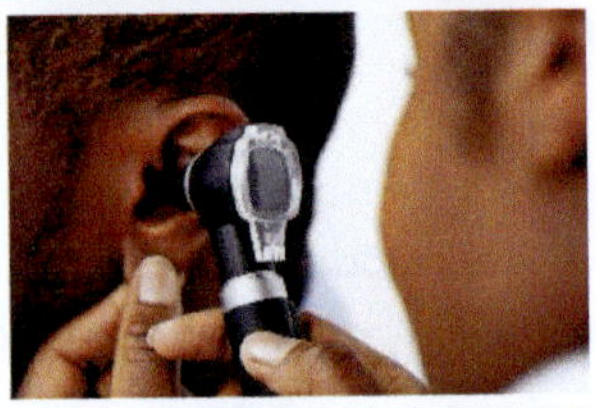
Audioscope	The tool used to screen patients for hearing loss. The audioscope is placed in the patient's ear and makes a serious of tones to which the patient can respond to.	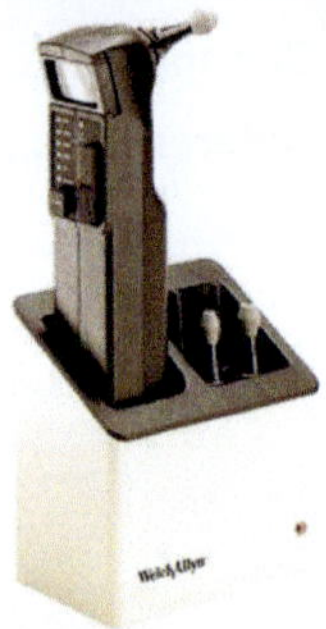
Ophthalmoscope	The tool used to examine the interior structures of the eye. The ophthalmoscope has a light, magnifying lens and opening for the physician to view the eye.	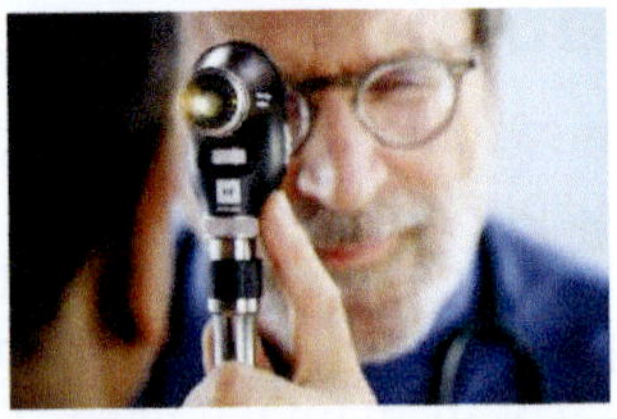

9.1. Clinical Methods in ENT

The clinical method is the basic instrument and procedure that must be applied in the therapeutic setting to gather the data and other elements required for the treatment of individuals.

9.1.1. Equipment, History Taking and General Setup

A meaningful history must be obtained from the patient, and the examination of the patient's darker cavities in the ear, nose, pharynx, and larynx demands expert dexterity. This is something that a student should practice frequently in ENT clinics.

9.1.1.1. Equipment

Safe surgical and procedural care is essential to guaranteeing the provision of high-quality healthcare in international contexts. A costly infrastructure is needed for the procurement, sterilization, and upkeep of critical equipment as well as reliable support services like imaging, laboratory testing, histopathology, and blood banking in order to provide effective surgical care. Otolaryngology-head and neck surgery (OHNS) covers a wide range of diseases and surgical procedures, making a large range of equipment necessary to deliver critical care. The accessibility of resources and the infrastructures of health systems cause variations in the availability of equipment by region and practice setting.

Surgical subspecialties, like pediatric surgery, have developed tools and health service frameworks that are vital to the advancement of surgical infrastructure quality, resource advocacy, and the ability of surgeons to provide standard surgical care in a variety of contexts.

9.1.1.1.1. Prioritizing Equipment and Ancillary Services in Surgery

Treatment for operable conditions—which account for 28–32% of the global burden of disability and mortality—requires surgical, anesthetic, and ancillary medical services. For a variety of reasons, including the perceived high cost of surgical infrastructure and the complexity of surgical care delivery, surgery has not received enough attention in global health initiatives. Not only is it morally right to provide access to high-quality healthcare, but surgery has also shown to be a financially sensible course of action. For instance, a 2014 systematic review of cost-effectiveness studies conducted in low- and middle-income countries (LMICs) found that, when compared to currently recommended public health interventions, surgical intervention can be very cost-effective or cost-effective based on World Health Organization (WHO) criteria. Surgical care cannot be provided satisfactorily if the prioritization of surgical equipment in some subspecialties—like OHNS—is not taken into account.

Specialized tools and facilities are essential to the provision of surgical care. The World Health Organization (WHO) initiated the Global Initiative for Emergency and Essential Surgical Care in 2005. The initiative published guidelines for public district hospitals to support the provision of basic intensive care units, well-equipped operating rooms, and the capacity to treat a number of severely incapacitating and potentially fatal surgical conditions. To this end, the WHO collaborated with stakeholders in clinical, biomedical engineering, government, and medical devices to enhance the accessibility of critical surgical equipment in low- and middle-income countries. Since then, many inventories have been created to evaluate surgical capacity, such as the International Assessment of Capacity for Trauma (INTACT) index, the Personnel, Infrastructure, Procedures,

Equipment, and Supplies (PIPES) tool, and the WHO Tool for Situational Analysis to Assess Emergency and Essential Surgical Care (SAT). These inventories have shown glaring shortages of surgical equipment in several sub-Saharan African, Asian, and Central/South American nations, underscoring the necessity of government engagement in the development of surgical capacity, both in terms of people and infrastructure.

The differentiation of surgical equipment lists outside the scope of general and trauma surgery has been a defining characteristic of the next generation of surgical equipment appraisal. The International Standards for a Safe Practice of Anesthesia, developed by the World Federation of Societies of Anesthesiologists and the WHO, introduced specific guidelines for anesthetic supplies and staff at different care levels. Consensus guidelines on the best supplies and equipment for treating pediatric surgical conditions in low- and middle-income countries (LMICs) were developed by the Global Initiative for Children's Surgery, an independent consortium of pediatric surgical providers. Surgical subspecialty groups have expanded the use of current assessment tools by adapting the PIPES tool to allow for the assessment of pediatric surgery and neurosurgical capacity. These lists of surgical equipment are used not only for evaluating the infrastructure but also for internal quality control, the creation of surgical policies by health ministries, and the determination of investment priorities for advocacy and humanitarian endeavors.

9.1.1.1.2. Essential Equipment and Services for OHNS Care

Despite OHNS conditions representing a substantial disease burden, they are still comparatively understudied in terms of the worldwide delivery of surgical care. According to the Global Burden of Disease study conducted by the Institute for Health Metrics and Evaluation, 1.57 billion people worldwide suffer from hearing loss, which is the third leading cause of disability (with a threshold of ≥20 dB for mild hearing loss). The incidence of otitis media, one of the most frequent and avoidable causes of hearing loss in children, is estimated to be between 471 and 709 million cases annually. 5% of cancer-related deaths worldwide are caused by head and neck cancers, with low- and middle-income countries (LMICs) suffering from a notably higher death rate and consequent economic loss than high-income countries (HICs). Other OHNS conditions that have a high global disease burden include deep neck space infections, pediatric foreign bodies, head and neck trauma, cleft lip/palate, and upper respiratory infections. One significant obstacle to providing care for OHNS conditions has been found to be the expense of purchasing and maintaining subspecialty-specific equipment. The COVID-19 pandemic has brought to light the difficulties faced by otolaryngologists operating in low- and middle-income countries (LMICs). These challenges included a shortage of surgical and personal protective equipment, which made it difficult for them to continue performing surgeries. There is currently no description of the critical surgical equipment required for the provision of high-quality OHNS care globally, despite the high global burden of OHNS conditions. The Global OHNS Initiative created an expert-driven list of necessary supplies and services to close this gap and provide top-notch OHNS surgical care.

9.1.1.1.3. The Global Otolaryngology–Head and Neck Surgery Initiative: Essential Equipment and Services

The goal of the Global OHNS Initiative is to provide "universal access to high-quality, safe, timely, and affordable care for those with OHNS conditions." It is an international alliance of OHNS clinical providers, trainees, and researchers. Prioritizing OHNS conditions and procedures that all national health systems should be able to handle was determined by the group using the Delphi methodology in order to start defining the role of OHNS care within comprehensive health systems. These results were then utilized by the initiative to create an expert-driven list of the minimal equipment required for the surgical and medical treatment of the priority conditions. As a result, equipment that was included in the majority of general surgery equipment checklists was not included in this list, which was developed with the supposition that a facility offering OHNS care would already have the resources necessary for general surgery care. When adding new services or equipment that they routinely use in their clinical practice, OHNS providers from a range of practice settings were consulted.

An internal survey was distributed to OHNS providers and advanced-level trainees involved in the initiative after a preliminary list was compiled. Professionals from 11 nations, including the US, Uganda, Israel, Pakistan, Kenya, Lebanon, Chile, Myanmar (Burma), the UK, India, and Austria, participated in the survey. The OHNS subspecialties of general otolaryngology, otology, head and neck surgery, rhinology, skull base surgery, and pediatric otolaryngology were among those whose equipment was covered by the survey. The following criteria were used to define primary and tertiary care levels, and providers were asked to rate the usefulness of each type of equipment and service.

- Primary = ENT (ear, nose, and throat) treatment given in a community hospital or clinic.
- Tertiary = a referral-only facility for ENT care from specialists or subspecialists that is not typically handled in the community.
- Three classifications were used to group equipment and auxiliary services:
    - "Essential" – This service, which is essential to the treatment of ENT conditions encountered at the appropriate care level, needs to be available internally.
    - "Aspirational" – This equipment might be helpful for ENT needs, but it might not be required to provide care at this particular level of healthcare. It would be used frequently if it were available.
    - "Nonessential" – The management of ENT conditions at the appropriate care level does not require the use of this equipment or service. There might be adequate alternatives that serve the same purpose as this machinery or service.

Multiple group consensus meetings were used to compile and review the results of the internal survey. For baseline OHNS care, a final list of necessary supplies and supplemental services was created (Table 9.1 and 9.2). The development of high-quality OHNS care in diverse healthcare settings and the provision of a high standard of care for all patients with OHNS conditions may be aided by consulting this list of necessary OHNS supplies and services.

Table 9.1: A list of essential equipment for baseline care in otolaryngology-head and neck surgery as compiled by the Global OHNS Initiative

General care		
	Primary	Tertiary
Essential	Headlights 512Hz turning fork Laryngeal mirror Otoscope and ear speculum Suction aspirator Ear forceps Ear curettes Nasal speculum Flexible endoscopy Bipolar/diathermy Bone-cutting drill Operating microscope (suitable for OHNS procedures)	Headlights 512Hz turning fork Laryngeal mirror Otoscope and ear speculum Suction aspirator Ear forceps Ear curettes Nasal speculum Flexible endoscopy Bipolar/diathermy Bone-cutting drill Operating microscope (suitable for OHNS procedures) Loupes Bedside/POC ultrasound Facial nerve monitoring
Aspirational	Loupes Bedside/POC ultrasound Facial nerve monitoring	
Non-essential		
Endoscopy		
	Primary	Tertiary
Essential	Endoscopy tower (light source and video processor) Hopkin's rod (rigid telescope) Rigid bronchoscope Rigid bronchoscope accessory instruments Direct laryngoscopy and biopsy set Esophagoscope	Endoscopy tower (light source and video processor) Hopkin's rod (rigid telescope) Rigid bronchoscope Rigid bronchoscope accessory instruments Direct laryngoscopy and biopsy set Esophagoscope Flexible bronchoscope

Aspirational	Flexible bronchoscope	
Non-essential		
Otology		
	Primary	Tertiary
Essential	Otologic drill Hammer and gauge Otology set (or equivalent supplies) Myringotome (surgical knife for paracentesis of eardrum) Tympanostomy set (or equivalent supplies) Cutting diamond-head drill burrs Alligator ear forceps	Otologic drill Hammer and gauge Otology set (or equivalent supplies) Myringotome (surgical knife for paracentesis of eardrum) Tympanostomy set (or equivalent supplies) Cutting diamond-head drill burrs Alligator ear forceps Otoendoscope Bone pate Cochlear implant Jeweler forceps
Aspirational	Otoendoscope Bone pate	
Non-essential	Cochlear implant Jeweler forceps	
Head and neck surgery		
	Primary	Tertiary
Essential	Neck dissection set (or equivalent supplies) Tracheotomy tubes of different sizes	Neck dissection set (or equivalent supplies) Tracheotomy tubes of different sizes Endovascular microscope and loupes Maxillofacial plating set Microsurgical/microdissection set (or equivalent supplies) Tracheoesophageal voice prosthesis
Aspirational	Endovascular microscope and loupes Maxillofacial plating set	
Non-Essential	Microsurgical/microdissection set (or equivalent supplies) Tracheoesophageal voice prosthesis	

Rhinology and sinus surgery		
	Primary	Tertiary
Essential	Straight (0-degree) nasal endoscope Angled (30-degree) nasal endoscope Sinus surgery set (or equivalent supplies) Rhinology, rhinoplasty, septoplasty set (or equivalent supplies)	Straight (0-degree) nasal endoscope Angled (30-degree) nasal endoscope Angled (45-degree) nasal endoscope Angled (70-degree) nasal endoscope Sinus surgery set (or equivalent supplies) Rhinology, rhinoplasty, septoplasty set (or equivalent supplies) Rotation (suction) microdebrider Endoscopic dissection tools (miniature forceps, dissectors, etc.) Anterior skull base dissection set
Aspirational	Angled (45-degree) nasal endoscope Angled (70-degree) nasal endoscope Rotation (suction) microdebrider Endoscopic dissection tools (miniature forceps, dissectors, etc.)	Computer-assisted navigation for skull base surgery
Non-essential	Anterior Skull Base Dissection Set Computer Assisted Navigation for Skull Base Surgery	
Pediatric otolaryngology		
	Primary	Tertiary
Essential	Mouth gag Suction electrocautery Tonsillectomy set (or equivalent supplies) Adenoidectomy set with adenotomes Pediatric airway set (with airway dilators, balloons, choanal atresia perforators)	Mouth gag Suction electrocautery Tonsillectomy set (or equivalent supplies) Adenoidectomy set with adenotomes Pediatric airway set (with airway dilators, balloons, choanal atresia perforators) Coblation (cold ablation)
Aspirational	Coblation (Cold Ablation)	
Non-Essential		

Source: Tarika Srinivasan, Alexander Cherches, Amina Seguya, Valerie Salano, Rolvix H. Patterson, Mary Jue Xu, Blake C. Alkire, Samuel N. Okerosi, and Sharon Ovnat Tamir, "Essential equipment and services for otolaryngology care: a proposal by the Global Otolaryngology-Head and Neck Surgery Initiative," doi: 10.1097/MOO.0000000000000885

Each column indicates a different category for services at the primary and tertiary care levels. For every care level, services can be classified as essential, aspirational, or nonessential.

Table 9.2: A list of essential services for baseline care in otolaryngology-head and neck surgery as compiled by the Global OHNS Initiative

	Primary	Tertiary
Essential	Audiology Histopathology and cytology Microbiology Blood serology Blood bank Equipment sterilization Biomedical equipment maintenance X-ray radiography Computerized tomography (CT) Ultrasonography (with specialist ultrasonographer and radiologist interpretation)	Audiology Histopathology and cytology Microbiology Blood serology Blood bank Equipment sterilization Biomedical equipment maintenance X-ray radiography Computerized tomography (CT) Ultrasonography (with specialist ultrasonographer and radiologist interpretation) Magnetic resonance imaging (MRI) Positron emission tomography (PET) Speech-language pathology Medical oncology consult Radiation oncology consult
Aspirational	Magnetic resonance imaging (MRI) Positron emission tomography (PET) Speech-language pathology Medical oncology consult Radiation oncology consult	
Non-essential		

Source: Tarika Srinivasan, Alexander Cherches, Amina Seguya, Valerie Salano, Rolvix H. Patterson, Mary Jue Xu, Blake C. Alkire, Samuel N. Okerosi, and Sharon Ovnat Tamir, "Essential equipment and services for otolaryngology care: a proposal by the Global Otolaryngology-Head and Neck Surgery Initiative," doi: 10.1097/MOO.0000000000000885

The arrangement of services and equipment according to primary and tertiary facility levels enables a more comprehensive comprehension of the resources required for proper OHNS care. Equipment was also divided into "essential" and "aspirational" categories to show relative importance. Aspirational equipment has become more and more common in high-resource settings to enhance patient safety and overall quality of care. It frequently included items that are not absolutely necessary for the provision of OHNS care. Respondents to the survey gave global standards of care a higher priority than newer technologies for the "essential" category in order to establish a more equitable benchmark that a larger percentage of OHNS providers, facilities, or hospital systems could meet.

The evolution of training standards, equipment availability, and disease burden all affect these categorizations. Responses to the survey brought to light differences in how equipment is used due to training requirements and resource limitations. Laryngeal mirrors for indirect laryngoscopy were considered necessary at the primary level in the general otolaryngology care section. However, due to patient comfort and the comprehensiveness of laryngeal examination, clinicians in HICs have shifted away from using laryngeal mirrors and toward using fiberoptic laryngoscopy (FOL) or rigid laryngeal endoscopy for visualization of the supraglottic and glottic regions. Therefore, it was thought that both laryngeal and FOL mirrors were necessary to cover the range of infrastructure accessibility and changing training requirements across socioeconomic classes.

Respondents classified a rigid bronchoscope as necessary for primary endoscopy and a flexible bronchoscope as aspirational. In the discussion that followed, participants said that a rigid bronchoscope can be used to treat nearly any tracheal foreign body, lesion, or tumor. Nevertheless, recent research indicates that in situations where rigid bronchoscopic examination is unclear or unable to reach more distal locations in the airway, flexible bronchoscopy may be able to help definitively rule out foreign body aspiration. Even though pulmonologists and thoracic surgeons usually use this equipment as a tool, OHNS providers are increasingly using it, which suggests that future iterations of these lists may reclassify some equipment as essential.

A small number of survey participants mentioned different ways to use the equipment to provide care outside of its original intended purpose in open-ended responses. For instance, two respondents mentioned that nasal endoscopes were often used for pediatric airway foreign body removal and otologic procedures. One more respondent mentioned that pediatric anterior skull base surgery at their institution was performed using otologic instruments. The COVID-19 pandemic led to a shortage of equipment, which sparked interest in creating economical surgical capacity strategies, such as equipment reuse and repurposing. According to a recent study on the advantages of repurposing equipment, endoscopic middle ear procedures exhibit better anatomic visualization along with surgical and audiometric results comparable to those of binocular procedures. Furthermore, compared to the otologic microscopic surgical setup, the endoscopic surgical setup has significantly fewer logistical and financial obstacles, which makes the endoscope a practical choice for otologic surgical teaching in low- and middle-income countries. As a result, when classifying equipment priority for the lists, the variety of applications for particular equipment items was taken into account.

An operating microscope for microsurgical work in head and neck operations was considered essential at the primary level, while loupes were classified by survey respondents as aspirational. For microsurgical anastomosis, loupes-only magnification has been used in a number of applications; however, the term "aspirational" may refer to the requirement that loupes be fitted to a specific surgeon rather than universally available microscopes that can be adjusted for magnification.

Other surgical services that need an operating microscope may also share an operating microscope. Otoendoscopes were also considered aspirational at the primary level (Table 9.1), even though research showed that they produced comparable results to traditional microscopic ear surgery and had ergonomic advantages. This may be because it is a relatively new addition to the otology toolkit and requires a significant learning curve for individuals who have only been trained with operative microscopes to consistently reap the benefits of using otology equipment.

It should be mentioned that only computer-assisted navigation for skull base surgery was considered aspirational at the tertiary level. This technology, which offers real-time computed tomography-based surgical guidance, may have been viewed as aspirational because of its exorbitant cost, the paucity of conclusive data demonstrating better results, and the requirement for skilled personnel to operate it.

In order to characterize the need for OHNS services and equipment across economic strata, this survey included the opinions of OHNS providers from both HICs and LMICs. This collection of necessary tools and services have a wide range of applications. Initially, this list could be used to gauge the availability of resources, increasing the possibility that OHNS care will be included in the present surgical capacity evaluations. Precise evaluations of capacity are essential for both the internal evaluation of health systems and the more general objectives of academic global surgery. Second, ministries of health, health systems, and facilities can use this list as a guide when making equipment purchases related to OHNS. National surgical plans have not placed enough emphasis on OHNS conditions, but the list of necessary supplies and services could help shape future policy that will enhance OHNS treatment. Third, this list can be used to support the philanthropic donation of necessary equipment to nations without access to the supplies required for high-quality OHNS care. Similar lists have been used to persuade nongovernmental organizations, medical equipment manufacturers, and HIC academic centers to contribute "essential equipment kits" to clinical centers with low funding. When combined, these lists can be used to maximize the use of available resources and promote improved OHNS care for patients worldwide.

OHNS care is still significantly hampered by a lack of ancillary support services and equipment in health systems all over the world. In order to meet the demands for focused resource investment and infrastructure capacity assessment, surgical providers have created essential resource checklists. This list of crucial OHNS tools and services, compiled by experts, serves as a starting point for other frameworks that can be modified for purposes such as internal quality evaluation, implementation studies, creating health policies, and determining financial priorities. In the end, we anticipate that these lists of necessary tools and services for healthcare delivery will enhance health outcomes for people everywhere and establish standards of excellence for OHNS care delivery.

9.1.1.2. Principles of Patient History Record in ENT

Maintaining good history taking throughout your training is a crucial skill. You can help the patient feel more at ease about discussing their symptoms by developing a strong rapport with them. It offers the chance to investigate a patient's expectations and worries. You ought to have a solid notion of the most likely differential diagnosis after finishing a comprehensive history.

- Before Starting:
  - Wash your hands
  - Make an introduction, then check on the patient's comfort.
  - Make sure to maintain eye contact and keep in mind how important it is to build a rapport with the patient (and the parents, if they are present).
- Structure of History Taking:
  - Making a complaint (chief or presenting concern (CC or PC)) and asking, "How may I help you today?"
  - History of complaint presentation (HPC): "When did this problem start?"
  - Ask specific questions about the complaint that is being presented, as well as about the pertinent risk factors. Do you have a specific set of inquiries for PCs concerning the "Ear," "Nose," and "Throat/ Head Neck"
  - Past episodes: Hospitalization, severity, and reaction to prior care.
  - Past medical history (PMH)
  - Birth History – especially crucial for pediatric ear conditions.
  - Drug history (DH) – Including vaccinations and over-the-counter drugs.
  - Allergies
  - Family History
  - Social history (SH) – Remember to ask about the effect the complaint is presenting has had on your quality of life.
  - Systems review – Ask about any propensity to bleed or bruise easily as well.
- At the End of the History:
  - Give the patient a brief overview of their past. Confirm that you have understood them correctly and ask if they have any other questions.

9.1.2. Examination of the Ear

This involves evaluating both the ear's appearance and hearing.

9.1.2.1. History

The following issues should be included:

- Deafness, tinnitus, discharge (otorrhoea), pain (otalgia), fullness in the ear, vertigo, dizziness, and unsteadiness are typical signs of ear disease.
- Associated symptoms: fever, nausea, vomiting, headache.
- Previous ear surgery
- Previous head injury.
- Family history of deafness.
- Systemic disease (e.g., stroke, multiple sclerosis, cardiovascular disease).
- Ototoxic drugs (antibiotics (e.g., gentamicin), diuretics, cytotoxics).
- Continuous exposure to noise or abrupt loud noise exposure (such as

when shooting or using a pneumatic drill).

- History of atopy and allergy.
- Neurological symptoms.

9.1.2.2. Inspecting the External Ear

Examine the external ear using an otoscope prior to examination. Wipe away any wax and any discharge. Seek out any overt indications of abnormality.

- Size and shape of the pinna.
- Extra cartilage tags/pre-auricular sinuses or pits.
- Signs of trauma to the pinna.
- Suspicious skin lesions, such as neoplasia, on the pinna.
- Skin disorders affecting the external canal and pinna.
- Discharge-producing external ear canal infection or inflammation.
- Scars or indicators of prior surgery.
- Obvious masses or lymph node enlargements.

9.1.2.3. Palpation

If there are any enlarged lymph nodes, measure their size, location, and tenderness. Before doing an otoscopy, move the pinna and press the tragus if acute otalgia is reported. This is usually painful in cases of otitis externa but not in cases of otitis media. Additionally, check behind the ear; in a patient presenting with fever and ear pain, post-auricular fluctuant tenderness is suggestive of mastoiditis.

9.1.2.4. Inspecting the Ear Canal and Eardrum

In order to straighten the ear canal and examine the TM, the examination technique entails grasping the pinna and pulling it up and backward (posteriorly and superiorly). When examining a baby, only pull the pinna posteriorly rather than superiorly. Reducing the patient's discomfort caused by hand movements that are exaggerated in the ear is possible by holding the otoscope close to the eyepiece as opposed to at the end. Speculums used in otoscopes are disposable. To get the best view, the speculum must be fitted correctly in size. Although it may be tempting to use a small piece for ease of insertion, doing so will only limit the image that can be seen. Small speculums are generally best left for young children or people with small ear canals.

Take note of the wax, foreign tissue, and discharge levels, as well as the state of the canal skin. An otoscope-mounted pneumatic speculum can be used to assess the eardrum's mobility. As the balloon is squeezed, the drum ought to move.

9.1.2.5. Inspecting the Tympanic Membrane

It is possible to see multiple views of the drum by moving the otoscope; however, it is not always feasible to view the entire drum in a single view. The drum measures approximately 1 centimeter in diameter.

The following structures can be found in a typical drum:

- Handle the malleus's lateral process.
- Umbo – the malleus's attachment to the TM's center.
- Light reflex / cone of light.
- Pars tensa and pars flaccida (attic).

There are times when a thin, healthy drum exhibits the following:

- Long process of the incus.
- Chorda tympani.
- Eustachian opening.

- Promontory of the cochlea.

Common ear-related pathological conditions include:

- Note the size, position, and site of the perforations.
- Tympanosclerosis, especially in those with a history of middle ear infections or grommet insertion.
- Glue ear/middle-ear effusion.
- Retractions of the drum.
- Haemotympanum, or middle ear blood.

If any ear pathology is found, examine the function of the facial nerve.

9.1.2.6. Basic Hearing Tests

Audiology clinics are typically where comprehensive hearing tests are conducted.

A person with normal hearing should be able to hear in both ears equally well.

- **Tuning Fork Tests:** The tests by Weber and Rinne. Tune a fork to 512 Hz while performing
  - o Weber 's test – This is carried out in tandem with the Rinne test. The ball of the hand or a cushioned surface is struck by the vibrating fork. Next, position the vibrating fork in the center of the forehead for four seconds. The patient is asked if the tone is heard in the center, to the right, or to the left. Central hearing is indicative of symmetrical hearing. Hearing this in the afflicted ear suggests that you may have conductive hearing loss. Additionally, this indicates an asymmetric sensorineural hearing loss if heard in the unaffected ear.
  - o Rinne's test – Tap a tuning fork on the examiner's elbow or knee. Hold it vertically, with the patient's external auditory meatus approximately 1 centimeter away from the nearest prong. Then, move it right away to the mastoid process and hold it there for two seconds while exerting counterpressure on the other side of the head. Whichever of the two positions was louder, the patient is asked to report. In general, the patient should be able to hear the air conduction (i.e., the first position better than the second position) more clearly than the bone conduction. This Rinne's test result is positive. It is a sensorineural issue rather than a conductive one if the Rinne's test is positive and hearing impairment is present. A conductive issue is present if the Rinne's test results indicate hearing loss (Figure 9.1).

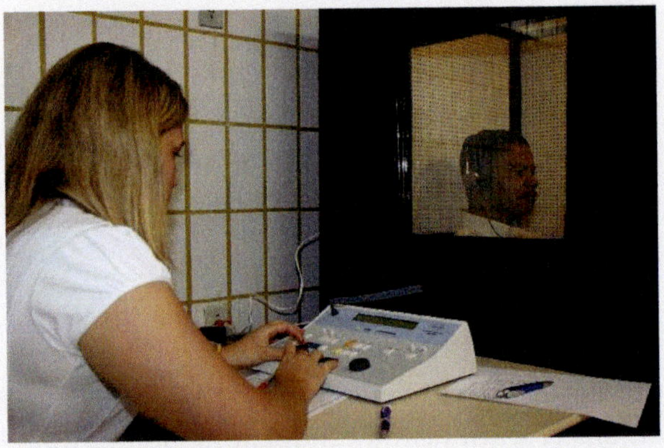

Figure 9.1. *A hearing health professional conducting an audiometric hearing test in a sound-treated testing booth.*

Source: By Flávia Costa – http://www.agenciaminas.mg.gov.br/admin/fotos/25112008061145imagem%2001%2009.jpg, CC BY 3.0, https://commons.wikimedia.org/w/index.php?curid=5610368.

9.1.3. Examination of the Nose

Examining the entire nose includes evaluating its function, airway resistance, and sometimes its sense of smell. It involves peering into the pharynx and mouth.

Nasal diseases often present with the following symptoms:

- Airway obstruction.
- Rhinorrhoea (runny nose).
- Sneezing.
- Loss of smell (anosmia).
- Facial pain caused by sinusitis.
- Snoring (associated with nasal obstruction).

History

The following issues should be covered:

- Allergies/atopic disease.
- Smoking.
- Pets at home.
- Occupation.
- History of previous nasal surgery.
- Previous trauma.
- General medical history.
- Seasonal or daily variation in symptoms.

Inspection of the Nose

Examine the external nose first. Request that the patient take off any eyewear. Check the nose for any indications of the following conditions from the front and side. Note and look for the following:

- Size and shape.
- Any obvious deformity: It is usually best to view a deviated nose from above.
- Swelling.
- Scars or abnormal creases.
- Redness (evidence of skin disease).
- Discharge or crusting.
- Offensive smell.

Examining the anterior nares from the front requires raising the nose tip and peering inside without the use of a speculum. Assess the patient's patency on both sides and request a sniff. Hold a cold metal tongue compressor beneath the patient's nose as they exhale, observing any condensation under both nostrils. Alternatively, cover one nostril while the patient sniffs to get a good sense of the patency of their nasal airway.

Endoscopy is now used by the majority of otolaryngologists for additional examination. Nonetheless, the conventional approach of using a head mirror or bright glasses with a Thudichum speculum to open the nose allows for a more precise examination of the nasal cavity and is better suited for primary care. It may take some time to get the hang of holding the instrument comfortably. Gently insert the Thudichum speculum and locate the nasal septum medially, turbines laterally, inferior turbinate (which is almost always visible), and the middle turbinate, which is frequently small and hard to see. Examine the area for inflammation (rhinitis), the septum's position, and the presence of polyps (feet should be insensitive to touch). In secondary care, the nasopharynx—the postnasal space containing the pharyngeal recess, Eustachian tube orifices, and possibly adenoids or nasopharyngeal cancer—is viewed using a flexible nasal endoscope. Lastly, check the palate. Seek for tumors originating from the soft palate and large nasal polyps.

9.1.4. Examination of the Throat

This entails a comprehensive assessment of the oral cavity.

9.1.4.1. History

Ask about:

- Sore throat.
- Odynophagia (pain on swallowing).
- Dysphagia (difficulty swallowing).
- Hoarseness and changes in voice quality.
- Halitosis.
- Snoring, mouth breathing, or disturbed sleep.
- Trismus (spasm of the jaw muscles).

9.1.4.2. Inspection

Request that the patient take out any dentures before using a bright torch to thoroughly examine the following areas of the patient's mouth: the tongue, hard and soft palate, tonsillar fossa, gingivolabial and gingivobuccal sulci, floor of the mouth, and undersurface of the tongue. Follow the following steps:

- Look into the mouth and observe the state of the tongue.
- Examine the tonsils and back of the tongue (use a tongue depressor to press down on the tongue).
- Evaluate the overall state of the dentition.
- Feel the base of the tongue for any lumps that might not be immediately apparent.
- Inspect the uvula and soft palate.
- Examine the area between the cheek and gums, known as the gingivobuccal sulcus, as well as the buccal region.
- Examine the floor of the mouth and ask the patient to stick their tongue out to look for lumps or stones in the submandibular duct.
- Use a flexible fiberoptic nasendoscope or a mirror to examine the larynx and nasopharynx.

9.2. Neck Masses

In clinical practice, neck masses are common. With organized, effective diagnostic techniques, the family physician should be able to identify the cause of a mass. The primary objective is to diagnose a benign or malignant mass; malignancies are more common in adult smokers over 40. Etiologies can be classified based on whether they have an acute onset or duration (e.g., contagious), subacute (e.g., such as squamous cell carcinoma), or long-term (e.g., thyroid), and further restricted by the patient's characteristics. Imaging and surgical tools are useful if a clear cause cannot be found by a physical examination and history. For adults, contrast-enhanced computed tomography is the preferred initial diagnostic test. The assessment of pulsatile neck masses is best served by computed tomography angiography rather than magnetic resonance angiography. A fine-needle aspiration biopsy can be carried out to rule out the involvement of underlying vital structures. This biopsy provides diagnostic information through the use of cytology, Gram stain, and cultures of bacteria and acid-fast bacilli. When it comes to identifying cancer, fine-needle aspiration biopsy has a sensitivity and specificity range of 77% to 97% and 93% to 100%, respectively.

9.2.1. Normal Anatomy

It takes an understanding of normal structures to make an accurate diagnosis of a neck mass. It is possible to differentiate between true pathology and normal anatomical variations with experience and practice, obviating the need for further testing or subspecialist consultation.

Central to the neck region are the hyoid bone, thyroid cartilage, and cricoid cartilages. Under the thyroid cartilage, the thyroid gland is typically palpable in the midline. Pulsatile carotid arteries have the potential to be highly noticeable in the presence of atherosclerotic disease. The entire sternocleidomastoid muscles should be palpated, paying particular attention to the lymph nodes in the deep jugular.

The preauricular region on either side of the lateral neck is home to the parotid glands. Every parotid gland has a tail that extends inferior to the ear lobe and below the mandibular angle. The sternocleidomastoid muscle, the posterior belly of the digastric muscle, and the mandibular body form a triangle that contains the submandibular glands. These glands may become ptotic and become more noticeable in elderly patients. The most common locations for neck masses are lymph nodes, which are found all over the head and neck area. Additional assessment is necessary for lymph nodes larger than 1.5 cm and those that are matted, firm, or fixed.

9.2.2. History

An in-depth medical history can offer crucial hints for the diagnosis of a cervical mass. The most important indicators of neoplasia are the patient's age as well as the mass's size and duration. The most crucial factor is the patient's age, as the chance of cancer increases with age. It is also necessary to ascertain when symptoms start and how long they last. Adenopathy brought on by an upper respiratory tract infection is suggested by acute symptoms like fever, sore throat, and cough. Chronic dysphagia, hoarseness, sore throat, and altered voice quality are frequently linked to structural or functional changes in the larynx or pharynx.

An infectious or inflammatory cause for a neck mass is suggested by recent travel, head and neck trauma, insect bites, and contact with domestic or farm animals. A prior radiation treatment history, heavy alcohol consumption, or a history of smoking increases the risk of cancer. To narrow the differential diagnosis and create a suitable treatment plan, a review of related medical conditions and prior treatments is helpful.

9.2.3. Acute Neck Masses

In general, neck masses that develop gradually are symptomatic. A hematoma may result from blunt or sharp trauma that damages the vasculature and tissue. Small hematomas usually go away on their own, but large, quickly growing hematomas need to be treated right away and may need to be surgically explored. The development of pseudoaneurysms or arteriovenous fistulas, which are characterized by soft, pulsatile masses with a thrill or bruit, is exacerbated by similar trauma mechanisms in addition to the addition of shearing forces. The extent of any potential vascular injury is determined by computed tomography (CT) angiography, and surgical ligation is typically the course of treatment.

Cervical lymphadenopathy is primarily caused by infection or inflammation resulting from various odontogenic, salivary, viral, and bacterial etiologies. These lymph nodes can be warm and erythematous, and they are frequently swollen, tender, and mobile. Common virus-induced upper respiratory symptoms typically resolve in one to two weeks, while lymphadenopathy usually goes away three to six weeks later. While 20–30% of upper respiratory infections in adults occur twice or four times a year on average due to unknown viruses, rhinoviruses, coronaviruses, and influenza are more frequently occurring viral pathogens. When an abnormal node does not go away after four to six weeks, a biopsy is warranted. It should also be done right away in patients who have other symptoms that point to cancer, like fever, weight loss, night sweats, or a rapidly expanding mass. A thorough lymph node evaluation is essential because certain infectious etiologies, such as Epstein-Barr virus, cytomegalovirus, toxoplasmosis, and HIV, can lead to generalized lymphadenopathy.

Neck and head bacterial infections are the main cause of cervical lymphadenopathy. The sites of lymph node inflammation in lymphadenopathy resulting from group A beta *Streptococcus* or *Staphylococcus aureus* are unpredictable. The cervical chain is frequently impacted by HIV infection or disseminated Epstein-Barr virus. Amoxicillin/clavulanate (Augmentin), clindamycin, and first-generation cephalosporins are common antibiotics used for lymphadenopathy.

The symptoms of a Bartonella henselae infection are similar to those of staphylococcal and streptococcal infections in that they are characterized by isolated, erythematous, tender, and mobile lymph nodes. When B is transferred by a flea or a kitten, cat scratch disease develops. *Henselae*, typically in the vicinity of the injection site, resulting in a localized lymphadenopathy.

Cervical lymphadenopathy is the result of Mycobacterium tuberculosis infection in its extrapulmonary form. Situated in the posterior triangle/cervical chain, the diffuse, bilateral lymph nodes are characterized by their multiple, fixed, firm, and nontender masses. Those who have recently moved to or left tuberculosis-endemic regions like India, Southeast Asia, or sub-Saharan Africa should be closely watched, and purified protein derivative testing should be carried out in these patients. It is still important to take into account the possibility of atypical mycobacterial infections even in cases where purified protein derivative testing yields a negative result. If the lymphadenopathy does not improve after initial diagnosis and treatment, a head and neck surgeon referral or a fine-needle aspiration biopsy (FNAB) of the lymph nodes may be necessary. Acute salivary gland inflammation (also known as sialadenitis) frequently happens in elderly, disabled people who have recently had dental work done or are dehydrated. Affected salivary glands can cause swelling and pain that develops quickly or gradually. Localized edema, erythema, and tenderness or fluctuation that is indicative of an abscess can also occur. Purulent discharge may be released into the oral cavity by bimanual compression in the direction of the duct opening. To confirm this diagnosis and rule out other contributing etiologies like a dental abscess or local tumor compression, a neck CT scan with intravenous contrast media may be necessary.

9.2.4. Subacute Neck Masses

It takes weeks or months to detect subacute masses. These masses may grow fairly quickly, but because they are asymptomatic at first, they frequently go undetected. Until proven differently, a neck mass that persists without symptoms in an adult should be diagnosed as malignant. It is critical for family physicians to identify common presentations of head and neck cancers because delayed diagnosis lowers survival in conditions like laryngeal cancer. The most frequent primary neoplasms of the head and neck are squamous cell carcinomas of the upper aerodigestive tract, which frequently cause cervical lymphadenopathy of unknown etiology through their metastases. Nonhealing ulcers, dysarthria, dysphagia, odynophagia, loose or misaligned teeth, globus, hoarseness, hemoptysis, and oropharyngeal paresthesias are among the frequently occurring presenting symptoms. Typically, firm, fixed, and matted lymph nodes are linked to cancer. Nonetheless, additional research is necessary if there is persistent cervical lymphadenopathy or symptoms combined with risk factors, an unclear etiology, or a nonresponse to antibiotics.

Male sex and the use of alcohol, tobacco, or betel nuts—which Southeastern Asians are known to chew—are risk factors for upper aerodigestive tract cancers. Poor oral hygiene and a family history of squamous cell carcinoma of the head and neck are two additional risk factors for oropharyngeal cancer.

Human papillomavirus infections (particularly high-risk HPV 16 and 18) are a subset of squamous cell carcinomas that are becoming more common. The symptoms of these lesions include pharyngeal bleeding, dysphagia, lingual tonsillar asymmetry, rapidly expanding, lateral, cystic lymph nodes, and persistent cervical nodal hypertrophy. White men aged 35 to 55 who have a history of smoking, heavy drinking, and having multiple sexual partners—especially those involving orogenital contact—are the most vulnerable demographic.

The parotid gland is the site of about 80% of benign salivary gland tumors. In contrast to malignant tumors, which can have rapid growth, skin fixation, pain, or involvement of cranial nerves (particularly cranial nerve VII [facial]), these tumors are unilateral, asymptomatic, slow-growing, mobile masses. Another possibility for diagnosis is an isolated pre-auricular lymph node, or intraparotid lymph node. After reviewing the results of FNAB or contrast-enhanced CT scans, excisional biopsy is the recommended diagnostic procedure for these tumors. A hypertrophied, fibrotic gland may indicate chronic sialadenitis brought on by a duct stone (sialolith) or stenosis, while persistent glandular enlargement accompanied by xerophthalmia and xerostomia symptoms may indicate Sjögren syndrome.

Local lymph nodes are another site of metastasis for skin cancers, particularly melanoma. If a primary head and neck cancer is not clearly the cause of the regional lymphadenopathy, doctors should look for melanoma in the mucosal areas of the nose, paranasal sinuses, oral cavity, and nasopharynx. Lymphadenopathy is an uncommon side effect of squamous and basal cell carcinoma metastases. Fever, chills, night sweats, and weight loss are constitutional symptoms that may indicate distant metastases. In over 50% of cases, FNAB indicates a malignancy when metastases present as supraclavicular lymphadenopathy, with age older than 40 years being the main predictor of malignancy. The most frequent primary malignancy sites that result in cervical lymphadenopathy are the pancreas, ovaries, uterine cervix, breasts, lymphomas, and gastroesophageal region.

Lymphoma often manifests as a painless lymph node in the neck, which may grow quickly and then become painful. Diffuse lymphadenopathy and splenomegaly frequently develop before the onset of early constitutional symptoms. The lymph nodes linked to lymphoma are typically rubbery, soft, and mobile in contrast to the metastatic disease-associated lymph nodes described above. Hodgkin lymphoma is more common in older adults and is more likely to present extranodally in the tonsillar ring located in the pharynx. On the other hand, non-Hodgkin lymphoma has a bimodal age distribution and rarely presents extranodally in the tonsillar ring. Stage the lymphoma and identify potential biopsy sites with contrast-enhanced computed tomography scans of the neck, chest, abdomen, and pelvis. Rheumatologic conditions represent 4% of disorders presenting with cervical lymphadenopathy and 3% of disorders presenting with enlarged salivary glands. The two rheumatic conditions that most frequently result in enlargement of the salivary glands or cervical nodes are sarcoidosis and Sjögren syndrome.

9.2.5. Chronic Neck Masses

Although they are more common in children, congenital masses can grow slowly and last into adulthood. The most prevalent congenital cyst, thyroglossal duct cysts, are located midline, next to the hyoid bone, and they rise with deglutition. Most of these cysts are detectable by the age of five, and 60% are found by the age of 20. Nonetheless, 7% of adults in one autopsy series had thyroglossal duct cysts, the majority of which were not clinically noticeable. Branchial cleft cysts account for 22% of congenital neck masses and typically manifest anterior to the sternocleidomastoid muscle. Patients frequently report recurrent upper respiratory symptoms in conjunction with a distinct, tender, erythematous mass. Less common than thyroglossal or branchial cleft cysts, dermoid cysts are soft, doughy, painless masses that enlarge with entrapment of epithelium in deeper tissue. They are usually found in the submental triangle.

Empiric antibiotic coverage for staphylococcal, streptococcal, and gram-negative anaerobe pathogens using first-generation cephalosporins, amoxicillin/clavulanate, or clindamycin is appropriate in the initial management of a presumed congenital cyst infection, much like the treatment for bacterial lymphadenopathy previously discussed. After recurrent infections, excision—the only effective treatment for these cysts and tracts—may be an option.

The majority of chronic anterior neck masses are caused by thyroid pathology, and these masses are frequently subtle. In addition to goitrogenic exposures like lithium, diffusely enlarged thyroid glands can result from Graves' disease, Hashimoto thyroiditis, or iodine deficiency. With an estimated prevalence of 4–7% in adults, thyroid nodules are common; only 5% of these are malignant. For nodules smaller than 1 cm, physical examination is not a reliable method of detection. A laryngocele may also develop in the anterior triangle as a traumatic neck mass created by chronic coughing or repetitive blowing (e.g., from nose blowing or blowing into a musical instrument), which causes herniation of the laryngeal diverticulum through the lateral thyrohyoid membrane.

An intermittent, air-filled swelling of the neck that resonates to percussion is brought on by increased airway pressure. The swelling may develop into an airway obstruction called a laryngopyocele. Laryngoscopy or contrast-enhanced CT scans can be used to confirm laryngocele or laryngopyocele, which need to be surgically excised. Neuroendocrine tumors known as paragangliomas affect the chemoreceptors in the lateral neck of the carotid body, jugular vein, or vagus nerve. Tumors of the carotid body and glomus jugulare typically appear as a pulsatile, compressible mass with a bruit or thrill in the upper anterior triangle, close to the carotid bifurcation.

These tumors are fixed in the cranial to caudal plane, despite being mobile from medial to lateral directions. Although they are typically asymptomatic, when they do function, the release of catecholamines can result in flushing, palpitations, and hypertension. Plasma or 24-hour urine collection is used for diagnostic testing to measure catecholamines and metanephrines. Lipomas are common subcutaneous adipose tumors that are soft, mobile, and distinct. Though they can appear anywhere on the neck, they typically affect the trunk and extremities. They frequently appear in patients who are posttraumatic or older than 35.

9.2.6. Evaluation of the Neck Mass

A common clinical finding that affects patients of all ages is a mass in the neck. The differential diagnosis may be very wide, and while benign processes account for the majority of masses, malignant disease should not be disregarded.

For this reason, it is critical that doctors create a methodical process for arriving at a diagnosis and creating a treatment plan for their patients.

9.2.6.1. General Considerations

The patient's age group ought to be taken into account first. It is necessary to take into account three primary age groups: pediatrics (0–15 years), young adults (16–40 years), and late adults (>40 years). Children's neck masses are typically more inflammatory or congenital than neoplastic. In the young adult, this distribution is comparable. Neoplasia, however, ought to be taken into account first in late adulthood. The "rule of 80"—which states that 80% of adult non-thyroid neck masses are neoplastic and 80% of these masses are malignant—is frequently applied. On the other hand, a child's neck mass has a 90% chance of being benign. The mass's location ought to be taken into account next. Usually benign, a midline location is a thyroglossal duct cyst or dermoid cyst. The location of metastatic neck masses may be crucial in identifying the original tumor, since lymph node drainage patterns in the upper aerodigestive tract are relatively consistent.

9.2.6.2. Diagnostic Steps

A careful and comprehensive history and a comprehensive head and neck examination are essential first steps in the evaluation of a patient with a neck mass. A detailed examination of its developmental trajectory, accompanying symptoms, individual habits, and history of trauma, radiation, or surgery is crucial. Asking about alcohol and tobacco use, fever, pain, weight loss, nocturnal sweats, and tuberculosis exposure is important. If the patient is a late adult and has a history of smoking, dysphagia, otalgia, and/or hoarseness, these symptoms most likely indicate a neoplastic process.

The examiner shouldn't ignore the full examination of the head and neck in favor of giving the neck mass undue attention. It is recommended to visualize all mucosal surfaces of the larynx, nasopharynx, oropharynx, using either direct examination or fiberoptic visualization. In addition to the neck mass, digital palpation should be used to assess the oral and pharyngeal surfaces. Focusing on the neck mass's location, mobility, and consistency can frequently classify it into a broad etiologic category, such as vascular, salivary, nodal/ inflammatory, congenital, or neoplastic. A clinical trial of antibiotics and observation lasting no more than two weeks with close monitoring may be necessary if there is a tender, moving mass or if there is a strong suspicion of inflammatory adenopathy with an otherwise negative examination.

9.2.6.3. Diagnostic Studies

9.2.6.3.1. Fine Needle Aspiration Biopsy (FNAB)

The current gold standard for diagnosing neck masses is FNAB, which should be used for any neck mass that does not appear to be an obvious abscess and continues to grow despite taking prescribed antibiotics. FNAB distinguishes benign or malignant neoplastic lesions from inflammatory and reactive processes, which typically do not necessitate surgical intervention. Additionally, it could calm the patient's concerns about cancer and assist the doctor in telling a carcinoma from a lymphoma, avoiding the need for an unnecessary panendoscopy. FNAB has no contraindications, and the fine needle gauge minimizes the risk of hemorrhage. Today's fine needles do not pose a risk for tumor needle-track seeding.

9.2.6.3.2. Ultrasonography

When combined with guided FNAB, this study could be helpful in locating difficult or deep anatomic areas. It can occasionally be helpful in distinguishing congenital cysts from solid lymph nodes, solid tumors, and cystic masses.

9.2.6.3.3. CT, MRI/MRA, and PET

Neck CT scanning has emerged as a very useful diagnostic tool in cases that are difficult to diagnose. When combined with contrast, it can identify the origin and entire extent of deep, ill-defined masses, differentiate between cystic and solid lesions, and show blood flow or vascularity. To identify an unknown primary lesion and aid in staging, CT should be performed on patients with metastatic carcinoma to the neck from an unknown primary. Metastatic carcinoma is frequently indicated by lentient changes within nodes, size greater than 1.5 cm, and loss of sharpness of nodal borders. In order to prevent the administration of iodinated material that might subsequently interfere with radioactive-iodine imaging studies or therapy, contrasted CT should be withheld in cases of suspected thyroid lesion.

MRI and CT share a lot of the same information. Because of the motion artifact on CT, it is currently preferable for upper neck and skull base masses. When combined with contrast, MRA can even be used in place of arteriography for vascular delineation in pulsatile masses or masses exhibiting bruits or thrills. While PET scanning is still relatively new, it is very useful in evaluating the extent of metastatic disease and identifying unknown primary sites in the workup of head and neck masses.

9.2.6.3.4. Open Biopsy

An open excisional biopsy of the cervical lymph node may be carried out if a negative or ambiguous FNAB is obtained but suspicion of malignancy endures. Depending on the findings of the frozen sections, the patient and the surgeon should be ready to move forward with a full neck dissection. Should the biopsy solely reveal granulomatous or inflammatory alterations, tissue culture is necessary. Closing the wound, doing additional workups, and staging procedures are determined by the presence of lymphoma or adenocarcinoma before treatment decisions are made.

A Closer Look

Carotid Body Tumor

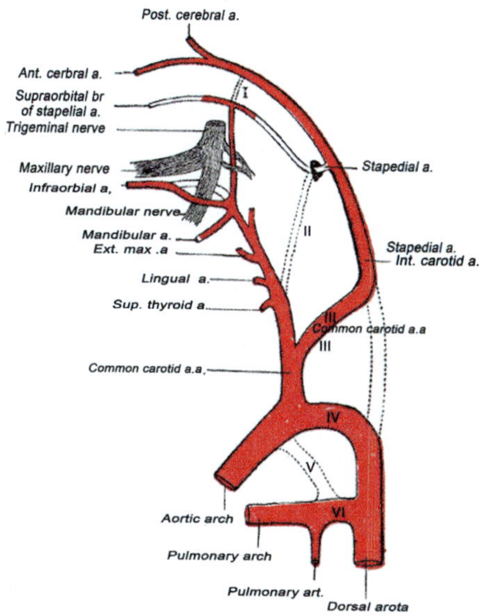

Source: By Henry Vandyke Carter – Henry Gray (1918) Anatomy of the Human Body (See "Book" section below)Bartleby.com: Gray's Anatomy, Plate 474, Public Domain, https://commons.wikimedia.org/w/index.php?curid=567241.

A mass that develops in the blood vessels close to the major arteries on either side of your neck, known as the carotid arteries, is called a carotid body tumor. Your head and brain receive blood flow from your heart via these arteries. Another name for a carotid body tumor is a carotid body paraganglioma or chemodectoma. Most tumors of the carotid body are benign (not cancerous). Less than 10% of carotid body tumors are thought to be malignant (cancerous) according to certain studies. A carotid body tumor can occur to anyone. The condition typically affects adults over the age of 20, and it appears to affect women and those assigned to the female gender at birth more frequently than men and those assigned to the male gender at birth. Although carotid body tumors usually don't hurt, your doctor might still want to remove it if it gets big enough to damage your neck's blood vessels or cause other symptoms.

Symptoms: A carotid body tumor may not show any symptoms at first, but as it enlarges, it may put pressure on blood vessels and nearby nerves. There could be a lump on your neck. Additional signs of a carotid body tumor may be:

- Hoarseness.
- Numbness in your tongue.
- Sore throat.
- Swallowing problems (dysphagia).

Causes: Although the exact cause of carotid body tumors is unknown, hypoxic individuals are more likely to develop them. Since about 90% of cases are sporadic, anyone can be affected, regardless of family history. 10% of cases are familial, which means that there is a genetic component and that the condition may run in families.

Diagnosis and Tests: Your healthcare provider will first conduct a physical examination of your head and neck to check for any signs of a carotid body tumor. If any potential signs are found, they may recommend further tests to confirm the diagnosis. Imaging tests commonly used to diagnose carotid body tumors are:

- CT scan.
- Magnetic resonance angiography (MRA).
- MRI.
- Ultrasound.

Management and Treatment: You will discuss your symptoms with your healthcare provider. They might advise you to do the following.

- Surgery to remove the tumor.
- Radiation therapy.

Transcatheter embolization to stop blood flow to the tumor, which you may have before surgery to help shrink the tumor.

During the surgical removal of large carotid body tumors, a hole in the carotid artery may be left behind. To fix this, a surgeon may choose to use a patch or a graft to close the hole and restore normal functioning of the artery during the procedure.

Complications: Many patients with treatment for a carotid body tumor experience no side effects. Yet, the treatment of carotid body tumors may involve numerous blood vessels. Following their therapy, some patients might have:

- Difficulty swallowing (dysphagia).
- Injury to their cranial nerves.
- Problems with healing at the surgical incision site.
- Stroke.

Summary

- The clinical method is the basic instrument and procedure that must be applied in the therapeutic setting to gather the data and other elements required for the treatment of individuals.
- Safe surgical and procedural care is essential to guaranteeing the provision of high-quality healthcare in international contexts.
- Maintaining good history taking throughout your training is a crucial skill. You can help the patient feel more at ease about discussing their symptoms by developing a strong rapport with them. It offers the chance to investigate a patient's expectations and worries.
- In clinical practice, neck masses are common. With organized, effective diagnostic techniques, the family physician should be able to identify the cause of a mass. The primary objective is to diagnose a benign or malignant mass; malignancies are more common in adult smokers over 40.
- Neck masses in children are typically more inflammatory or congenital than neoplastic. In the young adult, this distribution is comparable.

References

1. Al-Dajani, N., & Wootton, S. H. (2007). Cervical lymphadenitis, suppurative parotitis, thyroiditis, and infected cysts. *Infectious Diseases Clinics of North America, 21*(2), 523–541.
2. Al-Khateeb, T. H., & Al Zoubi, F. (2007). Congenital neck masses: A descriptive retrospective study of 252 cases. *Journal of Oral and Maxillofacial Surgery, 65*(11), 2242–2247.
3. Brown, J. R., & Skarin, A. T. (2004). Clinical mimics of lymphoma. *The Oncologist, 9*(4), 406–416.
4. Crozier, E., & Sumer, B. D. (2010). Head and neck cancer. *Medical Clinics of North America, 94*(5), 1031–1046.
5. D'Souza, G., Kreimer, A. R., Viscidi, R., et al. (2007). Case-control study of human papillomavirus and oropharyngeal cancer. *New England Journal of Medicine, 356*(19), 1944–1956.
6. Glass, C. (2008). Role of the primary care physician in Hodgkin lymphoma. *American Family Physician, 78*(5), 615–622.
7. Goffart, Y., Hamoir, M., Deron, P., Claes, J., & Remacle, M. (2005). Management of neck masses in adults. *B-ENT, 1*(suppl), 133–140.
8. Hawke, M. M. (2002). *Diagnostic Handbook of Otorhinolaryngology*. Martin Dunitz.
9. Heikkinen, T., & Järvinen, A. (2003). The common cold. *The Lancet, 361*(9351), 51–59.
10. Knopf, A., Bas, M., Chaker, A., et al. (2011). Rheumatic disorders affecting the head and neck: Underestimated diseases. *Rheumatology (Oxford), 50*(11), 2029–2034.
11. Knox, M. A. (2013). Thyroid nodules. *American Family Physician, 88*(3), 193–196.
12. Koch, W. M. (2012). Clinical features of HPV-related head and neck squamous cell carcinoma: Presentation and work-up. *Otolaryngologic Clinics of North America, 45*(4), 779–793.
13. Lee, J., & Fernandes, R. (2008). Neck masses: Evaluation and diagnostic approach. *Oral and Maxillofacial Surgery Clinics of North America, 20*(3), 321–337.

14. Miller, M. C. (2010). The patient with a thyroid nodule. *Medical Clinics of North America, 94*(5), 1003–1015.

15. O'Donoghue, G. M. (2000). *Clinical ENT: An Illustrated Textbook* (2nd ed.). Singular Publishing Group.

16. Paleri, V., & Hill, J. (2010). *ENT Infections: An Atlas of Investigation and Management*. Clinical Publishing.

17. Rosenberg, T. L., Brown, J. J., & Jefferson, G. D. (2010). Evaluating the adult patient with a neck mass. *Medical Clinics of North America, 94*(5), 1017–1029.

18. Vasileiadis, I., Kapetanakis, S., Petousis, A., Stavrianaki, A., Fiska, A., & Karakostas, E. (2012). Internal laryngopyocele as a cause of acute airway obstruction: An extremely rare case and review of the literature. *Acta Otorhinolaryngologica Italica, 32*(1), 58–62.

19. Wippold, F. J. II, Cornelius, R. S., Berger, K. L., et al. (2012). *American College of Radiology ACR Appropriateness Criteria*. Retrieved from: http://www.acr.org/~/media/ACR/Documents/AppCriteria/Diagnostic/NeckMassAdenopathy.pdf (accessed on 4 September 2024).

Chapter

OPERATIVE SURGERY

10

Contents

Introduction

Surgery is a branch of medicine that diagnoses and treats pathological conditions (such as e.g., trauma, illness, injury, or cancer), to change how the body functions (i.e., malabsorption brought on by bariatric procedures like gastric bypass), to restore or enhance beauty and appearance (cosmetic surgery), or to remove foreign objects or undesired tissues like body fat, glands, scars, or skin tags. Surgery treats acute injuries and illnesses differently from chronic, slowly developing diseases, with the exception of patients who require surgery for the latter kind of condition.

Orientation and Directional Terms

Term	Definition	Illustration
Myringotomy	A myringotomy is a procedure to create a hole in the ear drum to allow fluid that is trapped in the middle ear to drain out.	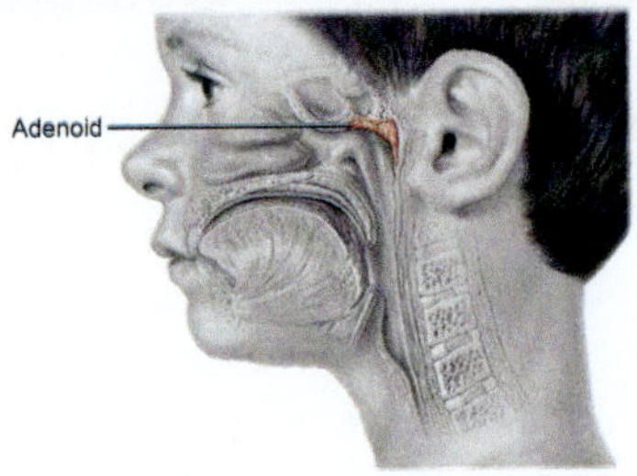
Mastoidectomy	Mastoidectomy is a surgical procedure of the temporal bone that opens postauricular air cells by removing the thin bony partitions between them.	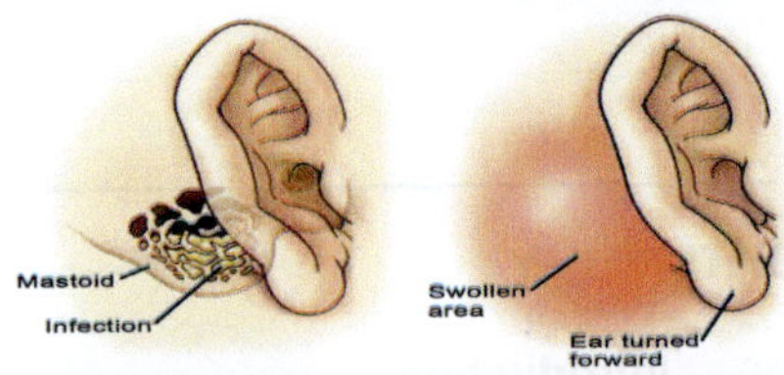
Myringoplasty	A myringoplasty is a surgery performed by an otolaryngologist to repair a hole in the eardrum. In this surgery, the hole is repaired by placing a graft made of either a small piece of tissue from elsewhere on the body, or a gel-like material.	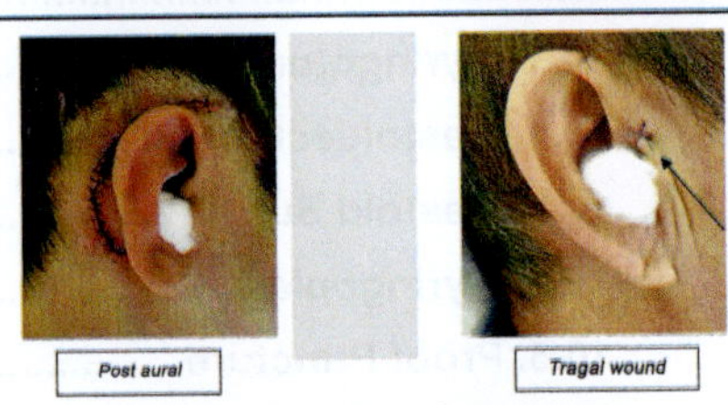
Septoplasty	Septoplasty is a surgery to correct a deviated septum. It improves airflow through your nasal passages, helping you breathe better.	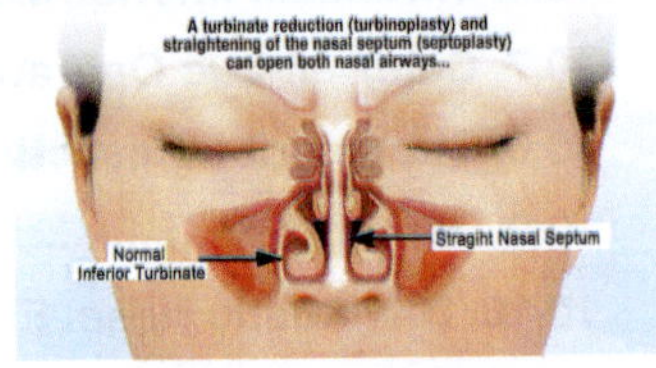
Bronchoscopy	Bronchoscopy is a procedure that lets doctors look at your lungs and air passages. It is usually performed by a doctor who specializes in lung disorders (a pulmonologist). During bronchoscopy, a thin tube (bronchoscope) is passed through your nose or mouth, down your throat and into your lungs.	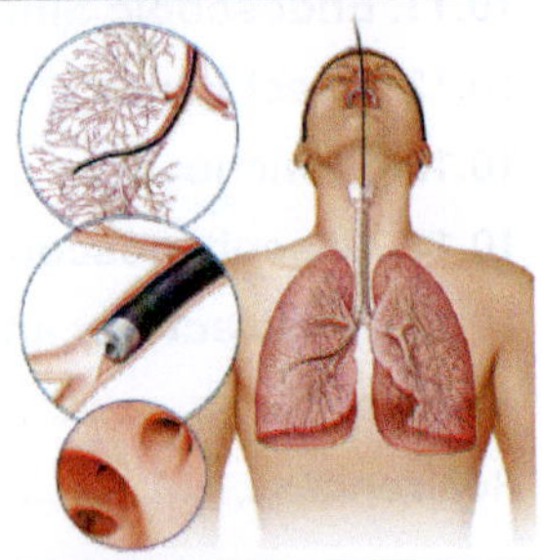
Laryngoscopy	Laryngoscopy is when a doctor uses a special camera to look down the throat to see the voice box (larynx) and vocal cords.	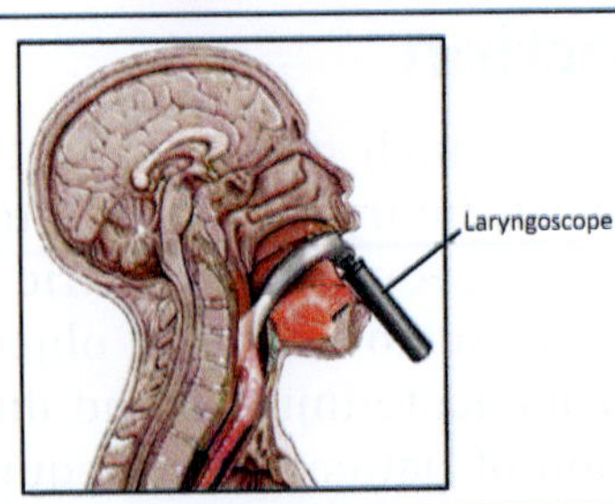

10.1. Myringotomy

A surgical procedure known as a myringotomy involves making an incision in the tympanic membrane, or eardrum, in order to drain pus from the middle ear or relieve pressure brought on by an excessive accumulation of fluid. To maintain the aeration in the middle ear for an extended period of time and to stop fluid from reaccumulating, a tympanostomy tube may be placed through the eardrum. In two to three weeks, the incision usually heals on its own without the need for a tube to be inserted. The tube is either removed during a minor procedure or naturally extrudes in 6 to 12 months, depending on the type. Individuals in need of a myringotomy typically have a blocked or malfunctioning eustachian tube, which makes it unable to carry out normal ventilation or drainage functions. Prior to the development of antibiotics, a common treatment for severe acute otitis media (middle ear infection) was myringotomy without the insertion of a tube.

10.1.1. Indications

In the pediatric age group, tympanostomy has many indications; the most common ones are recurrent otitis media and chronic otitis media with effusion (OME), which is resistant to antibiotics.

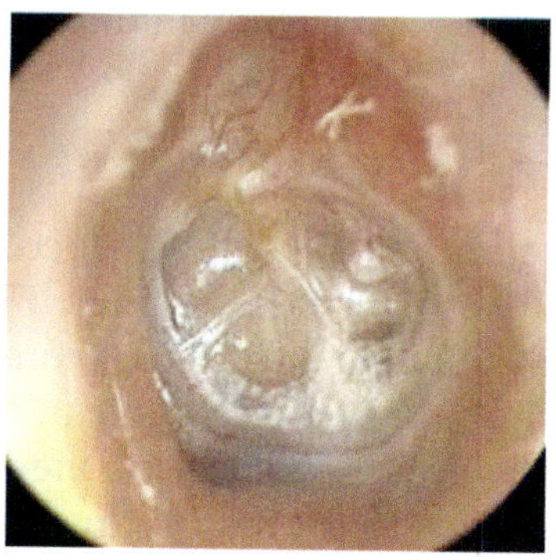

Figure 10.1. *Retracted eardrum.*

Source: By Adrian L James – Own work, CC BY-SA 3.0, https://commons.wikimedia.org/w/index.php?curid=17774654.

The symptoms in adults are a little different and include recurrent signs and symptoms of Eustachian tube dysfunction, such as vertigo, tinnitus, fluctuating hearing loss, and a severe retraction pocket in the tympanic membrane. Recurrent barotrauma episodes should be taken into consideration, particularly if they occur during flying, diving, or hyperbaric chamber treatment (Figure 10.1).

10.1.2. Procedure

Typically, myringotomy is done as an outpatient procedure. For children, general anesthesia is the preferred method, whereas local anesthesia is adequate for adults. The eardrum is lightly incised after the ear is cleaned. After aspirating any fluid that may be present, the preferred tube is inserted, and the ear is packed with cotton to stop any minor bleeding that may happen. This procedure, called a conventional myringotomy or cold knife myringotomy, typically takes one to two days to heal.

A new technique, known as tympanolaserostomy or laser-assisted tympanostomy, employs a CO_2 laser that is computer-driven and guided by a video monitor to create a precise hole in the eardrum. The laser can make the opening in just one-tenth of a second, without causing damage to the surrounding skin or other structures. This perforation remains open for several weeks, allowing for ventilation of the middle ear without the need for the insertion of tubes. Although laser myringotomies maintain the opening slightly longer than traditional cold-knife methods (two to three weeks versus two to three days without tubes), they have not been proven to be more effective in treating fluid buildup in the ear. One study found that laser myringotomies are safe but not as effective as ventilation tubes for chronic OME. Factors such as frequent ear infections in children, a history of allergies, thick mucoid effusions, and previous tube insertions make laser tympanostomy less likely to be successful.

Tympanostomy tubes come in a variety of sizes. The more common silicon, titanium, polyethylene, gold, stainless steel, or fluoroplastic tubes have supplanted traditional metal tubes. The more modern ones have phosphorylcholine and antibiotic coatings.

10.1.3. Aftercare

The care of the ear following the insertion of tubes is not well supported by science. There is a small but statistically significant benefit to wearing ear protection when swimming, according to a single randomized trial. The general consensus has been against the use of ear protection devices in the absence of compelling evidence. To avoid ear infections, it is advised to wear protective gear when swimming in untreated pools, rivers, lakes, or oceans, such as cotton balls covered in petroleum jelly, earplugs, or ear putty. No ear protection is advised when bathing, shampooing, or swimming in chlorinated pools on the surface.

10.1.4. Complications

Installing tubes does not provide a cure. There's a good chance the child will continue to experience episodes of middle ear inflammation or fluid collection if the middle ear disease has been severe or persistent enough to warrant the placement of a tube. About 15% of patients may experience tube otorrhea, or early tube drainage, in the first two weeks following insertion, and 25% may experience it more than three months later. This condition is typically not a long-term issue. It is believed that bacterial colonization is the primary cause of otorrhea. *Pseudomonas aeruginosa* is the most frequently isolated organism, whereas Methicillin-resistant Staphylococcus aureus (MRSA) is the most problematic. Research indicates that while some practitioners apply topical antibiotic drops during the postoperative phase, the bacterial biofilm is not eliminated by this approach. Although no research has been done on humans yet, a lab study revealed that tubes coated with the antibiotic vancomycin inhibited the formation of MRSA biofilm in vitro when compared to noncoated ones. The incidence of post-operative otorrhea, tube blockage, and extrusion did not differ statistically significantly between fluoroplastic tympanostomy tubes coated with phosphorylcholine and those that were not.

10.1.5. Efficacy

Research suggests that children with simple OME who do not have any other significant medical issues benefit only temporarily from tympanostomy tubes. No impact on the development of speech and language has yet been demonstrated. Approximately 50% of patients with CO_2 laser myringotomy-treated otitis media recovered after six months, according to a retrospective analysis of success rates in 96 adults and 130 children. There are no published systematic reviews as of yet. A novel treatment for OME caused by eustachian tube dysfunction has shown promise: balloon dilation eustachian tuboplasty (BDET). The extremely small number of patients in the cited studies—22 and 8, respectively, and 18 in the tympanometric study—merely emphasizes the necessity for larger, carefully monitored studies.

10.2. Mastoidectomy

A mastoidectomy is a surgical procedure used to remove diseased mastoid cells. The hollow spaces in your mastoid, the honeycomb-shaped bone that sits just behind your ear, are where these air cells grow. When otitis media, an ear infection, spreads to the skull, a mastoidectomy is required. Cholesteatoma, a noncancerous growth that develops behind the eardrum and is frequently a consequence of recurrent ear infections, is another condition for which the procedure is used. Mastoidectomy is frequently done in conjunction with cochlear implant surgery. Your surgeon will do a mastoidectomy with tympanoplasty if your eardrum has burst. A procedure called a tympanoplasty fixes your eardrum. Even in cases where your eardrum doesn't require repair, tympanoplasty refers to surgery performed behind your eardrum.

10.2.1. Procedure Details

The extent of the procedure is determined by your particular circumstances. Your ear canal and middle ear structures will remain fully intact while the disease in your mastoid is treated with a straightforward mastoidectomy. More bone is removed during a tympanomastoidectomy or canal-wall-up mastoidectomy than during a standard mastoidectomy. This is done to allow your surgeon to access your ossicles, which are the three tiny bones inside your ear that transmit sound waves, as well as the middle-ear space behind your eardrum. Your ear canal remains entirely unaltered after this procedure.

When the disease has irreversibly damaged your ear canal or when the removal of your ear canal is necessary to eradicate the disease completely, a canal-wall-down mastoidectomy or tympanomastoidectomy is carried out. Your mastoid bone and ear canal are combined during this procedure to create a large, open area known as the mastoid cavity, or mastoid bowl. To make future cleaning of your mastoid cavity easier, your ear canal opening is usually enlarged. Sometimes referred to as a radical or modified mastoidectomy, this procedure is only used when a more limited surgery has failed to treat an extensive disease or recurrent (repeating) disease.

10.2.1.1. Before a Mastoidectomy

You will receive a list of preoperative instructions from your healthcare provider, which you should carefully adhere to. You might occasionally need to take certain medications for a short period of time. Since a mastoidectomy is done while under general anesthesia, you'll also need to make plans for a reliable family member or friend to drive you to and from the procedure.

10.2.1.2. During a Mastoidectomy

To guarantee your comfort during the procedure, general anesthesia will be administered to you. Your surgeon will then:

- Make a cut to reach your mastoid bone from behind your ear. Your surgeon will make this incision with precision to minimize the visible scar from your mastoidectomy.
- Proper tools should be used to open your mastoid bone.
- Take out the infected mastoid air cells.
- Stitch the surgical site closed.
- Use gauze to clean the surgical wound.

The average duration of a mastoidectomy procedure is two to three hours.

10.2.1.3. After

During your mastoidectomy, you shouldn't experience any pain. A mastoidectomy can, however, cause some minor discomfort following the procedure, just like any other surgery. You might experience pain from the incision behind your ear and a full or stuffy feeling in your ear. Over-the-counter (OTC) painkillers like acetaminophen or ibuprofen can help you manage these side effects. To keep you comfortable during the healing process, your surgeon will also provide you with post-operative instructions.

You will awaken in recovery following your mastoidectomy. Your healthcare team will keep an eye on your recovery, and you'll be allowed to return home when you're ready. Particular postoperative instructions will be provided by your surgeon. It is critical that you adhere to these.

10.3. Mastoid Surgery

Even though a middle ear infection is already extremely painful, untreated cases may result in mastoiditis. When the mastoid bone becomes infected, it can cause mastoiditis, which can lead to bone loss if treatment is delayed. Loss of hearing may also result from the infection's spread to the brain. Should antibiotics prove ineffective, mastoid surgery might become imperative.

10.3.1. Causes of Mastoiditis

Ear infections are the main cause of mastoiditis. Fluid cannot properly drain because the bacteria from the middle ear infection travel to the air cells of the mastoid bone. This blockage of drainage causes fluid to accumulate and causes mastoiditis. Mastoiditis mostly affects children, but if caught early enough, it usually goes away without causing any long-term issues. Cholesteatoma is another condition that can lead to mastoiditis. One kind of cyst that appears in the middle ear is called a cholesteatoma.

10.3.2. Symptoms of Mastoiditis

The symptoms of mastoiditis include:

- Tenderness, redness, and swelling in the earlobe and behind the ear.
- Fluid draining from the ear
- Fever
- Irritability
- Lethargy

10.3.3. Diagnosis and Quick Treatment of Mastoiditis is Important

Mastoiditis can be hazardous and potentially fatal if left untreated. It can even spread to the brain and result in long-term problems like hearing loss. The good news is that antibiotics are usually effective in treating most cases, and our doctors at ENTACC are skilled in diagnosing and treating all ear conditions. To check for any infections, our doctor will first perform a thorough ear examination. To rule out any more conditions, they might then prescribe additional tests like an MRI or CT scan. Our doctors will determine that you have mastoiditis and then create a personalized treatment plan for you. If antibiotics are ineffective, some chronic cases may need to be treated with frequent ear cleanings or surgery.

10.3.4. Mastoid Surgery: Mastoidectomy

If the severity or recurrence of your mastoiditis are too high, mastoid surgery might be necessary. A mastoidectomy involves drilling a hole in the mastoid bone to extract the infection. The procedure is performed under general anesthesia, and most patients can return home the same day.

Following surgery, your ear will probably be bandaged, you will probably have stitches, and you might have the following symptoms.

- Headaches
- Ear pain
- Numbness

You will be prescribed antibiotics and painkillers, and you will be given an appointment to return for a check-up and stitch removal. The instructions following surgery include avoiding physically demanding activities, preventing water from getting inside your ears, and avoiding activities that put pressure on your ears, like flying. While not frequent, complications can include tinnitus, vertigo, sensorineural hearing loss, facial nerve paralysis, and taste changes.

10.4. Myringoplasty

Myringoplasty is the procedure used to seal the tympanic membrane's pars tensa perforation. Tympanoplasty is the term for myringoplasty plus scar tissue excision. The patient is positioned supine with their face turned to the side during the procedure. Temporalis fascia is the most frequently utilized graft material in this surgical procedure. Some surgeons also use the tragal cartilage and tragal perichondrium as the graft. In some tinnitus cases, myringoplasty restores hearing loss. Following surgery, there is a decreased risk of re-infection and persistent discharge. Myringoplasty should not be done in patients with uncontrolled nasal allergies, those with active middle ear discharge, those whose other ear is dead, or children younger than three years old. Although it can also be done under local anesthesia, myringoplasty is typically performed under general anesthesia.

10.4.1. Technique of Surgery

10.4.1.1. Underlay Technique

A graft is made of the temporalis fascia. An incision is made on the perforation's edge, and an epithelium ring is extracted. A mucosal layer strip is extracted from the perforation's inner side. An antibiotic-soaked gel foam is packed into the middle ear. The graft edges ought to protrude beneath the perforation's margins, with a tiny portion of them also covering the posterior canal wall. After that, the tympanomeatal flap is changed.

10.4.1.2. Overlay Technique

The removal of the temporal fascia entails elevating the medial meatal skin with tympanic membrane epithelium, an incision is made. A slit is made to tuck the graft under the malleus handle after it has been placed on the outer surface of the tympanic membrane. The incision is closed and the ear is packed with gelfoam and antibiotics. Mastoid dressing is done at the end.

10.4.2. Advantages

- Restores the tinnitus and hearing loss in certain situations.
- Examines the recurrence of infections from the eustachian tube and external auditory canal.
- Checks for aeroallergens that could cause a persistent ear discharge by penetrating the exposed middle ear mucosa.

10.4.3. Contraindications

- Middle ear discharge that is active.
- Controlling nasal allergies is important before surgery.
- When the other ear is deaf or incapable of receiving sound.
- Otitis externa
- Children below 3 years

10.5. Proof Puncture

Antral irrigation, also known as proof puncture, is a procedure used to treat and diagnose sinusitis. It involves making an incision in the inferior meatus to insert a canula into the maxillary sinus.

10.5.1. Medical Uses

It can be used as a therapeutic procedure for:

- Maxillary sinusitis, both acute and chronic, not improving with medication.

- Treatments for persistent infections are not working.
- Irrigating the gathered purulent secretions and cleaning them up.
- Dental maxillary sinusitis.
- Oro-antral fistula in the event that sinusitis is present.
- Viral rhinosinusitis in acute form. However, it should not be used as a routine treatment and should only be used in extreme circumstances.

It can be also used as a diagnostic procedure for:

- If the returning fluid in a case of chronic sinusitis is mucopurulent or purulent, a culture and sensitivity test should be performed.
- Exfoliative cytology of the fluid that is returning to exclude any cancer.

10.5.2. Contraindications

- **Age:** Under the age of 3 years because the maxillary sinus is underdeveloped.
- **Bleeding Disorders:** May lead to epistaxis.
- **Fracture of the Maxilla:** Fluid may escape via fracture lines as a result of antral lavage.
- **Febrile Stage of Acute Maxillary Sinusitis:** May cause osteomyelitis of Maxilla.
- Patients with hypertension and diabetes should not undergo this procedure.

10.5.3. Instruments

The procedure makes use of the following instruments:

- Tilley's Forceps
- Lichtwitz Antral Trocar Cannula
- Higginson's Rubber Syringe
- Nasal Speculum

10.5.4. Diagnosis of Antral Pathology

1. The presence of a cyst is indicated by watery, amber-colored fluid that immediately flows from the cannula upon puncture and contains cholesterol crystals.
2. Mucopus blobs in washings are an indication of hyperplastic sinusitis.
3. The presence of strong-smelling pus that easily mixes with irrigation fluid is a sign of suppuration. In these cases, an antral wash may be repeated once or twice a week.
4. The most precise non-invasive technique for identifying aneurysm is plain radiological X-rays (Water's view) of the sinuses.

10.5.5. Difficulties

During antral lavage, the following challenges could occur:

- **Hard Bone:** The procedure may be challenging due to the possibility of a hard maxillary sinus wall. When the cannula tip comes into contact with the sinus's posterior wall, it could become blocked and the fluid wouldn't return when the Higginson syringe is pumped. The cannula gets patent and is slightly withdrawn.
- **Blocked Ostium:** If the sinus's ostium is obstructed, fluid cannot return through it. To avoid the ostium, an additional trocar and cannula are placed where the first

one was, and a fluid is redirected through the second cannula.

10.5.6. Complications

1. Vasovagal shock: The patient may become pale, faint, and fall, and their pulse rate may drop as a result of excessive vagus nerve stimulation.
2. At the puncture site, bleeding may happen; this will stop quickly with a cotton wool plug.
3. False entrances into the orbit or cheek that result in emphysema, or fluid seeping into the orbit, lower eyelid, or cheek. Hemorrhage and a cerebrospinal fluid leak are possible side effects.
4. It is common to have a maxillary sinus infection.
5. Adverse effects from anesthesia can happen.
6. Air embolism.

10.5.7. Repetition

After a week, the puncture is repeated if the fluid that is returning is purulent. If the patient has more than three punctures and the returning fluid is consistently purulent, functional endoscopic sinus surgery (FESS) and occasionally a Caldwell-Luc operation may be necessary. Antral Washout can be performed as an outpatient treatment for Subacute Maxillary Sinusitis because it is a far less complicated process than FESS. FESS is still the preferred method of treating chronic maxillary sinusitis, nevertheless.

10.5.8. Post Operative

1. An hour after the procedure, the patient is taken out of the pack and lies down for 10 to 15 minutes.
2. In cases of suppuration, antibiotics should be administered for 5–7 days, depending on the culture and sensitivity.
3. To increase ostium patency, decongestants are administered orally and locally.
4. For post-operative headaches, analgesics might be necessary.

10.6. Intranasal Inferior Meatal Antrostomy

The procedure known as an intranasal inferior meatal antrostomy involves creating an intranasal orifice in the nasoantral wall of the inferior meatus. This procedure has been replaced by functional endoscopic sinus surgery, which is now infrequently needed.

10.6.1. Indications

Chronic purulent maxillary sinusitis

10.6.2. Contraindications

1. Permanent alteration in the mucous lining of the sinuses, such as polypoidal hypertrophy.
2. Presence of osteitis.
3. Suspicion of malignancy

10.6.3. Anesthesia

Local or general anesthesia.

10.6.4. Technique

A sizable periosteal elevator is present in the medially and upwardly fractured inferior turbinate. The inferior meatus's nasoantral wall is punctured using a curved hemostat, and the opening is then made larger by using forceps to cut through it straight through in the back and punch the bone forward using a Kerrison bone punch or reverse backbiting forceps. The opening should be as near to the nose's floor as feasible, with a diameter of 1–2 cm. By suction, intrasinus debris and pus are removed. A biopsy may also be performed. Severe bleeding may necessitate packing into the sinuses and nose.

10.6.5. Postoperative Care

Within 24–48 hours, the nasal and sinus pack are removed.

10.6.6. Complications

Few complications.

1. Postoperative bleeding.
2. Injury to nasolacrimal duct.

Note: The middle meatus is used for intranasal antrostomy these days. Using nasal endoscopes and other surgical tools used in functional endoscopic sinus surgery, middle meatal antrostomy is a more physiological procedure.

10.7. Caldwell-Luc Operation

An external approach is used in the Caldwell-Luc operation to surgically treat the severely diseased maxillary sinus. It is an alternative to endonasal endoscopic surgery for middle meatal antrostomy, which was the main method for entering the maxillary sinus prior to the development of endoscopic sinus surgery. Selected patients with extensive maxillary diseases, especially those with massive polyposis or fungal disease, are eligible for the Caldwell-Luc operation. An early postoperative recurrence of the disease could occur if the maxillary mucosa is not cleared completely. Endoscopic access to the anterior and inferior regions of the maxillary antrum presents unique challenges.

10.7.1. Indications

- Complex rhinosinusitis, either acute or chronic, typically following endoscopic sinus surgery (ESS).
- Surgery on the pterygomaxillary space.
- trauma, e.g., maxillary floor fractures
- foreign body retrieval
- benign tumor removal
- combined with ESS: orbital decompression and inverting papilloma removal.

10.7.2. Technique

- Vasoconstrictor-soaked pledgets are inserted into the nasal cavity and a lidocaine-epinephrine solution is injected into the gingivobuccal sulcus while the patient is under general anesthesia.
- incisione effettuata nel sulcus gingivobuccale sopra la fossa del cane.
- The infraorbital nerve was identified after the incision proceeded through the periosteum, which was then elevated superiorly.
- window cut using an osteotome into the maxillary antrum.
- You can use punch forceps to make the window larger.
- To create an antrostomy, a curved hemostat is passed into the sinus beneath the inferior nasal concha.
- At this point, both windows show the maxillary sinus, and debridement starts.
- Absorbable sutures are then used to seal the gingival incision.

10.7.3. Caveats

- An antrostomy should be made at least 1 centimeter posterior to the anterior edge of the inferior concha in order to protect the nasolacrimal duct.
- An incision should be made above the secondary dentition in children. It is possible to prevent damage by using CT visualization or even just plain radiography.

10.7.4. Post-Treatment and Aftercare

Following a Caldwell-Luc procedure, recovery is comparatively easy. You can return home right away after treatment if you receive local anesthesia prior to the procedure. You cannot go home until the effects of general anesthesia wear off; you must stay in a recovery room during this time. Your doctor should answer any questions you may have about post-treatment issues and provide you with information about your recovery before you leave the surgical office. In order to relieve any mild to moderate discomfort you may have for about a week following Caldwell-Luc surgery, they may also prescribe you pain medication. In order to help prevent any infections, they might also include antibiotics in their prescription.

Following the Caldwell-Luc procedure, you should be prepared for the following typical side effects:

- Mild discomfort and pain following surgery for one to two weeks.
- The possibility of infection (which would be treated by antibiotics).
- The appearance of a black eye or mild bruises.
- Momentary facial weakness or numbness.
- The gums next to the upper teeth may hurt or become numb.

After a Caldwell-Luc procedure, the majority of patients recover in a matter of days. However, it might take a few weeks for every side effect to go away.

There are actions you can do to expedite the healing process, such as:

- Drink plenty of fluids.
- Sleep with your head elevated.
- Throughout your recuperation, stay in contact with your physician for check-ins and support with any issues you may have.

It is crucial to consult your doctor on a regular basis. Although Caldwell-Luc complications are uncommon, your doctor should keep an eye on your healing process in case they arise.

10.7.5. Complications

- recurrent nasal obstruction (most common)
- recurrent sinusitis
- recurrent polyposis
- facial numbness
- facial asymmetry
- wound dehiscence
- Oro-antral fistulae
- dacryocystitis
- devitalized teeth

The canine fossa puncture (CFP) technique, which performs debridement through a 4 mm trocar under direct visualization, has largely replaced the Caldwell-Luc operation. Because CFP is less invasive, there is a decreased likelihood of complications.

10.8. Submucous Resection of Nasal Septum (SMR Operation)

Submucosal resection (SMR) and septoplasty are surgical procedures commonly used to treat a deviated septum in the nose. While SMR involves the removal of large portions of tissue, septoplasty is a tissue-sparing procedure. Most ENT surgeons use these terms interchangeably due to their goal of correcting a deviated septum.

10.8.1. Issues Associated with a Deviated Septum

The wall that splits the nose in half is called the septum. It is mostly made up of bone and cartilage. Although the septum is not perfectly centered in about 80% of cases, this is typically not an issue. Breathing issues through the nose or issues with sinus drainage may result from a deviated septum. In addition to these issues, a deviated septum may cause persistent sinus infections, nosebleeds, or facial pain. A cold may make your symptoms worse. Although many people have a deviated septum from birth, facial trauma can also be the cause of this condition. In actuality, septal deviation may begin mildly and become more severe over time.

10.8.2. Indications for Submucosal Resection

In certain cases, SMR is not required when treating a deviated septum. But if you have recurring sinus infections that are not improving after trying other treatments, you and your doctor might want to take this into consideration. It might also be taken into consideration if your septal deviation is making it difficult for you to breathe or if it is causing chronic nosebleeds. In addition, this procedure might be performed if your deviated septum is preventing your surgeon from easily accessing other areas of your nose or sinuses during nasal sinus surgery. SMR is occasionally used in conjunction with cleft palate repairs.

10.8.3. The Procedure

Nasal SMR is typically done as same-day surgery. Both a local and a general anesthetic can be used for it. An hour to an hour and a half is how long the procedure takes on average. Some of the septum may be readjusted or removed completely during the procedure. The entire procedure of SMR is carried out through the nostrils, leaving the nose looking the same from the outside. There won't be any visible scars or incisions following the procedure. Since the septum is still growing, people under the age of 18 should not typically have this procedure done.

10.8.4. Risks

Bleeding, infection, septal perforation (hole), saddle nose deformity (if too much septum is removed), and anesthesia-related complications are among the risks associated with SMR of the nose. After surgery, you might experience some nosebleeds for about 24 hours. Due to swelling, you might also have a stuffy nose for a few days following this procedure. A cool-mist humidifier may be beneficial and help avoid nasal crusting.

10.9. Septoplasty

In the fields of plastic surgery and otorhinolaryngology (ENT), nasal septoplasty is one of the most often done procedures. The main reason for this functional surgery, rather than just cosmetic one, is typically a septal deviation that causes a significant and symptomatic obstruction of the nasal airway. Many surgical approaches and techniques, such as endoscopic, open, and endonasal procedures, have been described. In order to improve surgical exposure and access, septoplasty can also be done in conjunction with or in addition to turbinoplasty, rhinoplasty, or functional endoscopic sinus surgery. Serious complications are rare, and surgical recovery typically lasts a few weeks. Choosing the right patients is essential to improving patient outcomes.

10.9.1. Anatomy and Physiology

In order to perform a successful septoplasty, one must have a solid understanding of nose anatomy, particularly with regard to the nasal septum. The nasal dorsum, columella, and nasal tip are all supported by the septum, which is the primary structural component of the external nose. Additionally, it divides the nasal cavity into two separate nasal passageways, which allow laminar airflow and warm and humidify inspired air. Septal deviation can cause the nasal valve's cross-sectional area to decrease, obstructing the airway in the process. This may result in nasal obstruction symptoms and, in certain cases, exacerbate obstructive sleep apnea symptoms. Septal deviation-related bony spurs can cause facial pain, headaches (such as Sluder syndrome or rhinogenic headaches), and epistaxis.

10.9.1.1. Septal Structures

The membranous, cartilaginous, and bony components make up the septum's three main parts. The most anterior part of the septum, between the medial crura of the lower lateral cartilages and the caudal end of the quadrangular cartilage (the cartilaginous septum), is composed of fibrous tissue and is known as the membranous septum. The quadrangular cartilage, as its name implies, is shaped like a quadrangle and is positioned behind this membranous septum. It attaches inferiorly to the maxillary crest, superiorly to the upper lateral cartilages, and posteriorly to the bony septum. Usually, a thin, cartilaginous tail measuring one to two centimeters in length rests on one side of the bony septum. The vomer, which rests inferior-posterior to the cartilage, and the perpendicular plate of the ethmoid (PPE), which rests superiorly and posteriorly, combine to form the bony septum. The middle and superior turbinates are located in the ethmoid bone, which is also adjacent to the sphenoid and base of the skull. The nasal bones are connected to the superior aspect of the upper lateral cartilages and are positioned on the medial dorsal aspect of the upper nose, above the PPE.

The nasal valve, also known as the "internal" nasal valve, is a critical anatomical concept located in the narrowest part of the nasal passage. It is a triangular area positioned just under the middle of the nasal vault and is defined by the dorsal septum, the caudal border of the upper lateral cartilage, and the head of the inferior turbinate. While the traditional nasal valve angle is considered to be around 15 degrees, it is often closer to 30 degrees. In approximately 50% of individuals, there is a cluster of submucosal glandular and vascular tissue called a septal swell body or "septal turbinate" at the internal nasal valve level, making it appear wider than usual. Although the swell body may seem like a septal deviation when viewed from one side, it typically appears symmetrically on both sides.

The septum's junctions with the keystone area and the anterior nasal spine of the maxilla are its two surgically important points of articulation. The keystone area, which is where the nasal bones, quadrangular cartilage, upper lateral cartilage, and PPE converge, is an essential area for stability and structure. During septoplasty, it must be handled carefully to prevent upsetting the support system for the nasal dorsum. The rhinion, a cephalometric point, is directly beneath the keystone area. A saddle nose deformity may occur if the keystone area is disturbed, and repair may be technically difficult. Mucoperichondrium and mucoperiosteum, which cover the cartilaginous and bony components of the septum, respectively, offer innervation and a plentiful vascular supply. The blood vessel network in the nasal cavity facilitates the warming and humidification of the air. Predominantly, pseudostratified respiratory epithelium makes up the surface mucosa. The nasal cavity's olfactory cleft region is closer to the olfactory epithelium, which is situated more superiorly and contains basal, supporting, and olfactory cells.

10.9.1.2. Blood Supply

A group of arteries that originate from the internal and external carotid arteries supply blood to the nasal septum. The anterior and posterior ethmoidal arteries, which supply the superior aspect of the septum, are derived from the internal carotid artery through the ophthalmic artery. The facial and maxillary arteries originate from the external carotid, and their terminal branches supply the remaining vascular supply. The branches of the facial artery form the superior labial artery, which supplies blood to the anterior aspect of the nose. The inferior and posterior septum are supplied by the greater palatine and sphenopalatine arteries, which are branches of the maxillary artery. These five arteries (anterior and posterior ethmoid, superior labial, greater palatine, and sphenopalatine) anastomose anteroinferiorly at Little's area on the septum to form Kiesselbach's plexus, which is the most common site of epistaxis.

10.9.1.3. Innervation

The internal and external noses are innervated by the ophthalmic (CN V1) and maxillary (CN V2) branches of the trigeminal (CN V) nerve. The anterior and posterior ethmoid nerves, which supply the anterior-superior and posterior-superior aspects of the septum, respectively, are specifically derived from the nasociliary branch of CN V1. The posteroinferior aspect of the septum receives its supply from the nasopalatine branch of CN V2. The anterior septum is supplied by the superior alveolar nerve, which is a branch of the maxillary nerve. Sensory data from the olfactory epithelium to the olfactory bulbs is transmitted via the olfactory nerve (CN I).

10.9.2. Indications

A nasal septal deformity is the primary indication for a septoplasty. This typically results in a reduction in cross-sectional area, obstruction of airflow, and a feeling of nasal blockage. It is caused by the cartilaginous and/or bony portions of the septum deviating into one or both of the nasal passages. Patients may specifically complain of obstruction symptoms when exerting themselves or during physical activity. Trauma is the most frequent reason for the deviation. Neural obstruction symptoms must be present in order for functional surgery to be justified. There are numerous methods for grading symptoms of nasal obstruction. A validated tool for assessing the degree of obstruction is the Nasal Obstruction Symptom Evaluation (NOSE) scale. Surgery is unlikely to be beneficial for those with low scores. To determine whether concurrent conditions like trauma, rhinosinusitis, allergies, vasculitis, illicit drug use, chronic decongestant use, autoimmune disease, or cancer may exacerbate or cause obstruction, a complete history is crucial. In these cases, adequate medical therapy (e.g., intranasal corticosteroids for chronic allergic rhinitis) should be offered prior to considering surgery.

Additional indications for septoplasty comprise of sinusitis, recurrent epistaxis, obstructive sleep apnea, and facial pain and/or headaches resulting from contact between septal spurs and a turbinate, also known as Sluder's syndrome. To improve access to target structures, septoplasty might also be required in addition to endoscopic sinus, skull base, or orbital surgery.

10.9.3. Contraindications

There are various situations in which surgery should not be performed. These comprise coexisting conditions like vasculitis or rhinosinusitis, as well as situations where appropriate medical treatment has not been tried. Although nasal sprays cannot correct a deviated septum, they can reduce chronic inflammation and alleviate symptomatic nasal obstruction to the point where surgery is not necessary. Additionally, if conservative therapy has not been tried to no avail, third-party payers are unlikely to approve a costly surgical procedure. It is strongly discouraged to use recreational drugs actively during the perioperative period, especially intranasal cocaine. Cocaine's mucosal-damaging and vasoconstrictive properties can lead to complications like septal perforation, delayed healing, and, in the end, dorsal collapse with saddle nose deformity. Prior to surgery, it is recommended that patients have abstained for a minimum of 6 to 12 months. Toxicology screening may also be required to verify compliance. In patients exhibiting symptoms of medicamentosa rhinitis, similar measures ought to be implemented. Although they can help reduce bleeding during and after surgery, vasoconstrictive decongestant nasal sprays should also be avoided for a considerable amount of time prior to the procedure. Although smoking is generally harmful to patients' health, there is not much evidence at this time to suggest that smoking has a negative effect on how well nose surgery goes.

Surgery should not be recommended to patients who have unreasonable expectations for the functional or cosmetic results of a septoplasty without first providing thorough preoperative counseling. This is especially true for people who are having rhinoplasty procedures done concurrently. Achievable expectations between the patient and the surgeon are essential to enhancing post-operative satisfaction for both parties. In a similar vein, patients with limited functional symptoms but septal deviation and deformity may not benefit much from surgery. To assess whether a general anesthetic would be safe and whether patients could handle the post-operative recovery process, factors such as patient co-morbidities, age, and functional status (ASA grade) must be taken into account.

10.9.4. Equipment

Typical components of a standard septoplasty set are as follows. Be aware that depending on their preferred methods, surgeons might only utilize a portion of these tools during the procedure.

- Headlight
- Hartmann/Vienna nasal speculum
- Cottle nasal speculum
- Killian nasal speculum (3 sizes)
- Killian retractor
- Hills elevator
- #15 blade on a #7 Bard-Parker scalpel handle
- Cottle curved scissors
- Gorney nasal shears
- Jansen-Middleton forceps
- Blakesley nasal forceps
- Takahashi nasal forceps
- Blakesley-Wilde nasal forceps
- Lubet-Barbon nasal dressing forceps
- Ferguson or Frazier suction tip
- Bipolar diathermy forceps
- Adson-Brown forceps
- Cushing-Brown bayonet forceps
- Jansen nasal dressing forceps
- Cottle lower lateral forceps
- Cotton applicator
- McKenty raspatory

- Freer chisel
- Freer elevator
- Freer septal knife
- Pierce elevator
- Cottle elevator
- Woodson elevator
- Cottle chisel
- Cottle metal mallet
- Backhaus towel forceps
- Needle holder
- Medicine cup
- Hopkins rod, light source, and stack (if endoscopic)
- Silastic splints
- 5-0 and 4-0 chromic gut suture
- Mupirocin ointment

10.9.5. Personnel

Septoplasty procedures are typically performed by ENT surgeons. Most ENT surgeons perform simple septoplasties among otolaryngologists. Experts in rhinology or facial plastic surgery may perform more involved procedures such as revision surgery, either in conjunction with or apart from rhinoplasties. Septoplasties are also performed by certain plastic surgeons. The following staff members are needed to finish the procedure: coordinators, anesthetists, scrub nurses, surgical technologists, and nurses for the operating room and recovery.

10.9.6. Preparation

10.9.6.1. History

It is important to get a thorough history that describes the type and severity of nasal symptoms. It is important to assess symptoms of any other systemic or sinonasal pathologies, including allergies. It is possible to grade symptoms of nasal obstruction by using scoring systems like the NOSE scale. A thorough medical history should be acquired, paying special attention to intranasal decongestants and corticosteroids, as well as any recreational drug use. Smoking cessation should be considered if the patient smokes, even though there is no conclusive evidence linking smoking to worse outcomes following nasal surgery. Clarifying the patient's history of bleeding disorders, problems with previous anesthetics, and nasal or sinus surgery is helpful.

10.9.6.2. Physical Examination

In the outpatient clinic, patients should receive a comprehensive examination. A thorough examination of the head and neck should be done, and then an anterior rhinoscopy using a nasal speculum should be performed. When the results of an anterior rhinoscopy do not match the patient's history, flexible nasendoscopy can be used to search for masses in the posterior nasal space or indications of sinonasal disease (e.g., severe symptoms of nasal blockage when there are normal-looking turbinates and a midline anterior septum). The surgeon should examine the mucosa's quality and any indications of inflammation, as well as the size and composition of the turbinates, especially the inferior turbinates, when assessing the nasal septum. A turbinoplasty might also be necessary if the excessively large turbinates are causing poor access.

When assessing the size, location, and type of deviation, the septum should be palpated. It is important to note whether the deviation appears to be cartilaginous or bony as well as any septal perforations, dislocations, or bony spurs. Septal palpation using a cerumen curette or cotton-tipped applicator to assess the amount of cartilage still present in the septum is crucial if a previous septoplasty has been carried out. An external examination should be performed, and the degree of nasal tip support, the dynamic collapse of the alae with inspiration, and any additional deformity should be noted. Finally, Cottle's maneuver ought to be used to evaluate stenosis of the internal valve. Determining whether surgery is necessary, how difficult it would be, and which method and technique would be best for the patient all depend on a thorough examination.

10.9.7. Technique or Treatment

10.9.7.1. Endonasal (Figure 10.2)

Preparation:

- The head of the supine patient is inclined slightly in the direction of the surgeon.
- Prominent nasal hairs are trimmed.
- Certain surgeons would rather use Moffatt's solution or oxymetazoline to clear the nose.
- Using a 1:1,000,000 ratio of 1% lidocaine to epinephrine, a local anesthetic is injected bilaterally into the submucoperichondrial plane until the mucosa is thoroughly blanched. In addition to providing analgesia and hemostasis, this aids in the hydro-dissection of the planes.

Raising Mucoperichondrial Flaps:

- The cartilaginous septum's caudal edge is made visible using a nasal speculum. To expose the cartilage, a 15-blade incision is made along this caudal edge. Usually, a Killian's incision, which is a vertical incision made more posteriorly over the quadrangular cartilage, or a hemi-transfixion, which is a vertical incision through one side of the membranous septum, are used. When a septoplasty is combined with an open rhinoplasty, the upper lateral cartilage and dorsal quadrangular cartilage are separated, allowing for an approach to the septum from above.
- After creating a sub-mucoperichondrial plane and dissecting posteriorly to expose the quadrangular cartilage, PPE, and vomer, dissecting scissors and Freer or Cottle elevators are utilized. In order to guarantee that the mucoperichondrial flap is robust and well-vascularized, it is crucial to expose the bare cartilage. The quadrangular cartilage typically has a pearly white or blue appearance. It is important to take caution not to pierce the mucosa, particularly if dissection is required over bony spurs or deviations. The same incision may then be used to raise a second flap on the contralateral side. Extreme caution must be exercised to prevent perforating the contralateral side if a mucosal perforation has occurred on one side. Bilateral, opposing perforations may result in a septal perforation after surgery. Longer nasal specula will be needed to achieve good visualization as the surgeon reaches farther posteriorly, unless an endoscope is used.

Septal Deviation Correction:

- An assessment is conducted regarding the deformity's location, direction, and nature (bony or cartilaginous).
- To incise the septum, a variety of tools can be used; occasionally, these

are combined. The deviated cartilage piece is removed using a blade, a Freer elevator, Jansen-Middleton forceps, or Takahashi forceps for example. An L-strut shape of quadrangular cartilage (dorsal and caudal edges) is preserved to maintain nasal dorsum and tip stability; consequently, the posterior aspect of the cartilage is frequently removed. If the deviation affects the L-strut, either an open approach with grafting or an extracorporeal septoplasty might be necessary. To ensure that the external nose has enough support, the L-strut's dorsal and caudal limbs, as well as the points where they attach to the bone, should continue to measure 10 to 15 mm in width. To remove sections of bone or cartilage, a twisting motion is frequently used; however, extreme twisting outside of the anterior-posterior axis can fracture the cribriform plate and possibly leak cerebrospinal fluid. Additionally, when removing the septum's deviated portions, caution should be exercised to prevent disturbing the keystone region.

- Conserving removed cartilage requires either regular saline or a surgical gauze sponge moistened with regular saline. Reshaped native cartilage fragments can be used as graft material for rhinoplasty procedures or as reinforcement for the L-strut when needed.

Closure:

- Repositioning the mucoperichondrial flaps against the septum is done. Utilizing absorbable suture material, interrupted stitches (e.g., chromic gut) are utilized to seal the wound.
- Quilting, also known as running mattress sutures, is frequently used to close any dead space in the septum and bring the flaps back together to prevent hematoma accumulation after surgery. Some surgeons will make a tiny incision inferiorly in one mucoperichondrial flap if the flaps are fully intact at the conclusion of the procedure. This is done to help any fluid that may have accumulated inside the septum escape. When placing a quilting suture, some surgeons would rather use a septal stapler than do it by hand.
- Sometimes, elastic splints are necessary. These are easily removed in the outpatient clinic by being cut to size, positioned next to the septum, and sutured transseptally if needed. If the turbinates are hypertrophied or if turbinoplasties have also been done, the purpose of the splints is to prevent adhesions to the turbinates.
- An antibiotic cream can be applied intranasally.

Post-Operative Care:

- Most of the time, patients can leave the hospital that same day.
- Oral analgesics and topical antibiotic cream are prescribed.
- Saline sprays and oxymetazoline may also be helpful in creating a hygienic intranasal environment while the wound heals.
- The patient must return in one

to two weeks for a post-operative evaluation and, if necessary, to have any splints removed.

- Usually, antibiotics are not necessary. Antibiotics may be necessary if gauze packing is used to stabilize comminuted bone fragments in order to prevent staphylococcal toxic shock.

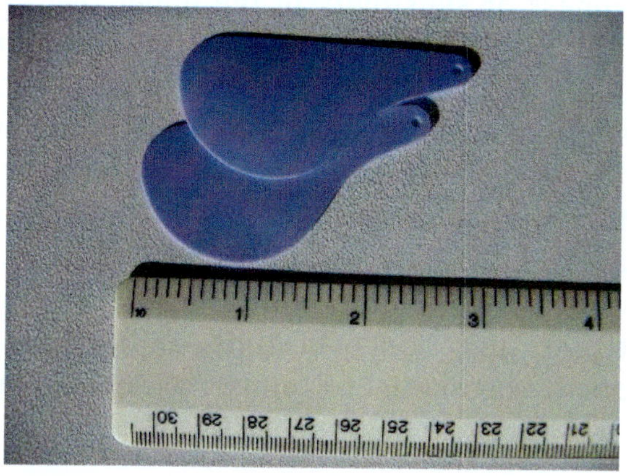

Figure 10.2. *Typical flexible splints that may be used in septoplasty. They are held in place in the nose with a stitch through the hole, and are typically removed seven to 10 days after surgery.*

Source: By I.K. Brown, Public Domain, https://commons.wikimedia.org/w/index.php?curid=2821757.

10.9.7.2. Endoscopic

The different procedures and methods are comparable to the conventional endonasal approach. To view the nasal structures and septum, however, a 0-degree Hopkins rod endoscope is utilized instead of a nasal speculum and headlight. The endoscope can be positioned in between mucosal flaps to guarantee sufficient resection. This technique is more frequently used in conjunction with functional endoscopic sinus surgery (FESS), in which endoscopic techniques are already in place and the necessary septoplasty may be limited to opening up a specific area of the nasal cavity for access or visualization. An isolated septal deformity can be accessed more easily with the endoscopic method by making a Killian incision, which can be made just anterior to a bony spur. This avoids elevating entire mucoperichondrial flaps all the way back from a hemi-transfixion incision.

Endoscopic techniques offer improved visibility and a closer look at the anatomy, making it beneficial for training junior surgeons. Observing endonasal procedures can be challenging, especially with scarring or adhesions in revision cases. Endoscopic visualization can assist in identifying correct dissection planes in these situations. However, performing endoscopic septoplasties may be more complex compared to endonasal methods. It may take experienced surgeons around 60 procedures to achieve satisfactory operative times and reduce the risk of complications in endonasal and FESS surgery. Correcting anterior defects endoscopically can be particularly difficult, as the surgeon may need to use a free-hand technique without the ability to stabilize the endoscope easily.

10.9.7.3. Extracorporeal

Using the previously mentioned techniques may be extremely difficult or impossible in cases of complex septal deformities in all three areas (quadrangular cartilage, PPE, and vomer) or prior comminuted fractures. Extracorporeal techniques, which involve removing the entire septal cartilage, correcting the deviation, and replacing the septum, might be required in this situation. This can be done as a closed procedure using an extended hemi-transfixion incision, or it can be done as an open procedure using a rhinoplasty approach or as part of a septorhinoplasty. Several methods can be employed to straighten the septum after it has been removed. These include drilling and filing portions of the septum, attaching grafts to overlap and splint the deviated cartilage, making partial-thickness scoring incisions on the concave side of the deviation, and incising fracture lines and re-suturing component parts together. Another method that is especially helpful when there is little cartilage left in the septum is to suture the removed pieces of septal cartilage to a polydioxanone scaffolding plate. If replacing the cartilage in a different orientation results in better structural support, it may be rotated and replaced. The anterior nasal spine and lateral cartilages must then be sutured and reimplanted.

When there is little cartilaginous septum left (because of necrosis or prior surgery), a neoseptum can be created using autologous material or pieces of the patient's own septal cartilage e.g., cartilage of the costa. It is also possible to employ homologous grafts, which are made of costal cartilage taken from cadaveric donors.

10.9.8. Complications

Informed consent discussions with the patient should include a thorough explanation of any potential complications that may arise after septoplasty. Excessive bleeding is the most common; some leaking is normal, but larger bleeding can be controlled with nasal packing and, in rare cases, cautery. In order to avoid infection, septal perforation, and/or saddle nose deformity, bleeding beneath the mucoperichondrium can result in septal hematomas, which need to be drained or aspirated. Revision surgery may be required if a perforation nears the keystone area, as it may result in a saddle nose deformity. Perforations can also arise from bilateral, opposing mucosal lacerations that occur during surgery.

A percentage of patients may experience prolonged healing, nasal obstruction, and infection. Most patients recover completely in a matter of weeks from infections, which are uncommon and typically treatable with oral antibiotics. Some patients (more often those who have concurrent turbinoplasty procedures) have been reported to experience hyposmia; this typically goes away in six months. Although intranasal adhesions are possible, their risk is reduced when using silastic splints. Finally, due to intraoperative manipulation of the nasopalatine nerve, patients may experience numbness or sensitivity of the upper teeth or lip; this issue is typically transient, returning normal sensation within a few months. The most frequent long-term complaint following septoplasty, with or without turbinoplasty, is that there is not enough improvement in nasal breathing. There are several possible causes for this, including weight gain, repeated trauma, cartilage migration over time, and technical errors. It is essential to counsel patients about this risk prior to surgery.

10.10. Diagnostic Nasal Endoscopy

Endoscopy is a minimally invasive medical diagnostic procedure. Using it, doctors can see the inside surfaces of a tissue or organ, giving them access to parts of the body that they would not typically be able to see during a routine examination. Nasal endoscopy, also known as rhinoscopy, is usually carried out in the ear, nose, and throat (otolaryngologist) office, where the physician can examine your sinuses and nasal passages with direct, high-quality, magnified vision.

A nasal endoscope is a device made up of fiber-optic cables attached to a thin, rigid tube. It is connected to a light source and a video camera so that enlarged images can be projected onto a screen. After that, the otolaryngologist takes and documents the endoscopic pictures for every patient. The ear, nose, and throat doctor views images of the area they are examining while inserting the instrument into your nose and guiding it through your sinuses and nasal passages during a nasal endoscopy procedure. The process aids in the diagnosis and treatment of various medical disorders. Occasionally, the doctor may use tiny instruments to carry out specific duties, such as collecting microscopic tissue samples.

10.10.1. Indications for a Nasal Endoscopy

Nasal endoscopy indications may include:

- Diagnosing illness in patients exhibiting sinonasal symptoms, such as pain or pressure in the face, mucopurulent drainage, diminished sense of smell, or congestion or blockage in the nose.
- Evaluating unilateral disease.
- Assessing the patient's response to medical treatment, including the resolution of polyps, purulent secretions, inflammation, and mucosal edema following administration of antibiotics, antihistamines, oral steroids, or topical nasal steroids.
- Assessing patients who have sinusitis-related or imminent complications.
- After functional endoscopic sinus surgery, clearing the blocked sinus and nasal cavities of mucus, crust, and fibrin.
- Obtaining a purulent secretion culture.
- Assessing possible recurrence of pathology following functional endoscopic sinus surgery (FESS).
- Assessing the nasopharynx for nasal obstruction, lymphoid hyperplasia, and Eustachian tube issues.
- assessing and biopsying nasal masses or lesions.
- Evaluating anosmia or hyposmia.
- Evaluating cerebrospinal fluid leak (CSF).
- Evaluating and treating nasal foreign bodies.
- Evaluating and treating epistaxis.

10.10.2. Side Effects of Nasal Endoscopy

In general, a nasal endoscopy is a low-risk operation. Like with any procedure, there is always a chance of potential bleeding and mucosal trauma side effects or complications from nasal endoscopy, especially in individuals who already have a higher risk of bleeding, such as those taking anticoagulant medications (Coumadin, Plavix, etc.) or aspirin. Adverse reactions to anesthetics or topical decongestants administered prior to the procedure may occur. Therefore, prior to applying a topical medication, your healthcare provider will confirm whether you have any allergies.

Make sure you ask your doctor if you need to stop taking any medications, like blood thinners, before your procedure. You will probably receive detailed instructions from your doctor regarding what to do and what not to do prior to your procedure. For example, prior to your procedure, you might be asked to fast for a predetermined amount of time. The procedure is rarely painful, but you might feel some slight discomfort if your nasal cavity is unusually narrow or if your nasal lining is swollen.

Prior to your nasal endoscopy, your otolaryngologist will spray your nose with a local anesthetic that temporarily numbs your nose and reduces the chance that you will sneeze because of sensitivity. He or she will also use a nasal decongestant. This helps the endoscope pass through your nose more easily by gradually reducing any swelling of the nasal membranes. To ensure that there is no discomfort, they might use an additional numbing spray or an endoscope that is sized for a child.

10.10.3. Uses of a Nasal Endoscopy Procedure

If your doctor needs additional information about any of the following, they may do a nasal endoscopy on you.

- Nasal blockage
- Nasal congestion
- Nosebleeds
- Nasal polyps
- Rhinosinusitis (sinus and nasal infection)
- Nasal tumors
- Cerebrospinal fluid leak
- Loss of ability to smell

The endoscopy may provide the doctor with specific information, such as the location of nasal tissue swelling or bleeding. They might also examine a growth that might be cancer. A nasal endoscopy may occasionally be used by the doctor as a treatment. For example, they could use it on a child to extract something from their nose. To monitor the effectiveness of a treatment for a sinus or nasal issue, such as the shrinking of nasal polyps, they might do an endoscopy. In other instances, the Vivaer Nasal Airway Remodeling procedure, which is intended to help with numerous nasal congestion issues, comes after the endoscopy.

10.10.3.1. Other Nasal Endoscopy Uses

Rhinosinusitis is one of the most frequent reasons for undergoing a nasal endoscopy procedure. Symptoms like facial pain, blocked nose, and yellow or greenish nasal fluid could be experienced. A nasal endoscopy can be used by the physician to look for swelling and polyps. To identify the cause of the infection and the most effective course of treatment, they might collect pus from an affected area. In a hospital or surgery center, your doctor may use a nasal endoscope to perform minimally invasive surgery. They treat diseases like nasal polyps, sinus infections, and nasal tumors with this procedure. It is not even necessary for your doctor to make an external incision.

Make sure you are aware of everything you need to know before consenting to the procedure, including:

- The procedure name
- The rationale behind your procedure.
- The expected outcomes and their significance.
- The procedure's advantages and disadvantages.
- The credentials of the doctor conducting the operation.
- The possible adverse effects or complications.
- Where and when the surgery is scheduled to be performed.
- What potential consequences could arise if the procedure is not completed?

10.10.4. Using Nasal Endoscopy Instruments

In order to keep the cavities open, your doctor might occasionally perform a nasal endoscopy and clean your sinuses and nasal cavity in the weeks following your sinus surgery. To accomplish these tasks, they will use various smaller instruments, such as forceps or suctions in certain cases. These and other smaller instruments are made especially for use in the nose and sinuses during a nasal endoscopy procedure. Otolaryngologists are typically very proficient with endoscopy and nasal instruments. Certain instruments, like these, are curved, which facilitates the doctor's ability to reach around the corners of the nose more easily. These kinds of tools are frequently used by the physician with angled endoscopes. They might use them in the operating room or in the office while doing a routine surveillance check with your otolaryngologist.

During the nasal endoscopy, your ENT physician can gather vital data that will help them create a personalized treatment plan for you. After your endoscopy, they will probably sit down and discuss the course of treatment with you. Make sure you adhere to your doctor's instructions regarding all prescriptions and follow-up appointments. Most of the time, your doctor will want to schedule a follow-up appointment to see how your treatment is going. Attendance at all follow-up appointments is important as they guarantee your health and well-being, unless you are unable to do so.

10.11. Endoscopic Sinus Surgery

Long-term infection and inflammation of the sinus and nasal linings are the hallmarks of chronic sinusitis. Numerous symptoms, such as facial pressure, nasal congestion, discolored nasal discharge, and "post-nasal drip," are experienced by patients with chronic sinusitis. Sinusitis should only be diagnosed after a thorough examination by your physician. The majority of sinusitis patients respond well to medication treatment for infections. However, even after lengthy courses of medication, infections recur or persist in a small percentage of patients. Surgery is often beneficial for these patients. Your ear, nose, and throat specialist can assess whether you are a good candidate for surgery after looking over your medical history and X-ray results.

The goal of endoscopic sinus surgery is to restore the health and function of the sinuses by opening their natural drainage pathways. The inflammation of the limited drainage pathways in chronic sinusitis prevents the sinuses from draining properly. Consequently, nasal secretions may get stuck in the sinuses and develop a persistent infection. The purpose of surgery is to carefully remove the mucous membranes and thin, delicate bone that obstruct the sinuses' drainage pathways. The word "endoscopic" describes how tiny fiberoptic telescopes are used to perform all surgery through the nose, negating the need for any skin incisions. The majority of endoscopic sinus surgeries are done as outpatient procedures (Figure 10.3).

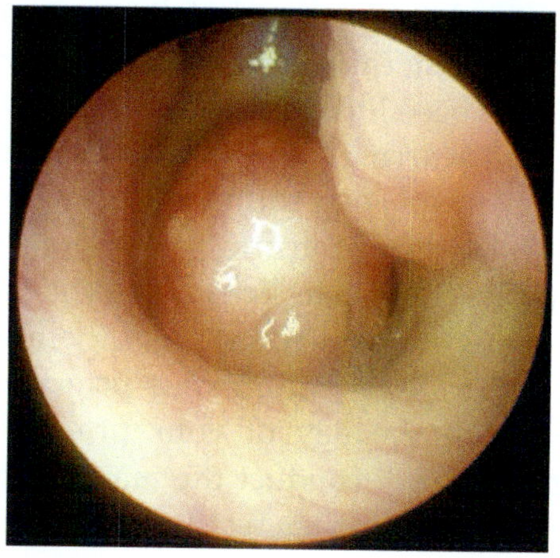

Figure 10.3. *Large nasal polyp (round mass, center), which is commonly treated and removed by FESS.*

Source: By Michael Hawke MD – Own work, CC BY 4.0, https://commons.wikimedia.org/w/index.php?curid=40803949.

10.11.1. Procedure

Prior to Surgery: To ensure that your sinuses

are in optimal condition for surgery, your doctor may prescribe preoperative medications. Oral steroids and/or antibiotics are possible medication options. Kindly make sure to take any preoperative medications exactly as prescribed and start them on the right day. Aspirin, ibuprofen (Motrin/Advil), naproxen (Aleve), other non-steroidal anti-inflammatories (NSAIDS), vitamin E (multivitamin is OK), gingko biloba, garlic (tablets), and ginseng should also be avoided for at least fourteen days prior to surgery. Certain drugs have the potential to thin the blood and cause excessive bleeding. Tylenol is safe and may be taken anytime up to the day of surgery. St. John's wort should also be avoided for 2 weeks prior to surgery because of possible interactions with anesthesia medications. If you take the blood thinner Coumadin, please discuss discontinuation of this medication with your surgeon.

It is imperative that smokers give up their smokes for at least four weeks following surgery and for at least three weeks before surgery. Smoking has been linked to surgical failure, poor healing, and scarring. You can find resources to help you stop smoking from your primary care physician. Lastly, it is critical that you let your primary care physician know that you intend to have sinus surgery. You can get the medical clearance for surgery from your primary care physician. On the day of your preoperative visit, Stanford will conduct the majority of the required pre-operative testing; however, on rare occasions, we may ask your primary care physician for previous records. Before and after your surgery, we will do everything in our power to keep your primary care physician updated on your health.

- **During Surgery:** You will typically be put under general anesthesia, which will keep you unconscious the entire time. Please let your doctor know if you would rather receive local anesthesia, though, as this may also be an option in some circumstances. You will spend approximately one hour in the recovery room following your surgery, and then another one to two hours recovering in the second stage recovery unit. Most patients are well enough the day after surgery to return home. Most likely, you won't have nasal packing when you return home.
- **After Surgery:** Following surgery, you should anticipate mild bleeding for one to two days and a general feeling of exhaustion for one to two weeks. Narcotic or non-narcotic drugs can generally be used to effectively manage pain. A successful outcome from your surgery depends on a number of postoperative visits. During every appointment, your physician will conduct a nasal endoscopy to monitor the sinus healing process. To clear blood from the sinuses and stop the early formation of scar tissue, a second procedure known as debridement may be required. Typically, during the first six weeks of your appointment schedule, you will have three visits. After that, the frequency of your visits will vary based on how quickly your sinuses heal, usually a few months apart.

10.11.2. Risks of Surgery

There are risks involved with endoscopic sinus surgery just like with any surgical procedure. Even though there is very little chance of a complication, it is still important that you are aware of the potential risks and discuss any concerns you may have with your surgeon.

- **Bleeding:** The majority of sinus surgeries result in some blood loss, which the patient can usually tolerate. But occasionally, severe bleeding might necessitate stopping the treatment. While the majority of patients don't need nasal packing, some will need their tissue spacer or tiny nasal pack removed after a week. Transfusions of blood are only administered in an emergency and are rarely necessary.
- **Recurrence of Disease:** Surgery is not a treatment for sinusitis, even though endoscopic sinus surgery significantly improves symptoms for the great majority of patients. It is therefore expected that even after a successful sinus surgery, you will still need to take your sinus medications, though generally speaking, your need for them should decrease. To maximize your surgical outcome, you might occasionally need more "touch-up" or revision surgery.
- **Spinal Fluid Leak:** There is an extremely slim possibility of causing a spinal fluid leak—the fluid that lines the brain—or harming the brain because the sinuses are situated close to the brain. In the unlikely event that a spinal fluid leak develops, it could open the door for an infection that could lead to meningitis. Hospitalization and surgical closure would be necessary in the event of a spinal fluid leak.
- **Visual Problems:** There have been cases of visual loss following sinus surgery as a result of optic nerve or eye damage. In these kinds of situations, there is little chance of recovery. Fortunately, this kind of issue is incredibly uncommon. Double vision could be the result of damage to the eye muscles. Another issue that could arise is continuous eye tearing. Tearing issues often go away on their own, but sometimes more surgery is needed.
- **Other Risks:** A change in the resonance or quality of the voice, swelling or bruising around the eye, persistence and/or worsening of sinus symptoms and facial pain, and altered sense of taste or smell are other unusual risks associated with surgery.

Some patients require a quick surgery known as a septoplasty to straighten their "deviated septum," which is a crooked nasal septum. Dissolvable stitches that are concealed in the nasal area are used during this procedure, which is carried out through a tiny hidden incision. If you need a septoplasty, there are more risks involved in the process. The main risks include infections or bleeding near the septum; numbness in the front teeth; septal perforation, or rupture of the septum; brain fluid leak; or recurrence of septal deviation. There is an extremely slim chance that these incidents will change the nose's outward look.

10.11.3. Restrictions During Postoperative Recovery Period

You should avoid blowing your nose for the first week after surgery. Furthermore, avoid bending, straining, or lifting more than 20 pounds in the first week. Anytime after surgery, light walking and routine household tasks are acceptable. After a week, you can start exercising again at 50% intensity, and after two weeks, at 100% intensity. Plan to take a week off from work, and on your first day back, try to schedule a half-day.

10.12. Direct Laryngoscopy

A direct laryngoscopy makes the larynx visible. It is employed in resuscitation, general anesthesia, and surgeries involving the larynx. This tool can be used in the operating room, intensive care unit, and emergency department, among other hospital settings. It is easier to perform endotracheal intubation when the larynx is visualized. For many patients, including those with altered mental status and those undergoing surgery, who are unable to maintain their own airway, this is a crucial step. A physician must be well-versed in the anatomy, indications, contraindications, preparation, equipment, proper technique, personnel, and complications of successful endotracheal intubation before using direct laryngoscopy to secure a patient's airway.

10.12.1. Anatomy and Physiology

Situated directly beneath the pharynx is the larynx. It is made up of the intrinsic muscles, three unpaired cartilages, and three pairs of smaller cartilages. The arytenoids, corniculate, and cuneiform are the three paired cartilages. The cricoid, thyroid, and epiglottis cartilages are the three unpaired cartilages. The only cartilage covering the trachea's circumference is the cricoid cartilage. For direct laryngoscopy, the epiglottis—which is situated above the cricoid cartilage—is a crucial landmark. The glottis is covered by a lid formed by the epiglottis, which is situated at the base of the tongue. The larynx is shielded from stomach contents aspiration by the epiglottis. The vallecula is a pocket of cartilage located at the base of the tongue, anterior to the epiglottis. Equally significant as a landmark is the vallecula, where some direct laryngoscopy blades, like the curved or Macintosh blade, are inserted to manipulate the region and enhance vocal cord visualization. In the vallecula, the laryngoscope blade presses against the hyoepiglottic ligament, which holds the epiglottis in place above the hyoid bone.

10.12.2. Indications

Endotracheal intubation via direct laryngoscopy is recommended in emergency, perioperative, or critical care situations. Acute respiratory failure, impending airway collapse indicated by hypoxia or hypercapnia, airway protection in patients with altered or depressed mental status, upper gastrointestinal bleeding, or hematemesis secondary to bleeding from esophageal varices are among the emergency room indications for direct laryngoscopy to perform endotracheal intubation. Endotracheal tubes can be inserted during perioperative care using direct laryngoscopy in patients under general anesthesia, during surgeries involving the airway or regions nearby, or during unusually positioned procedures like spinal surgery that necessitates prone positioning. In cases of intracranial hemorrhage, tumors, or masses, patients in the intensive care unit may require short-term hyperventilation, or direct laryngoscopy for endotracheal intubation in the event of impending airway collapse. In the intensive care unit, intubations are also used to control excessive secretions.

10.12.3. Contraindications

Rarely are there complete contraindications for direct laryngoscopy. Absolute contraindications refer to lesions of the supraglottis and glottis that would not allow the advancement of the endotracheal tube (ETT), such as complete obstruction caused by supraglottic or glottic tumors or high-grade subglottic or glottic stenosis. Furthermore, traction from the laryngoscope blade, the placement of the ETT, or pressure from the ETT stylet can exacerbate blunt trauma to the larynx that results in laryngeal fracture or disruption of the laryngotracheal junction. These conditions can encourage the formation of a false lumen in the trachea or cause perforation through the trachea. These patients need to have their airways surgically opened.

In the event of penetrating trauma to the upper airway, direct laryngoscopy for the placement of an ET is likewise contraindicated because manipulation of the area with a laryngoscope or ET may result in a hematoma or partial or complete transection of the airway. When dealing with such suspected cases, non-invasive methods of ventilation and oxygenation should be used until a definitive surgical airway is established. Although direct laryngoscopy is rarely possible with grade II trismus, it is absolutely contraindicated in cases of grade III trismus (inter-incisoral distance of less than 1 cm). Apart from severe and blunt airway trauma, other relative contraindications for direct laryngoscopy include infections, burns, and anaphylaxis, which can cause severe swelling and edema of the larynx or supralarynx. This is due to the possibility of not being able to visualize the vocal cords and airway entrance, as well as the possibility of airway swelling and edema exacerbating trauma and irritation from the laryngoscope blade and/or ETT, which may reduce the effectiveness of bag-mask valve ventilation and oxygenation. In these situations, direct laryngoscopy ought to be tried only in cases where plans are in place for an expedient surgical airway in the event that intubation fails.

Among the relative contraindications for laryngoscopy are patients with difficult airways (i.e., those who pose a challenge to the procedure, micrognathia, macroglossia, elevated Mallampatti score), trauma, and injury to the larynx, throat, or neck. Furthermore, patients with airborne infections that need to have their airway secured—tuberculosis, COVID-19, Ebola, to name a few—should avoid direct laryngoscopy if at all possible because it can spread the infection to medical professionals. Video laryngoscopy is advised for those patients, or a modified protocol to reduce aerosolization.

10.12.4. Equipment

Prior to starting a direct laryngoscopy, the patient needs to be placed on cardiac monitoring and have a continuous pulse oximeter. The suctioning device also needs to be ready and readily available, and the patient needs to be positioned and lit appropriately. Proper patient and equipment preparation is crucial to the procedure. A laryngoscope handle, blades (Macintosh or curved, Miller or straight with a curved end, Jackson-Wisconsin or straight), an appropriate sized ETT with a stylet, and an ETT one size bigger and one smaller are required for direct laryngoscopy and the subsequent endotracheal intubation. The majority of adult tracheal intubations in an emergency or perioperative context can be performed using 7.5 mm cuffed tubes. Larger tubes are preferred in the critical care environment because they facilitate flexible bronchoscopy and tracheal suctioning through the endotracheal tube (ETT). Additionally, larger tubes reduce airflow resistance through the ventilator; however, the tube shouldn't be so big as to raise the risk of subglottic stenosis or arytenoid injury. The right tools include a laryngoscope, blade, and ETT in addition to sterile lubricant for the ETT balloon and cuff and at least a 10 cc syringe for inflating the device after it has been successfully inserted.

The equipment for direct laryngoscopy includes various adjunct airway management devices like a "Bougie" ETT introducer, oral and nasal airways, and rescue airway devices such as a Combitube or supraglottic airway tubes. A capnography monitor is necessary to confirm the correct placement of the ETT. Additionally, back-up devices such as video laryngoscopes, laryngeal mask airways, and a cricothyrotomy or tracheostomy tray are also included in the equipment. In cases where a difficult airway is anticipated, the instruments for a surgical airway should be available before starting the laryngoscopy procedure.

10.12.5. Personnel

The hospital's staff who perform direct laryngoscopy may come from different departments. It can be used by emergency department doctors to intubate patients who are in critical condition. This method is frequently used in the operating room by anesthesiologists for endotracheal intubations. This technique is also used by critical care doctors to safeguard their patients' airways. If the need for surgery to open an airway becomes more probable, otolaryngologists or general surgeons may be required.

10.12.6. Preparation

Prior to the procedure, the patient needs to be evaluated. Certain patients might show to be more challenging candidates for direct laryngoscopy-assisted endotracheal intubation success.

The following characteristics can all make a patient a less-than-ideal candidate for direct laryngoscopy by making it more difficult to visualize the larynx:

- The gap between the interincisors of less than 4 cm.
- A thyromental separation of under 6 centimeters.
- A distance between the sternomental bones of less than 12 cm.
- Less than 30 degrees of head and neck extension from neutral.
- Mallampati class 3 or 4
- Mandibular retraction, also known as true retrognathia or micrognathia.
- A neck circumference that is higher than 40 cm
- Submental compliance
- History of cervical spinal fusion
- Radiation or neck burn contracture

The patient needs to be pre-oxygenated after receiving a proper assessment. Apneic oxygenation is a useful pre-oxygenation technique if a patient is difficult to intubate or at risk of rapidly desaturating. Passive oxygen insufflation through a nasal cannula at a rate of 15 liters per minute is how apneic oxygenation is accomplished. Preparing by keeping a bag-valve-mask and a working suction device close by is crucial. It is important to connect monitoring devices to patients properly, including capnography, continuous cardiac monitoring, pulse oximetry, and blood pressure. The establishment of intravenous access should come next. Making sure that induction agents, neuromuscular blocking agents, adjunctive medications, emergency medications, and surgical airway instruments are ready for use in the event that the patient has a suspected difficult airway is the last stage of preparation.

10.12.7. Technique or Treatment

Successful direct laryngoscopy involves multiple steps summarized below:

1. The patient must first be positioned correctly. The traditional "sniffing" position involves elevating the head three to seven centimeters using the atlanto-occipital extension; however, head and neck manipulation should not be done on patients who have suffered cervical spine injuries.
2. The patient's mouth must then be opened with the right hand. One useful approach is to apply the scissor technique. To do this, flex the thumb and middle finger past one another, applying pressure to the maxillary dentition with the middle finger and the mandibular dentition with the thumb.
3. After inserting the laryngoscope

into the right side of the mouth, the tongue is swept to the left with the blade, and the epiglottis is smoothly advanced with the blade. When using a Macintosh blade, the cutting edge advances to the vallecula; when using a Miller blade, the cutting edge advances past the epiglottis to the tracheal entrance, which is closest to the vocal cords.

4. The vocal cords are then visible by moving the laryngoscope anteriorly.

An assistant can help visualize the airway in cases of very anterior airways by applying mild to moderate cricoid pressure while lifting the laryngoscope.

10.12.8. Complications

Complications can occur, just like with many procedures. The laryngoscope can lacerate the lips, chip teeth, or cause blunt or penetrating trauma to the larynx, trachea, and oropharynx. Dislocation of the arytenoid cartilage and potential damage to the vocal cord are risks associated with direct laryngoscopy. To prevent these issues, careful technique is needed at all times. A sore throat is the most frequent side effect of this procedure, occurring in 14% to 57% of patients undergoing intubation for general anesthesia, according to reports. Pain, discomfort, hoarseness of voice, dysphagia, and dry throat are all included in the broad definition of sore throat and can happen separately or in combination. The majority of sore throats are mild and transient, going away in 48 hours or less. There are two types of complications following direct laryngoscopy and ETT placement: traumatic and non-traumatic. Traumatic injuries can result from direct blunt or penetrating trauma from the laryngoscope blade, the ETT style, or the ETT itself to the trachea, larynx, or oropharynx. The lips, tongue, pharynx, esophagus, and teeth may also sustain harm. One serious issue to be cautious of is broken and chipped teeth caused by poor technique. Furthermore, the ETT may result in dislocation of the arytenoid cartilages, damage to the vocal cords, paralysis, and glottic trauma. Rarely, patients with risk factors such as unstable cervical spinal column fractures, severe rheumatoid arthritis, or atlantoaxial instability may experience cervical spinal cord injuries as a result of extreme flexion or extension of the neck during direct laryngoscopy. In rare cases, dislocating the mandible for a laryngoscopy with excessive force can result in temporomandibular joint dislocation.

Aspiration of stomach contents, bronchospasm, and hypoxic brain injury from an extended attempt at intubation without sufficient oxygenation are nontraumatic consequences of direct laryngoscopy and ETT placement. The laryngoscopy blade can stimulate the highly innervated glottis, which can result in a sympathetic surge that causes tachycardia, dysrhythmias, myocardial ischemia, infarction, and/or hypertension. Similarly, the laryngoscopic blade can cause profound bradycardia by stimulating the vagus nerve, especially in younger patients. Another well-known side effect of direct laryngoscopy that is typically promptly detected and treated is esophageal intubation. Other well-known atraumatic consequences of direct laryngoscopy include barotrauma, pneumothorax, pneumoperitoneum, and hypotension. Because tracheal intubation causes tissue irritation and scarring, there may be long-term and chronic complications. These complications can result in laryngomalacia, tracheomalacia, or laryngeal stenosis (both glottic and subglottic).

10.13. Bronchoscopy

A bronchoscopy allows medical professionals to examine your airways and lungs. Usually, a pulmonologist—a medical professional who specializes in lung disorders—performs it. A tiny tube called a bronchoscope is inserted into your mouth or nose, down your throat, and into your lungs during a bronchoscopy. The most popular tool used for bronchoscopy procedures is a flexible bronchoscope. A rigid bronchoscope, however, might be required in specific circumstances, such as when there is significant bleeding in the lungs or when a large object becomes lodged in the airway.

A persistent cough, an infection, or something unusual seen on a chest X-ray or other test are common reasons for requiring a bronchoscopy. In addition, bronchoscopy can be used to treat lung issues, remove foreign bodies or other obstructions from the lungs or airways, and collect tissue or mucus samples. Finding the source of a lung issue is typically the goal of a bronchoscopy. For instance, if you have an abnormal chest X-ray or a persistent cough, your doctor may recommend a bronchoscopy.

Reasons for doing a bronchoscopy include:

- Diagnosis of a lung problem
- Identification of a lung infection
- Biopsy of tissue from the lung
- Elimination of mucus, a foreign object, or any other blockage in the lungs or airways, like a tumor.
- Insertion of a tiny tube (a stent) to maintain an open airway.
- Interventional bronchoscopy is used to treat lung conditions like bleeding, abnormal airway narrowing (stricture), or collapsed lung disease (pneumothorax)

Special instruments, such as a biopsy tool, an electrocautery probe to stop bleeding, or a laser to shrink an airway tumor, may be passed through the bronchoscope during certain procedures. To guarantee that the desired area of the lung is sampled, specific techniques are employed to guide the collection of biopsies. A bronchoscope with an integrated ultrasound probe can be used to examine the chest lymph nodes in patients with lung cancer. This is known as an endobronchial ultrasound, or EBUS, and it aids medical professionals in choosing the best course of action. When assessing whether a cancer has spread, EBUS can be utilized for different kinds of cancer.

10.13.1. Risks

Bronchoscopy-related complications are rare, typically minor, and very seldom severe. If a disease damages or inflames the airways, complications could be more likely. Adverse effects could stem from the procedure itself, the sedative, or the topical anesthetic. These include:

- **Bleeding:** If a biopsy was done, bleeding is more likely to occur. Usually, bleeding is not severe and goes away on its own.
- **Collapsed Lung:** An airway might occasionally be damaged during a bronchoscopy. A punctured lung may allow air to build up in the area surrounding it, potentially leading to lung collapse. Although this issue is typically easily resolved, hospitalization may be necessary.
- **Fever:** Fever is not always an indication of infection, but it is rather common following bronchoscopy. Usually, no treatment is required.

10.13.2. How You Prepare

Food and medication restrictions are typically part of the bronchoscopy preparation process, along with a discussion of extra safety measures.

- **Food and Medications:** A few

days prior to the bronchoscopy, you might be asked to cease taking blood-thinning drugs like aspirin, clopidogrel (Plavix), and warfarin (Coumadin, Jantoven). Additionally, you will be instructed to fast for four to eight hours prior to the procedure.

- **Clothing and Personal Items:** You will be asked to remove any removable bridges, partial dentures, and complete dentures on the day of the procedure and to change into a gown. In addition, you might be asked to take off your contacts, glasses, or hearing aids.
- **Other Precautions:** You will need a friend or family member to drive you home if you plan to leave the procedure. Due to the aftereffects of the medications used during the procedure, you will not be able to drive. Having someone stay with you for the remainder of the day is also a smart idea.

10.13.3. What You Can Expect

Bronchoscopy is typically performed in an operating room of a hospital or in a clinic procedure room. Preparation and recovery time included, the entire process usually takes about four hours. The actual bronchoscopy procedure typically takes 30 to 60 minutes.

10.13.3.1. Before the Procedure

You will be instructed to place your arms by your sides as you sit or lie back on a table or bed. Throughout the procedure, you will be hooked up to monitors that will allow the medical staff to keep an eye on your blood pressure, heart rate, and oxygen saturation.

To help you relax, a sedative medication will be injected intravenously (via a vein). Even though you'll feel drowsy, you'll be conscious, breathing on your own, and able to respond to any questions your doctor may pose while the procedure is happening. When a bronchoscopy is finished, sedative drugs frequently leave you with very little memory of the procedure.

An anesthetic, a numbing drug, will be sprayed into your throat. Occasionally, your nose is rubbed with an anesthetic gel. When the bronchoscope is inserted into your throat, these drugs numb the affected areas, which helps minimize coughing and gagging. The medication may taste bad at first, but that taste will pass.

10.13.3.2. During the Procedure

The bronchoscope is inserted into your mouth or nose during a bronchoscopy. The bronchoscope is equipped with a tiny camera and light at the tip that projects images onto a monitor to assist your doctor in carrying out the procedure. The bronchoscope is gently moved through the vocal cords, into the airways, and down the back of your throat. Although it might hurt, it shouldn't feel uncomfortable. Your medical team will make every effort to ensure your comfort. Devices passed through the bronchoscope may be used to perform procedures and take tissue and fluid samples. Your physician might inquire about shoulder, back, or chest pain. You shouldn't be in pain generally.

10.13.3.3. After the Procedure

Following the bronchoscopy, you will be observed for some hours. For a few hours, your throat and mouth will most likely be numb. Food and liquids won't be permitted to you until the numbness subsides. This aids in preventing liquids and food from getting into your lungs and airways. You can resume drinking when the numbness in your mouth and throat goes away and you can swallow and cough normally. Take small sips of water first. After that, you could have soft foods like soup and applesauce. As soon as you feel comfortable, add more food items.

You might be experiencing muscle aches, hoarseness, a cough, or a mild sore throat. This is typical. Lozenges and gargles with warm water can help ease the discomfort. Make sure the numbness completely subsides before attempting to gargle or suck on lozenges.

Call your doctor right away if you:

- Have a fever that lasts more than 24 hours
- Have increasing chest pain
- Have trouble breathing
- More than a few tablespoons of blood should come out.

10.13.4. Results

One to three days following the procedure, you will typically speak with your doctor about the results of the bronchoscopy. Your physician will discuss any procedures performed or determine how to treat any lung issues discovered based on the results. It is also possible that additional tests or procedures are required for you. If a biopsy was performed during the bronchoscopy, a pathologist will need to examine it. There are differences in the turnaround times for the results because the tissue samples require special preparation. It will be necessary to send some biopsy specimens for genetic testing, which could take up to two weeks.

10.14. Oesophagoscopy

An endoscope, which is a long, narrow tube-like device with a light and a camera, is inserted into your esophagus during an esophagoscopy procedure. A long, muscular tube called the esophagus aids in moving food and liquids from your mouth to your stomach. Your doctor looks for abnormalities in your esophagus with an endoscope or performs a biopsy to test for specific conditions on a sample of tissue. To treat or operate on you, your doctor may also use instruments that are attached to the endoscope.

There are several types of esophagoscopy:

- During a rigid esophagoscopy, a firm, unbending tube is manually inserted through the mouth into the esophagus. The tube typically contains an eyepiece, a light, and multiple lenses to enable the doctor to visualize the throat. This procedure can assist in conducting minor esophageal surgeries or identifying specific conditions like esophageal cancer.
- A thin, flexible tube is inserted into your esophagus during a flexible esophagoscopy. Through a network of fibers, tiny electrical cables are threaded through the endoscope tube to transmit images to a monitor and shine light into the esophagus.
- An endoscope is inserted through your nose, into your nasal cavity, down the back of your throat and into your esophagus during a transnasal esophagoscopy. This kind is typically regarded as the least intrusive. It can be completed quickly, and anesthesia is typically not required.

An esophagoscopy may be performed during a routine physical exam or if you exhibit any of the following symptoms:

- nausea
- vomiting
- trouble swallowing

- persistent sensation of a lump in your throat known as globus pharyngeus.
- a persistent cough that persists for an extended period
- long-term heartburn that hasn't gone away with changes to your diet or by taking antacids
- Acid reflux from the stomach travels up the esophagus and into the throat.

An esophagoscopy may be used to:

- Determine the cause of the unusual symptoms in the stomach, intestines, or throat.
- Obtain a tissue sample (biopsy) in order to diagnose disorders like dysphagia or gastroesophageal reflux disease (GERD) or cancer.
- Any sizable accumulation of food (referred to as a bolus) or a foreign object lodged in the esophagus should be removed.
- observe your upper gastrointestinal tract during surgery.

It may also be used with other GI imaging procedures, such as:

- gastroscopy to examine your stomach
- enteroscopy to examine your small intestine
- colonoscopy to examine your large intestine

10.14.1. Preparation

To get ready for an esophagoscopy, follow these steps:

- Before the esophagoscopy, wait six to eight hours before consuming any food or liquids. This helps your doctor see inside your upper gastrointestinal tract more easily by emptying your stomach. Clear liquids like water, juice, coffee, or soda are still acceptable to consume.
- Give up using aspirin and warfarin (Coumadin), among other blood thinners. In the unlikely event that your doctor needs to take a tissue sample or perform surgery, this lowers your risk of bleeding.
- Ensure that your doctor is aware of all other medications you take. Add vitamins or dietary supplements.
- Get a ride or a walk to and from the procedure from a friend or family member. This will guarantee your safe return home. You are free to drive yourself home after the procedure if you are not using any anesthetic or sedatives.

10.14.2. Procedure

Depending on the type, esophagoscopy procedures can change. The process may require as little as 30 minutes to as much as three hours. You can typically return home the same day because the procedure is performed as an outpatient.

To perform the procedure, your doctor does the following:

1. Uses anesthesia through an intravenous (IV) tube to keep you asleep or applies a substance, such as lidocaine, to numb your nose or throat so that the endoscope doesn't feel uncomfortable.
2. Gently and slowly insert the endoscope through the mouth or nose, into the throat.
3. Observes the inside of your esophagus by looking through an eyepiece or at a

screen that projects images from the endoscope. In order to make viewing easier, your doctor might also inject a tiny amount of air into your esophagus.

4. Uses instruments to remove a mass, remove a tissue sample, or suction out any blockages in the esophagus, such as forceps or a hollow suction tube.
5. Carries out any necessary esophageal conditions treatment procedures. This may consist of:
    - injections to aid in swallowing or to reduce enlarged veins, also known as varices.
    - application of heat or lasers to eliminate malignant tissue.
    - veins can be sealed with bands to stop bleeding.

10.14.3. Risks

Esophagoscopies are thought to be extremely safe and carry very little risk. The majority of complications are transient and resolve fast.

Possible risks include:

- throat soreness, discomfort, or pain
- hoarse voice
- a slight swallowing difficulty for a few days.
- irritation, damage, or tearing (perforation) of the tissue lining the esophagus
- Air trapped beneath the skin, also known as subcutaneous surgical emphysema.
- internal bleeding (hemorrhage)
- infection
- fever

10.14.4. Recovery

Following this procedure, bear in mind the following:

- After the procedure, especially if you were given anesthesia, you probably won't feel well. Anesthesia usually wears off after a day or two.
- You will be required to remain in the hospital for a minimum of 30 minutes and a maximum of several hours, during which time your doctor will monitor your vital signs, including heart rate and breathing, and your condition, until they determine that you are well enough to return home. Make sure you have someone who can drive you or accompany you home at this point.
- For a few hours or days afterward, it is common to experience some drowsiness, bloating or cramping in the abdomen, and soreness or pain in the throat.
- The procedure's pain and discomfort should progressively subside. See your doctor straight away to make sure there are no complications if they don't.

In the event that you experience any of the following symptoms, get emergency care.

- pain or discomfort getting worse over time
- vomiting or pooping blood
- difficulty breathing
- pain in your chest
- fever

10.14.5. Outlook

The esophagoscopy procedure is extremely safe. The prognosis is dependent upon what your physician is looking into or treating at the time of the procedure. You might be able to get the results immediately, or you might need to wait a few days for the laboratory to test tissue samples. Find out from your doctor when you can expect your results.

10.15. Tonsillectomy and Adenoidectomy

The surgical removal of the tonsils, which are two oval-shaped tissue pads at the back of the throat, one on each side, is known as a tonsillectomy. Tonsillitis, or infection and inflammation of the tonsils, was traditionally treated with a tonsillectomy. Currently, tonsillectomy is most often done for sleep disorders, but it can also be used as a treatment for tonsillitis that keeps coming back or doesn't go away. In addition, a tonsillectomy might be required to treat uncommon tonsil diseases as well as breathing and other issues linked to enlarged tonsils. Following a tonsillectomy, recovery typically lasts between 10 days and 2 weeks.

10.15.1. Anatomy and Physiology

As part of Waldeyer's ring of lymphoid tissue, the palatine tonsils function. Additional elements consist of the lingual tonsils, tubal tonsils, and adenoids. The pharyngobasilar fascia gives rise to a fibrous capsule that serves as a barrier between the lymphoid tissue and the surrounding muscle.

Perineurosillar space is the term used to describe the potential gap between the muscle and capsule. The muscles that make up the anterior and posterior pillars, respectively, the palatoglossus and palatopharyngeal, are where the tonsils are located. A muscle located lateral to the tonsil is the superior constrictor. The glossopharyngeal nerve, which is close to these muscles and vulnerable to damage during tonsillectomy, is situated there. Taste changes and referred otalgia may result from temporary swelling surrounding this nerve. Blood vessels of various sizes supply the vasculature of the tonsils. Main arteries: the lingual, facial, ascending pharyngeal, and internal maxillary arteries are branches of the external carotid artery. Exiting the tonsillar branch is the lingual artery. Two branches originate from the facial artery: the tonsillar and the ascending palatal. Through the descending palatal artery, the internal maxillary artery supplies the tonsil. This architecture may contain several anomalies (Figure 10.4).

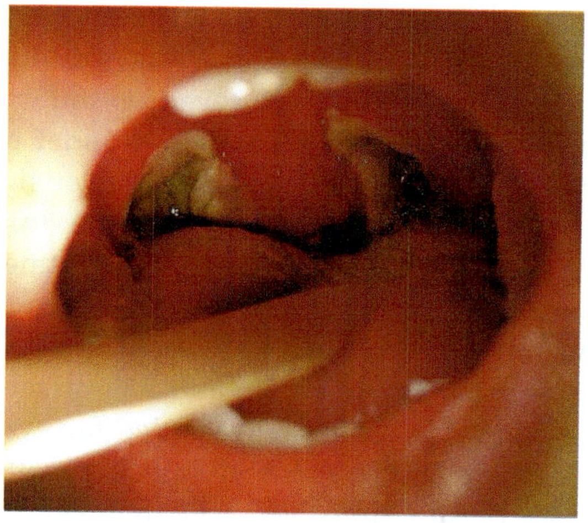

Figure 10.4. *Typical appearance of the back of the throat three days post-tonsillectomy.*

Source: By James Heilman, MD – Own work, CC BY-SA 3.0, https://commons.wikimedia.org/w/index.php?curid=8838676.

10.15.2. Indications

As was previously mentioned, sleep-disordered breathing and recurrent tonsillitis are the two most common reasons for tonsillectomy. An upper airway blockage that occurs repeatedly during sleep, either partially or completely, disrupting normal breathing and sleep patterns is known as sleep-disordered breathing. A physical examination and history can be used to diagnose it. SBD symptoms include aggression, fatigue during the day, and hyperactivity. Heroic snoring, observed apnea, restless sleep, growth retardation, inadequate academic performance, and nocturnal enuresis are indicators of sickle cell disease (SBD). Compared to children without SDB, children with SDB have much higher rates of antibiotic use, 40% more hospital visits, and a 215% increase in healthcare utilization due to increased upper respiratory infections. Hypertrophies of the tonsils and adenoids are the most frequent cause of SDB. Polysomnography can be used to further assess patients who exhibit signs and symptoms of SDB but do not have tonsillar hypertrophy. Tonsillar size is not always a reliable indicator of the severity of SDB. In patients with recurrent tonsillitis who have had fewer than seven episodes in the previous year, fewer than five episodes per year in the previous two years, or fewer than three episodes per year in the previous three years, watchful waiting is advised. Treatment recommendations may include tonsillectomy if the frequency of infections is higher than these figures. A sore throat and one or more of the following should be recorded for every infection: a temperature greater than 38.3 degrees Celsius, tonsillar exudates, cervical adenopathy, or a positive GABHS. In patients with recurrent tonsillitis, modifiable factors like antibiotic allergy or intolerance, PFAPA (periodic fever, aphthous stomatitis, pharyngitis, and adenitis), or peritonsillar abscess may call for early surgical intervention. Malignancy and tonsillar asymmetry are additional reasons for tonsillectomy (to rule out malignancy). The two most frequent cancers of the palatine tonsils are lymphoma and squamous cell carcinoma. The majority of childhood malignant neoplasms are lymphomas.

10.15.3. Contraindications

There are currently no known absolute contraindications to tonsillectomy. The two main risks associated with tonsillectomy are bleeding and anesthesia. For this reason, individuals having an adenotonsillectomy should be aware of any risk factors for these side effects (i.e., bleeding disorders, and a family history of malignant hyperthermia) were recognized and the appropriate safety measures were taken prior to surgery.

10.15.4. Equipment

Depending on the technique employed, different equipment is needed for tonsillectomy. Using an Allis clamp, Crowe-Davis or McIvor mouth gag, a "cold" tonsillectomy is carried out. A scalpel, Fisher tonsil knife/dissector, curved Metzenbaum scissors, Tyding snares, curettes for adenoidectomy, and a St. Forceps for adenoids, Clair-Thompson. Monopolar cautery is used to perform "hot" tonsil dissections. Bipolar ablation via radiofrequency (i.e., coblation) is an additional choice. Additionally, mircodebrider techniques are applied (particularly in the context of intracapsular tonsillectomies).

10.15.5. Personnel

A tonsillectomy requires the following personnel: a circulating nurse, anesthesiologist, surgical technician, and surgeon.

10.15.6. Preparation

Any method can be used to induce anesthesia in the same way. The patient receives an oral intubation while lying supine. Oral RAE endotracheal tubes are preferred by most surgeons. The midline of the tube is taped. The surgeon can then sit or stand at the head of the bed and place the shoulder roll after the bed has been rotated by 45 to 180 degrees. A mouth gag such as a McIvor or Crowe-Davis mouth gag keeps the patient's mouth open.

10.15.7. Technique or Treatment

There are two types of tonsillectomy: extracapsular and intracapsular. In the US, the most widely used method is the "hot" extracapsular technique using monopolar cautery. The tonsil is medialized once the Allis clamp is used to grasp its superior pole. Submucosally, the tonsil's lateral edge is recognized. If a conventional tip is used, about 20W of power is needed to incise the superior pole. The tonsil and musculature are located in the avascular plane. It is customary to remove the entire palatine tonsil from the superior to the inferior pole. Hemostasis can be maintained with packing, suction cautery, or ties.

Sharp dissection is used during a "cold" tonsillectomy. Using the Allis clamp, the tonsil is grasped and medialized. A number 12 scalpel is once more used to identify and incise the tonsil's lateral aspect. The avascular plane is then identified using a Metzenbaum scissors. A Fisher tonsil dissector works inside the plane to extract the tonsil from the fossa until the tonsil attachment is limited to the inferior pole. The tonsil is then separated from its inferior pole using a Tyding snare. Suction cautery, ties, or pressure from a tonsil sponge are methods for maintaining hemostasis. Coblation is a tonsil removal procedure that employs a method akin to monopolar cautery. Coblation is a technique that breaks down tissue molecules by converting saline irrigation into an ionized plasma layer. This is a common technique for partial tonsillectomies, with minimal heat generation. A partial tonsillectomy can also be carried out with a micro-debrider.

The benefits of one technique over another are still up for debate. Overall, a benefit is determined by its cost, lower rates of complications (i.e., bleeding rates), length of stay in the operating room, and pain following surgery. While some studies indicate that "hot" tonsillectomy reduces intraoperative blood loss and surgical time, "cold" tonsillectomy is thought to cause less pain after surgery. The surgeon's comfort level and experience determine the technique to be used.

10.15.8. Complications

One of the most frequent and feared side effects after tonsillectomy, whether or not an adenoidectomy is bleeding. In a 2009–2013 study involving more than 100,000 children, it was found that 2–8% of children had unscheduled follow-up visits due to bleeding after tonsillectomy, 1–6% of patients visited the emergency room, and 0–8% of patients needed surgery. With 50% of bleeding happening between 10 p.m. and 1 a.m. and 6 a.m. and 9 a.m., the frequency is higher at night. This is believed to be due to circadian rhythm abnormalities, vibratory effects of snoring on the oropharynx, or drying of the oropharyngeal mucosa from mouth breathing. Patients with established coagulopathies may be at considerably increased risk of bleeding.

Another frequent side effect after tonsillectomy is postoperative nausea and vomiting (PONV). Up to 70% of patients who did not receive prophylactic anti-emetics experience it. PONV can result in higher admission rates, more intravenous hydration requirements, a greater need for painkillers, and lower patient satisfaction. It is advised to give intraoperative dexamethasone during tonsillectomy as a single dose to combat these side effects. Since PONV is most likely to occur within the first 24 hours following surgery, some doctors regularly prescribe a single dose of ondansetron for outpatient surgeries. Pain is the main cause of morbidity after tonsillectomy, which can result in decreased oral intake, dehydration, dysphagia, and weight loss. It is crucial that caregivers are capable of keeping an eye out for symptoms of dehydration and persistently reminding their child to drink plenty of water. Using acetaminophen and ibuprofen at scheduled intervals can help reduce oropharyngeal pain.

Additionally, velopharyngeal insufficiency can develop after adenoidectomy and tonsillectomy. Hypernasal speech and regurgitating food through the nasal passage during feeding are possible symptoms.

A Closer Look

CT Sinuses

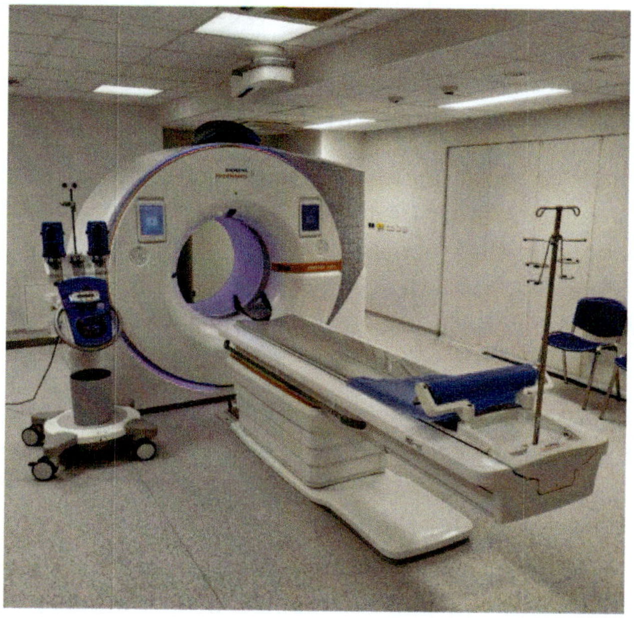

By Tomáš Vendiš – Own work, CC BY-SA 4.0, https://commons.wikimedia.org/w/index.php?curid=115330626.

- **CT Sinuses:** A diagnostic medical imaging test called computed tomography, or CT or CAT scan, is more widely used. Similar to conventional X-rays, it generates several images or pictures of the internal organs. Images produced by a CT scan can be resized in several planes. Even three-dimensional images can be produced by it. Your physician may view these photos on a computer screen, print them out on film or with a 3D printer, or store them on a CD or DVD. Compared to traditional X-rays, CT images offer more detail on internal organs, bones, soft tissue, and blood vessels. Particularly for blood vessels and soft tissues, this is accurate.

The paranasal sinus cavities of a patient are visible in the images obtained from a CT scan of their face. The nasal cavity is a network of air channels that connects the nose and the back of the throat. The paranasal sinuses are hollow, air-filled spaces that surround this system of channels inside the face's bones. The nasal cavity is connected to each of the four pairs of sinuses through tiny apertures.

CT of the sinuses is primarily used to:

- help diagnose sinusitis.
- evaluate sinuses that are filled with fluid or thickened sinus membranes.
- detect the presence of inflammatory diseases.
- provide additional information about tumors of the nasal cavity and sinuses.
- plan for surgery by defining the anatomy.

Preparation: For your test, dress comfortably and loosely. For the procedure, you might need to change into a gown. Metal items such as hairpins, eyeglasses, dentures, and jewelry can alter the CT pictures. Take them off before your exam, or leave them at home. You may be asked to take out your dental work and hearing aids for certain CT exams. Ladies will have to take off underwired bras made of metal. If it is feasible, you might need to take out any piercings.

If your exam will involve contrast material, your doctor might advise you to avoid eating or drinking anything for a few hours prior to the procedure. Inform your physician of all the medications you take and any allergies you may have. Your doctor may recommend medication (usually a steroid) to lower the risk of an allergic reaction if you have a known allergy to contrast material. Make sure to get in touch with your doctor well in advance of the exam date to avoid needless delays.

Additionally, let your doctor know about any recent illnesses or other medical conditions, as well as any past instances of thyroid issues, diabetes, asthma, heart disease, or kidney disease. Any of these circumstances could make a negative outcome more likely. If a woman suspects she might be pregnant, she should always let the CT technologist and her doctor know.

Equipment: A large, donut-shaped device with a short tunnel in the center is the typical CT scanner. On a small table that slides in and out of this brief tunnel, you will lie. The electronic X-ray detectors and X-ray tube rotate around you in a ring known as a gantry, opposite each other. In a different control room sits the computer workstation responsible for processing the imaging data. Here, the technologist runs the scanner and keeps a close eye on your examination. Using a speaker and microphone, the technologist will be able to speak with you and hear you.

Procedure: A CT scan functions much like a standard X-ray examination. The amount that different body parts absorb X-rays varies. On an X-ray or CT scan, this distinction enables the physician to identify different body parts from one another. A small amount of radiation is directed through the body part being examined during a traditional X-ray exam. The image is taken using a specialized electronic image recording plate. The X-ray shows white bones. The liver and heart are examples of soft tissue that appears in grayscale. Air seems to be dark.

A number of rotating X-ray beams and electronic X-ray detectors surround you during CT scanning. These gauge how much radiation is being absorbed by different parts of your body. Occasionally, during the scan, the exam table will move. This massive amount of data is processed by a specialized computer program to produce two-dimensional cross-sectional images of your body. The images are shown on a computer monitor by the system. There is a comparison made between CT imaging and slicing open a loaf of bread to look inside. The outcome of the computer software's reconstruction of the image slices is a multidimensional, incredibly detailed view of the inside of the body. Multiple slices can be obtained in a single rotation by almost all CT scanners. These CT scanners with multiple slices (multidetector) produce thinner slices faster. This yields more specific results. Large body sections can be imaged by modern CT scanners in a matter of seconds, and in younger patients, even faster. All patients benefit from this kind of speed. Children, the elderly, and those in critical condition—anyone who finds it difficult to remain motionless, even for the brief period of time required to obtain images—benefit greatly from speed. To lower the radiation dose for children, the radiologist will modify the CT scanner technique based on the size of the child and the area of interest. A contrast agent is sometimes used during CT scans to improve visibility in the body part being examined.

- **Before the Procedure:** Patients are first positioned on the CT examination table by the technologist. The most common position for a patient undergoing a CT scan of the sinuses is flat on their back. It is also possible to place the patient facedown with their chin up. During the examination, the patient may be assisted in holding still and maintaining the proper position with the use of pillows and straps. For some patients, a contrast material injection is necessary to improve the visibility of specific tissues or blood vessels. An intravenous (IV) line will be inserted by a nurse or technologist into a small vein in the patient's hand or arm if contrast material is needed. This line will be used to inject the contrast material.

After that, the table will swiftly pass through the scanner to ascertain the ideal place for the scans to begin. The table will then gradually pass through the apparatus to undergo the CT scan. The machine may perform multiple passes, contingent on the type of CT scan. During the scanning process, the technologist might ask you to hold your breath. Artifacts on the images can result from any motion, including breathing and body movements. This reduction in image quality may resemble the blurring that appears in photos taken of moving objects. After the exam is over, the technologist will ask you to wait while they confirm the quality of the images is sufficient for the radiologist to interpret them correctly. In most cases, the entire procedure takes 10 minutes, with the CT scan taking less than a minute.

- **During and After the Procedure:** In general, CT scans are quick, simple, and painless. The patient needs to lie still for a shorter period of time thanks to multidetector CT. While the scanning process is painless, having to stay motionless for a few minutes might be uncomfortable. A CT scan could be uncomfortable for you if you have chronic pain, have trouble staying still, or are claustrophobic. To help you endure the CT scanning process, the technologist or nurse, working under the supervision of a doctor, might prescribe you some medication.

In the event that iodinated contrast is used during the examination, your physician will screen you for acute or chronic kidney disease. You may experience a pinprick when the nurse puts the needle into your vein to administer contrast material intravenously (by vein). Warmth or flushing may be experienced during the contrast injection. It is also possible that you taste something metallic. This too shall pass. You might have the urge to go potty. These are merely the side effects of the contrast injection, though, and they go away fast.

Your body may be covered in unique light lines when you enter the CT scanner. You can make sure that you are positioned correctly on the exam table by following these lines. Modern CT scanners may make faint clicking, whirring, and buzzing noises. During the imaging process, these happen as the internal components of the CT scanner—which are typically invisible to you—rotate around you. Unless there are unusual circumstances, you will be the only patient in the examination room during the CT scan. For instance, a parent with a lead shield on may occasionally remain in the room with their child. Nonetheless, an integrated intercom system will allow the technologist to see, hear, and communicate with you at all times. Parents of young patients might be permitted in the room, but in order to reduce radiation exposure, they might need to wear a lead apron. Your intravenous line will be removed by the technologist following a CT scan. They will apply a tiny dressing to the tiny hole the needle created. You can get right back to your regular activities.

Benefits

- One of the safest means of studying the sinuses.
- The most reliable approach.
- Help in surgery planning.
- Particularly when compared to magnetic resonance imaging (MRI), computed tomography (CT) of the sinuses is now widely accessible and can be completed quickly.
- Painless, noninvasive, and accurate.
- A major advantage is its ability to image bone and tissue at once.
- Can be used in emergencies.
- Cost-effective and offers real-time images.
- A diagnosis via a CT scan may eliminate the need for exploratory surgery and surgical biopsy.
- The X-rays used for CT scanning should have no immediate side effects.

Risks

- There is a risk of radiation exposure but the benefits are more.
- Women should always tell their doctor and X-ray or CT technologist if there is any chance they are pregnant.
- Doctors do not generally recommend CT scanning for pregnant women unless medically required.

Limitations: When a sinus tumor is suspected, CT is typically the first test ordered. Magnetic resonance imaging (MRI) could prove useful if more data is required to ascertain the tumor's soft tissue extent. A large person might not be able to fit through the opening of a standard CT scanner. Alternatively, they might weigh more than the moving table's weight limit, which is typically 450 pounds.

Summary

- A surgical procedure known as a myringotomy involves making an incision in the tympanic membrane, or eardrum, to drain pus from the middle ear or relieve pressure brought on by an excessive accumulation of fluid.
- A mastoidectomy is a surgical procedure used to remove sick mastoid cells. The hollow spaces in your mastoid, the honeycomb-shaped bone that sits just behind your ear, are where these air cells grow.
- Even though a middle ear infection is already extremely painful, untreated cases may result in mastoiditis. When the mastoid bone becomes infected, it can cause mastoiditis, which can lead to bone loss if treatment is delayed. Loss of hearing may also result from the infection's spread to the brain. Should antibiotics prove ineffective, mastoid surgery might become imperative.
- Myringoplasty is the procedure used to seal the tympanic membrane's pars tensa perforation. Tympanoplasty is the term for myringoplasty plus scar tissue excision. The patient is positioned supine with their face turned to the side during the procedure.
- Antral irrigation, also known as proof puncture, is a procedure used to treat and diagnose sinusitis. It involves making an incision in the inferior meatus to insert a canula into the maxillary sinus.
- The procedure known as an intranasal inferior meatal antrostomy involves creating an intranasal orifice in the inferior meatus's nasoantral wall. This procedure has been replaced by functional endoscopic sinus surgery, which is now infrequently needed.
- An external approach is used in the Caldwell-Luc operation to surgically treat the severely diseased maxillary sinus. It is an alternative to endonasal endoscopic surgery for middle meatal antrostomy, which was the main method for entering the maxillary sinus before the development of endoscopic sinus surgery.
- Submucosal resection (SMR) and septoplasty are surgical procedures commonly used to treat a deviated septum in the nose. While SMR involves the removal of large portions of tissue, septoplasty is a tissue-sparing procedure. Most ENT surgeons use these terms interchangeably due to their goal of correcting a deviated septum.
- In the fields of plastic surgery and otorhinolaryngology (ENT), nasal septoplasty is one of the most often done procedures. The main reason for this functional surgery, rather than just a cosmetic one, is typically a septal deviation that causes a significant and symptomatic obstruction of the nasal airway.
- Endoscopy is a minimally invasive medical diagnostic procedure. Using it, doctors can see the inside surfaces of a tissue or organ, giving them access to parts of the body that they would not typically be able to see during a routine examination. Nasal endoscopy, also known as rhinoscopy, is usually carried out in the ear, nose, and throat (otolaryngologist) office, where the physician can examine your sinuses and nasal passages with direct, high-quality, magnified vision.

- Long-term infection and inflammation of the sinus and nasal linings are the hallmarks of chronic sinusitis. Numerous symptoms, such as facial pressure, nasal congestion, discolored nasal discharge, and "post-nasal drip," are experienced by patients with chronic sinusitis.
- A direct laryngoscopy makes the larynx visible. It is employed in resuscitation, general anesthesia, and surgeries involving the larynx. This tool can be used in the operating room, intensive care unit, and emergency department, among other hospital settings. It is easier to perform endotracheal intubation when the larynx is visualized.
- A bronchoscopy allows medical professionals to examine your airways and lungs. Usually, a pulmonologist—a medical professional who specializes in lung disorders—performs it. A tiny tube called a bronchoscope is inserted into your mouth or nose, down your throat, and into your lungs during a bronchoscopy.
- An endoscope, which is a long, narrow tube-like device with a light and a camera, is inserted into your esophagus during an esophagoscopy procedure. A long, muscular tube called the esophagus aids in moving food and liquids from your mouth to your stomach.
- The surgical removal of the tonsils, which are two oval-shaped tissue pads at the back of the throat, one on each side, is known as a tonsillectomy. Tonsillitis, or infection and inflammation of the tonsils, was traditionally treated with a tonsillectomy.

References

1. Balikci, H. H., Ozkul, M. H., Uvacin, O., Yasar, H., Karakas, M., & Gurdal, M. (2012). Antrochoanal polyposis: Analysis of 34 cases. *European Archives of Oto-Rhino-Laryngology, 270*(5), 1651–1654. https://doi.org/10.1007/s00405-012-2274-2.
2. Chand, G., Shafiq, M., & Khan, A. (2012). The comparative study of submucosal resection of nasal septum under local and general anesthesia. *Journal of the Pakistan Medical Association, 62*(10), 1020–1022.
3. Cummings, C. W. (2014). *Cummings Otolaryngology: Head and Neck Surgery* (3 volume set). Elsevier Saunders.
4. Datarkar, A. N., Dhawad, M., & Deshpande, A. (2012). Unusual foreign body in mid face. *Journal of Maxillofacial and Oral Surgery, 14*(S1), 96–99. https://doi.org/10.1007/s12663-012-0341-2.
5. Dong, J., Lu, M., Zhou, H., Zhang, W., Li, Y., & Dong, W. (2015). Clinical analysis of primary nasal sinus osteoma. *Zhonghua Er Bi Yan Hou Tou Jing Wai Ke Za Zhi = Chinese Journal of Otorhinolaryngology Head and Neck Surgery, 50*(1), 8–13.
6. Fettman, N., Sanford, T., & Sindwani, R. (2009). Surgical management of the deviated septum: Techniques in septoplasty. *Otolaryngologic Clinics of North America, 42*(2), 241–252, viii. https://doi.org/10.1016/j.otc.2009.01.005.
7. Flint, P. W. (2014). *Cummings Otolaryngology–Head & Neck Surgery*. Elsevier Saunders.
8. Gleeson, M. (2008). *Scott-Brown's Otolaryngology, Head and Neck Surgery* (7th ed.). Hodder Arnold.
9. Gustafson, L., et al. (2000). Flexible versus rigid esophagoscopy: A practical comparison for otolaryngologists. *Current Opinion in Otolaryngology & Head and Neck Surgery*. Retrieved

from: https://journals.lww.com/co-otolaryngology/Abstract/2000/06000/Flexible_versus_rigid_esophagoscopy__a_practical.18.aspx (accessed on 4 September 2024).

10. Kapadiya, M., & Tarabichi, M. (2019). An overview of endoscopic ear surgery in 2018. *Laryngoscope Investigative Otolaryngology, 4*(3), 365–373. https://doi.org/10.1002/lio2.276.

11. Kennedy, K. L., & Lin, J. W. (2021). *Mastoidectomy*. StatPearls Publishing.

12. Kuo, B., et al. (2006). Esophagus–Anatomy and development. Retrieved from: https://www.nature.com/gimo/contents/pt1/full/gimo6.html (accessed on 4 September 2024).

13. Laryngopharyngeal reflux (LPR). (2012). Retrieved from: https://my.clevelandclinic.org/health/diseases/15024-laryngopharyngeal-reflux-lpr (accessed on 4 September 2024).

14. Lotfi, A. R., Zarrintan, S., Naderpour, M., Sokhandan, M., Fakhrjou, A., Bayat, A., & Salehpour, F. (2014). Primary hydatid cyst of the right maxillary sinus: A case report. *Iranian Journal of Otorhinolaryngology, 26*(77), 257–261. https://doi.org/10.3287/ijor.2014.777.

15. Low, W. K., & Willatt, D. J. (1992). Submucous resection for deviated nasal septum: A critical appraisal. *Singapore Medical Journal, 33*(6), 617–619.

16. McGarey, P. O. Jr., et al. (2016). Rigid esophagoscopy for head and neck cancer staging and the incidence of synchronous esophageal malignant neoplasms. *JAMA Otolaryngology–Head & Neck Surgery*. Retrieved from: https://jamanetwork.com/journals/jamaotolaryngology/fullarticle/2482994 (accessed on 4 September 2024).

17. Schneider, J. S., Day, A., Clavenna, M., Russell, P. T., & Duncavage, J. (2015). Early practice. *Otolaryngologic Clinics of North America, 48*(5), 839–850. https://doi.org/10.1016/j.otc.2015.05.010.

18. Teixeira, J., Certal, V., Chang, E. T., & Camacho, M. (2016). Nasal septal deviations: A systematic review of classification systems. *Plastic and Reconstructive Surgery International, 2016*, 7089123. https://doi.org/10.1155/2016/7089123.

19. Walton, B., et al. (2011). *Esophagology and Esophagoscopy*. Retrieved from: https://www.utmb.edu/otoref/Grnds/esoph-2011-10-27/esoph-slides-2011-10-27-B.pdf (accessed on 4 September 2024).

20. Xu, W., Zhao, C., Jin, L., & Ge, R. (2015). Clinical analysis of simple orbital blowout fracture. *Lin Chuang Er Bi Yan Hou Tou Jing Wai Ke Za Zhi = Journal of Clinical Otorhinolaryngology, Head, and Neck Surgery, 29*(5), 418–421.

INDEX

C

D

E

F

G

H

N

O

V

W

X

Printed and bound by CPI Group (UK) Ltd, Croydon, CR0 4YY
18/09/2026
14965065-0003